Clinical Cardiology
Fifth Edition

Elliot Chesler

Clinical Cardiology

Fifth Edition

With 276 Illustrations

Springer-Verlag
New York Berlin Heidelberg London Paris
Tokyo Hong Kong Barcelona Budapest

Elliot Chesler, M.D. (Rand.) F.R.C.P. (Edin.) F.A.C.C.
Chief, Cardiovascular Division
Professor of Medicine
University of Minnesota
Veterans Administration Medical Center
One Veterans Drive
Minneapolis, MN 55417, USA

Library of Congress Cataloging-in-Publication Data

Chesler, Elliot.
Clinical cardiology.—5th ed. / by Elliot Chesler.
p. cm.
Rev. ed. of: Schrire's Clinical cardiology. 4th ed. / by Elliot Chesler, 1981.
Includes bibliographical references and index.
ISBN-13: 978-1-4613-9185-2 e-ISBN-13: 978-1-4613-9183-8
DOI: 10.1007/978-1-4613-9183-8
1. Heart—Diseases. 2. Cardiology. I. Chesler, Elliot. Schrire's clinical cardiology. II. Title.
[DNLM: 1. Heart Diseases. WG 200 C524c]
RC681.C423 1992
616.1′2—dc20
DNLM/DLC
for Library of Congress 91-5131

Printed on acid-free paper.

Production coordinated by Chernow Editorial Services, Inc., and managed by Terry Kornak.
Manufacturing supervised by Rhea Talbert.
Typeset by Asco Trade Typesetting Ltd., Hong Kong.

9 8 7 6 5 4 3 2 1

ISBN-13: 978-1-4613-9185-2

Dedicated to

Velva Schrire (1916–1972)
M.Sc., Ph.D., M.D. (Cape Town), F.R.C.P.E., F.R.C.P., F.A.C.C.
Founder of the Cardiac Clinic Groote Schuur Hospital and University of Cape Town, South Africa (1955)

Preface and Acknowledgments

Although the text of the fifth edition has been extensively revised to include advances in the management of dysrhythmias and ischemic heart disease, the original purpose remains unchanged. It presents a bedside approach to cardiology, where an adequate history and physical examination supported by the electrocardiogram, chest X-ray, and, more recently, the echocardiogram, are the most important aspects of diagnosis. Cardiac catheterization and other investigations are used in many instances for confirmation of the clinical diagnosis. It was this approach, so ably practiced by Professor Schrire, that made my stay at the University of Cape Town so rewarding, and motivated me to undertake the fourth and fifth editions as an expression of appreciation.

I am indebted to many colleagues for their discussions and help with the illustrations: Dr. Jesse E. Edwards, The Charles T. Miller Hospital, Saint Paul, Minnesota; Dr. James Møller, Department of Pediatric Cardiology, University of Minnesota; and Drs. Stephen Archer, Charles C. Gornick, Arthur From, E. Kenneth Weir, and Gordon L. Pierpont, of the Department of Cardiology, Veterans Administration Hospital, Minneapolis, Minnesota.

Many of the illustrations were prepared by Mr. Brett Hansen, Medical Illustrator at the V.A. Medical Center, and photographed in the associated Department of Photography; their valuable assistance is gratefully acknowledged.

Finally, I am profoundly grateful to Mrs. Brenda Tisdale, Secretary in the Department of Cardiology at the V.A. Medical Center, for her dedicated typing and preparation of the manuscript. Ms. Linda Chadwick's organizational skill was of great help.

Elliot Chesler

Contents

1
The History

A well-taken history provides the cardiologist not only with the initial step toward diagnosis but also with an assessment of disability. These are the prerequisites for successful patient management. Taking a good history is akin to a cross-examination and is a difficult technique, acquired by experience, patience, and skill. Additionally, a certain amount of tolerance is necessary. Giving a good qualitative and temporal account of symptoms is not always easy, even for the educated and sophisticated. All too often patients are labeled "poor historians" or "poor witnesses" when they provide an inadequate or garbled account of their illness. Yet, how often do we hear brief histories and concise case descriptions from our medical colleagues?

Early in the course of the interview an assessment should be made of the patient's level of intelligence, emotional state, and credibility. When it is recognized that the patient is unable to describe with accuracy the nature and time course of the symptoms, relentless questioning will accomplish little. With experience one learns when to pursue the history, when to give up, what to accept as reliable, and what to discard.

Symptoms produced by anxiety, hysteria, or malingering should be recognized *positively* by good interrogation and observation of the patient during the interview, not by retrospective exclusion of organic disease following a barrage of tests, which are so readily available to the modern cardiologist.

There is usually one symptom that dominates the patient's history, and the patient should be allowed to present this in a general way. After this has been done and a tentative diagnosis suspected (or, alternatively, when the description is inadequate) leading or "closed-end" questions should be skillfully interjected to corroborate the story.

It must be expected that a patient may be completely unaware of the presence of heart disease even when it is advanced. (Congenital heart disease is frequently discovered during routine examination by a school doctor, and systemic hypertension, valvular disease, and ischemic heart disease during examination for life insurance.) This may be because there are genuinely no symptoms or because the patient has learned to adjust automatically to the disability and is therefore unaware of any limitations. The latter is exemplified by the marked improvement noted in an apparently symptomless subject following corrective surgery for congenital or rheumatic heart disease. On the other hand, the examiner must be aware of deliberate suppression of symptoms because of the fear of the diagnosis and the consequences of heart disease.

Many patients are unaware of the symptoms of heart disease. It is easy to associate dysuria with urinary tract disease, but more difficult to attribute symptoms such as hemoptysis, edema, peripheral embolism, pain, and even dyspnea to heart disease. Compounding the problem, the increasing publicity accorded to heart disease among the lay public, and the frequent occurrence of heart disease in relatives, gives rise to a great deal of unnecessary fear and psychological suffering from symptoms such as left chest pain, headache, and fatigue, which are erroneously attributed to coronary artery disease or hypertension.

The assessment of disability, which is so important in making the decision to proceed with coronary artery bypass surgery, valve replacement, or commissurotomy, is particularly difficult. Even after successful operation, the cardiologist is again faced with the assessment of disability in relation to insurance claims, worker's compensation, and so on. An assessment of disability should clearly analyze the effect of effort on a particular symptom, the effect that the symptom has on the customary life-style, and a determination of whether the disabling symptom is stable or progressive. Usually, this information can be obtained only through leading questions.

It is unnecessary to stress here the importance of taking a general history and of eliciting the facts about past history, family history, occupation, and socioeconomic background. Evaluation of the patient's past history should be made with certain reservations. At least 40% of patients with well-established rheumatic heart disease give no history of an acute episode of acute rheumatic fever, and a negative response in this respect should not influence the results of physical examination. A history of a murmur in childhood is generally of little value since most murmurs in this category are of the innocent variety. The patient's family history may be extremely helpful when there is a history of sudden death (e.g., idiopathic hypertrophic subaortic stenosis, hereditary prolongation of QT interval, and the premature onset of coronary artery disease, particularly with the hyperlipidemic syndromes) or hypertension. Only the salient symptoms relating to the heart and great vessels will be considered here.

Dyspnea: This is the commonest symptom of heart disease. The duration of dyspnea, the speed with which it has progressed, and the degree of disability should be determined. For dyspnea to be significant it must be out of the ordinary, since everyone develops dyspnea, depending on the amount of effort undertaken and the person's physical fitness. Dyspnea may be graded in accordance with the New York Heart Association Classification: Class I patients have heart disease and are asymptomatic. Class II patients have dyspnea with the ordinary activities of everyday life. Class III patients are not dyspneic at rest but are symptomatic with less than ordinary activity, such as walking a few steps and performing minor household activities. Class IV disability is associated with loss of all cardiac reserve, so that symptoms are present at rest, and, in fact, the patient usually has evidence of congestive cardiac failure.

Dyspnea at rest must be distinguished from hyperventilation. This may be evident to the examiner during history-taking, but if necessary, leading questions should probe for the associated symptoms, such as paraesthesia of the extremities, carpal pedal spasm, and fainting attacks.

Orthopnea is the term applied to dyspnea occurring at rest in bed, forcing the subject to sit upright to breathe comfortably. It is an important sign of advanced heart disease but is significant only when this change in sleeping habit has been noticed spontaneously by the patient. Sleeping propped up on pillows obviously has no relevance if this is the normal sleeping habit.

Paroxysmal cardiac dyspnea (cardiac asthma, paroxysmal nocturnal dyspnea) characteristically occurs at night between 1 and 2 A.M., coming on suddenly and waking the patient from sleep. A feeling of suffocation forces the patient to sit upright in bed. Unlike orthopnea, however, sitting up does not afford immediate relief. Acute dyspnea may persist for 10 minutes or more and may then recur. Frequently, the victim gets out of bed, walks about, or opens a window in an attempt to alleviate the distress. When bronchospasm is superimposed, wheezing and expiratory difficulty added to the dyspnea. Cough is frequently present and may be associated with a little blood-stained frothy sputum. When acute pulmonary edema supervenes, extreme dyspnea results in the production of copious frothy blood-stained sputum. Attacks of paroxysmal nocturnal dyspnea are usually spontaneous but occasionally may be precipitated by the occurrence of a tachyarrhythmia.

Cough: Chronic pulmonary congestion frequently gives rise to cough, particularly disturbing at night. Also, there is a predisposition to infection, resulting in recurrent attacks of winter bronchitis, encountered particularly in mitral stenosis. On the other hand, chronic cough and sputum production may be associated with primary lung disease, which is a potent cause of heart failure (chronic cor pulmonale). Cough precipitated by walking or sexual intercourse is encountered in critical mitral stenosis. Tracheal obstruction produced by an aortic aneurysm produces a characteristic paroxysmal "brassy" cough, often with wheezing and stridor.

Hemoptysis: This may vary from slight blood- tinging of the sputum to massive hemorrhage. Fresh blood may emanate from rupture of a pulmonary vein (pulmonary apoplexy), rupture of bronchial collateral vessels, or necrotic lung tissue in pulmonary infarction. Usually, the underlying cardiac condition is easily recognizable, but occasionally, noncardiac causes such as tuberculosis and carcinoma of the lung may have to be excluded.

Chest pain: There are three important sources of chest pain in heart disease: the myocardium, the pericardium, and the great vessels. By and large, each has its individual highly characteristic quality, distribution, and associated features, so that a diagnosis can often be made by careful interpretation of this symptom alone. Typically, ischemic pain is pressing, squeezing, gripping, constricting, or heavy. It is situated in the center of the chest and may or may not radiate widely. Radiation may include the neck, the jaws, the arms, the epigastrium, and the back. It is commonly precipitated by the stress of exercise, by excitement, and by cold weather. The pain of angina pectoris lasts for a few minutes, but when myocardial infarction has supervened the pain may persist for hours.

Great care must be taken to distinguish cardiac from noncardiac chest pain, which is frequently psychogenic. The latter is often "knife-like," sharp, stabbing, vaguely dull, and frequently pinpointed to the area below the nipple. It does not have the same clear association with exercise that is so highly characteristic of ischemic chest pain.

Pericardial pain is usually sharp and stabbing, lasting for hours or days, situated centrally and to the left of the chest. It rarely radiates to the neck and arms and is unrelated to exercise. The pain may be relieved by sitting up and leaning forward, and may be aggravated by lying down and by inspiration.

Aortic pain, such as occurs with dissecting aneurysm, is sudden, tearing, and intense, persisting with the same intensity for hours, and associated with shock. It is usually felt in the upper chest but radiates through to the back, where it may be the most intense. It may radiate extensively, depending on involvement of the various arterial branches and spinal nerves. Frequently, it is unresponsive to morphine. Chronic aortic pain arises from an aortic aneurysm expanding and eroding surrounding structures. When bones are affected, pain is localized to the back and is persistent, boring, and nocturnal.

The heart has no monopoly of pain in the chest. Most thoracic and some abdominal structures may produce chest pain that must be differentiated from cardiac pain. Most important are local musculoskeletal chest wall pain, referred pain from spinal nerves, esophageal pain, and pain referred from the stomach and gallbladder.

Hepatic pain (hepatic angina) is associated with systemic venous hypertension and may be mistaken for cardiac pain, particularly when related to effort. *Right ventricular angina* may occur in severe pulmonary hypertension (as in mitral stenosis) or in acute pulmonary infarction.

Palpitation: An unpleasant awareness of the heart's action gives rise to this symptom. Frequently, it occurs during excitement, nervous tension, or violent exercise in the unfit, and is therefore physiological. In psychoneurosis, however, this sensation of forceful cardiac action is frequently described as "palpitations" and is a common complaint. It is also, however, associated with organic heart disease and is produced by vigorous ventricular contraction and typically may occur with aortic or mitral incompetence, thyrotoxicosis, and occasionally hypertension.

The most common causes of irregular palpitation are premature systoles and atrial fibrillation. The sudden interruption of regular rhythm gives rise to the sensation of palpitation, which may be a result of the premature beat itself, or the larger beat following the postectopic pause. Episodic regular palpitation occurs with paroxysmal supraventricular or ventricular tachycardia.

The patient should be encouraged to give an accurate verbal description of palpitation, supplemented by tapping the finger on the table. In this way, the rapidity of onset and offset, the duration, and the regularity or irregularity may provide good evidence of whether the sensation is a result of ectopic beats, paroxysmal tachycardia, or atrial fibrillation.

Fatigue: Since fatigue is such a common complaint in functional and organic disease in general, it is very difficult to attach too much significance to this symptom. It is more usually a result of noncardiac disease. However, fatigue on effort is a specific symptom arising from impaired cardiac output and is frequently observed among patients with pulmonary hypertension and right heart failure.

Syncope: This is a frequent symptom in cardiac and noncardiac disease. A cardiac cause of syncope is suggested by a dramatic onset, absolute loss of consciousness, followed by rapid recovery. The common faint, or vasovagal attack, occurs more gradually, rarely leads to complete loss of consciousness, and is seldom accompanied by injury. Neurological causes of syncope, such as ischemic caroticovertebral disease, are frequently followed by a state of semiconsciousness and residual neurological defect. Syncope on effort is usually the result of a cardiac cause and is a common symptom in aortic stenosis, primary pulmonary hypertension, and hypertrophic cardiomyopathy.

In the evaluation of syncope every effort should be made to interrogate an eyewitness whose evidence may provide diagnostic information.

Neurologic Symptoms: In dealing with diseases such as mitral stenosis, chronic atrial fibrillation, and left ventricular aneurysm, which are known to be complicated by systemic embolism, specific inquiry should be made for a history of transient disturbances of vision and speech, stroke, and weakness of the extremities.

Edema: This is one of the commonest manifestations of heart failure. Prior to the onset of edema, there is a subtle gain in weight; when sufficient fluid has accumulated, edema first appears at the end of the day, disappearing after a night's rest. Eventually, the lower extremities become permanently edematous, and later there is effusion into the serous cavities and swelling of the soft tissues of the face. The face is characteristically involved early in the course of acute nephritis, but this may also occur in cardiac failure, and is seen particularly in constrictive pericarditis and beriberi.

Sweating: This is an important manifestation of heart failure in infants and children. In adults, thyrotoxicosis and infective endocarditis must always be considered.

Weight loss: Weight loss and cardiac cachexia are encountered in protracted, inadequately treated congestive cardiac failure or constrictive pericarditis. They are a result of by nausea and vomiting (gastric congestion or digitalis intoxication), protein-losing enteropathy, or infective endocarditis.

2
Physical Examination

While the history is taken, the patient is under examination. This becomes automatic with experience. Thus, thyrotoxicosis may be suspected because of the general appearance, the manner of speech, nervousness, and sweating. In a young man, pulsating neck arteries may suggest aortic incompetence or coarctation of the aorta. Cyanosis, wheezing, and dyspnea in an elderly person suggests chronic car pulmonale. The patient's coloring, nutritional state, temperament, and bodily habitus are noted.

Discussion will be confined to examination of the cardiovascular system. It is assumed that the other systems have been adequately examined. At first it is best to adopt a fixed routine to avoid omissions; diagnosis often rests on apparently small observations, so that the technique must be meticulous and thorough. Once this has been mastered, however, examination need not be stereotyped. For example, if thyrotoxicosis is suspected, the neck and hands should be examined first; if heart failure is suspected, the liver can be palpated.

There should be no hesitation about reassessing a physical sign, especially if there is conflicting evidence. For example, the pulse might be regarded as normal, but if after auscultation aortic stenosis is suspected, the pulse should be reassessed. Eliciting and interpreting physical signs is very subjective; accuracy comes only with constant methods available for checking most bedside observations. For example, internal and external pulse recordings can be used for arterial and venous pulsations, phonocardiography for auscultatory findings, and electrocardiography for disturbances of rhythm. The patient should be stripped, at least to the waist, and examined in a good light, standing and lying.

The Arterial Pulse

Counting the heart *rate* at the pulse is convenient and generally accurate. When an arrhythmia is present, however, the rate must be counted by auscultation. For example, if a ventricular extrasystole occurs early, the aortic valve does not open, so that a beat is dropped at the pulse. If bigeminy is present, the pulse rate may be halved, so that bradycardia may be diagnosed incorrectly. In atrial fibrillation, a pulse deficit is frequently present, especially if the rate is fast. In an infant a heart rate of 130 beats per minute is normal, whereas in an adult the rate usually lies between 60 and 90. By feeling the pulse the *rhythm* is generally easily determined, particularly whether it is regular or not. Sinus arrhythmia and atrial fibrillation can be recognized and the diagnosis confirmed by auscultation.

It should be stressed that the *carotid arteries* are large vessels closest to the aortic valve and their character therefore most closely resembles central aortic pulsation. The anacrotic pulse of aortic stenosis is best detected in the carotid artery. The femoral arteries are far removed and their contour is more affected by reflected waves.

All the accessible arteries in the limbs and neck should be palpated routinely. In practice, first the right radial or brachial pulse is felt, simultaneously with the right femoral, to exclude the small, delayed femoral pulse of coarctation of the aorta. The femoral pulses may be absent, raising the possibility of atherosclerosis, arteritis, embolism, or dissection of the abdominal aorta. Both arm pulses are then felt simultaneously. A discrepancy between the two occurs in coarctation of the aorta, aortic arteritis, atherosclerosis, and aneurysm, as well as in supravalvular aortic stenosis. Absence of the right upper limb pulse is often a result of anomalous origin of the subclavian artery, but any of the above-named causes may be responsible.

Palpation of the right innominate and common carotid arteries reveals whether they are kinked and tortuous. A kinked carotid is frequently found in hypertensive women and is not a sign of aneurysm. Unlike an aneurysm, it becomes smaller, or invisible, with deep inspiration. Very rarely, the arch of the aorta may present itself as a pulsatile swelling in the neck. Narrowing or occlusion of a carotid artery is most commonly a result of local atherosclerosis but occasionally is evidence of the "aortic arch syndrome," which is usually caused by aortic arteritis, atherosclerosis, syphilis, or aneurysm.

Since examination is made from the patient's right side, the right thumb is placed on the patient's right brachial artery and the fingers of the left hand on the radial pulse. Compression of the brachial artery until the pulse is obliterated gives an idea of the *force* (systolic pressure) and *tension* (diastolic pressure), but these are measured more easily and accurately with a sphygmomanometer. At the same time, the vessel wall can be felt. When arteriosclerotic or calcified, the artery is abnormally tortuous and the vessel wall becomes palpably thickened. There is no relation, however, between the degree of peripheral arteriosclerosis and the state of the coronary or cerebral arteries.

The most useful information obtained by feeling the pulse is the determination of its quality. Gross deviations from normal are readily appreciated, but finer abnormalities test the most experienced examiner. For this reason, it is advisable to return to the pulse when the rest of the examination has been completed.

The Normal Pulse

The arterial system is a very complex structure, consisting of a series of muscular and elastic tubes of various diameters filled by an incompressible fluid. At one end, the left ventricle supplies the pumping force, and at the other, the arterioles and capillaries control the runoff. The normal pulse contour will therefore vary with the size and structure of the vessel and its proximity to the heart.

It should be emphasized that when the pulse is palpated, it is a transmitted pressure wave that is felt, not blood traversing the vessel. When blood is ejected into the aorta, an initial *percussion wave* is inscribed 110 msec from the time of onset, which in young people with compliant vessels forms the peak of the pulse (Fig. 2.1). The second systolic wave is the *tidal* or *reflected wave*, which is of lesser amplitude. In elderly paients with rigid vessels, however, the tidal wave may form the peak of the pulse. In proximal arteries, such as the carotids, the two waves are separate. Distally, in the femorals, there is fusion and summation of the percussion and tidal waves to produce a pulse of larger amplitude. For this reason, the blood pressure is normally higher in the legs than in the arms, a phenomenon known as *peripheral amplification*.

The central pulse contour closely follows the left ventricular pressure curve, but as left ventricular pressure falls and the distended elastic vessels recoil, the aortic valve closes (dicrotic notch) and a secondary wave is produced that is usually impalpable. Under certain conditions (see below), this wave may become palpable to form the dicrotic pulse.

A small pulse with narrow pulse pressure is frequently encountered in vasoconstriction and conditions associated with low cardiac output. This may be physiological (cold) or pathological (hypertension, mitral stenosis). A large bounding pulse with a wide pulse pressure, on the other hand, is associated with vasodilatation, which may be physiological (heat) or pathological (fever, anemia).

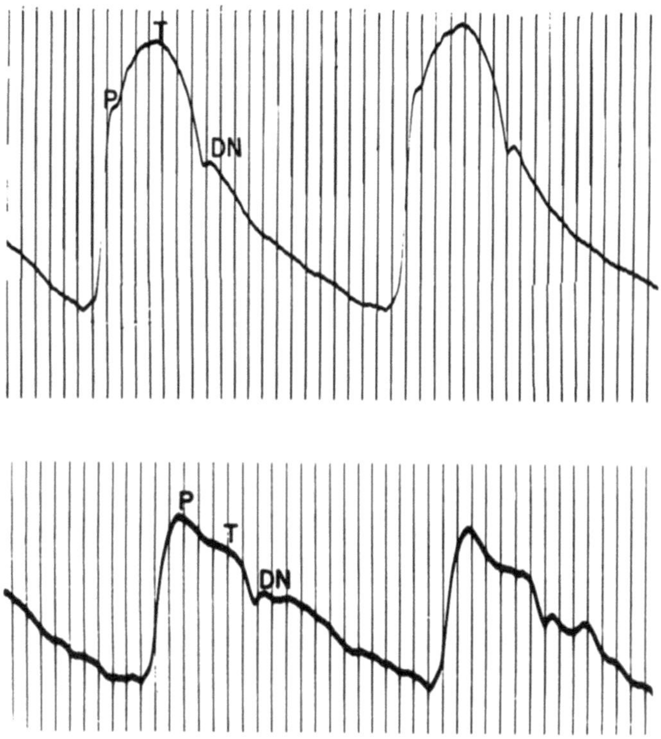

FIGURE 2.1. In the normal carotid pulse in the young (lower trace), the percussion wave (P) forms the peak and the tidal (reflected) wave (T) is smaller. In the elderly (top trace) the peak is formed by the tidal wave. DN, dicrotic notch.

Collapsing Pulse

This is associated with a large aortic runoff. There is an abrupt rise in the pulse wave, since the arterial system is lax and relatively empty. The tidal wave is reduced and there is a fairly abrupt fall in the pulse wave to the dicrotic notch, which is situated low down, because of the low diastolic pressure (Fig. 2.2).

Associated with this collapsing pulse (waterhamer pulse) is marked, visible pulsation in the peripheral vessels [e.g., pulsating carotid arteries (Corrigan's sign) and nodding of the head with each pulse beat (deMusset's sign)]. On auscultation over large arteries, a "pistol shot" sound can be heard. The best way of appreciating a collapsing pulse is to elevate the patient's arm above the head while feeling the brachial and radial arteries as described.

A valuable sign of aortic runoff is Duroziez's sign, which is a systolic and diastolic bruit detected by applying mild pressure with the stethoscope over the femoral artery. In normal subjects, only a systolic bruit is audible. The diastolic bruit is a result of retrograde flow toward the heart.

Causes of a Collapsing Pulse

1. *Aortic runoff into the heart.*
   a. Aortic valve incompetence is the most common condition.

   Less frequent causes are

   b. Ruptured sinus of Valsalva into a cardiac chamber.
   c. Aortico-left ventricular tunnel (congenital communication between aorta and left ventricle).
   d. Fistula between the coronary arteries and the right ventricle or right atrium.

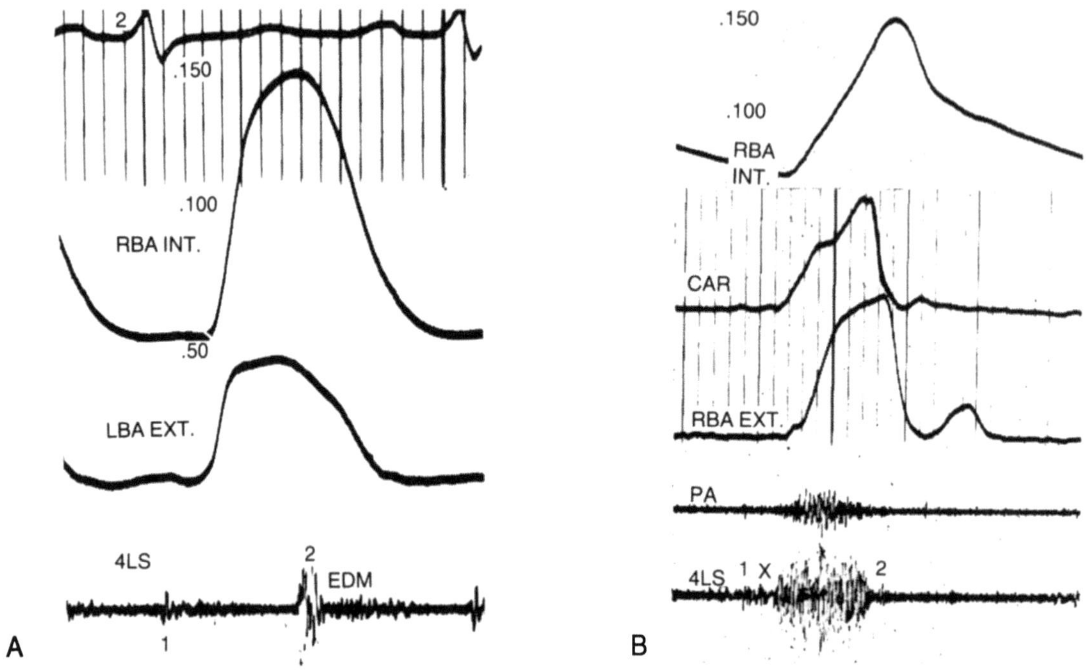

FIGURE 2.2. Synchronous internal and external brachial pulses from a patient with syphilitic aortic incompetence (A) and in a patient with severe aortic stenosis (B). In aortic incompetence the pulse is collapsing with a blood pressure of 150/50 mm Hg. The early diastolic murmur (EDM) is shown at the fourth left intercostal space (4LS). In aortic stenosis the pulse is slow rising, with an anacrotic shoulder and prolonged upstroke time. The phonocardiogram shows the typical aortic ejection systolic murmur and ejection click (X).

2. *Aortic runoff into the pulmonary arteries.*
   a. Patent ductus arteriosus.
   b. Aortopulmonary window without pulmonary hypertension.
   c. Surgical shunts.
3. *Aortic runoff into the peripheral vessels.*
   a. Physiological: heat, alcohol, pregnancy, extreme bradycardia.
   b. High output states: anemia, thyrotoxicosis, beriberi, cor pulmonale, and hepatic failure.
   c. Arteriovenous communication: vascular malformations, trauma, Paget disease, and fibrous dysplasia of the bones.

Stenotic Pulse

In aortic valve stenosis of sufficient severity, obstruction to outflow leads to prolongation of the left ventricular ejection time (Fig. 2.2B). The maximum rate of rise of the pulse is reduced and the pulse becomes *anacrotic* with a recordable and sometimes palpable anacrotic "shoulder." This is best felt in the carotid arteries and is a reliable sign of severe aortic stenosis in young people. In the elderly subject, however, the vascular tree is frequently arteriosclerotic and noncompliant. This produces deceptively brisk carotid pulses in the presence of severe aortic stenosis.

Jerky Pulse

This refers to a combination of a small volume pulse with collapsing quality. It is not sustained and has a rapid upstroke and quick falloff early in systole. Characteristically, it occurs when the left ventricle empties rapidly, in early systole. This may be due to leak into a low-pressure area such as the left atrium, as in

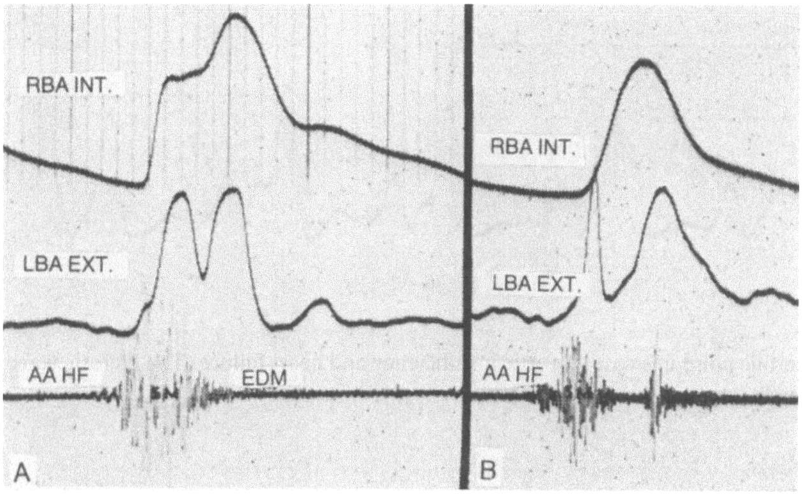

FIGURE 2.3. Synchronous internal and external brachial arterial pressures with phonocardiogram in syphilitic aortic incompetence, demonstrating pulsus bisferiens. The bisferiens pulse is partly artifactual, due to compression of the brachial artery by the recording device. The double pulse is present in the intraarterial tracing in (A) but not in (B). The aortic ejection murmur and early diastolic murmur are shown at the aortic area (AA).

severe mitral incompetence. It is less common in ventricular septal defect. It also occurs in obstructive and nonobstructive cardiomyopathy, due to rapid ejection of blood from the hypercontractile left ventricle.

Bisferiens Pulse

This is found when aortic stenosis is combined with significant aortic incompetence or in pure incompetence. In part, it is artifactual (as confirmed by comparing internal and external tracings (Fig. 2.3), produced by partially compressing the brachial artery so that two peaks are felt, because the percussion and tidal waves are separated. The character of the pulse is influenced by the condition of the arterial wall, the diastolic blood pressure, and the stroke volume. Normally, the percussion wave is produced by the sudden, relatively large increase in the volume of blood ejected into the arterial system and the tidal wave by the distensibility of the arterial walls. Significant stenosis prevents sudden arterial distension, so that a sharp percussion wave does not occur. Little diagnostic value can be attached to the presence of a bisferiens pulse, other than the presence of a marked aortic runoff. It is also encountered in hypertrophic obstructive cardiomyopathy, in which case the second (tidal) wave has a slow upstroke. In aortic insufficiency the upstroke of the tidal wave is rapid.

Dicrotic Pulse

This occurs when the normally impalpable dicrotic wave becomes accentuated (Fig. 2.4). Two pulse waves become palpable with every systole. It is not uncommonly observed in the early postoperative period following aortic valve replacement for aortic incompetence. It is a sign of myocardial failure with low cardiac output, low stroke volume, and increased peripheral resistance. It may also occur in debilitating fevers such as typhoid when the peripheral vascular resistance is low and the cardiac output normal.

Pulsus Alternans

This is encountered in severe myocardial disease, usually ischemic, hypertensive, or in-

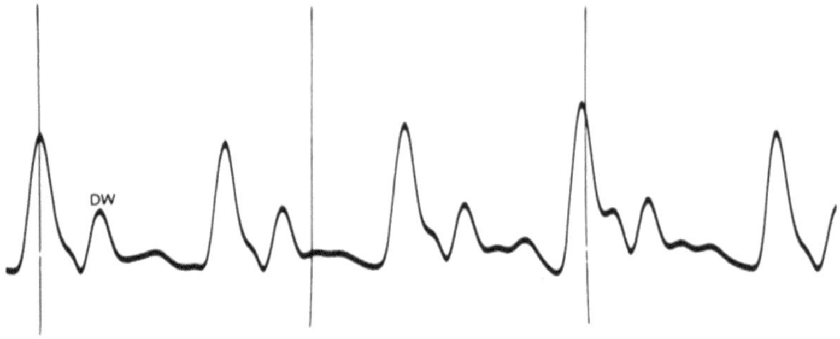

FIGURE 2.4. Dicrotic pulse in a case of aortic insufficiency and heart failure. The dicrotic wave (DW) follows a low dicrotic notch (arrow).

flammatory. The rhythm is regular and a weak beat alternates with a strong one (Fig. 2.5); it may be maintained for months or rarely years. Occasionally, it is transient for a few beats and is precipitated by a premature systole. The prognosis is extremely poor when encountered in the clinical context, except during paroxysmal tachycardia, because of the underlying conditions with which it is associated.

Left ventricular alternans is commonly encountered in the catheterization laboratory when a ventricular ectopic beat occurs either spontaneously or provoked. Normally, the postectopic pause is followed by a beat of the same or smaller magnitude. In left ventricular disease, however, the first few postectopic beats are increased in magnitude and return gradually to the preectopic level. When left ventricular dysfunction is more pronounced, however, the first postectopic beat may be followed by alternation of the succeeding beats.

Pulsus aternans is usually detected only during careful recording of the blood pressure with a sphygmomanometer, since the difference in

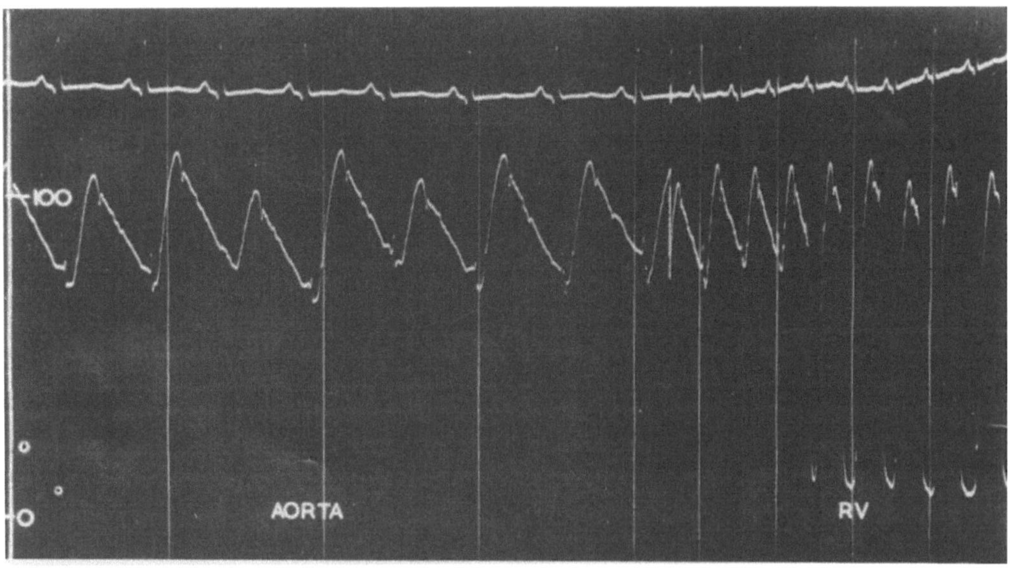

FIGURE 2.5. Pulsus alternans: Intraaortic pressure tracing from a patient with left ventricular failure. There is a 20-mm Hg variation in peak arterial pressure from beat-to-beat.

pressure from beat to beat is merely a few mm Hg. Rarely, a marked difference exists, and this may be palpable. Alternans of the heart sounds, usually of the second sound, can sometimes be heard, but occasionally all three sounds may alternate in intensity. Right ventricular alternans can be detected during cardiac catheterization, and both ventricles do not necessarily alternate together. Pulsus alternans must be differentiated from alternans due to tachypnea, when the respiratory rate is half the pulse rate.

Pulsus Paradoxus

Normally, there is a fall in systolic blood pressure with inspiration and a rise on expiration. This is due in part to the effects of increased negative pressure on the great vessels, and in part to the fact that the left ventricle lags a little behind the right, since it takes a few beats to transfer the increased right ventricular output that occurs with inspiration to the left side. There is little change, however, in the actual pulse pressure, so that the effects of respiration are not normally detected at the pulse.

In cardiac tamponade and *effusive* constrictive pericarditis, the pulse is palpably reduced during inspiration; it may, in fact, disappear. In cardiac tamponade the venous return to the right heart increases and the ventricular septum bulges into the left ventricle. Left ventricular stroke volume diminishes abruptly on inspiration, due to reduced flow from the pulmonary veins to the left atrium to the left ventricle; this is responsible for the reduced pulse so characteristic of pulsus paradoxus.

Pulsus paradoxus must be looked for during quiet respiration while palpating several arteries, particularly the femorals. Bracing the shoulders during inspiration can mechanically obstruct the subclavian arteries and produce a fictitious pulsus paradoxus. After examining the pulse on quiet respiration the patient can be asked to take a deep breath, which will exaggerate the abnormality.

A paradoxical pulse is found in conditions other than pericardial effusion. It commonly occurs in airway obstruction, for example, asthma, chronic bronchitis, and emphysema.

Valsalva Maneuver

This has been used as a bedside test for cardiac failure. After a deep inspiration the patient expires forcibly against the closed glottis for 10–15 seconds. The arterial pressure response is detected by palpating the pulse or, more accurately, with a sphygmomanometer. Normally, there are four phases: (1) a rise in systolic and diastolic pressures at the onset of straining, (2) a slow fall in pulse pressure and mean arterial pressure, (3) an abrupt fall in pressure when straining ceases due to drop in intrathoracic pressure, and (4) an increase or overshoot of systolic blood pressure and pulse pressure, with an associated bradycardia mediated through the baroceptors.

In heart failure, a square-wave response occurs. There is a persistent elevation of systolic and diastolic pressures with no change in heart rate during the forced expiration, no overshoot of blood pressure, and no bradycardia when straining is stopped. The easiest sign to detect at the bedside is the absence of bradycardia at the end of the procedure.

The Blood Pressure

The blood pressure is usually measured from the right arm. It should be measured in both arms whenever aortic aneurysm, arteritis, arteriosclerosis, or coarctation is suspected. Normally, a small difference in pressure between the two arms is not uncommon, but if it is greater than 10 mm Hg, one of the foregoing conditions should be suspected. When coarctation of the aorta is suspected, the pressure in the limbs must always be recorded in sequence (i.e., first the right arm, then the left leg, then the right arm again). The leg pressure is considerably higher than the arm pressure normally, because of the greater muscle mass that has to be compressed by the cuff and because of peripheral amplification. Leg pressures are measured most easily with the patient in the prone position.

The two most popular instruments in use are the mercury and aneroid sphyymomanometers. Cuffs of various sizes are available for adults, children, and infants, and blood pressures are recorded with the patient lying or sitting. The cuff must be firmly applied high around the completely relaxed arm and inflated until the pulse is obliterated. The pressure is gradually released and the level at which the pulse suddenly becomes palpable is the systolic pressure obtained on palpation, and gradually released. The level at which sounds first appear is the sytolic pressure, and this corresponds fairly closely to the systolic pressure on palpation. As the cuff pressure is reduced, a murmur replaces the sounds, and this in turn is replaced by loud clear sounds, which suddenly become muffled as the pressure is slowly reduced. A few mm Hg below this, the sounds usually disappear, although occasionally, even in health, sounds may continue down to zero. There is no universal agreement as to whether to record the point of muffling or the point of disappearance of sounds as the diastolic pressure. The former should be taken, and should there be a significant difference, both figures are expressed (e.g., BP 130/80/60).

If the pressure is determined by auscultation alone, the cuff must always be inflated to the maximum pressure recordable by the manometer and then deflated to avoid missing the auscultatory gap. This gap, during which no sounds or murmurs are audible, is often found in hypertension, so that if the cuff is insufficiently inflated, a falsely low systolic pressure may be found.

In infants, the blood pressure is often difficult to record by the technique described above. The "flush" method can then be used. The limb is emptied of blood by elevation and compression of the arterial supply until it becomes pallid. The cuff is then applied and inflated. It is then deflated and the systolic pressure is noted at the point where sudden flushing of the palm or sole is observed.

At best, the sphygmomanometer is an indirect and approximate measure of the arterial blood pressure. Readings should therefore be expressed only to the nearest 5 mm Hg.

The normal limits of blood pressure are discussed in Chapter 15. In infants the blood pressure averages 90 systolic, in children 100/60, and in adults 95–150 systolic and 60–90 diastolic. Over the age of 50, higher values are accepted in the Western world. Several studies among racial groups living under more primitive conditions have shown no rise in blood pressure with advancing age.

Pulsus alternans and pulsus paradoxus should be looked for routinely during recording of the blood pressure. Pulsus alternans can usually be detected only by lowering the pressure 1–2 mm Hg at a time until the sounds first come through. The patient then holds his breath in expiration and the pressure is dropped another 1–2 mm Hg. Pulsus paradoxus is detected by measuring the pressure when the sounds come through on inspiration and expiration during quiet breathing. In health, with a pulse pressure of approximately 40 mm Hg the difference in pressure seldom exceeds 8–10 mm Hg. In cardiac tamponade this figure is often exceeded and one beat may actually disappear. Often the pulse pressure is only 20 mm Hg in which case a difference of 10 mm Hg is highly significant.

Jugular Venous Pressure and Pulsation

Venous pulsation in the neck can be differentiated from arterial pulsation as follows (Fig. 2.6):

1. *Position*. The external jugular vein lies superficial to the sternomastoid muscle and is easily narrowed or compressed by the superficial fascia, muscles, or tendons of the neck. Communication with the right atrium is less direct, and therefore pulsations are not as well marked as in the internal jugular vein; pulsations are damped, so that the pressure approaches the mean right atrial pressure.

The internal jugular vein, on the other hand, runs parallel with the carotid artery, medial to the sternomastoid, communicates directly with the superior vena cava, and pulsates freely. When the internal carotid artery divides, the major branches lie deep in the sternomastoid, whereas the internal jugular vein remains superficial in the parotid near the earlobe. Pulsation behind the mandible and of the

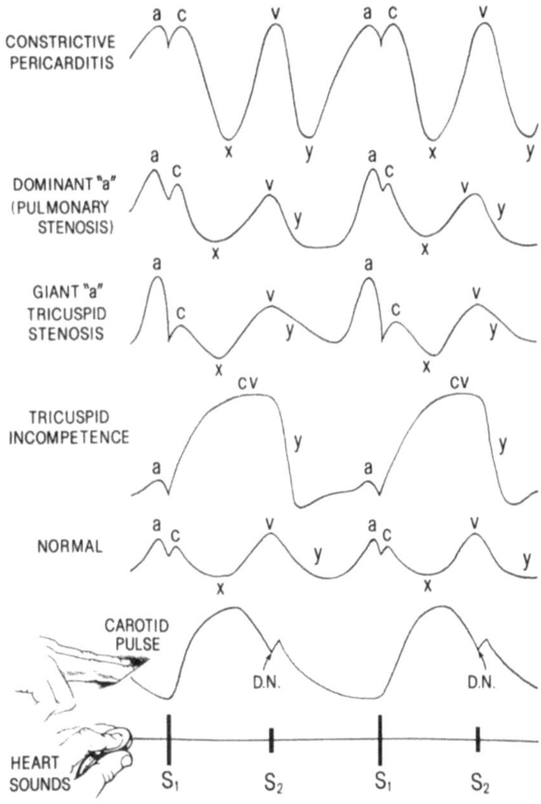

FIGURE 2.6. Diagrammatic respresentation of various abnormalities of the jugular venous pulse. These are best elucidated by inspection and simultaneous palpation of the carotid pulse or auscultation of the heart sounds.

earlobe is therefore venous. Venous pulsation is markedly altered by changes in position. Venous pulsation is vigorous, extending to the earlobes, when lying flat; in the seated position, the level drops. Arterial pulsation, on the other hand, is more marked in the upright position. Pressure on the liver or abdomen, or elevation of the legs, temporarily amplifies venous pulsation.

2. *Wave form*. Venous pulse waves are multiple, with at least two peaks and two troughs for every arterial pulse beat when the heart rate and rhythm are normal. With increasing rate the peaks become fused: With rapid rhythm it may become difficult to differentiate arterial from venous pulsations. However, venous pulse waves are usually impalpable and gentle pressure obliterates all waves, unlike arterial pulsation. Venous pulsations, moreover, are slow rising and more diffuse.

3. *Timing*. The first venous wave precedes the first heart sound and the upstroke of the carotid pulse when sinus rhythm is present, whereas the second venous wave succeeds the arterial upstroke.

Jugular Venous Pressure

The internal jugular vein communicates directly with the right atrium and accurately reflects atrial pulsation and pressure. Since it is not a rigid container, lateral pulsation occurs, in addition to pulsation at the summit of the venous column. Therefore, when the pressure is estimated, it is important to measure the top of the oscillating column.

The patient is examined with the head and shoulders at an angle of 30°, 60°, or 90°, respectively, and the height of the venous column is measured from the angle of Louis (sternal angle), which is the best clinical reference point. Because of gravity, the position of the patient is important, the venous pressure being lower in the neck in the upright than in the recumbent position. When properly estimated, the jugular venous pressure accurately measures right atrial pressure.

The normal jugular venous pulse is not seen above the sternal angle at an inclination of 45°. Exercise, amyl nitrite, and vasodilators slightly elevate the pressure by increasing venous return and transmitting arterial pressure to the venules.

Inspiratory filling of the veins (Kussmaul's sign) is an exaggeration of normal venous filling with inspiration. In health, the compliance of the right heart is such that the increased venous return during inspiration is accepted without significant pressure change. In constrictive pericarditis and severe congestive cardiac failure, however, the right heart compliance is reduced, so that increased venous return produces increased venous filling of the neck veins, with distension and elevation of the pressure in these structures.

Hepatojugular reflux Slow, continuous pressure on the liver or elsewhere on the abdomen for about 1 minute will aggravate venous congestion or make it evident when latent. During pressure, the patient must continue to breathe quietly and normally. In health, the right ventricle copes adequately with the increased systemic venous return. In right ventricular failure, latent or manifest, the increased systemic venous return is held up and distends the neck veins.

Causes of Elevated Pulsating Jugular Veins

1. Congestive cardiac failure is by far the commonest cause.
   a. Right heart failure secondary to left heart failure is usually responsible.
   b. Right heart failure secondary to pulmonary hypertension or right–sided valve disease.
2. In high output states (anemia, thyrotoxicosis, beriberi, arterioaneurysms) the jugular venous pressure is moderately elevated, and it is controversial whether this is part and parcel of the hyperkinetic circulation. It may well be due to arteriolar dilatation, resulting in less damping effect of the arterial pulse, transmission of more pressure to the venous system, and increased blood flow. When liver distension and other signs, such as edema, develop, it is clearly due to cardiac failure.
3. When the volume capacity of the right ventricle is restricted, it cannot accept a normal venous return, resulting in venous distension. The common causes are pericarditis (effusion or constriction), tumor of the right ventricle, and obstructive cardiomyopathy.
4. Increased blood volume, especially when acutely produced (e.g., by overtransfusion, excessive sodium retention, steroid administration, acute nephritis, pregnancy, hepatic disease).
5. Raised intrapleural and abdominal binders and pregnancy produce a raised jugular venous pressure, which can be relieved immediately when the cause is removed.

Causes of Elevated Nonpulsating Jugular Veins

The only genuine cause is complete obstruction of the neck veins, either because of thrombosis of the superior vena cava or its main tributaries, or because of external compression by conditions such as superior mediastinal glands, aneurysm, and so on. The external jugular vein is commonly obstructed for purely local anatomical reasons, and this can often be relieved by altering the position of the neck. Partial obstruction of the veins (e.g., by a tight collar) does not completely obliterate all pulsations.

In constrictive pericarditis the neck veins are often so distended that lateral pulsation does not occur. Distended, nonpulsating veins have been wrongly regarded as a feature of this condition. If the top of the oscillating column is carefully sought (e.g., behind the ears) in the upright posture or in the temporal veins, definite pulsation will always be found.

Jugular Venous Pulsation

The normal venous pulse (Fig. 2.6) consists of two positive ("a" and "v") and two negative ("x" and "y") waves. With atrial contraction the "a" wave is produced, and with ventricular contraction the "v" wave is formed. The "v" wave is due to pressure buildup in the venous reservoir, while the tricuspid valve is closed. Between the "a" and "v" waves is the "x" descent, which is associated with atrial relaxation. The "x" descent is partly interrupted by a small positive "c" wave. The "c" wave is produced by tricuspid valve closure. Between the "v" wave and the succeeding "a" wave is the "y" descent, produced by emptying of the venous reservoir into the right ventricle.

When the compliance of the right ventricle is reduced, or the right ventricle is overdistended, as in severe right heart failure, the ventricle fills rapidly and early in diastole. After this the pressure mounts in the venous system, producing a sharp "h" wave following the "y" descent and preceding the succeeding "a" wave. Normally, the "h" wave is absent or diminutive.

Abnormalities of the "a" Wave

In *normal sinus rhythm* the "a" wave precedes ventricular systole and therefore the first heart sound and carotid pulsation. By timing the carotid upstroke with the finger and auscultating the first heart sound the venous wave can be seen to precede arterial pulsation and the first heart sound by a very short interval. When the P-R interval is prolonged, the interval between "a" and carotid upstroke is prolonged correspondingly. "A" waves disappear in atrial fibrillation.

Giant "a" Waves Are Produced by a Hypertrophied Right Atrium.

A hypertrophied right atrium is associated with a dominant or giant "a" wave (5–10 or over 10 mm Hg, absolute figures, respectively). Unless properly timed they may be mistaken for an arterial pulsation, because the wave is rapid, forceful, and often palpable. Giant "a" waves are most commonly encountered in pulmonary stenosis, especially when severe, and pulmonary hypertension. When present it is an important sign but no inferences can be drawn when it is absent.

In tricuspid stenosis, a dominant or giant "a" wave is almost always present, even when the degree of stenosis is mild. Presystolic pulsation of the liver is the equivalent of a giant "a" wave. A loud presystolic "knocking" sound is often audible in the neck when a giant "a" wave is present. Inspiration accentuates the "a" wave and intensifies this sound.

"Cannon a waves" occur when atrial contraction occurs during ventricular systole. They occur when there is A-V dissociation. The force of atrial contraction is transmitted back to the venous system because the tricuspid valve is closed (Fig. 2.7). Isolated cannon "a" waves occur most commonly with ventricular ectopics. Regular cannon "a" waves at a normal heart rate occur in nodal rhythm or sinus rhythm with a long P-R interval. Regular cannon waves at rapid heart rates occur in supraventricular tachycardia, especially nodal.

Irregular cannon "a" waves occurring at a slow heart rate suggest heart block, particularly complete heart block, whereas at fast heart rates the diagnosis is paroxysmal ventricular tachycardia.

Abnormalities of the v Wave

In tricuspid incompetence the "c" and "v" waves are characteristically fused and prominent. When the incompetence is severe, as in rheumatic tricuspid valve disease, the pulsation in the neck may become palpable. It can be recognized, however, by the slow prolonged nature of the wave. A similar pulsation is felt in the distended liver. Prominent "cv" waves are encountered in heart failure from any cause, particularly when atrial fibrillation is present. In atrial fibrillation without heart failure the *v* wave is abnormally age.

Abnormality of the "x" Descent

When the "c" and "v" waves are fused the "x" descent disappears, as in tricuspid incompetence. In the absence of atrial activity (e.g., atrial fibrillation), "x" is generally absent. A

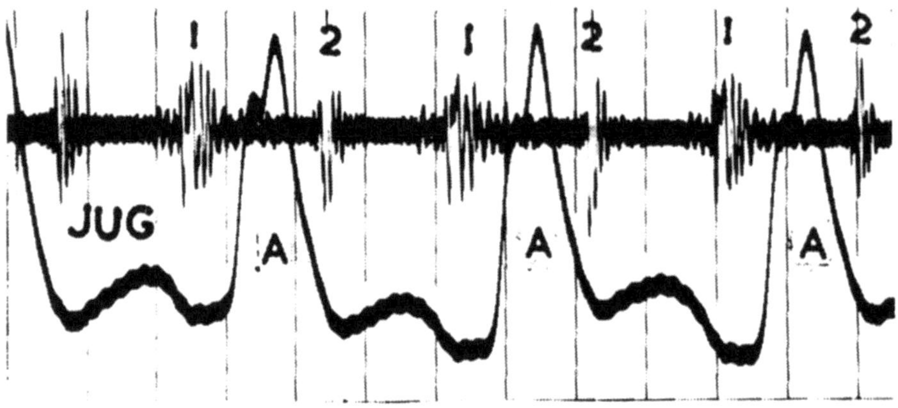

FIGURE 2.7. Phonocardiogram and jugular venous tracing demonstrating cannon "a" waves produced by atrial contraction occurring during ventricular systole in a case of paroxysmal supraventricular tachycardia.

prominent "x", even in the presence of atrial fibrillation, has, however, been described in constrictive pericarditis. In this condition the venous pulsation is often highly characteristic. The pressure is generally markedly elevated, with prominent "x" and "y" descents of short duration (i.e., the negative waves rather than the positive dominate the venous pulse).

Abnormalities of the "y" Descent

A slow "y" descent with a high mean venous pressure is characteristic of tricuspid stenosis, (raised venous pressure, giant "a" wave and slow "y" descent). The "y" descent is precipitous in constrictive pericarditis (Friedreich's sign) and in severe heart failure, due to sudden release of blood dammed back in the right atrium during ventricular systole. Equally characteristic is the sharp "h" wave that succeeds "y" descent (see above).

Examination of the Heart

Inspection of the *chest cage* may disclose various abnormalities. These include (1) the barrelshape of emphysema, (2) a depressed sternum, or scoliosis, which often displaces the heart, producing fictitious cardiomegaly and abnormal murmurs, (3) a central chest bulge, frequently associated with large ventricular septal defect, or (4) left chest bulge, often seen with large atrial septal defects.

Dilatation of the veins over the chest is produced by superior mediastinal obstruction. Visible arterial pulsations, particularly posteriorly, in the interscapular and intercostal spaces indicate coarctation of the aorta. Pulsations in the first and second intercostal spaces to the right of the sternum occur with aneurysm of the ascending aorta.

The apex beat can frequently be localized by inspection. Abnormal pulsations due to left or right ventricular enlargements, aneurysm of the aorta, or pulsation of the pulmonary artery may be observed. Gallop rhythm is often better seen and felt than heard.

Palpation: By definition the apex beat is the farthest point of cardiac pulsation downward and outward, although some authorities regard the point of maximum thrust as the apex. Diffuse pulsation may be present in the region of the apex, but the apex, being a point, cannot be diffuse. Localization of the apex beat is important in assessing cardiac size and, within certain limits, is a most accurate guide. The normal apex beat is usually felt within the midclavicular line in the fifth intercostal space. When displaced, the position is expressed in relation to the intercostal space and the midclavicular, anterior, mid- or posterior axillary lines (e.g., sixth space midaxillary line).

False conclusions about cardiac size may be

drawn if conditions displacing the apex are not recognized. Usually, when the heart is displaced and not enlarged, it is moved laterally and upward; downward and outward displacement is rare. Pleural or pulmonary pathology, scoliosis, and sternal depression are the common causes of cardiac displacement. Occasionally, the heart is pushed forward and the apex displaced outward by an aneurysm of the descending aorta, producing an apparent cardiomegaly. More rarely, the aneurysm itself may produce a pulsation, giving rise to a double apex beat. The pulsation produced by the aneurysm follows the apex beat by a fraction of a second.

The heart may be central in position (mesocardia), in which case the apex is nearer the sternum than normal. Mirror-image dextrocardia or dextroversion may be present when the apex beat is in the right midclavicular line.

The character of the *apex beat* and of the cardiac pulsations provides important evidence of chamber enlargement. Palpation should always be performed first with the patient on the back, propped up at an angle of about 45°.

In health, the left ventricle strikes the anterior chest wall and forms the apex. The portion of the heart underlying the parasternal area is the anterior wall of the right ventricle. Early in systole the left ventricle moves forward, then retracts away from the chest wall. The normal apical impulse therefore consists of an outward thrust that is short and ends well before the second sound.

In *high output states* such as thyrotoxicosis, anxiety, and anemia, the normal impulse is exaggerated but remains rapid and short, and this is particularly well noted in children with thin chest walls. The same rapid short impulse occurs with diastolically overloaded left ventricles, associated with aortic and mitral incompetence. However, pulsation is more diffuse, hyperdynamic, and forceful, the thrust having increased amplitude.

Left ventricular hypertrophy associated with systolic overload is characterized by a sustained pansystolic, localized, heaving thrust (Fig. 2.8). The ventricular septum is rotated to the right and the apical impulse is actually formed by the anterolateral wall of the left ventricle. The left ventricle no longer retracts away from the chest wall but may actually move forward, accounting for prolongation of the pulsation. Where both systolic and diastolic left ventricular overload are present, a combination of an overactive and a sustained impulse is present.

Attention should now be paid to the left parasternal and epigastric regions. In health, movement of the anterior surface of the right ventricle is associated with little pulsation and there may be a visible retraction. *Systolic overload of the right ventricle* (pulmonary stenosis or pulmonary hypertension) produces a heaving sustained pulsation formed by the hypertrophied right ventricle. The parasternal lift of right ventricular hypertrophy is usually not of great magnitude. In severe right ventricular hypertrophy, the heart may be so rotated that the right ventricle comes to form the apex. The heaving apex of right ventricular hypertrophy may then be mistaken for left ventricular hypertrophy.

Diastolic overload of the right ventricle produced by tricuspid incompetence or atrial septal defect produces a palpable diastolic lift in the parasternal region. In severe tricuspid insufficiency a "tricuspid rock" may be evident. This is produced by systolic pulsation to the left of the sternum produced by the right ventricle (Fig. 2.9). This must be distinguished from the left parasternal lift of mitral insufficiency ("left atrial lift") (Fig. 2.8).

In ischemic heart disease, ectopic sustained systolic pulsations may be palpable over the precordium and are a result of aneurysm or dyskinesis. They may be transient and evident only during an attack of angina pectoris.

The base of the heart must now be palpated. In the presence of increased pulmonary flow (left to right shunts, particularly atrial septal defects) a diastolic lift can be felt over the right ventricular outflow tract and a systolic pulsation over the pulmonary artery. In pulmonary hypertension, palpable closure (diastolic shock) of the pulmonary valves occurs.

Presystolic pulsation (double apical impulse) must always be looked for carefully at the apex. It is a result of powerful left atrial contraction and can often be more readily felt than

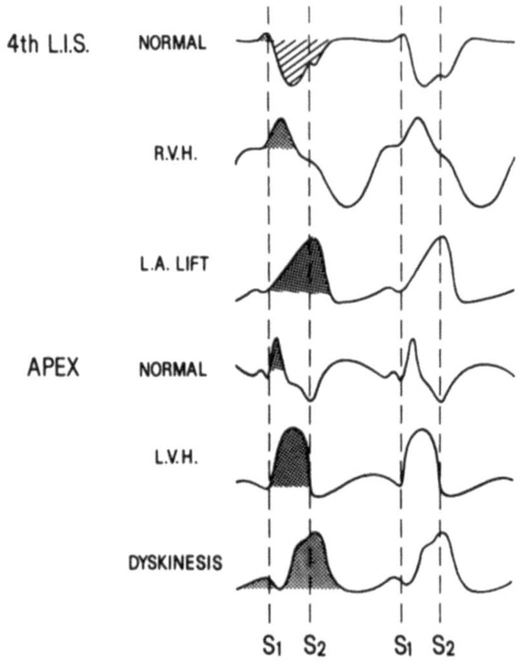

FIGURE 2.8. Diagrammatic representation of precordial impulses palpable in the fourth left intercostal space (4th LIS) and at the apex. The shaded positive areas represent palpable lifts. The lined negative area in the 4th LIS is a visible (but not palpable) retraction.

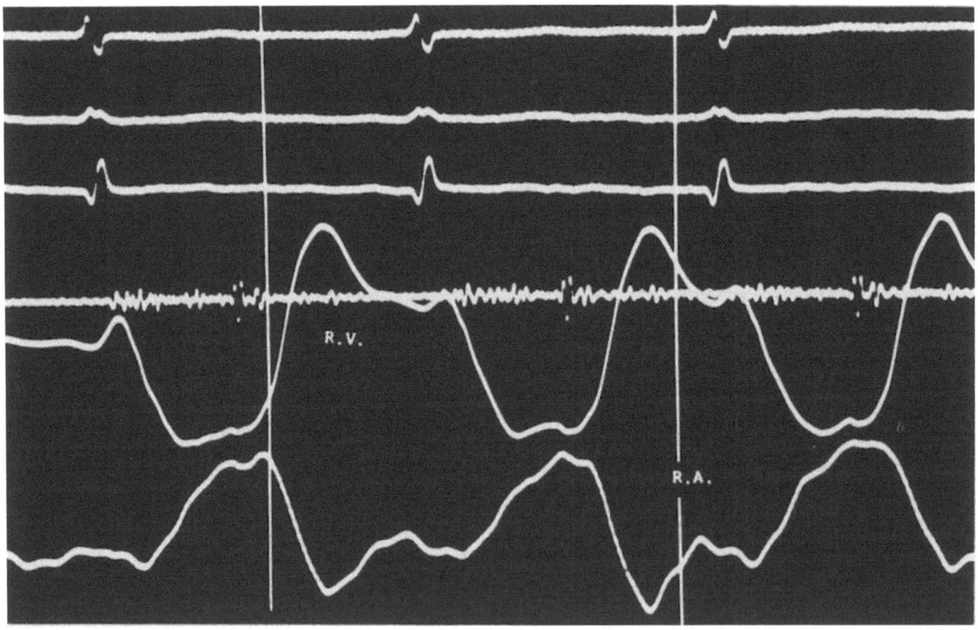

FIGURE 2.9. Kinetocardiograms demonstrating a "tricuspid rock" produced by systolic pulsation of the right atrium (R.A.) to the right of the sternum, and diastolic pulsation to the left of the sternum produced by right ventricular filling. R.V. right ventricle; R.A. right atrium. (Courtesy of Dr. T.G.A. Armstrong.)

the fourth sound heard. It accompanies left ventricular hypertrophy with diminished compliance and is common in systemic hypertension, aortic stenosis, and obstructive cardiomyopathy. In the latter condition, the apex beat may have three impulses: a presystolic pulsation and an ensuing bifid systolic pulsation produced by left ventricular hypertrophy, complicated by midsystolic outflow tract obstruction.

The patient should now be turned onto the left side (left decubitus position) and the apex palpated again. Palpation in this position brings the left ventricular wall nearer the chest wall, due to change in the position of the heart, elevation of the diaphragm, and shift of the mediastinum to the left. It is a particularly good position for feeling a presystolic pulsation and for appreciating diastolic left ventricular filling and the third heart sound. The sustained nature of the left ventricular thrust of left ventricular hypertrophy is also observed more easily.

With *mitral stenosis* the first heart sound is frequently felt as a sharp, short tap, replacing the normal apical pulsation, and the left ventricular lift is impalpable. What one actually feels is the sensation imparted by the sudden closure of the thickened and diseased mitral valve.

With *constrictive pericarditis* retraction occurs late in systole and is frequently overlooked because it is overshadowed by the rapid outward pulsation that occurs early in diastole. The latter corresponds to the rapid filling of the ventricles. This diastolic pulsation may be misinterpreted as systolic unless timing is precise. This is an important physical sign. Congestive cardiomyopathy may mimic constrictive pericarditis quite closely. When the diastolic lift is improperly timed as systolic (particularly when a third heart sound is present), cardiomyopathy may be erroneously diagnosed.

Thrills are the expression of loud murmurs, systolic or diastolic. They are best felt in held expiration. Aortic thrills are felt at the base, with the patient sitting up, leaning forward, and holding the breath in expiration. Mitral diastolic thrills are best felt after exercise, with the patient in the left decubitus position during held expiration.

Percussion is of limited value. Cardiomegaly can generally be better determined by other means. It may be, useful in detecting pericardial effusion when cardiac pulsations are absent. On rare occasions, dullness beyond the apex beat is found in pericardial effusion. The most useful sign of pericardial effusion is dullness to percussion over the lower sternum. Similar dullness is encountered only in gross right atrial enlargement. Dullness to percussion is found over an aneurysm and pleural effusion.

The Hands

Examination of the hands is rewarding. Warm, sweaty hands, with a coarse or fine tremor, suggest *thyrotoxicosis*; cold, moist hands suggest anxiety or nervousness; and dry hands with a rough skin suggest *hypothyroidism.* Long, tapering hands and fingers indicate arachnodactyly and *Marfan syndrome. Osler nodes* are painful, tender, reddish-brown areas in the pulps of the fingers; like *splinter hemorrhages* under the fingernails, they suggest infective endocarditis. Only splinter hemorrhages at the base of the nail, particularly when they are red and fleshy looking, are significant. Linear brown streaks at the nail tips are extremely common in healthy individuals, particularly manual workers.

Spoon-shaped nails or koilonychia accompany iron-deficient anemia. Telangiectasia of the fingers and nails, with atrophy of the fingers, suggests systemic lupus erythmatosus, and nodules on the tendons of the fingers suggest rheumatic fever or rheumatoid arthritis. Scleroderma not uncommonly involves the fingers and has several cardiovascular associations.

Clubbing of the fingers with cyanosis suggests congenital cyanotic heart disease, the degree paralleling the intensity of the cyanosis. Clubbing without cyanosis suggests pulmonary disease or infective endocarditis.

Hot, moist hands in congestive cardiac failure suggest cor pulmonale, thyrotoxicosis, or beriberi; when cyanosis is also present, cor pulmonale is more likely. Cyanosis with a cold skin and a pink tongue indicates peripheral cyanosis. Pink palms with warm hands suggest liver disease, which may be primary or secondary to chronic venous hypertension. Capillary pulsation indicates peripheral vascular dilatation, especially aortic incompetence.

The Eye

The Orbits

Hyperteleorism (wide separation of the orbits) has a common association with pulmonary valve stenosis. *Exophthalmos* is a classical complication of thyrotoxicosis but may also be found in euthyroid patients with protracted heart failure. This is a result of elevated intraorbital pressure, which causes orbital protrusion and a stare produced by weight loss (cardiac exophthalmos).

The Conjunctivae

Conjunctival hemorrhages occur frequently in infective endocarditis. A velvety dusky appearance is characteristic of polycythemic congenital cyanotic heart disease. Suffused, congested conjunctivae in chronic lung disease is often suggestive of respiratory acidosis. Jaundice is recognized most easily in the bulbar conjunctivae. *Arcus senilis* (which is neither an arc nor a manifestation of senility, in most cases), better called arcus cornealis, is produced by a collection of cholesterol and other lipids in the corneal membranes. The prevalence increases with advancing years and it appears earlier and more frequently in men than in women. It has long been regarded as an accompaniment of hypercholesterolemia and thus a sign of ischemic heart disease. Its appearance under the age of 40 suggests an increased susceptibility to coronary artery disease, but over 40 it has no clinical significance.

The Iris

The disturbance of connective tissue, fundamental to the pathology of Marfan syndrome, can be detected in the eyes by laxity of the lens. In milder forms, iridodonesis ("iris wobble") is present. This is elicited by asking the patient to look to one or the other side suddenly and observing the iris. *Dislocation of the lens* is a more advanced manifestation. Pupillary abnormalities (irregularity, altered responses to light) may indicate syphilis.

The Fundi

In hypertension the state of the retinal arteries should always be determined. Changes vary from a slight increase in the light reflex (grade 1) to papilledema with exudates and hemorrhages (grade 4). In health, the arterial diameter should be no less than two thirds the venous. In hypertension, the arterial diameter is narrowed, and tortuosity, kinking, and venous compression develop. Severe cor pulmonale with polycythemia may be associated with papilledema but without arterial changes. Hemorrhage and exudates in the fundi are commonly found in hypertension, nephritis, diabetes, and blood diseases. They must be particularly sought for in infective endocarditis. Hemorrhages with pale centers (Roth spots) suggest infective endocarditis or leukemia. Tortuous arterioles around the disc margin have been described in coarctation of the aorta.

Cyanosis

Cyanosis can be detected clinically when the arterial oxygen saturation is 85% or less. It is more readily recognized in nonpigmented patients. When mild, the presence or absence of cyanosis is frequently controversial, and considerable errors are made in both directions. Fluorescent light is particularly deceptive, producing a bluish tinge when cyanosis is in fact absent.

Under normal circumstances, blood leaving the lungs is almost fully saturated, so that 100 ml contains 15 g of oxyhemoglobin. By the time this blood returns to the lungs, it contains only 10 g of oxyhemoglobin. The tissues do not extract oxygen uniformly. For example, the heart muscle removes at least 70% of the oxygen, whereas kidneys and skin may remove as little as 10%. The bright blood in the capillaries and superficial skin vessels accounts for the normal skin color. When capillary blood contains 5 g or more of reduced hemoglobin, cyanosis becomes detectable in nonpigmented skins. Dilatation of the capillaries increases the ease with which the blue color can be detected. Vasoconstriction reduces the blue appearance. In polycythemia a small percentage drop in saturation may lead to a great deal of circulating reduced hemoglobin, hence the ease with which cyanosis is detected in the presence of polycythemia. Conversely, in anemia a large percentage drop in saturation is required before cyanosis becomes evident.

Cyanosis may be due entirely to local disturbance of skin circulation—fully saturated blood entering and markedly reduced blood leaving the skin (peripheral cyanosis)—or it may be due to central causes—reduced hemoglobin entering the skin, becoming more educed as it leaves it (central cyanosis). Both factors may be operative in the same patient.

Peripheral Cyanosis

Peripheral cyanosis is a result of stagnation and sluggish circulation of blood through skin. Most commonly it occurs when the extremities are exposed to cold and is of no pathological significance. It is seen, however, in shock, low output heart failure, and venous obstruction. Clinically, the condition is recognized by the presence of poor peripheral circulation and reduced cardiac output. The extremities are cold and blue, the heart rate rapid with small pulses, and sweating is often present. The internal mucosae, like the tongue, remain pink, unless circulatory failure is extreme, with shock. Peripheral cyanosis frequently coexists with central cyanosis, as in mitral stenosis. Peripheral cyanosis is also encountered in obstruction to the venous drainage of the extremities.

Central Cyanosis

Any condition that sufficiently reduces the arterial saturation below the normal 95–99% produces central cyanosis. It is produced by (1) right-to-left shunt, (2) admixture lesions where there is obligatory mixing of pulmonary and systemic venous blood, (3) Lung disease, and (4) abnormal hemoglobin.

1. *Right-to-Left Shunt*
   a. *At Atrial Level*: Reversed shunt through an atrial septal defect or stretched foramen ovale (pulmonary stenosis, pulmonary hypertension).
   b. *At Ventricular Level*: Ventricular septal defect with reversed shunt (Eisenmenger syndrome, Fallot tetralogy, pulmonary atresia).
   c. *At Aortopulmonary Level*: Reversed shunt through a patent ductus arteriosus or aortopulmonary window.
   d. *At Pulmonary Venous Level*: Pulmonary A-V fistula and vascular tumors (e.g.,

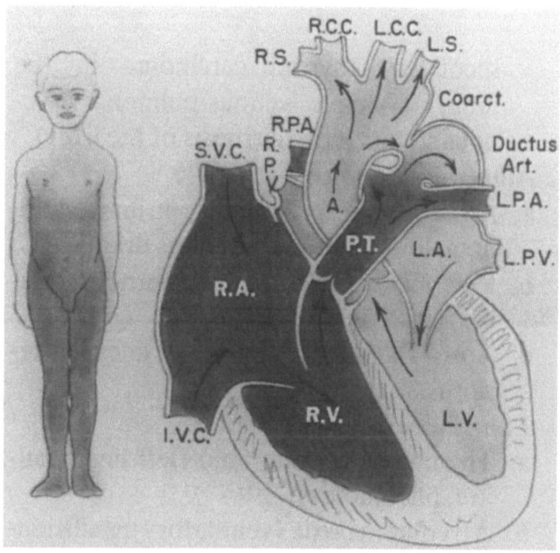

FIGURE 2.10. Diagrammatic representation of *differential cyanosis* evident in the trunk and lower extremities, produced by a right-to-left shunt through a patent ductus ateriosus and associated with a preductal coarctation of the aorta. R.S. and L.S. right and left subclavian arteries, respectively; R.C.C. and L.C.C. right and left common carotid arteries, respectively; S.V.C. and I.V.C. superior and inferior vena cava, respectively; L.P.A. and R.P.A. left and right pulmonary arteries, respectively; L.V. and R.V. left and right ventricles, respectively. Reprinted, with permission, from Chesler et al. Am J Cardiol 21:72, 1968.

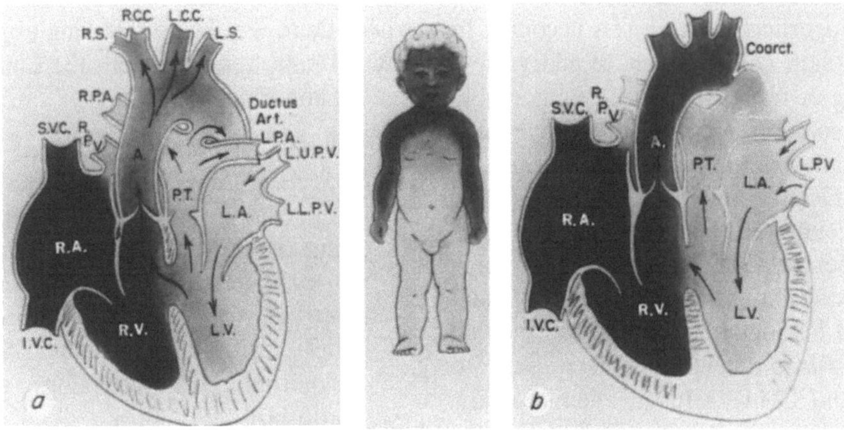

FIGURE 2.11. Diagrammatic representation of *reversed differential cyanosis*, where there is cyanosis of the head and upper extremities but not of the trunk and lower extremities, produced by (a) transposition of the great vessels, ventricular septal defect, and patent ductus arteriosus throughout which there is a right-to-left shunt leading to delivery of oxygenated blood to the lower extremities, and (b) with associated preductal coarctation of the aorta. Abbreviations as in Figure 2.10. Reprinted, with permission, from Chesler et al. Am J Cardiol 21:72, 1968.

secondary thyroid carcinoma in the lung), systemic venous-pulmonary venous shunts (e.g., cirrhosis of the liver).

2. *Admixture Lesions*:
   a. *Atrial Level*: Common atrium, total anomalous pulmonary venous drainage.
   b. *Ventricular Level*: Single ventricle, double outlet right ventricle.
   c. *Aorto-Pulmonary Level*: Truncus arteriosus.
3. *Lung Disease:*
   a. The alveoli contain fluid (left heart failure, pneumonia).
   b. Alveolar hypoxia (ventilatory insufficiency with poor distribution and mixing of air, alveolar hypoventilation, hyaline membrane disease).
4. *Abnormal Hemoglobin*: Methemoglobinemia and sulfhemoglobinemia prevent the uptake of oxygen by hemoglobin.

Differential Cyanosis

In patent ductus with reversed flow the toes are more cyanosed than the fingers and this is more marked after a hot bath. Rarely, the fingers are more cyanosed than the toes (e.g., transposition of the great vessels with coarctation and a patent ductus arteriosus) (Figs. 2.10 and 2.11).

The Skin

Pallor, cyanosis, sweating, and dryness have been discussed under examination of the hands. Of special significance to the cardiologist are *erythema marginatum* and subcutaneous nodules, which occur in acute rheumatic fever. Petechial hemorrhages and purpura occur in infective endocarditis. Pigmentation of the skin occurs in Addison disease and hemochromatosis. Attacks of *flushing*, particularly of the ace, occur in carcinoid tumors, in which the skin becomes blotchy and erythematous with a cyanotic tinge. A paroxysm of hypertension in pheochromocytoma is associated with pallor or flushing of the skin, sweating, headache, and abdominal or chest pain. Xanthomatous infiltration of the skin with nodules in the tendons of the calves and nodules over a bony prominence such as the elbow indicate primary xanthomatosis, in which the vessels, particularly the coronary arteries may be involved. Lentigenes, brown macules on the neck and trunk, are associated with pulmonary stenosis and hypertrophic cardiomyopathy.

Additional Reading

Armstrong TG, Meeran MK, Gotsman MS: The left atrial lift. Am Heart J 82: 764, 1971.

Bedford DE: The ancient art of feeling the pulse. Br Heart J 13:423, 1951.

Bordley J, Connor CAR, Hamilton WF, Kerr WJ, Wiggers CJ: Recommendations for human blood pressure determinations by sphygmomanometers. Circulation 4:503, 1951.

Eddleman EE, Hefner L, Reeves TJ, Harrison TR: Movements of the human heart. I. The genesis of apical impulses. Arch Int Med 99:401, 1957.

Hartman H: The jugular venous tracing. Am Heart J 59:698, 1960.

Hurst JW, Blackard E: Inspection and palpation on the front of the chest. Am Heart J 56:159, 1958.

Mounsey JPD: Inspection and palpation of the cardiac impulse. Prog Cardiovasc Dis 10:187, 1968.

Schrire V, Beck W, Chesler E: The heart and the eye. Am Heart J 85:122, 1973.

3
Auscultation

Accurate auscultation is a difficult discipline acquired by meticulous attention to detail. Repeated self-monitoring with sound and pulse tracings increases proficiency. The accomplished auscultator possesses a powerful diagnostic technique, particularly in the field of congenital heart disease.

It is insufficient to "pick up a murmur." A good examiner will determine its timing, frequency, configuration, site of maximal intensity, and radiation, and also reposition the patient to note the effect of various bedside maneuvers. Additionally, he or she will come away with a positive analysis and impression of the normal and additional heart sounds, having assessed each event carefully and independently.

A good stethoscope should be binaural, fitting snugly in the ears, with two tubes about 10 in. long made of rigid rubber so that they do not rub against each other. Both a bell and a diaphragm must be available, preferably incorporated into one piece. The bell should be applied lightly to the chest wall to prevent stretching of the skin. The greater the pressure on the bell, the more the skin tightens and the more the bell behaves as a diaphragm, damping out low-frequency sounds. The diaphragm is essential for the auscultation of high-frequency, and the bell for low-frequency sounds and murmurs. The bell is reserved for auscultation of the middiastolic murmurs of mitral and tricuspid stenosis and the third and fourth heart sounds; the diaphram is reserved for all other murmurs, clicks, and sounds.

The human ear can detect changes in pitch more easily than it can detect changes in intensity. Although high- and low-pitched tones may have the same intensity, the human ear interprets the higher pitched tone as the louder one. The sensitivity is poor for lower pitched vibrations and better for higher pitched vibrations; many cardiac vibrations are therefore inaudible. Should a loud sound or murmur be followed by a weaker or lower pitched sound, the latter may be masked.

Auscultation of the heart should always be carried out in a noise-free area. Patients should be examined from their right, lying on their back, then turned onto the left side, then sitting up. Under certain circumstances they should be standing or leaning forward or squatting. The examination is performed in held expiration; then the effects of respiration should be noted and, if necessary, vasoactive drugs may be used. It may be necessary to exercise the subject and then auscultate again, usually in the left decubitus position to best detect mitral events.

Concentrate on one event at a time. The first step is to identify the first heart sound by palpating the carotid artery. The upstroke of the carotid pulse coincides with the first heart sound in all areas. Having identified the first and second heart sounds, systole and diastole are then auscultated in turn, noting the intensity, quality, duration, and radiation of each sound or murmur. A mental note is made of the timing and the site of maximal intensity of all the auscultatory events. Both the front and the back of the chest, and the neck, should be carefully auscultated rather than just the pure

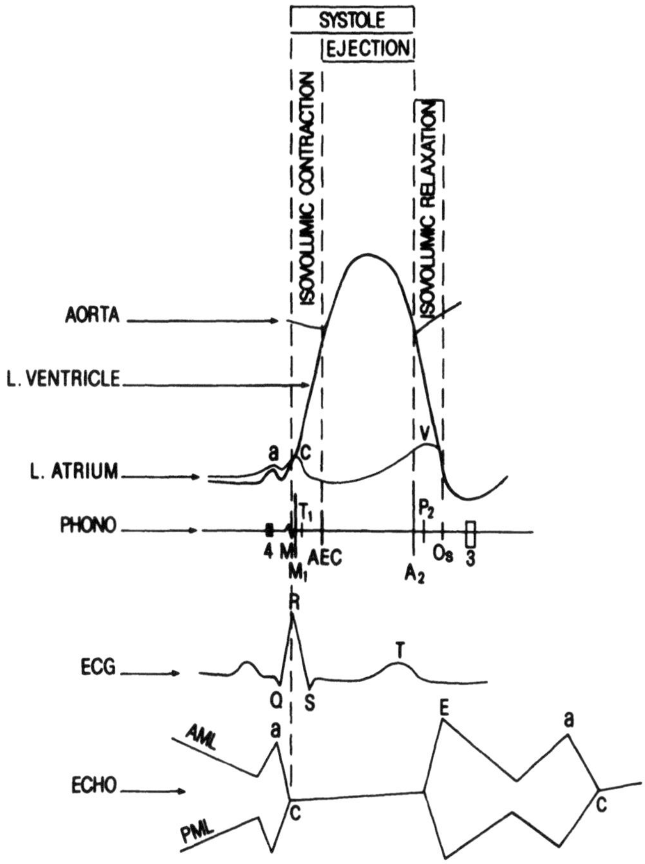

FIGURE 3.1. Diagrammatic representation of the left-sided hemodynamic events in the cardiac cycle related to a simultaneous phonocardiogram, echocardiogram, and electrocardiogram. The fourth heart sound follows left atrial contraction, the P wave of the electrocardiogram, and the reopening movement of the mitral leaflets echocardiographically. "M" occurs at the time of crossover of the left atrial and left ventricular pressure pulses, and is synchronous with the R wave of the electrocardiogram at the onset of preisovolumic systole. M1 follows "M" and is synchronous with the left atrial C wave and apposition of the anterior and posterior mitral leaflets. T1 (representing tricuspid valve closure) follows M1. An aortic ejection click (AEC) occurs at the time of crossover of aortic and left ventricular pressure pulses. A2 occurs when left ventricular pressure drops below that of aortic; it is followed by P2. The opening snap of the mitral valve (OS) occurs when the left atrial pressure drops below that of the left ventricle. The third heart sound occurs at the time of rapid ventricular filling.

localized prescribed areas. The prescribed areas are as follows: the apical or *mitral area* (MA); the *tricuspid area* (4LS), the fourth left intercostal space parasternally; and the *aortic area* (AA), the second right intercostal space parasternally.

The Heart Sounds

Closure of the atrioventricular and semilunar valves is (Fig. 3.1) responsible for the first and second heart sounds, respectively. Since right ventricular pressure is much lower than the left, the sounds produced by tricuspid (T1) and pulmonary valve closure (P2) are far softer than mitral (M1) and aortic closure (A2). They, therefore, do not radiate as widely.

Anatomically, the heart valves are very close to each other, but on the chest wall there are certain areas where the sounds produced by each valve are best heard. Thus pulmonary valve closure is most readily heard in the second left intercostal space—called the *pulmonary area* (PA); the sound is soft and is restricted to the second and third left intercostal spaces. Tricuspid valve closure is best heard at the fourth left intercostal space in the *tricuspid area* (4LS). The mitral and aortic closure sounds are heard at all areas, the former better at the apex in the mitral area (MA), the latter at the base of the heart.

The first heart sound at the apex is almost entirely a result of mitral valve closure, since Tl is too soft to radiate to the apex. In the second right intercostal space, the aortic area (AA), the second sound is produced entirely by aortic valve closure.

The First Heart Sound

This consists of a low-pitched, usually inaudible initial vibration called "M", which occurs at the very onset of isovolumic systole at the time of crossover of the left atrial and left ventricular pressures and the first forward movement of the apexcardiogram (Figs. 3.2 and 3.3). Initially thought to be a result of coaption of the leaflets of the mitral valve, it is more likely to result from a vibration set up by tensing of the ventricular walls at the very onset of systole. The sound is present and sometimes accentuated and even clinically audible when the atriorventricular valves have been replaced with a prosthesis and therefore cannot arise from leaflet coaption. M becomes louder during the short cycles of atrial fibrillation and may be the mechanism for "presystolic" accentuation of the middiastolic murmur in atrial fibrillation (Fig. 3.3).

The major component of the first heart sound, M1, occurs slightly later, at the peak of the left atrial C wave and is produced by leaflet apposition, which can be demonstrated echocardiographically (Fig. 3.4). For clinical purposes, therefore, apposition of the leaflets of the mitral valve is responsible for the mitral component of the first heart sound and apposition of the tricuspid leaflets for the tricuspid component of the first heart sound.

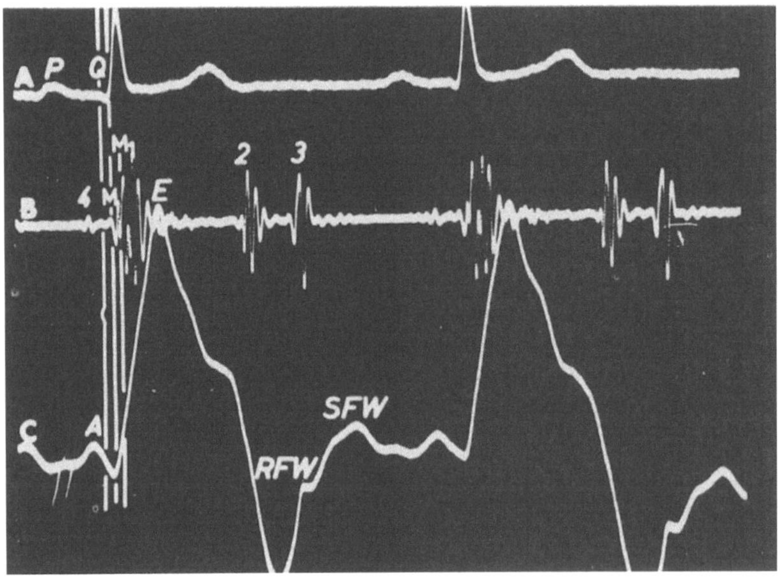

FIGURE 3.2. Phonocardiographic recording of the left-sided heart sounds (B) in relationship to the electrocardiogram (A) and apexcardiogram (C). "M" occurs at the very onset of isovolumic systole, represented by the first forward movement of the apexcardiogram after the nadir following the A wave. The fourth heart sound is synchronous with the peak of the angle between the rapid filling phase (RFW) and slow filling phase (SFW) of the ECG. Reprinted, with permission, from T.G.A. Armstrong et al. Echocardiographic and phonocardiographic observations on the initial low frequency component of the first heart sound. Heart J 40:750, 1978.

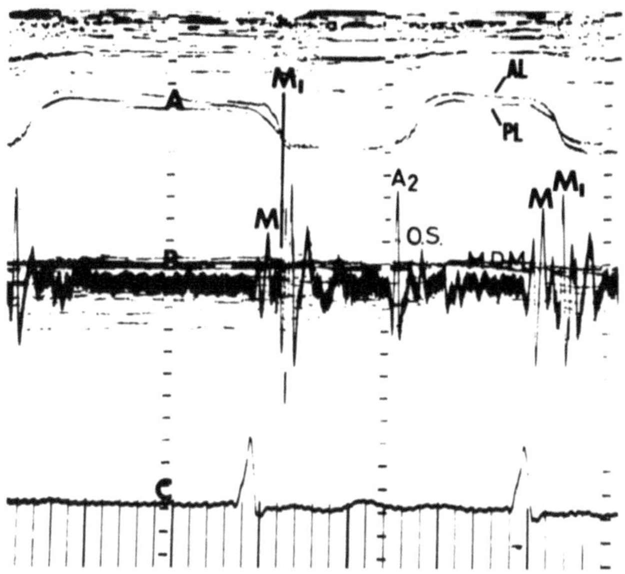

FIGURE 3.3. Echocardiogram (A), phonocardiogram (B), and electrocardiogram (C) in mitral stenosis demonstrating the initial low-frequency component of the first heart sound (M) occurring immediately before MI, the latter being synchronous with coaption of the anterior and posterior leaflets of the mitral valve (AL and PL, respectively). During the second shorter cycle of atrial fibrillation, M is increased in amplitude and may be responsible for the "presystolic" murmur of mitral stenosis, in the absence of atrial systole. Reprinted, with permission, from Armstrong et al. Echocardiographic and phonocardiographic observations on the initial low frequency component of the first heart sound. Br. Heart 40:750, 1978.

The intensity of the first heart sound is influenced by several factors, the most important of which is the position of the atrioventricular valves at the onset of ventricular systole. This is to a large extent determined by the length of the PR interval. When the PR interval is long and atrial systole occurs well before the first heart sound, the valve leaflets have sufficient time to float back and almost reach their closure position. During the ensuing ventricular systole, there is thus very little excursion of the leaflets to their point of apposition and the ensuing first heart sound is therefore soft. However, when the PR interval is short, the leaflets are displaced well into the left ventricular cavity at the onset of ventricular systole and their wide excursion therefore produces a loud first heart sound.

Variations in the intensity of the first heart sound will occur in any form of atrioventricular dissociation (e.g., complete heart block, paroxymal ventricular tachycardia). Under these circumstances, the first heart sound will be loud when a P wave precedes a QRS complex appropriately, and soft when the P wave is dissociated from the QRS complex. When there is atrial fibrillation and complete AV dissociation, the first heart sound will be constant in intensity.

The intensity of the first heart sound is characteristcally increased in mitral stenosis provided that the leaflets are mobile. This is because the obstruction produced by the stenotic valve results in prolonged ventricular filling thoughout diastole so that the leaflets are deeply displaced into the ventricular cavity at the onset of systole; ventricular systole then produces wide travel of the leaflets and a correspondingly loud first heart sound. A soft first heart sound in the presence of mitral stenosis is strongly suggestive of calcification and/or fibrosis of the leaflets. In tachycardia from any cause, especially in hyperkinetic states such as thyrotoxicosis, the intensity of the first heart

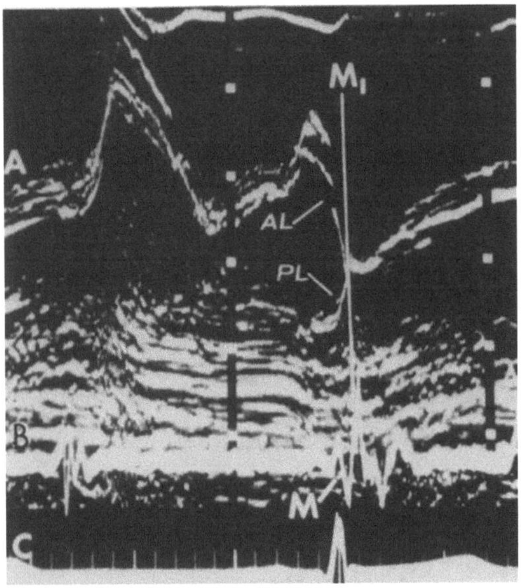

FIGURE 3.4. Echocardiogram (A), phonocardiogram (B), and electrocardiogram (C) in a normal subject demonstrating the high frequency mitral closure sound MI at the time of coaption of the anterior and posterior leaflets of the mitral valve. Reprinted with permission, from Armstrong et al. Echocardiographic and phonocardiographic observations on the initial low frequency component of the first heart sound. Br Heart J 40:750, 1978.

sound is increased because diastole is short and the leaflets are therefore still well within the left ventricular cavity at the time of onset of ventricular systole.

The rate of rise of pressure during the period of isovolumic left ventricular systole also influences the intensity of the first heart sound. A slow rise in left ventricular pressure during systole as occurs in myocarditis or myocardial infarction may produce softening of the first heart sound. Similarly, a soft first heart sound encountered with left bundle branch block is most likely a result of concomitant left ventricular disease, which leads to a slow rate of rise of left ventricular pressure and a slow rate of travel of the mitral valve to its closed position. A similar mechanism may be operative in aortic stenosis, where the first heart sound is often soft or absent and, indeed, often confused with an aortic ejection click.

The first heart sound is also not infrequently reduced in intensity in cases of aortic insufficiency, but in this instance is most probably a result of the long PR interval that is present in approximately one-third of cases. In the presence of emphysema or thick chest wall, the first heart sound is soft, but so are all the heart sounds.

Normal *physiologic splitting* of the mitral and tricuspid components of the first heart sound may be detected at the lower sternal edge. Wide splitting of the first heart sound in this area is usually a result of complete right bundle branch block, which produces a delay in the onset of right ventricular systole and therefore a delay in tricuspid valve closure. This effect is not seen in incomplete right bundle branch block since the onset of right ventricular systole is not delayed.

The same phenomenon pertains in left bundle branch block, where the first heart sound is usually normally split because the onset of left ventricular systole is not delayed. In any event, splitting is difficult to detect in left bundle branch block because the mitral component of the first heart sound is so frequently soft.

Wide splitting of the first heart sound is a characteristic feature of Ebstein anomaly, where delay in closure is produced by the redundant leaflets, resulting in the so-called "sail sound". Tricuspid valve closure may be audibly delayed in a right atrial myxoma, which mechanically delays leaflet position.

Splitting of the first heart sound must be distinguished from a preceding atrial sound, which is usually lower pitched, best heard with a bell, and varies with respiration. A pulmonary ejection click can be distinguished by the fact that it disappears almost completely with inspiration. Aortic ejection clicks occur later and are more widely heard over the precordium.

The Second Heart Sound

The aortic valve closes as the pressure in the aorta falls below that in the left ventricle. The sudden deceleration of blood sets up vibrations producing the aortic component of the second heart sound, which radiates widely and is audible at all areas. Similarly, pulmonary valve closure occurs when the pressure in the pulmonary artery drops below that of the right ventricle. The pulmonary component of the second heart sound is softer than the aortic component and has a restricted radiation.

Asynchronous closure of the semilunar valves is responsible for the normal *splitting of the second heart sound* (Fig. 3.5). With inspiration, the right ventricle is distended by the augmented venous return, prolonging right ventricular systole and delaying pulmonary valve closure. This means that P2 moves away from the first heart sound. With expiration, right ventricular filling is diminished and P2 moves closer to the first heart sound as the duration of right ventricular systole diminishes (Fig. 3.6). Respiratory changes in left ventricular volume lags a few beats behind that of the right. During inspiration, there is an increase in the pulmonary vascular capacitance leading to pooling of blood in the lungs and a decreased left atrial pressure. This leads to diminished left ventricular stroke volume and left ventricular ejection time, thus shortening the interval from the first heart sound to A2. When pulmonary venous return is augmented during expiration, A2 moves away from the first heart sound and approximates P2. The effect of respiration on the second heart sound is thus to produce constant variation in the degree of splitting, which is quite characteristic of health.

On expiration the second heart sound may be single but can remain split up to 40 msec, particularly in children and young adults. In the case of children and young adults it it important to listen in the upright position because the second sound in held expiration, then becomes single—an important differential point when the question of atrial septal defect arises.

Abnormally *wide splitting* of the second sound may occur when there is electrical delay in right ventricular activation. Thus, in right bundle branch block the delay in onset and

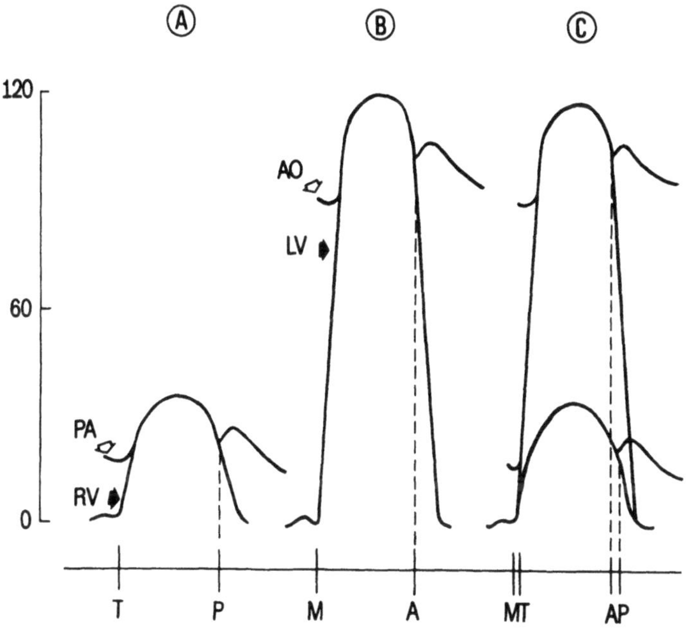

FIGURE 3.5. Asynchronous closure of the mitral and tricuspid, and aortic and pulmonary valves. In (A) the tricuspid valve closure sound (T) occurs at the onset of right ventricular isovolumic systole and the pulmonary valve closure sound (P), when the right ventricular pressure drops below that of the pulmonary artery. In (B) mitral and aortic closure sounds are related to similar events on the left side. Asynchrony is demonstrated in (C) with mitral valve closure preceding tricuspid valve closure because the left ventricle contracts first. Pulmonary valve closure follows aortic valve closure because the duration of the systolic ejection period is longer for the right ventricle than the left.

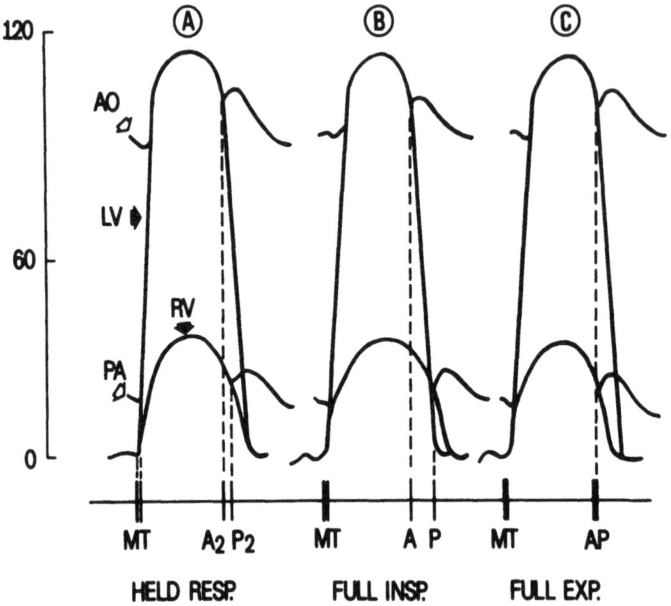

FIGURE 3.6. In held respiration (A) a steady-state is achieved and the asynchronous closure of the aortic and pulmonary valves produces splitting of the second heart sound. During inspiration (B) prolongation of right ventricular systole occurs, further separating P2 from A2. During expiration (C), left ventricular systole is prolonged and right ventricular systole shortened so that aortic and pulmonary valve closure sounds are superimposed.

duration of right ventricular systole produces a late P2 with resultant wide splitting of the second sound; however, the normal respiratory variation of the two components is usually detectable. For the same reason there is abnormally wide splitting of the mitral and tricuspid components of the first heart sound in right bundle branch block.

Wide fixed (little or no respiratory variation) splitting of the second heart sound is characteristic of atrial septal defect. P2 is delayed because of volume overloading of the right ventricle, and the split is fixed because the stroke volume of the two ventricles is the same. This is because both ventricles are filled from a functionally common atrium, so that respiratory changes in volume are transmitted equally to both ventricles. Some degree of splitting is retained even in the presence of severe pulmonary hypertension, and this is a valuable sign in the differential diagnosis of Eisenmenger syndrome.

Mechanical overloading of the right ventricle as occurs in pulmonary stenosis with intact septum produces a delay in pulmonary valve closure and wide splitting of the second heart sound. In pulmonary stenosis the delay in P2 corresponds roughly with the degree of prolongation of right ventricular systole, the height of the right ventricular pressure, and therefore the severity of the pulmonary stenosis. However, in Tetralogy of Fallot pulmonary artery pressure and flow is so low because of the right-to-left shunt that it is unusual to hear or even record P2.

Early closure of the aortic valve may also result in a widely split second sound. In mitral insufficiency, regurgitation into the left atrium shortens left ventricular systole to such an extent that the aortic valve closes early and wide splitting results.

In constrictive pericarditis a highly characteristic, abrupt, short-lived wide splitting of the second heart sound occurs at the onset of inspiration. The splitting is widest at the onset of inspiration and narrows to become single again within a few beats. Phonocardiographic analysis shows that the splitting is due to shortening of left ventricular systole whereas right ventricular systole remains relatively fixed (i.e., A2 moves in and P2 remains stationary). Shortening of left ventricular systole is the result of reduction in left ventricular stroke volume which occurs at the very onset of inspiration at the time of the weak beat in pulsus paradoxus.

Paradoxical splitting of the second heart sound (i.e, maximal splitting with expiration which disappears on inspiration) is the result of a delay in aortic valve closure so that P2 precedes A2. Therefore, at the onset of inspiration P2 is delayed and becomes superimposed on the later A2 and the splitting disappears. The usual cause for the delay in A2 is complete left bundle branch block, which prolongs left ventricular activation. Mechanical prolongation of left ventricular systole, as occurs in aortic stenosis or systemic hypertension, may also delay A2 and therefore result in paradoxical splitting of the second heart sound.

The *intensity of the second heart sound* may be altered because of

1. A genuine change in aortic or pulmonary artery pressure.
2. An alteration in conduction of heart sounds because of change in the structures between the chest wall and the heart.
3. An anatomical alteration in relation between aorta and pulmonary artery, as in transposition of the great vessels.

As long as splitting is present, the component responsible for increased intensification can be identified. Splitting tends to be abolished in essential hypertension and with increasing age. Prolongation of left ventricular systole delays aortic valve closure so that A2 and P2 are superimposed. In pulmonary hypertension, however, especially when advanced, splitting tends to persist, with accentuation of the pulmonary component.

The site of the intensification is also helpful. Accentuation of the second sound (sometimes with a "ringing" quality) in the aortic area and to the right of the sternum is commonly found in systemic hypertension and aortic aneurysm. In transposition and dextrocardia the loud sound at the aortic area is of pulmonary origin.

In the pulmonary area accentuation of the second sound is often palpable and produces a diastolic "shock". This is commonly found in pulmonary hypertension from any cause, particularly congenital heart disease and mitral stenosis. In Tetralogy of Fallot and transposition of the great vessels, accentuation of the second sound in the pulmonary area is aortic in origin because of the anteriorly situated aorta.

In ventricular septal defect and aortopulmonary shunts with equal resistances, or a single ventricle, where the two circulations are in free communication with equal pressures, the second sound is virtually single and loud. In atrial septal defect with pulmonary hypertension, the two circulations are separated and splitting persists, with accentuation of P2. Since P2 is louder than normal, it radiates more widely and is audible at the apex. P2 is rarely audible at the apex in the absence of marked pulmonary hypertension. A loud second heart sound with normal splitting is frequently encountered in healthy children when the chest is thin with little overlying lung tissue.

Reduced intensity of the second sound may be a result of a thick chest wall, emphysema, or pericardial effusion. Usually, it is P2 that is difficult to hear under these circumstances, leading to a mistaken diagnosis of a single second sound. A truly single second sound may be produced by absence of P2, absence of A2, or superimposition of A2 and P2.

P2 is characteristically absent in Tetralogy of Fallot, pulmonary atresia, and truncus arteriosus. A2 is characteristically absent in calcific aortic stenosis . It is present but is frequently obscured by the pansystolic murmurs of mitral regurgitation or ventricular septal defect or by the long ejection systolic murmur of pulmonary stenosis.

The Third Heart Sound and Diastolic Gallop Rhythm

A third heart sound occurs 12 to 18 msec after A2, in early diastole, toward the end of the rapid-filling phase. It is produced by sudden deceleration of rapid ventricular filling, which results in tautening and vibration of the myocardium and the atrioventricular valvular apparatus. Third sounds may arise from either the left or the right ventricle, or both.

A *physiological third sound* is a common auscultatory finding in normal young people. It is of low intensity and best heard in thin-chested individuals. In young children it is frequently accompanied by an innocent vibratory systolic murmur, and this combination not infrequently gives rise to the suspicion of heart disease. There are, however, no symptoms, physical signs, or abnormalities of the electrocardiogram and chest X-ray that would even arouse a suspicion of heart disease under these circumstances, even though the third sound has the same timing as the diastolic gallop.

A third heart sound is frequently associated with conditions in which there is rapid ventricular filling, such as mitral insufficiency and left-to-right shunts, and under these circumstances it is not referred to as a gallop rhythm, nor does it imply any impairment of left ventricular function.

For practical purposes a third heart sound, even when soft, cannot be regarded as a normal finding in a person above the age of 40. Abnormal accentuation of the physiological third sound produces a diastolic gallop rhythm and implies myocardial decompensation. It is commonly found in hypertension, myocardial infarction, myocarditis, and cardiomyopathy, where it implies a serious prognosis. It is frequently an early and more subtle sign of left ventricular disease in relatively asymptomatic patients.

A *diastolic gallop* is frequently readily palpable and is best heard with the bell lightly applied to the point of maximum cardiac impulse with the patient turned into the left lateral decubitus position. The circumstances under which diastolic gallop rhythm occurs may have prognostic value. When heard evanescently during the early clinical course of myocardial infarction it does not necessarily connote an adverse prognosis. Contrariwise, a gallop rhythm that appears late in the course of myocardial infarction and persists despite adequate medical treatment carries a poor prognosis because it indicates seriously disturbed left ventricular function.

As a sign of left ventricular failure diastolic gallop frequently occurs in association with pulsus alternans. When pulsus alternans is detected, a diastolic gallop rhythm is invariably present, but the reverse does not apply. Right ventricular gallops can be diagnosed with certainty only when a purely right-sided lesion is present, as in cor pulmonale.

In constrictive pericarditis, the third heart sound occurs earlier than in any of the foregoing conditions (8–12 msec after A2) and has a higher frequency than the physiological third heart sound. This sound has also been called the *pericardial knock* and the *early diastolic sound* of constrictive pericarditis. It occurs during the rapid-filling phase of ventricular diastole and is produced by the restraining action of the pericardium, preventing myocardial relaxation in diastole. It has no particular prognostic significance but is a useful additional diagnostic finding.

The Fourth Heart Sound (Presystolic Triple Rhythm)(Atrial S4)

Normally, the fourth heart sound or atrial sound is incorporated into the first heart sound and in normal hearts will become audible only when the PR, interval is long. Under these circumstances it is without pathological significance. However, a presystolic triple rhythm (or gallop) is usually pathological, being a sign of systolic overload and reduced ventricular compliance. On the left side it is commonly heard in systemic hypertension, aortic stenosis, myocardial infarction, and cardiomyopathy. Its presence signifies a stressed ventricle but not necessarily heart failure.

The added stretch given to the ventricle by atrial contraction in presystole enables it to perform more adequately. Any manipulation that reduces systolic overload, such as lowering the blood pressure in systemic hypertension, will make the sound disappear. The sound may disappear during carotid sinus pressure and may appear or become louder during exercise and amylnitrate inhalation. Naturally, it disappears with the onset of atrial fibrillation.

An atrial sound is heard almost universally during the acute episode of myocardial infarction and is usually of low intensity. During an attack of angina (which is associated with a reduction in ventricular compliance) the atrial sound becomes louder. In young patients with aortic stenosis the presence of a loud atrial sound is a fairly good indicator of severe disease. In elderly patients, however, the presence of an atrial sound is so frequent that its diagnostic specificity is markedly reduced. Right-sided atrial sounds are useful predictors of right ventricular systolic overload. They may be heard in severe pulmonary valve stenosis and are a frequent finding in acute pulmonary embolism.

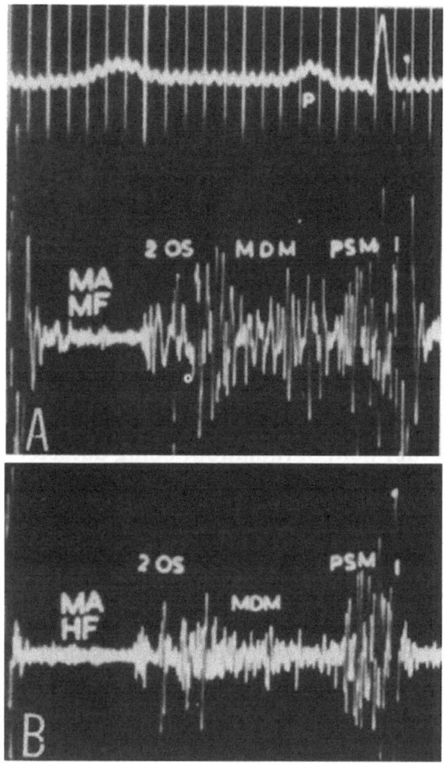

FIGURE 3.7. Phonocardiograms in pure mitral stenosis recorded at the mitral area (MA), medium frequency (MF) in A, and high frequency (HF) in B, demonstrating the opening snap (OS) occurring shortly after the second heart sound, and followed by a long rumbling middiastolic murmur with presystolic accentuation.

Summation Gallop

When third and fourth heart sounds are present in the same patient, the presence of a tachycardia may result in a fusion of these two sounds to produce a single loud sound called a *summation gallop*. Therefore, no special significance can be attached to the presence of a summation gallop. The existence of a summation gallop can be proved clinically if the heart rate can be slowed by carotid sinus pressure so that the two sounds can be separated and individually identified as third and fourth heart sounds; when tachycardia is resumed the summation gallop is evident once more.

Mitral and Tricuspid Opening Snaps

Normally, opening of the atrioventricular valves is silent. However, when there is commisural fusion, a snapping sound occurs at the time of maximum excursion of the leaflets when they are displaced downward into the left or right ventricular cavity (Fig. 3.7). A prerequisite for an opening snap is the presence of pliable, mobile leaflets. Tricuspid opening snaps are heard and recorded less frequently than are mitral opening snaps because tricuspid stenosis usually occurs concomitantly with mitral stenosis, and the snap is therefore rarely recognized.

A mitral opening snap is best heard between the left sternal border and the apex beat. Not infrequently, it is well heard in the second right interspace, in the aortic area. In general, the tighter the stenosis of the mitral valve, the closer is the opening snap to A2. This is a result of the high left atrial pressure opening the mitral valve early.

When the A2–OS interval is in excess of 80 msec, mitral stenosis is likely to be tight. There are, however, exceptions to this statement. Thus, a low cardiac output which reduces left atrial pressure and mitral flow may produced a long A2–OS interval. Contrariwise, tachycardia or a high cardiac ouput raises the left atrial pressure and thus shortens the A2–OS interval in the presence of relatively mild mitral stenosis. In atrial fibrillation this interval varies according to the preceding RR interval. As the RR interval shortens, so does the A2–OS interval. This is related to the fact that long diastolic filling periods reduce left atrial pressure and therefore shorten the A2–OS interval.

The opening snap is frequently mistaken for P2, particularly when the latter is delayed. Distinguishing points are that the opening snap has a wider field of radiation, being detected at the apex and the aortic area, unlike P2, which is strictly limited to the pulmonary area and the second and third left interspaces. Additionally, P2 changes its timing in relationship to A2 during the various phases of respiration, whereas the opening snap is constant in position. An opening snap may also be confused with a third heart sound, but the latter usually follows A2 by 12 msec or more, and in the presence of a middiastolic murmur of any length it would be unusual to detect a third heart sound.

In the presence of the other auscultatory findings of mitral stenosis, the absence of a mitral opening snap is a fairly good predictor of an immobile valve mechanism resulting from fibrosis and/or calcification. Following mitral valvotomy the opening snap may be reduced in intensity but rarely disappears.

Ejection Sounds

The Aortic Ejection Click

This sound arises from a stenotic aortic valve or a dilated ascending aorta. Therefore, it is encountered clinically among cases of congenital bicuspid valve, rheumatic aortic stenosis, aortic insufficiency, aneurysms of the ascending aorta, and Tetralogy of Fallot.

When associated with the other findings suggestive of aortic stenosis, it provides ancillary evidence that the stenosis is valvular in origin rather than supravalvular, subvalvular, or a result of idiopathic hypertrophic subaortic stenosis.

An aortic ejection click is heard well over

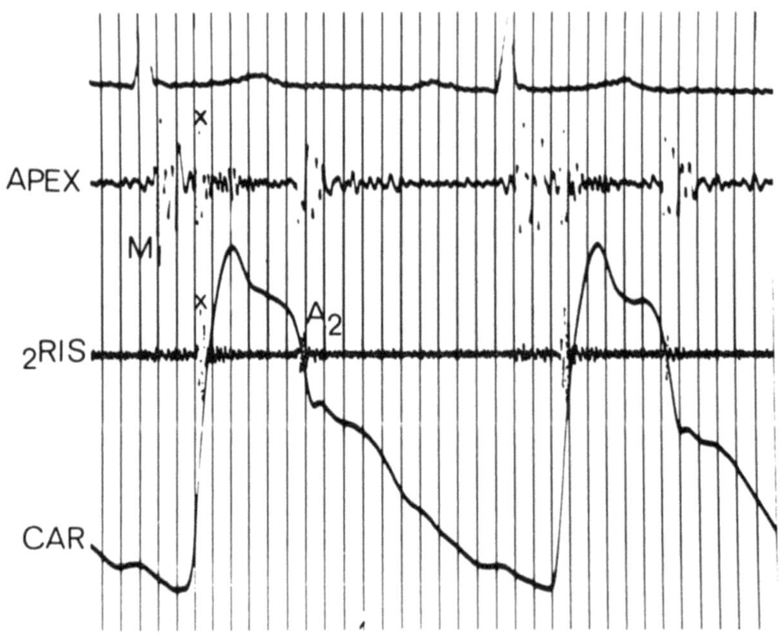

FIGURE 3.8. Electrocardiogram (top) high-frequency phonocardiograms recorded at the apex and the second right intercostal space (2 RIS) and the simultaneous carotid pulse demonstrating an aortic ejection click well recorded at the apex and commencing shortly after the onset of ventricular ejection.

the entire precordium and not infrequently is heard better at the apex than at the base. Its position in systole is not affected by the phases of respiration (Fig. 3.8).

The Pulmonary Ejection Click

Like the aortic ejection click, this emanates from a stenotic pulmonary valve or a dilated pulmonary artery. However, the pulmonary ejection click occurs later because isovolumic systole of the right ventricle is normally longer than that of the left. Its most characteristic feature, however, is its tendency to disappear or become markedly softer with inspiration. The latter is the result of augmented right ventricular filling during inspiration, which results in presystolic upward movement of the pulmonary valve to its fully open position. At the onset of systole the valve cannot move further and a click is therefore absent. This reverses during expiration, so that the valve opens at the onset of systole and the click therefore becomes audible.

Unlike the aortic ejection click, a pulmonary ejection click is strictly localized to the second and third left intercostal spaces and is not heard at the apex. Clicks may be detected in any cause of *pulmonary hypertension* but are also a characteristic feature of *idiopathic dilatation of the pulmonary artery* where the pulmonary artery pressure is normal. Pulmonary ejection clicks are absent in *infundibular stenosis* or in the rare form of pulmonary stenosis caused by *dysplastic pulmonary valve* tissue. In *valvular pulmonary stenosis*, the earlier the ejection click, the more severe is the pulmonary stenosis. In the most extreme examples of pulmonary stenosis where the right ventricular pressure is in excess of systemic, the pulmonary ejection click may be superimposed on the first heart sound.

Non-ejection Clicks

These sounds, which may be single or multiple, occur in middle to late systole and are unrelated to opening of the semilunar valves (Fig. 3.9). They arise from a myxomatous mitral valve apparatus in the *billowing mitral leaflet syndrome*. They are frequently followed by a late systolic murmur, which is the result of mild mitral insufficiency produced by billowing of the posterior (and occasionally the anterior) mitral valve leaflet into the left atrium. They are discussed more fully in Chapter 13.

Murmurs

Murmurs are produced when the normal laminar flow of blood becomes nonlaminar, that is, instead of all the particles in the bloodstream moving unidirectionally, particles move in different directions, thus creating vibrations. If these vibrations are in the range audible to the human ear, they are interpreted as murmurs. Whether turbulence or vortex formation is responsible for the vibrations is still controver-

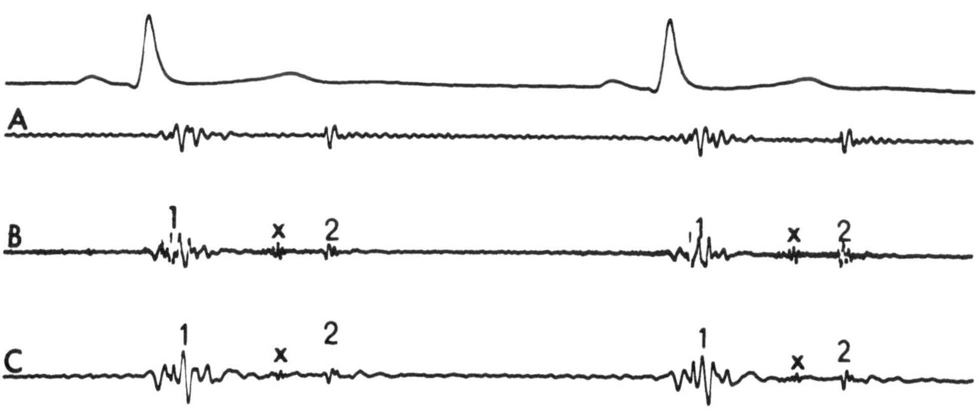

FIGURE 3.9. Nonejection click recorded in the billowing mitral leaflet syndrome. (A) Phonocardiogram at second LIS (B) and (C) high and low frequency phonocardiograms at the apex.

sial. A series of successive vibrations is termed a *murmur*; one or two vibrations is termed a *sound*. Murmurs are classified as *systolic*, *diastolic*, or *continuous*. Systolic and continuous murmurs may have an intracardiac or an extracardic basis.

Innocent murmurs are unassociated with any functional or structural abnormality. A murmur can be classified as innocent only following complete cardiological evaluation. If there is any doubt about the significance of the murmur it is better simply to describe the murmur and avoid any prognostic implications until further investigations have been done.

Flow murmurs are produced by torrential flow across normal semilunar or atrioventricular valves (e.g., a pulmonary ejection murmur in atrial septal defect or a short middiastolic murmur in pure mitral and tricuspid insufficiency).

Functional murmurs arise from an incompetent atrioventricular valve with normal leaflets when its annulus is stretched by a failing ventricle (e.g., mitral or tricuspid insufficiency) or from an intrinsically normal pulmonary valve, rendered incompetent by pulmonary hypertension. *Organic* murmurs arise from structurally abnormal valves.

Systolic Murmurs

The following factors should be assessed when a systolic murmur is encountered.

1. Intensity: grades 1 to 6.
2. Duration: holosystolic (pansystolic), ejection (midsystolic), late systolic, or early systolic.
3. Site of maximum intensity.
4. Radiation.
5. Quality: musical, blowing, rough, etc.
6. Response to breathing, and various maneuvers, including exercise, Valsalva maneuver, and the use of vasoactive drugs.

Intensity

A rough, quantitative, bedside assessment of loudness of a systolic murmur may be attained by using six grades of intensity. Although purely subjective, agreement between experienced observers is remarkably close.

A grade 1 murmur is barely audible, whereas a grade 6 murmur is so loud that it can be heard without applying the stethoscope to the chest. There are not many grade 6 murmurs! A grade 5 murmur is very loud with the stethoscope applied to the chest. Grade 2 is louder than grade 1, easily audible but not very intense. Grades 3 and 4 are usually associated with a thrill and are always abnormal. Murmurs of grade 1 and 2 in intensity are usually innocent.

Duration

Ejection murmurs commence with opening of the semilunar valves at the end of isovolumic systole (Fig. 3.10). Therefore, they begin shortly after the first heart sound, and because they closely mirror the rate volume of flow across these valves, they have a peak intensity during systole when the velocity of ejection is

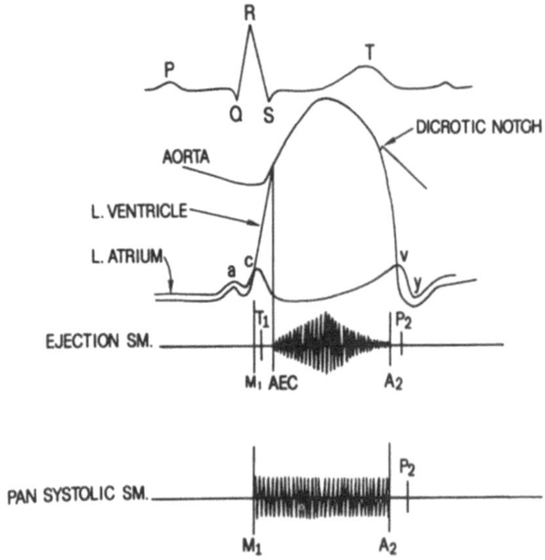

FIGURE 3.10. Diagrammatic representation of left ventricular systole. An aortic ejection murmur corresponds to the period of ejection from left ventricle into aorta, whereas a regurgitant systolic murmur commences with M1 and continues throughout systole beyond A2 when left atrial and left ventricular pressures equilibrate (see text).

at its maximum. The murmur then diminishes in intensity and ends before the semilunar valves close. Since left ventricular systole is generally shorter that right, aortic ejection murmurs are generally shorter than pulmonary.

Because ejection murmurs are frequently preceded by an ejection sound, there is no true auscultatory gap audible between the first heart sound and the onset of the murmur. Clinically, therefore, the diagnosis of an ejection murmur is more readily made by noting that the murmur ends before A2. There are, however, some exceptions to the last statement. In severe pulmonary stenosis where the right ventricular pressure exceeds that of the left ventricle, right ventricular systole is so prolonged that the pulmonary ejection murmur extends beyond A2 and may actually obscure the sound. The differential diagnosis of ejection systole murmurs is presented graphically in Figures 3.11 and 3.12.

Regurgitant murmurs are holosystolic (or pansystolic), starting with the first heart sound and continuing with an equal intensity throughout ventricular systole until, or even beyond, A2. Regurgitant murmurs are produced by insufficiency of the mitral or tricuspid valves or a left-to-right shunt through a ventricular septal defect. Thus, in mitral incompetence, the murmur commences with mitral valve closure (Ml) and extends throughout systole beyond aortic valve closure until the point where the left ventricular pressure drops below that of the left atrium. Similarly, in ventricular septal defect the murmur commences with M1, extends through left ventricular systole, and stops at P2. Regurgitant murmurs also occur with tricuspid insufficiency and communications between the aorta and pulmonary artery, such as patent ductus arteriosus. In the presence of pulmonary hypertension, however, there may not be a pressure gradient between the left and right ventricles throughout systole, so that all regurgitant murmurs need not necessarily be holosystolic.

In summary, a short murmur with midsystolic crescendo (diamond-shaped) usually indicates ejection across the aortic or pulmonary valves, whereas a holosystolic murmur indicates regurgitation either through an abnormal communication or through an incompetent atrioventricular valve.

Site of Maximum Intensity

An important clue to diagnosis is the site of maximum intensity of a murmur. Thus, in mitral incompetence the murmur is usually most intense at the apex. In tricuspid incompetence it is best heard at the lowermost portion of the sternum. A murmur of ventricular septal defect is best heard in the left third and fourth intercostal spaces. The murmur of pulmonary stenosis is best heard in the second and third left intercostal spaces, the murmur of aortic stenosis at the second right intercostal space, and that of a patent ductus arteriosus in the first left intercostal space. Unfortunately, there is considerable overlap. For example, the murmur of pulmonary and infundibular stenosis, aortic stenosis, and ventricular septal defect are often most intense in the third left intercostal space.

Radiation

Mitral incompetent murmurs radiate to the left axilla and the left chest posteriorly. The murmur of ventricular septal defect and tricuspid murmurs radiate from the fourth left space toward the apex and pulmonary area. Pulmonary systolic murmurs radiate from the pulmonary area down the left sternal border and into the left upper chest anteriorly. Aortic murmurs radiate into the vessels of the neck, to the right and left of the sternum, and down to the apex.

Quality

Insufficient attention is paid to the quality of murmurs, partly because description of such a purely tonal phenomenon is difficult. Thus, mitral systolic murmurs are characteristically blowing; aortic ejection murmurs rough, rasping, or musical; and tricuspid murmurs are

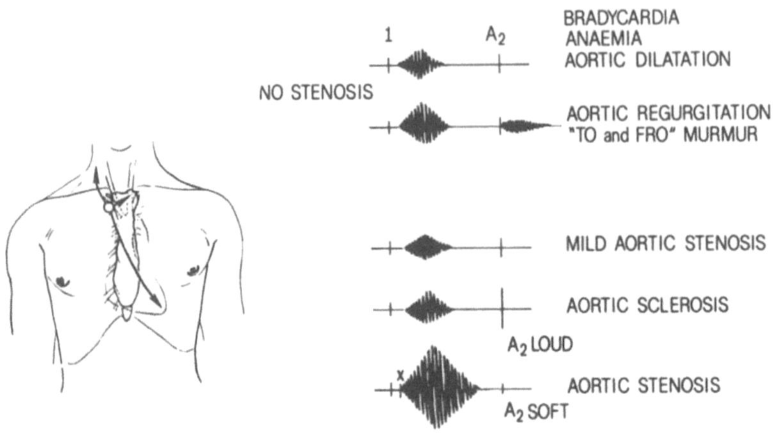

FIGURE 3.11. The differential diagnosis of aortic ejection systolic murmurs (see text). Aftr Dr. L. Vogelpoel.

usually blowing. Occasionally, "honking" murmurs may arise from incompetent mitral or tricuspid valves.

Response of Systolic Murmurs to Various Maneuvers

The simplest bedside test is the response of a systolic murmur to respiration. Right-sided murmurs tend to increase with inspiration, whereas left-sided murmurs are unaffected or may decrease with inspiration. Characteristically, tricuspid murmurs increase with inspiration, and this is readily appreciated, since the tricuspid area is not covered by lung tissue, so that sound conduction is unimpaired. The murmur of tricuspid insufficiency is augmented during inspiration because of the temporary in-

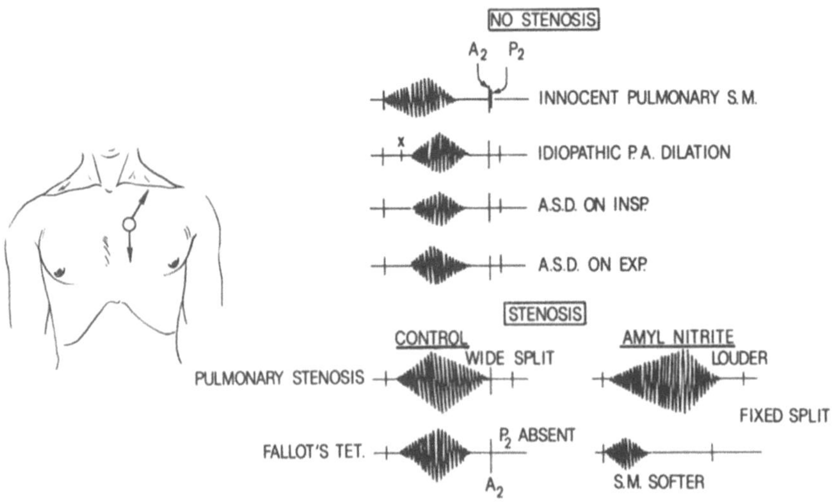

FIGURE 3.12. The differential diagnosis of pulmonary ejection systolic murmurs (see text). After Dr. L. Vogelpoel.

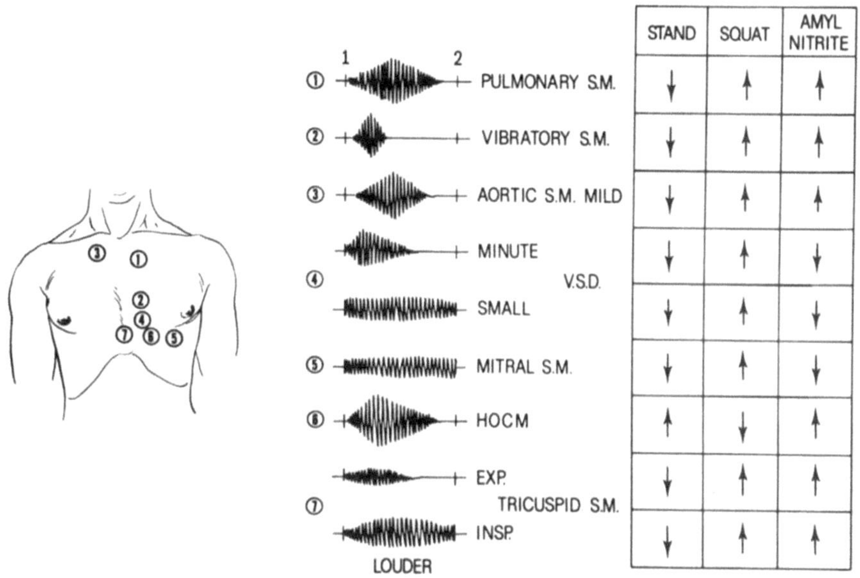

FIGURE 3.13. Differential diagnosis of left and right sided systolic murmurs and their response to standing, squatting, and amyl nitrite (see text). After Dr. L. Vogelpoel.

crease in right ventricular volume. Systolic ejection murmurs such as those of pulmonary stenosis or atrial septal defect usually show no inspiratory augmentation because the pressure- or volume-overloaded right ventricle is unable to change its stroke volume significantly.

Amyl nitrite is extremely useful in differentiating left-sided from right-sided murmurs (Fig 3.13). Inhalation of this drug produces systemic vasodilation and hypotension with tachycardia, leading to increased venous return to the right side of the heart. Left-sided regurgitant murmurs (mitral incompetence, ventricular septal defect) become softer and shorter because of the fall in systemic pressure. Right-sided regurgitant murmurs (tricuspid incompetence) and all ejection murmurs become louder because of the increased venous return and increased forward flow, provided that heart failure is absent. There is only one exception: Tetralogy of Fallot. In this condition, the ejection systolic murmur softens or disappears because reduction of the systemic vascular resistance increases the right-to-left shunt across the ventricular septal defect, thereby diminishing pulmonary blood flow. The test is extremely useful in making the distinction between a small ventricular septal defect and mild pulmonary stenosis, and between pulmonary valve stenosis with intact ventricular septum and acyanotic Tetralogy of Fallot. Similarly, in the case of left-sided murmur, amyl nitrite increases the intensity of the murmur of aortic stenosis and softens the murmur of mitral insufficiency.

Vasoconstrictor drugs such as phenylephrine elevate the systemic vascular resistance while scarcely changing that of the pulmonary circulation. These drugs intensify left-sided regurgitant murmurs. In Tetralogy of Fallot the systolic murmur is similarly intensified because the increased systemic vascular resistance decreases the right-to-left shunt across the ventricular septal defect, thereby increasing pulmonary blood flow.

Prompt squatting increases systemic vascular resistance and systemic pressure, thereby intensifying the murmur of mitral insufficiency and softening the murmur of idiopathic hy-

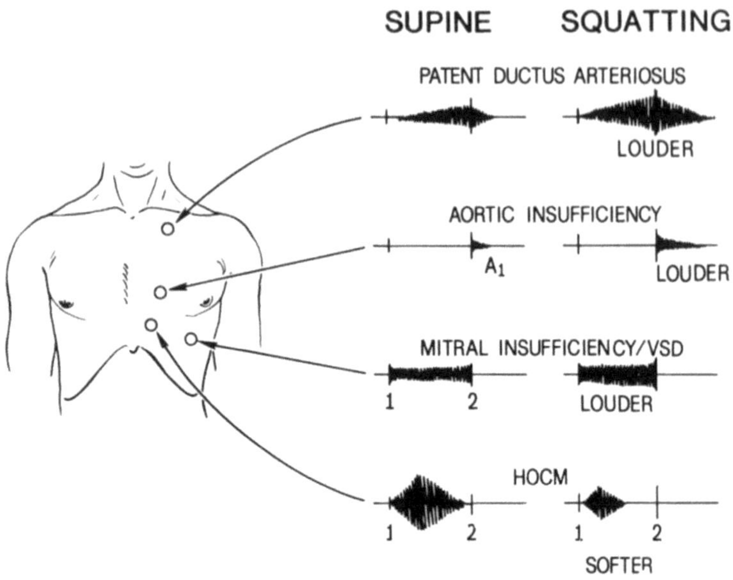

FIGURE 3.14. The response of various murmurs to squatting (see text). After Dr. L. Vogelpoel.

pertrophic subaortic stenosis (Fig 3.14). This is a useful bedside test for the diagnosis of the latter condition, but the findings may be inconclusive because IHSS is fairly frequently complicated by mitral insufficiency.

The *Valsalva maneuver* is useful in distinguishing left- and right-sided murmurs. During the straining phase, right-sided murmurs disappear rapidly, whereas those emanating from the left side of the heart soften a few beats later. When the maneuver is terminated, the return of blood flow to the right side of the heart results in immediate intensification of ight-sided murmurs and a delayed intensification of left-sided murmurs because of the time taken for the venous return to traverse the pulmonary circuit.

The test is particularly useful in identifying the murmur of IHSS, where there is a paradoxical response—the murmur intensifying during the straining period. This is the result of aggravation of left ventricular outflow tract obstruction because of diminished left ventricular filling. The murmur of mitral valve prolapse intensifies and may become holosystolic for the same reason.

Variations in cycle length (because of ectopic beats) produce characteristic alterations in murmurs that are easily detected at the bedside. This is particularly valuable in the distinction between mitral insufficiency and aortic stenosis when there is overlap in the site and radiation of the respective murmur. Systolic ejection murmurs intensify after long pauses, whereas regurgitant murmurs are unaffected. An ejection murmur is augmented because a postectopic pause is associated with an increase in ventricular stroke volume and a fall in pressure in the systemic and pulmonary circuits, leading to a prolonged ejection period and a longer systolic murmur. In the case of regurgitant murmurs, however, the long cycles are associated with increased atrial pressure, so that regurgitant flow is hardly altered.

Innocent Systolic Murmurs

Not infrequently, one of the most difficult problems encountered in cardiology is assessing the significance of a systolic murmur, particularly in children (Fig. 3.15). With the help of the features discussed above, most murmurs can be evaluated correctly.

1. *The Pulmonary Ejection Murmur*: This

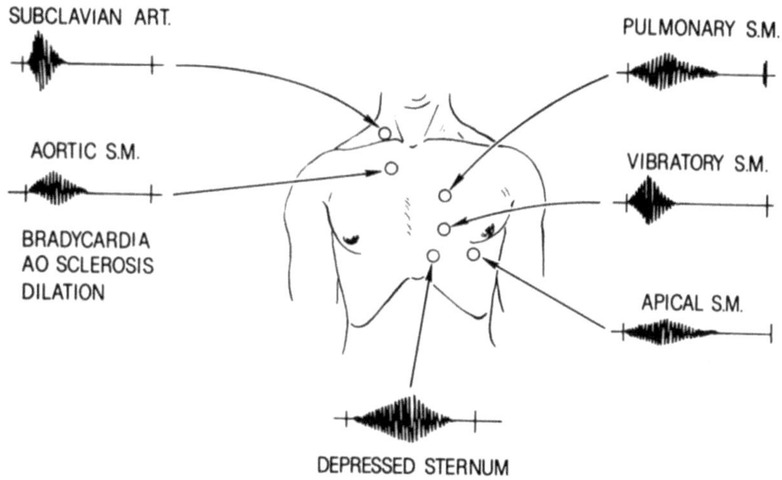

FIGURE 3.15. The differential diagnosis of innocent systolic murmurs (see text). After Dr. L. Vogelpoel.

murmur is commonly encountered in youth and young adults and is the result of flow across the pulmonary valve. The intensity is usually grade 3 or less and has a characteristic early systolic crescendo best heard in the pulmonary area and the third and fourth interspaces along the left sternal border. Its quality is blowing and it becomes louder with amyl nitrite.

These murmurs are particularly common during pregnancy and other high-output states, such as thyrotoxicosis. The second sound is physiologically split and the pulmonary component normal in intensity.

2. *The Vibratory Systolic Murmur (Still's Murmur)*: This is the most common innocent murmur encountered under the age of 10 and may be heard in 75 to 100% of normal children. It has the qualities of a soft grade 2 ejection systolic murmur with an early crescendo.

The murmur has a peculiar "twanging," "buzzing," or "groaning" quality. The murmur arises in the outflow tract of the left ventricle since the Valsalva maneuver demonstrates that it takes a few beats for the murmur to disappear and a few beats for the murmur to reappear during the straining and release phases of the test. A loud third heart sound frequently present at the apex frequently adds to the suspicion of heart disease. However, once the observer gains familiarity with the characteristic intonation of this murmur, it is readily identifiable and may be dismissed as innocent with great certainty. The majority of such murmurs disappear by the age of 20.

3. *Subclavian Bruit*: This murmur is best heard in the supraclavicular area or over the carotid artery. It is commonly detected in children and young adults and almost certainly arises from the subclavian, innominate, or carotid arteries. The murmur is short, occupying less than half of systole, and may be modified by compression of the subclavian vessels. It is better heard on the right side of the neck than on the left and is conducted poorly, if at all, to the aortic area and upper thorax. This contrasts with an aortic murmur, which is loudest at the base and is heard less well in the neck.

4. *Aortic Murmurs*: Innocent ejection murmurs may occur when the aorta is dilated, the cusps thickened by old age, or the flow increased by bradycardia.

5. *Depressed Sternum*: Innocent ejection murmurs are common and are related in some way to cardiac compression.

6. *Short Apical Systolic Murmurs*: These are heard occasionally in otherwise normal hearts.

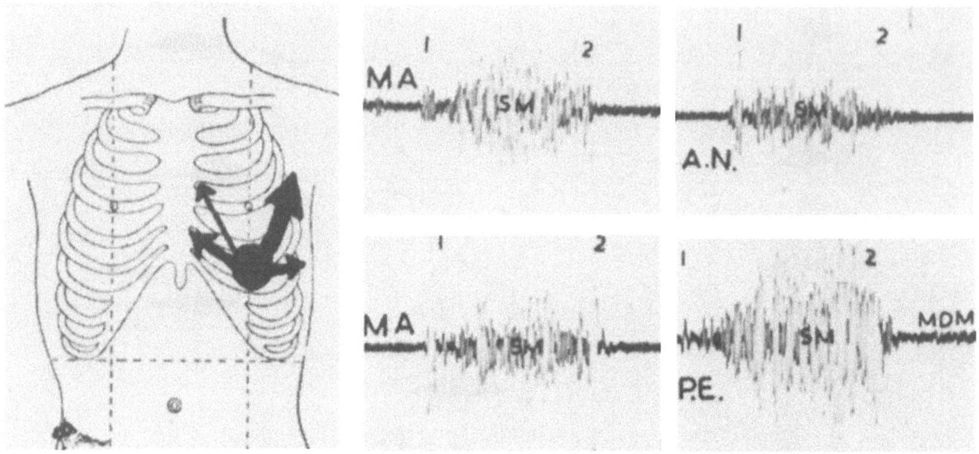

FIGURE 3.16. Mitral incompetence. The radiation of the murmur is shown in the diagram (left). The pansystolic murmur softens with amyl nitrite (A.N.) (upper right panel) but intensifies with phenylephrine (P.E.) phonocardiogram (lower right panel).

Mitral Insufficiency

The hallmark of mitral insufficiency is a pansystolic murmur with maximal intensity at the apex, plateau-shaped, or with a late systolic accentuation, radiating into the left axilla posteriorly and to the left infrascapular area (Fig. 3.16). The radiation of the murmur depends on whether the jet of mitral insufficiency is anteriorly or posteriorly directed. In *rheumatic mitral insufficiency*, the jet is usually directed posteriorly and the murmur radiates as described above.

However, when mitral insufficiency is the result of *rupture of the chordae tendinae* (whether spontaneous or the result of infective endocarditis) the regurgitant jet is frequently directed anteriorly and medially to strike the atrial septum, which is contiguous with aortic root. Therefore, the murmur radiates to the left sternal border, to the base, and even into the neck.

This type of mitral insufficiency is associated with marked elevation of the left atrial V wave, which may nearly equal the left ventricular systolic pressure. This results in diminution of incompetent flow in late systole, so that the murmur may closely resemble the ejection type of murmur of *aortic stenosis*. There are, however, helpful distinguishing clinical features. If the rhythm is irregular because of atrial fibrillation or ventricular ectopics, there is little change in intensity, whereas increase in intensity of the murmur after a long filling period is suggestive of an aortic ejection murmur. In aortic stenosis A2 may be inaudible, or alternatively, it may be paradoxically split. In mitral insufficiency the second sound is widely split and has normal respiratory variation. Vasoactive drugs are also helpful in making the distinction.

The murmur of ruptured chordae must also be distinguished from rheumatic mitral regurgitation. The latter is almost always associated with a middiastolic murmur and soft first heart sound, which are results of leaflet fusion. With ruptured chordae, the leaflets are mobile: The first heart sound is loud, an S3 is frequent, and a middiastolic murmur absent.

The *intensity* of the systolic murmur in mitral insufficiency varies but is usually grade 3 to 6. Generally, loud murmurs indicate severe insufficiency, and soft murmurs, as in acute rheumatic valvulitis, milder degrees of regurgitation. However, there are exceptions. Gross mitral insufficiency may on occasion have little or no murmur, especially if atrial fibrillation is present, whereas a loud murmur may be caused by a small jet with high velocity. Severe mitral insufficiency may be present in leaking prosthetic valves with little or no murmur. Although the classical and usual murmur of mitral insufficiency is pansystolic, the murmur on occasion may be short, early, and midsystolic. This applies particularly to the murmur produced by ischemic dysfunction of the papillary muscle, which determines how and where the mitral valve apparatus is distorted during left ventricular contraction. Mitral insufficiency is frequently a result of stretching and/or distortion of the annulus (left ventricular failure of any cause, papillary muscle dysfunction, left ventricular aneurysms, etc.) and under these circumstances the murmur is usually grade 1 to 3 in intensity unassociated with a middiastolic murmur, but frequently accompanied by a loud third sound. The absence of a middiastolic murmur in a case of mitral insufficiency points to a cause other than rheumatic involvement of the mitral leaflets.

The Late Systolic Murmur of Mitral Insufficiency (Mitral valve prolapse.)

This is found at any age but is particularly common in young people. The intensity is grade 3 or less, seldom louder. It is usually loudest at the apex and best heard in the left decubitus position. It may occasionally be musical, or even have a honking quality. It is louder in the standing than in the lying position, and its characteristic feature is its late onset and late crescendo.

This murmur is often accompanied by a mid- or late systolic click, both of which may vary spontaneously. The murmur softens with amyl nitrite inhalation and becomes louder after phenylephrine. It is a result of prolapsing of the mitral leaflets (particularly the posterior) in late systole at the time when the pressure in the left ventricle is falling off and when the gradient between the left ventricle and left atrium is decreasing. Maximal billowing of the posterior leaflet occurs in late systole and coincides with the late systolic click, when the chordae are maximally stretched.

Generally speaking, the degree of regurgitation is of no hemodynamic importance, but there may be a tendency for progressive elongation of the chordae, leading to their eventual rupture with severe mitral insufficiency. This type of murmur is associated with other characteristic clinical symptoms and electrocardiographic abnormalities, discussed in Chapter 12.

Tricuspid Insufficiency

The pansystolic murmur is usually grade 3 to 4 in intensity, but the loudness does not reflect the degree of insufficiency and gross tricuspid insufficiency may occasionally be silent. It is maximally intense at the fourth left interspace, radiates toward the apex, but rarely beyond, and is blowing and occasionally honking in quality.

It is important to appreciate that the systolic murmur of tricuspid insufficiency may be heard well at the apex, expecially when marked right-sided enlargement is present. It can then easily be misinterpreted as mitral in origin. Thus, in tight mitral stenosis with pulmonary hypertension and right heart enlargement, tricuspid insufficiency may be mistaken for mitral insufficiency. Also, in secundum atrial septal defect complicated by heart failure and tricuspid insufficiency, rheumatic mitral insufficiency or an ostium primum defect may be suspected erroneously.

Tricuspid systolic murmurs are often transient, evident during heart failure but disappearing rapidly after bed rest and diuretic therapy. Their characteristic feature is the marked accentuation on inspiration, with the murmur becoming loudest at the height of inspiration. However, when heart failure is advanced and the right heart overdistended, inspiration may have little effect on the intensity of the murmur. Sometimes, several inspirations are required to bring out the intensifica tion. Amyl nitrite inhalation accentuates this murmur. The murmur of tricuspid insufficiency is frequently well heard to the right of the sternum and in the epigastrium.

Tricuspid insufficiency is most commonly a result of stretching of the annulus in right ventricular failure consequent on any cause of pulmonary hypertension, in which case it is said to be *functional*. Rheumatic involvement of the tricuspid valve is much less common than mitral valve involvement, but the disease is still by far the commonest cause of organic tricuspid insufficiency. Other rare causes are endocardial cushion defect, Ebstein anomaly, infective endocarditis (particularly in drug addiction), carcinoid syndrome, endocardial fibroelastosis, and systemic lupus erythematosus.

Ventricular Septal Defect

Here the regurgitant murmurs are dependent on (1) the size of the defect, (2) the pulmonary arterial resistance, and (3) the presence or absence of pulmonary stenosis. In small to moderate-sized defects, a considerable gradient exists between the left and right ventricle throughout systole, so that a pansystolic, regurgitant murmur is heard. In large defects, pulmonary arterial resistance is elevated and systemic and pulmonary arterial pressures are the same. When there is very little left-to-right shunt, there is little murmur produced at the site of the defect, and when the shunt is reversed (right to left) there is no murmur. If the shunt is still dominantly left to right, a short early systolic murmur is present.

Most commonly, a grade 3 to 6 rough, harsh pansystolic murmur, often associated with a thrill, is present, with maximal intensity at fourth left intercostal space, radiating to the epigastrium and left sternal border, but less well to the apex (Fig. 3.17).

In some small ventricular septal defects, particularly the *supracristal variety*, the murmur is heard maximally at the pulmonary area and closely mimics severe pulmonary stenosis because of its length and midsystolic crescendo; the latter feature is probably related to regurgitant jet entering the pulmonary artery directly. It can be differentiated from pulmonary stenosis by the presence of a short middiastolic flow rumble at the apex, normal splitting of the second heart sound, softening with amyl nitrite, and a normal electrocardiogram.

Uncommonly, a late systolic murmur preceded by a midsystolic click may be present when a left-to-right shunt occurs through a small defect in an *aneurysm of the membranous ventricular septum*. The click is produced by bulging of the aneurysm.

The regurgitant murmur of ventricular septal defect softens with amyl nitrite inhalation and intensifies with vasopressor drugs, provided that the defect is isolated and pulmonary hypertension is absent. In the presence of a

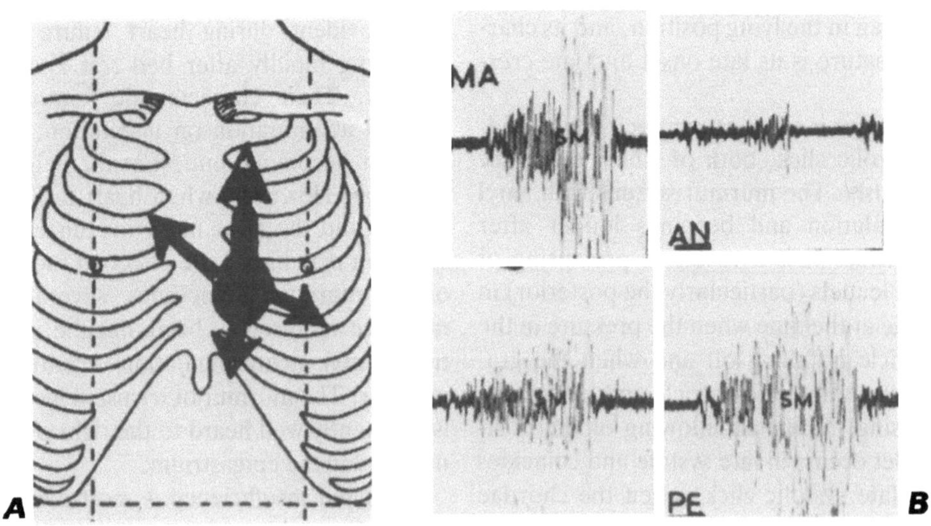

FIGURE 3.17. Ventricular septal defect. The site of maximum intensity of the murmur and the radiation (A). The typical pansystolic regurgitant murmur (B), promptly softening with amyl nitrite and intensifying with phenylephrine.

high pulmonary vascular resistance, particularly if the murmur is short, the reverse occurs because of the preferential and dominant effect of the drugs on the pulmonary arterioles.

Because of the variable configuration of the murmur of ventricular septal defect produced by changes in pulmonary artery pressure and pulmonary vascular resistance, the second sound should be carefully analyzed. The latter is influenced not only by the pulmonary artery pressure but also by the presence or absence of pulmonary outflow tract obstruction. It is single or narrowly split, but accentuated in pulmonary hypertension; it is widely split in outflow tract obstruction and small isolated defects with normal pulmonary artery pressures. In the absence of pulmonary hypertension, normal splitting also occurs. Because of the masking effect of very loud murmurs, P2 is often not appreciated by the ear, but readily demonstrated on the phonocardiogram.

Ejection Systolic Murmurs

Aortic Stenosis

The ejection murmur is usually grade 3 to 6 in intensity and the louder and longer the murmur, the more severe the stenosis, and the more likely it is to be associated with a thrill.

Phonocardiographically, the later the crescendo, the greater the severity; when the crescendo is 220 msec or more after the preceding Q wave of the electrocardiogram, severe aortic stenosis is almost certainly present. The murmur is typically ejection in type, starting after the first sound and stopping before A2, with a midsystolic crescendo (Fig. 3.18). As the stenosis increases, left ventricular systole become prolonged beyond right ventricular systole, so that *reverse splitting* of the second sound occurs. The murmur may therefore continue beyond P2, stopping before a softly audible, or inaudible A2.

When left ventricular failure supervenes in aortic stenosis the stroke volume drops and the murmur may soften and even disappear. It may be audible only at the apex, so that its significance may not be appreciated. Aortic stenosis is common in middle-aged and elderly men with thick chest walls or emphysema, in whom all sounds and murmurs are damped, so that a murmur, even if soft, must be carefully evaluated. In these patients, auscultation in the suprasternal notch and over the carotid artery is helpful but not totally reliable, since carotid bruits are frequently present. Furthermore, the carotid upstroke time in the elderly is deceptively brisk and the diagnosis of aortic stenosis is therefore extremely difficult.

Pulmonary Stenosis

The auscultatory findings depend on the severity of the stenosis and whether the ventricular septum is intact. If the septum is intact, the only exit from the right ventricle is through the pulmonary valve; the tricuspid valve usually retains its competency. The more severe the stenosis, the longer is right ventricular systole and the longer the murmur, so that in extreme stenosis, A2 is obscured. The murmur always remains ejection in type, starting after the first sound and ending before P2.

The intensity of the murmur usually varies from grade 3 to 6 in intensity, becoming louder as the severity of the stenosis increases. Like aortic stenosis, the murmur may be soft in the presence of heart failure. The site of maximal intensity is usually the pulmonary area or the first left interspace, since the stenosis is usually valvar.

In infundibular stenosis, the maximum intensity is lower down, and in transposition of the great vessels it may be to the right of the sternum. The murmur radiates down the left sternal border, is harsh in quality, and crescendo–decrescendo in shape. Respiration has a variable effect, but amyl nitrite produces prompt and marked intensification unless the right ventricle is unable to increase its output, or tricuspid incompetence is present. A pulmonary ejection click is present, particular in mild cases with poststenotic dilatation of the pulmonary artery. Splitting of the second sound is wide and an atrial gallop may be present (Fig. 3.12).

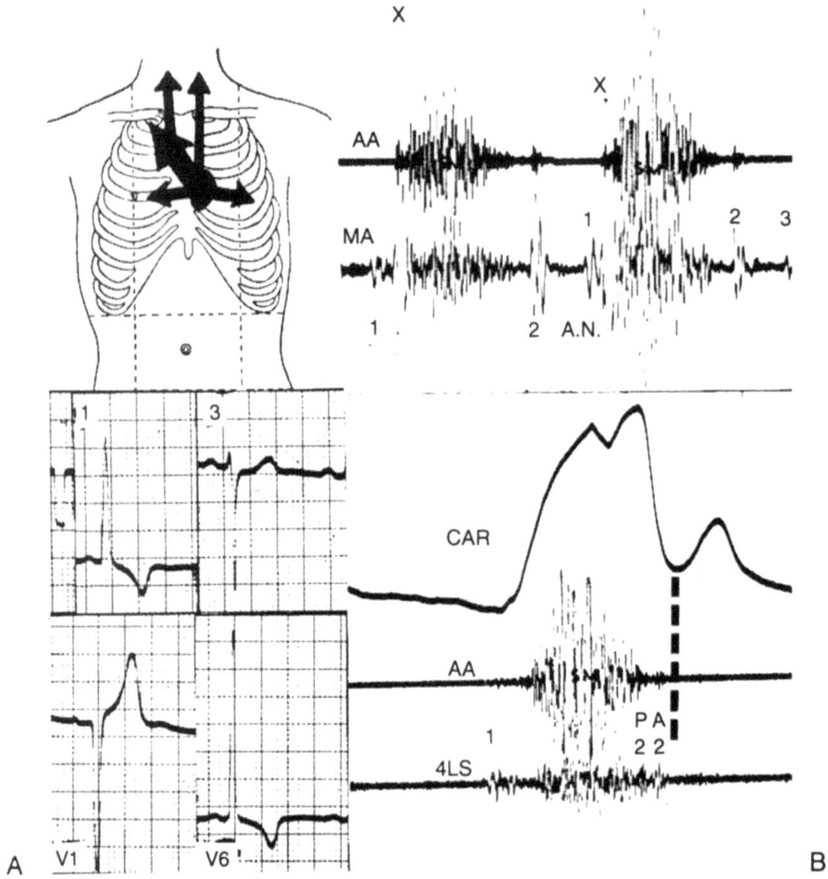

FIGURE 3.18. Aortic stenosis. The site of maximum intensity of the murmur and the radiation (A). The typical aortic ejection murmur with midsystolic crescendo is shown in the upper right panel. The first sound is soft and the loud aortic ejection sound (X) is immediately followed by by the murmur which stops before A2. After amyl nitrite (A.N.) inhalation, the murmur promptly intensifies. The electrocardiogram (B) shows severe left ventricular hypertrophy.. The aortic ejection murmur continues beyond P2 since "reversed splitting" is present. The carotid tracing shows a prolonged upstroke (anacrotic pulse) in the lower right panel.

Tetralogy of Fallot

The murmur arises from the stenotic pulmonary valve or infundibulum, or both. Because pressures in the ventricles are identical, a murmur does not arise from the ventricular septal defect.

The presence of the ventricular septal defect accounts for the behavior of the murmur in Tetralogy. The right venticle has two exits, so that the more severe the pulmonary stenosis, the greater is the right-to-left shunt reduction in pulmonary blood flow, and the murmur is therefore shorter. In most patients the murmur is short and stops before a single second sound composed of A2 only. In *acyanotic* subjects, the murmur is long, obscuring A2 and stopping before a soft P2. In *extremely severe* cases, the murmur is very short or absent and an aortic ejection click is present.

The maximum intensity of the murmur is usually the third or fourth left parasternal space, since the infundibular stenosis is usually present, and the intensity, quality, and radiation are similar to that of pulmonary stenosis. Amyl nitrite produces marked softening and shortening of the murmur (Fig. 3.12). Vasopressors intensify and lengthen the murmur.

Diastolic Murmurs

These are either *early diastolic* resulting from semilunar valve regurgitation, or *middiastolic* arising at the atrioventricular valves because of stenosis or abnormally high flow.

Aortic Diastolic Murmurs

When an aortic valve is incompetent, regurgitation occurs as soon as the left ventricular pressure drops below that of the aorta. Thus, the early diastolic murmur commences immediately after A2 (Fig. 3.19).

The murmur is high-pitched at the third and fourth left intercostal spaces, radiating along the left sternal border toward the apex. When the ascending aorta is dilated and elongated or aneurysmal, the murmur is often best heard at the aortic area and to the right of the sternum rather than the left. Clinical suspicion of an ascending aortic aneurysm is often aroused by detection of an early diastolic murmur louder to the right of the sternum than the left (Levine's sign).

The murmur is decrescendo, and, except in mild lesions, continues throughout diastole. In some patients it is best heard with the patient sitting up and leaning forward, after maximal expiration, using the diaphragm of the stethoscope firmly pressed to the chest wall. The larger the diaphragm the easier it is to hear the murmur. In other patients, the murmur is best heard with the patient lying completely flat. In our experience, the murmur is best heard with the patient standing and can be accentuated by prompt squatting.

Because of its high pitch and softness, an aortic diastolic murmur is the most commonly missed of all murmurs. Vasopressor drugs accentuate the murmur and amyl nitrite diminishes it. An aortic ejection sound and a systolic murmur often accompanies the diastolic murmur. When aortic stenosis is associated, the diastolic murmur is often rough and associated with a thrill, but this may also be found in syphilis, where there is no element of stenosis. A *cooing dove* musical murmur often denotes eversion of a cusp as in syphilitic aortitis, or perforation as a result of infective endocarditis.

A

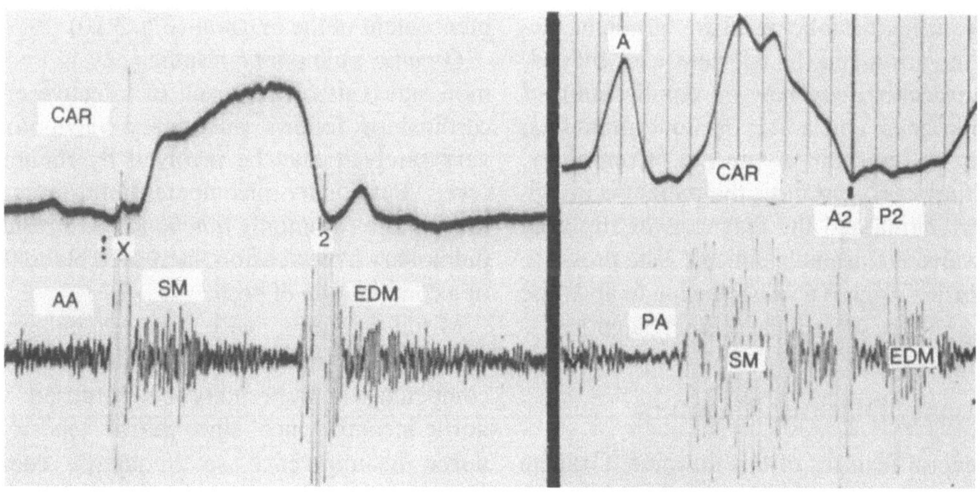

B

FIGURE 3.19. In aortic incompetence (A), the early diastolic murmur commences with A2 and, therefore, occurs early in diastole. In pulmonary incompetence (B), the diastolic murmur commences with P2 and the degree of splitting determines how soon in diastole it appears. Note the soft first sound and loud ejection click (x) in A. Note the coincidental recording of the a wave of the jugular venous pulse by the same transducer.

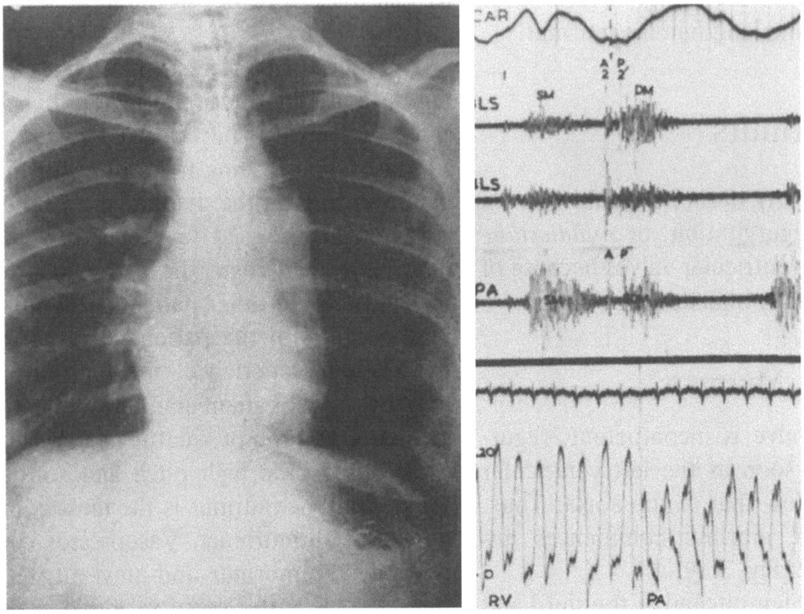

FIGURE 3.20. Idiopathic pulmonary artery dilatation and incompetence. The X-ray shows gross enlargement of the main pulmonary artery but no plethora. Phonocardiogram (upper right) shows the wide splitting of the second sound with a pulmonary systolic and diastolic murmur. The pressure trace in the lower right panel reveals a normal right ventricular pressure, a trivial gradient across the pulmonary valve, and a low pulmonary diastolic pressure.

In *acute sudden severe aortic insufficiency*, which occurs when infective endocarditis is complicated by cusp perforation, the early diastolic murmur is soft and short because there is very little diastolic pressure gradient between the aorta and the left ventricle. Indeed, in severe cases there may be equilibration of left ventricular and aortic diastolic pressures, so that no murmur is present. Commonly, under these circumstances the patient is in pulmonary edema and the diagnosis of ruptured aortic valve is extremely difficult. The presence of Duroziez's sign is a valuable clue to an aortic runoff and may suggest the correct diagnosis.

Pulmonary Diastolic Murmurs

The general features of this murmur (Graham Steel) are the same as those of aortic insufficiency, with which it is often confused. The most important clue is the site of maximum intensity, which is the pulmonary area, and the more limited radiation of the murmur. A pulmonary ejection sound is frequently associated. The murmur commences after closure of the pulmonary valve so that if P2 is delayed, there is an interval between A2 and the commencement of the murmur (Fig. 3.20).

Organic pulmonary insufficiency is uncommon and is usually a result of infective endocarditis, or follows pulmonary valvulotomy; very rarely it may be involved by rheumatic fever. Pulmonary incompetent murmurs are much more commonly *functional*, as a result of pulmonary hypertension, increased blood flow, or a combination of both.

Mitral stenosis with severe pulmonary hypertension complicated by pulmonary incompetence may readily be confused with aortic incompetence, since mitral stenosis and aortic incompetence so frequently coexist. However, a palpable second sound at the pulmonary area (diastolic shock), followed by an early diastolic murmur, most intense at the pulmonary area that radiates poorly and associated with an early, poorly radiating click, suggests pulmonary incompetence. Pulmonary hypertension associated with congenital heart disease is less readily confused with aortic incompetence.

Idiopathic dilatation of the pulmonary artery with dilatation of the valve ring may be associated with pulmonary incompetence (Fig. 3.20). Occasionally, pulmonary valve stenosis is complicated by mild pulmonary insufficiency and this usually signifies a previous attack of infective endocarditis.

Mitral Middiastolic Murmurs

Rheumatic mitral stenosis is the commonest cause of a mitral middiastolic murmur. In acute rheumatic endocarditis a transient middiastolic apical murmur is often heard (*Carey-Coomb's murmur*), but most murmurs are heard in chronic rheumatic valvulitis.

In mitral stenosis diastolic flow commences after mitral valve opening and ceases with mitral closure. Maximal flow occurs during early diastole and atrial systole adds the final increment, leading to maximal presystolic ventricular distention. The more obstructive the mitral valve, the longer the murmur, so that ultimately the murmur commences after opening of the valve (indicated by the opening snap), continuing throughout diastole with presystolic accentuation produced by atrial systole (Fig. 3.7). A full-length diastolic murmur with presystolic accentuation thus indicates critical stenosis. A presystolic murmur alone indicates established mitral stenosis, but this need not be severe. The length of the middiastolic murmur is the most reliably clinical sign for estimating the severity of mitral stenosis.

The murmur is low-pitched, rumbling in quality, usually localized to the apex, and best heard on expiration, after effort, and with the patient turned onto the left side. When there is both mitral stenosis and insufficiency, the length of the murmur helps determine which is the predominant lesion.

Predominant mitral insufficiency is associated with a pansysolic murmur and a short middiastolic murmur occurring at the time of the third heart sound and diminishing rapidly thereafter. When, however, there is significant

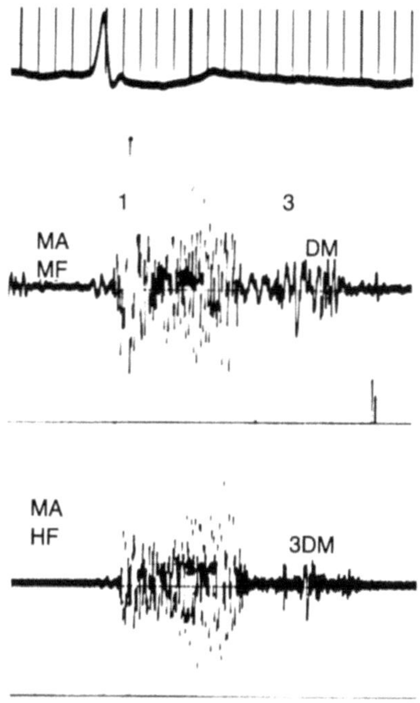

FIGURE 3.21. Phonocardiograms in rheumatic mitral regurgitation showing pansystolic murmur and short middiastolic rumble; medium frequency (MF) above and high frequency (HF) below.

mitral stenosis the murmur is long and indicates a significant pressure gradient across the valve. The length of the mid diastolic murmur is particularly easy to assess in the presence of a long pause during atrial fibrillation (Fig. 3.21).

Functional diastolic murmurs are heard in conditions associated with torrential flow across the mitral valve. They begin in middiastole, frequently following a loud third heart sound, and are characteristically short. They do not have presystolic accentuation.

Left-to-right shunts resulting from ventricular septal defect or patent ductus arteriosus and gross mitral incompetence are the most common causes. High output states such as anemia, thyrotoxicosis, and beriberi are occasional causes. Complete heart block may also be associated with excessive mitral flow and a short middiastolic mitral rumble.

A rumbling middiastolic apical murmur occurs in most cases of severe aortic incompetence without mitral stenosis and is called the *Austin–Flint* murmur. It is frequently found in syphilitic aortic incompetence, but is more difficult to diagnose when the incompetence is rheurmatic in origin. The murmur sounds exactly like that of mitral stenosis and may even have presystolic accentuation. Furtheremore, the first heart sound is not necessarily soft and may actually be accentuated. Only the opening snap is missing. Aortic incompetence is generally, but not always, severe. If clear-cut evidence of mitral valve disease such as calcification, or disproportionate enlargement of the left atrium, can be found, mitral valve disease can be diagnosed. An Austin–Flint murmur diminishes with the administration of amyl nitrite, whereas the murmur of true mitral stenosis is accentuated.

The Austin–Flint murmur is the result of the regurgitant jet striking the leaflets of the mitral valve, causing them to "flutter." This is readily recognized by echocardiography, which is the most reliable way of confirming the diagnosis of the Austin–Flint murmur.

Murmur of Organic Tricuspid Valve Disease

These are usually a result of rheumatic involvement. Mitral valve disease almost always coexists, but unlike mitral stenosis, pure tricuspid stenosis without incompetence is rare.

The murmur of *tricuspid stenosis* is best heard at the tricuspid area, starting after a tricuspid opening snap. Presystolic accentuation indicates well-established disease. The murmur frequently radiates toward the apex. It characteristically becomes louder during inspiration and following the inhalation of amyl nitrite.

The important differential diagnosis is from mitral stenosis; that is, the problem to be resolved is whether there is tricuspid plus mitral stenosis, or mitral stenosis alone. The auscultatory clues are the site of maximum intensity of the murmur, the fact that the murmur has a higher frequency than that of mitral stenosis, and the marked intensification with inspiration.

Because the murmur frequently has a high frequency and also starts surprisingly early, it may be confused with the early diastolic murmur of aortic insufficiency. Auscultation in the epigastrium under these circumstances is of particular value and points to a tricuspid origin. Tricuspid insufficiency frequently coexists and the accompanying systolic murmur, which also intensifies with inspiration, is an additional clue.

Congenital tricuspid valve disease, such as *Ebstein anomaly*, may be associated with a tricuspid opening snap and a short middiastolic murmur. The latter is a result of a mild degree of commissural fusion which occurs in this disease.

Functional tricuspid middiastolic murmurs are a result of torrential flow across the tricuspid valve: They are commonly heard in atrial septal defect and partial or total anomalous pulmonary venous drainage. The murmur is fairly high pitched, and may radiate to the apex. The commonest functional tricuspid diastolic murmur occurs with tricuspid insufficiency. When the latter is severe it can be impossible to determine whether the diastolic murmur is the result of organic valve disease or not. Functional diastolic murmurs with presystolic accentuation may be heard in severe pulmonary insufficiency and is the counterpart of the Austin–Flint murmur affecting the mitral valve.

Continuous Murmurs

These murmurs begin in systole, extend through the second heart sound, and occupy portions, or all, of diastole. They are produced by flow from a high- to a low-pressure area with a continuous pressure difference throughout systole and diastole.

The murmurs are continuous in a special sense: In mitral incompetence with coexisting aortic incompetence, a continuous murmur is present, in that the murmurs occupy all of systole and all of diastole, without a break. However, the murmurs are produced at two different sites. In fistulae, the continuous murmur is produced at one site, starting after the first heart sound extending throughout systole (often with a crescendo toward the end of systole), beyond the second sound and often continuing through the rest of diastole. The systolic component is usually harsher and radiates more widely than the diastolic component, which is more blowing or humming in character.

Arteriovenous Fistulae

The following communications between the high- and low-pressure systems are encountered:

1. *Aorta to Pulmonary Artery.* Patent ductus arteriosus is by far the commonest cause. The continuous nature of the murmur is maintained until the pulmonary artery pressure rises significantly in diastole. When the diastolic pressure in the pulmonary artery equals that of the aorta, the diastolic component of the continuous murmur may disappear, and when both sytolic and diastolic pressures are equal the ductus may be "silent".

An *aortopulmonary window* is a large communication between the ascending aorta and pulmonary arteries and, for the reason just given, a continuous murmur is uncommonly heard; usually it is confined to systole. Communications between the *bronchial arteries* and pulmonary arteries such as occurs in pulmonary atresia are heard in all areas of the chest. Surgically produced communications between the aorta and pulmonary artery for the relief of cyanosis in congenital heart disease are common causes of continuous murmurs (the Blalock–Taussig, Potts, and Waterston–Cooley operation).

2. *Systemic Artery to Systemic Vein.* These are less common and may be of the congenital or acquired variety. They may involve the coronary artery and coronary vein, any systemic artery to systemic vein, cerebral artery to cerebral vein, or anomalous origin of the coronary artery from the pulmonary trunk.

3. *Aorta to Vena Cava or Any Cardiac Chamber.* Fistulae between the aorta and the superior vena cava are usually traumatic. Rupture of a sinus of Valsalva may produce a fistula from the aorta to the right atrium or the right ventricle.

4. *Pulmonary Artery to Pulmonary Vein.* Congenital pulmonary arteriovenous fistulae and occasionally vascular tumors of the lung may be responsible for a continuous murmur.

Continuous Murmurs Not Produced by Fistulae

These murmurs may be heard in a systemic or pulmonary vein and are a result of torrential or turbulent flow. Often, diastolic accentuation of the murmur is present.

Jugular venous hum is common in the neck and the first intercostal spaces. When this murmur radiates below the clavicle, it may be mistaken for a patent ductus arteriosus. The distinction can be made quite simply by compression of the internal jugular vein on the side. A venous hum may be audible under either clavicle in total anomalous pulmonary venous drainage at the site of connection of the ascending vertical vein with the corresponding innominate vein. A venous hum may be heard in the epigastrium in cirrhosis of the liver associated with portal venous obstruction and collateral venous channels.

Continuous murmurs may also be heard over *dilated intercostal arteries* and the *internal mammary artery* in coarctation of the aorta and aortic arteritis. In *aortic coarctation*, the murmur is best heard between the scapulae at the site of obstruction. In *proximal branch pulmonary artery* stenosis the murmurs are heard below either or both clavicles and, being conducted along the pulmonary artery, are often well heard in the back. When the stenosis is mild or moderate the murmurs are systolic only, but when severe the murmur is continuous. In renal artery stenosis the murmur is best heard in the abdomen or paraspinally posteriorly.

Continuous murmurs are occasionally heard in atrial septal defect associated with mitral stenosis (*Lutembacher's syndrome*), where there is a continuous pressure difference across a restrictive atrial septal defect. A continuous murmur may be heard over the lactating breast (*mammary souffle*), but is unlikely to be confused with organic heart disease.

Pericardial Friction Rub

The typical pericardial friction rub has three separate components related to atrial systole, ventricular systole, and ventricular diastole, respectively. The quality of the rub is likened to the sound of two pieces of sandpaper rubbed together intermittently. However, a rub may be systolic or diastolic only.

The rub is best heard along the left sternal border and in the xiphoid area in held expiration with the patient leaning forward. It increases with inspiration and is accentuated by increasing pressure with the bell or diaphragm. It sounds more superficial than the other heart sounds. A pericardial friction rub is often transient so that if doubt exists, frequent observation over 1 or 2 days soon settles the question. Occasionally rubs may persist for months. Whenever heard it is diagnostic of pericarditis from any cause. In the presence of a pericardial rub, murmurs may be obscured.

When heard at the apex only, a pericardial rub may be difficult to differentiate from a pleuropericardial rub. The latter is usually heard near the apex when the left pleura is involved, and increases markedly on inspiration. A pleuropericardial rub extends beyond the heart border and is heard over the left lung.

Additional Reading

Barlow JB: The diagnosis and treatment of mitral incompetence. S Afr Med J 42:400, 1968.

Barlow JB, Pocock WA: The problem of nonejection systolic clicks and associated mitral systolic murmurs: Emphasis on the billowing mitral leaflet syndrome. Am Heart J 90:636, 1975.

Beck W, Schrire V, Vogelpoel L: Splitting of the second heart sound in constrictive pericarditis, with observations on the mechanism of pulsus paradoxus. Am Heart J 64:765, 1962.

Beck W, Schrire V, Vogelpoel L, Nellen M, Swanepoel A: Hemodynamic effects of amyl nitrite and phenylephrine on the normal human circulation and their relation to changes in cardiac murmurs. Am J Cardiol 8:341, 1961.

Leatham A: Auscultation of the heart. Lancet 2:703, 757, 1958.

Leatham A: Phonocardiography. Br Med Bull 8:333, 1951.

Nellen M, Gotsman MS, Vogelpoel L, Beck W, Schrire V: Effects of prompt squatting on the systolic murmur in hypertrophic obstructive cardiomyopathy. Br Med J 3:140, 1967.

Tavel ME: "Clinical Phonocardiography and External Pulse Recording" 4th Ed. Year Book Pulishers, Chicago, 1985.

4
Cardiac Radiology

Teleradiology of the heart includes one frontal, lateral, and two oblique views of the chest, with the films taken at a patient to tube distance of 6 feet. This distance ("tele-" at a distance) is chosen to avoid distortion since the X-rays are then nearly parallel and there is therefore minimum magnification of the heart size. In the anterior–posterior (AP) view the patient faces the tube and the X-rays penetrate the chest to the X-ray film behind.

Usually, the posterior–anterior (PA) view is chosen, with the patient's back to the tube and the sternum as close to the film as possible, to reduce distortion to a minimum. In the oblique views, the patient is rotated approximately 45°, so that the right shoulder faces the X-ray film (RAO view) or the left shoulder faces the film (LAO view). For routine purposes, a normally penetrated PA view, an overpenetrated PA view, and a lateral view with barium in the esophagus are frequently used.

The diagnostic value of chest radiography in clinical cardiology cannot be overemphasized. This applies not only in the initial assesment but also at subsequent examinations where comparison is made with previous films.

Before any assessment is made, however, careful attention should be paid to technique and film quality. The first step is to ascertain that the film has been adequately exposed. Overexposed ("hard") films make the assessment of the pulmonary vasculature extremely difficult and may lead to an erroneous diagnosis of pulmonary oligemia. However, underexposed ("soft") films may accentuate the pulmonary vascular markings and be misinterpreted as an increase in the pulmonary vasculature. Generally, adequate penetration is considered to be present when the spinal column is just obscured by the cardiac silhouette. Second, films should be checked for rotation that may distort the cardiac silhouette and lead to an incorrect diagnosis of enlargement of an individual chamber, or great vessel. When the film is properly centered, the tracheal shadow is central and the inner ends of the clavicles equidistant from the trachea.

Attention should be paid to the size and shape of the chest since these influence the radiological findings considerably. Scoliosis may produce considerable distortion of the cardiac silhouette. Similarly, marked depression of the sternum reduces the anteroposterior diameter of the chest and produces a false impression of cardiomegaly. Third, the position of the diaphragms should be checked to ensure that the films have been taken during an adequate inspiration. Underinflation of the lungs with high diaphragms produces false enlargement of the heart and an increase in the cardiothoracic ration.

The Heart Size

Many measurements have been devised, but none is entirely satisfactory. Perhaps the best known and most widely used is the cardiothoracic ratio (CTR). This is most coveniently expressed as a percentage:

$$\frac{\text{maximum transverse diameter of the heart}}{\text{maximum transverse diameter of the chest}}$$

Care should be taken not to include the apical epicardial fat pad in the measurement of the maximum transverse cardiac diameter. Normally, the cardiothoracic ratio should be less than 50%. Even with good radiological technique a false diagnosis of cardiomegaly may be made when films are exposed during a long diastolic pause when the heart is well filled.

Radiological Anatomy

The PA Projection

The right cardiac border is made up of the right atrium below and the superior vena cava above (Fig. 4.1). The right ventricle does not contribute to the right cardiac border in this projection. The left cardiac border consists of the left ventricle below with a small radiolucency in the left cardiophrenic angle produced by the epicardial fat pad. Above the outline of the left ventricle is the edge of the left atrium, which just extends to the left border of the heart. The main pulmonary artery segment lies above this and the most superior segment is made up of the aortic knuckle.

The Lateral View

The anterior heart border is made up of the right ventricle (Fig. 4.2). The posterior border is made up of the posterior wall of the left ventricle below; above this is the left atrium. The inferior vena cava may be visualized between the left ventricle and the left leaf of the diaphragm. Normally, the left ventricle does not extend posterior to the shadow of the inferior vena cava.

Left Anterior Oblique View

The left cardiac border from superior to inferior is made up of aorta, the right atrium, and the right ventricle (Fig. 4.3). The posterior cardiac border is made up of the left ventricle below with the left atrium above it.

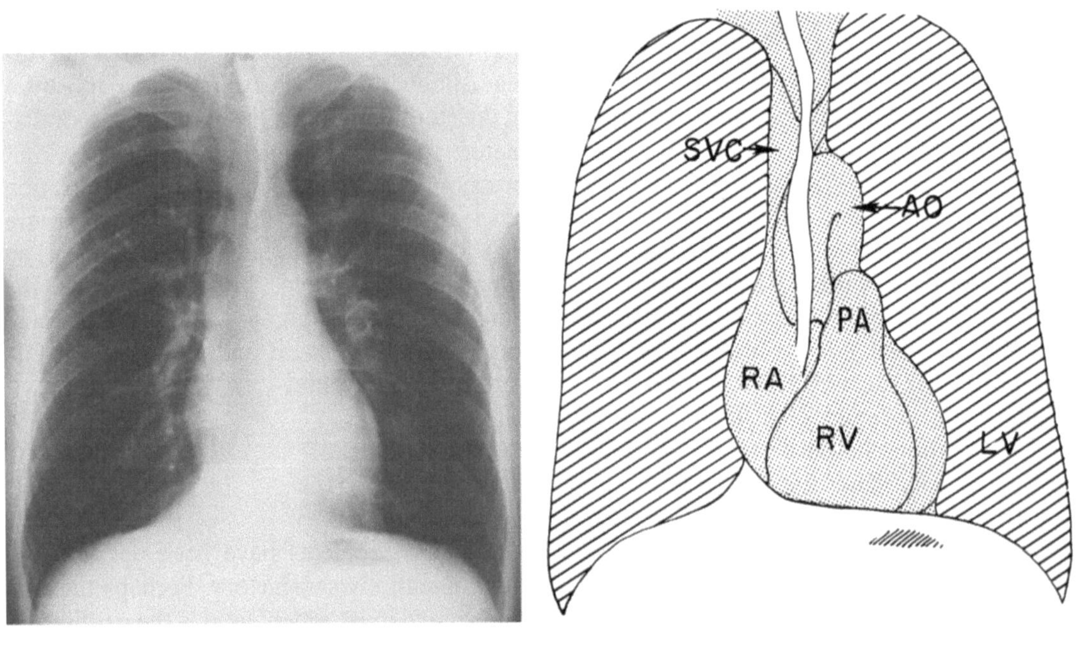

FIGURE 4.1. The normal cardiac silhouette, frontal projection, with the anatomy represented diagrammatically on the left. In this, and succeeding illustrations SVC, superior vena cava; Ao, aorta; PA, pulmonary artery; RA and RV, right atrium and right ventricle, respectively; LV, left ventricle.

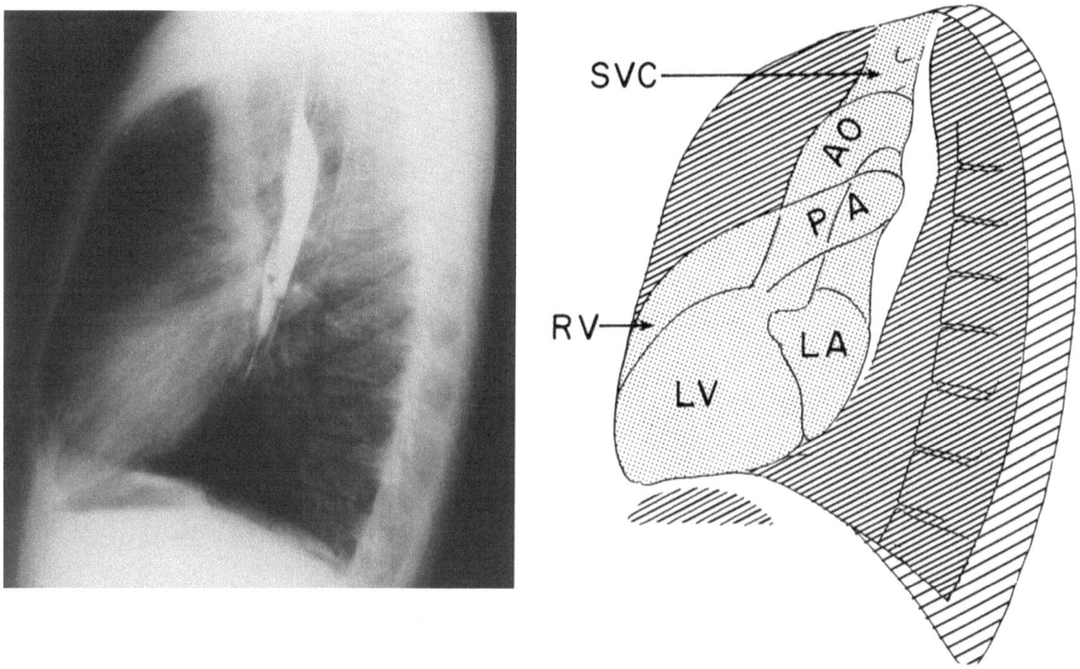

FIGURE 4.2. The normal cardiac silhouette, lateral view.

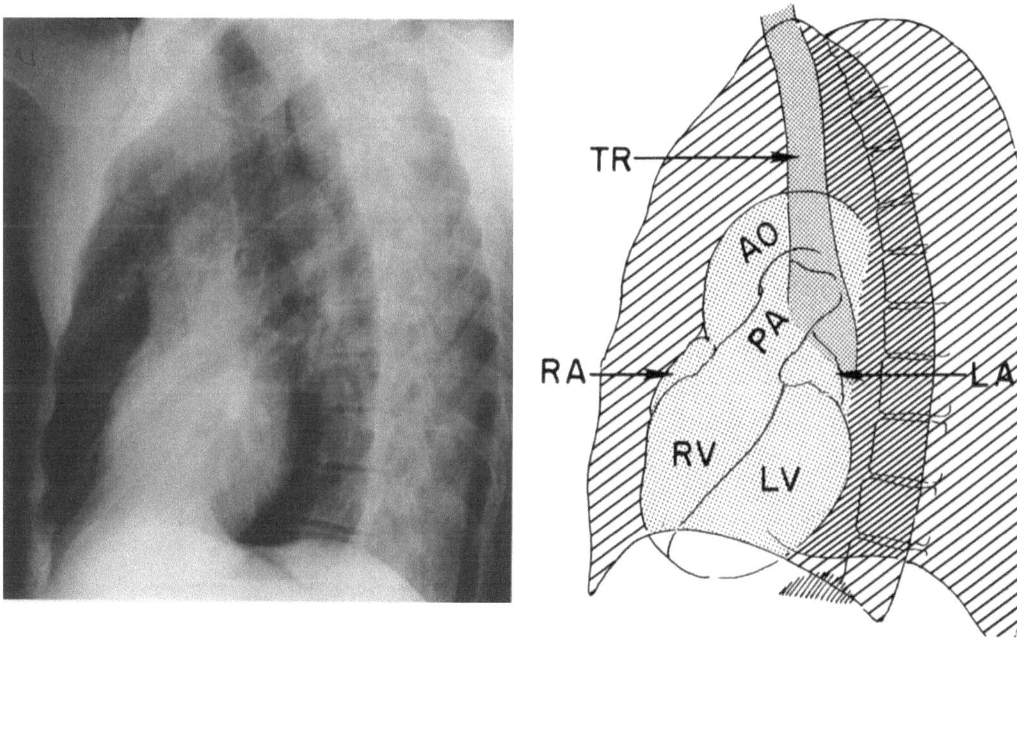

FIGURE 4.3. The normal cardiac silhouette, left anterior oblique view.

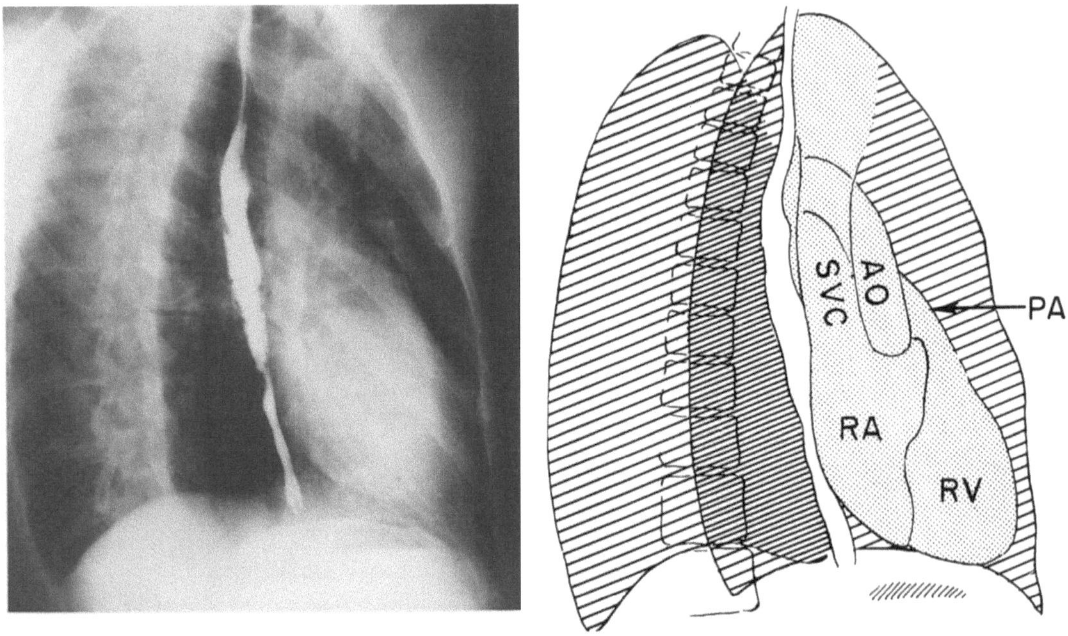

FIGURE 4.4. The normal cardiac silhouette, right anterior oblique view.

Right Anterior Oblique View

Anteriorly, the cardiac border is made up of the right ventricle below and the pulmonary artery above (Fig. 4.4). Posteriorly the cardiac border is made up of the inferior vena cava below with the right atrium and the superior vena cava successively above this.

Fluoroscopy

This is carried out with an image intensifier that provides great detail at little radiation hazard. It is most useful in detecting valvular and pericardial calcification, which may be difficult to recognize with standard X-ray pictures. It has little to offer, however, for the evaluation of overall heart size and individual chamber enlargement.

Generalized Enlargement of the Cardiac Silhouette

This may be a result of cardiac enlargement or pericardial effusion and the two may coexist (Figs. 4.5 and 4.6). The distinction between cardiomegaly and pericardial effusion may be extremely difficult. Certain points favor the diagnosis of pericardial effusion: In an effusion, fluid collects in the most dependent position

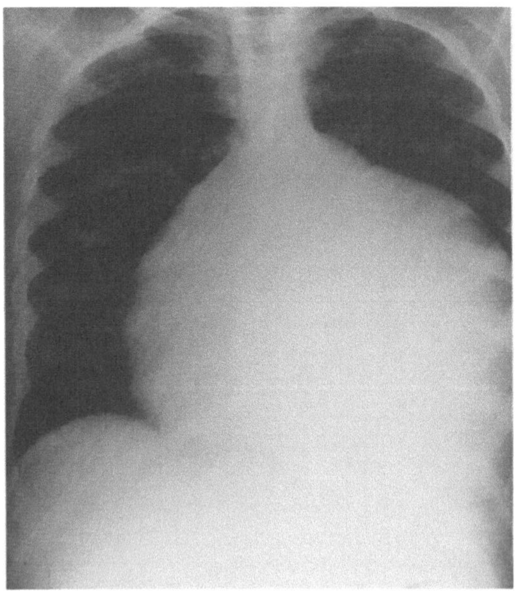

FIGURE 4.5. Chest X-ray in a case of severe Ebstein disease demonstrating massive cardiomegaly.

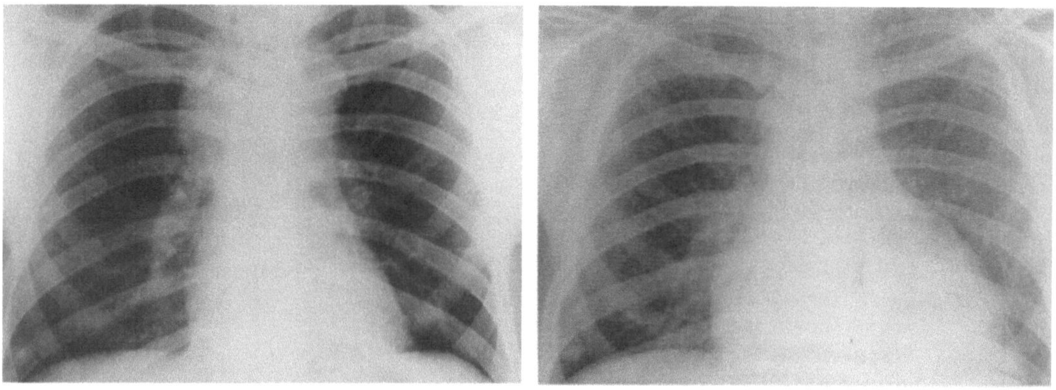

FIGURE 4.6. Chest X-rays demonstrating pericardial effusion in a case of Hodgkin's disease (left) before and (right) after pericardiocentesis. Following aspiration the heart size is normal and mediastinal lymphadenopathy is evident.

and retrosternally. The "waterbottle" appearance in the upright position becomes more globular in the lying position; in the lateral view, the enlargement is anterior and the cardiac shadow is less likely to overlap the spine; straightening of the cardiac border and the diaphragm is more acute; the angle of the bifurcation of the trachea is not increased; the lung fields are comparatively clear, but this is more apparent than real because the hila are usually obscured; cardiac pulsations are diminished or absent; and shrinkage of heart size does not occur with the Valsalva maneuver.

Unfortunately, none of these signs is absolutely diagnostic of pericardial effusion. For example, pulsation may be normal in pericarditis and absent in cardiomyopathy and pericardial effusion. However, the advent of echocardiography and nuclear angiography has made this distinction relatively easy.

Enlargement of Individual Chambers

Isolated Left Ventricular Enlargement

This is usually a result of hypertension, aortic valve disease, mitral insufficiency, cardiomyopathy, and ischemic heart disease.

In the PA projection this manifests as a rounding and bulging of the left lower cardiac border. In the LAO projection the enlarged left ventricle overlaps the spinal column and in the lateral projection the posterior border of the left ventricle extends beyond the shadow of the inferior vena cava (Fig. 4.7). These signs may be present, however, when there is a left ventricular aneurysm, pericardial effusion, or cyst. Additionally, severe right ventricular hypertrophy may displace the left ventricle laterally and posteriorly and therefore result in a false diagnosis of left ventricular enlargement.

The chest X-ray is not highly sensitive in detecting concentric left ventricular hypertrophy, and this has particular importance in the clinical assessment of valvular aortic stenosis. Critical aortic stenosis is not infrequently associated with a normal cardiothoracic ratio and a lack of posterior protrusion beyond the shadow of the inferior vena cava; the only radiological sign that may be present is a "rounding" of the left cardiac border. Therefore, the clinical suspicion of severe aortic stenosis should not be negated by the absence of the typical radiological finding of left ventricular enlargement. Radiology is much more sensitive in the detection of left ventricular dilatation encountered in aortic insufficiency, cardiomyopathy, and ischemic heart disease.

Left Atrial Enlargement

This is readily recognized when it exists as the only radiologic abnormality, such as occurs in

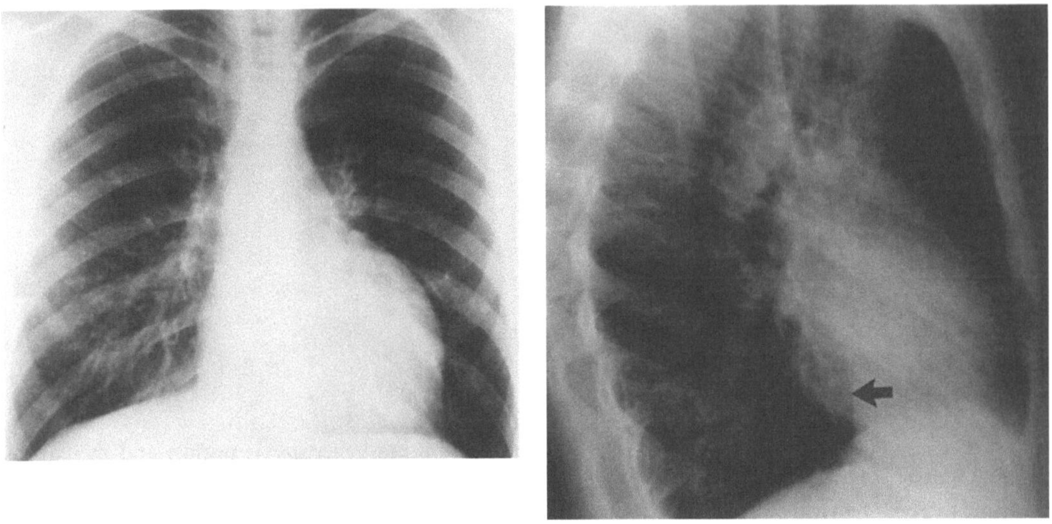

FIGURE 4.7. Chest X-ray in a case of hypertrophic obstructive cardiomyopathy demonstrating concentric left ventricular hypertrophy manifested by a rounding and bulging of the left cardiac border (left) and a posterior protrusion on the left ventricle beyond the inferior vena cava marked by an arrow in (right).

mitral valve disease. When, however, there is enlargement of other chambers (e.g., because of aortic valve disease, or severe pulmonary hypertension with tricuspid insufficiency) the recognition of left atrial enlargement is more difficult.

When significant cardiomegaly is present, the demonstration of well-marked left atrial enlargement is a good indicator for the diagnosis of organic mitral valve disease. For example, the Austin–Flint murmur complicating severe aortic insufficiency may be extremely difficult to differentiate from the auscultatory findings of mitral stenosis; radiological demonstration of left atrial enlargement disproportionate to left ventricular enlargement would strongly favor the diagnosis of organic mitral valve disease.

Left atrial enlargement produces filling in of the left cardiac border in the PA view. Subsequently, enlargement of the left atrial appendage forms a distinct bulge below the main pulmonary artery. Overpenetrated films in the PA projection show the round shadow of the enlarged left atrium whose right border is visible just internal to the right atrial shadow, forming the so-called "double-density."

Occasionally, left atrial dilatation is so extreme that it may protrude beyond the right cardiac border. Dilatation of the left atrium characteristically elevates the left main bronchus producing widening of the tracheal bifurcation. Backward displacement of the barium-filled esophagus is usually well demonstrated in the LAO and left lateral views (Fig. 4.8).

Right Ventricular Enlargement

This is recognized by anterior protrusion of the cardiac shadow toward the sternum resulting in obliteration of the retrosternal air space (Fig. 4.9). It is best observed in the lateral and RAP projections.

In the PA projection enlargement of the right ventricle may displace the right cardiac border to the right, but this represents displacement of the right atrium. Similarly, in this view, the left ventricle may be displaced toward the left, producing a false appearance of left ventricular enlargement; when in addition, the apex is tilted up the heart assumes the typical boot-shaped configuration of Tetralogy of Fallot.

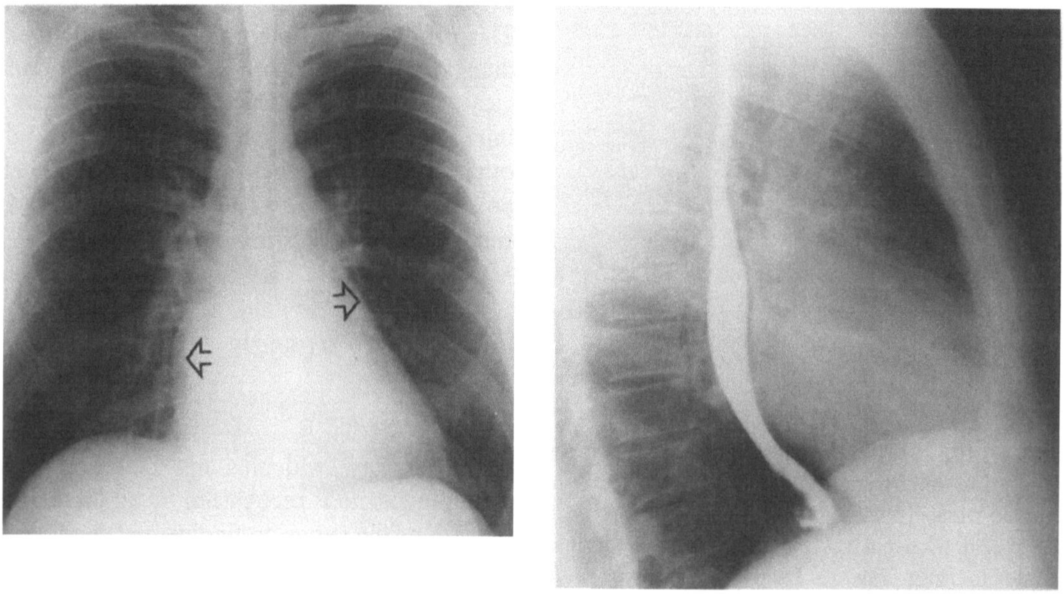

FIGURE 4.8. The X-ray in mitral stenosis demonstrating enlargement of the left atrium in the frontal view (left) manifested as a straightening of the left cardiac border and a double density within the right cardiac border (arrows). The upper lobe pulmonary veins are distended. In the lateral view (right) the barium column is displaced posteriorly by the enlarged left atrium.

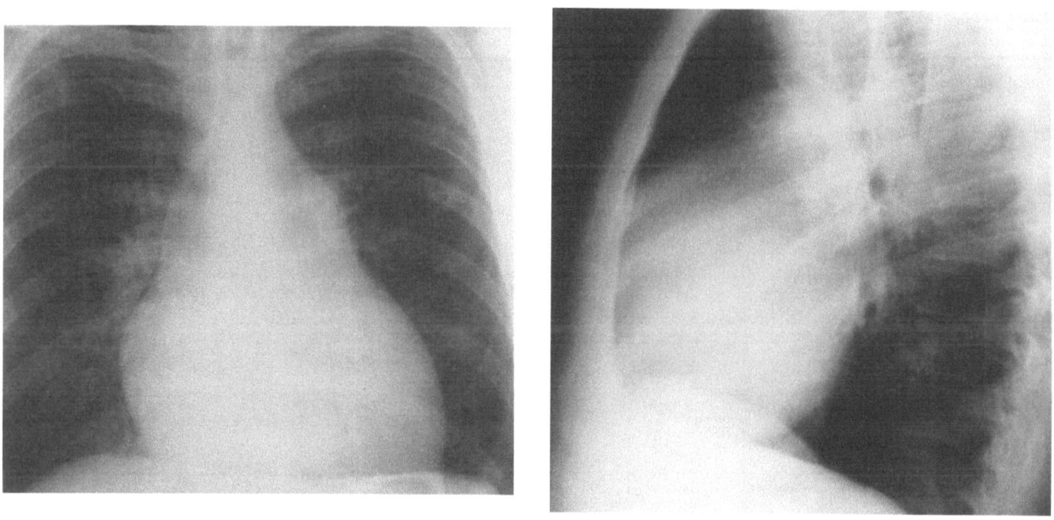

FIGURE 4.9. X-rays in a case of primary pulmonary hypertension. The main pulmonary artery is prominent and the peripheral vasculature is "pruned." The increased cardiothoracic ratio is the result of right atrial enlargement seen in the frontal view (left). Right ventricular enlargement manifested by filling in of the retrosternal air space in the lateral view (right).

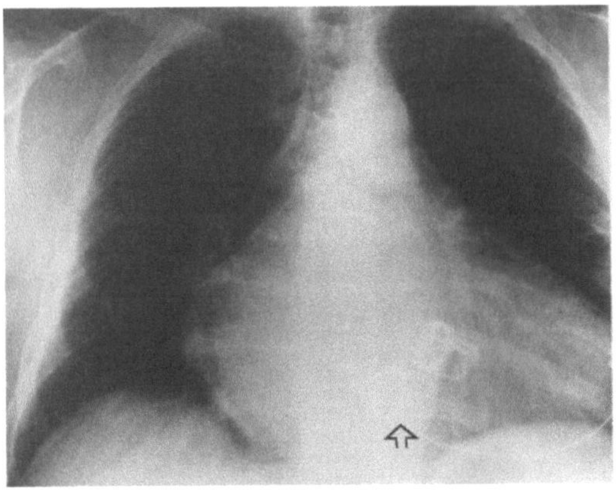

FIGURE 4.10. X-ray of the chest demonstrating gross right atrial enlargement as the result of an obstructed tricuspid valve prosthesis in a patient with mitral and tricuspid valve replacement. The right atrial dimension extends from the tricuspid valve prosthesis (arrow) to the right cardiac border.

Enlargement of the main pulmonary artery and its branches is an indirect sign of right ventricular hypertrophy. In general, the radiologic detection of pure concentric right ventricular hypertrophy is insensitive. The signs referred to above more usually reflect eccentric hypertrophy associated with dilatation of the chamber.

Right Atrial Enlargement

This produces a displacement of the right cardiac border to the right. However, the radiological diagnosis of right atrial enlargement is imprecise because it may be displaced by the other cardiac chambers and pure right atrial enlargement has to be quite marked before it is recognized (Fig. 4.10).

The Great Vessels

The Aorta

In the PA view, widening and dilatation of the ascending aorta is recognized by an increase in the size of the superior mediastinal shadow. In subjects under 40 years of age, rheumatic aortic valve disease or syphilitic aortitis is the usual cause. With advancing age, aortic atherosclerosis, with or without hypertension, is the major cause.

Arteriosclerosis characteristically produces an enlarged tortuous shadow, lifting the aortic knob toward the left sternoclavicular junction. Since the esophagus is adjacent, a barium swallow outlines the tortuous elongated kinked aorta. Poststenotic dilatation of the aorta occurs in aortic stenosis and this may be dis-

A

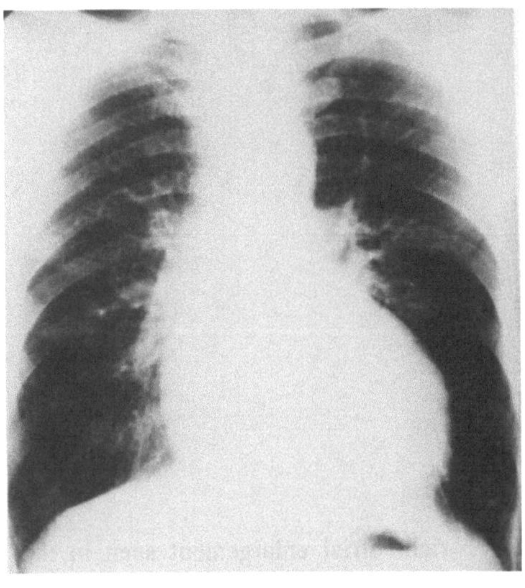

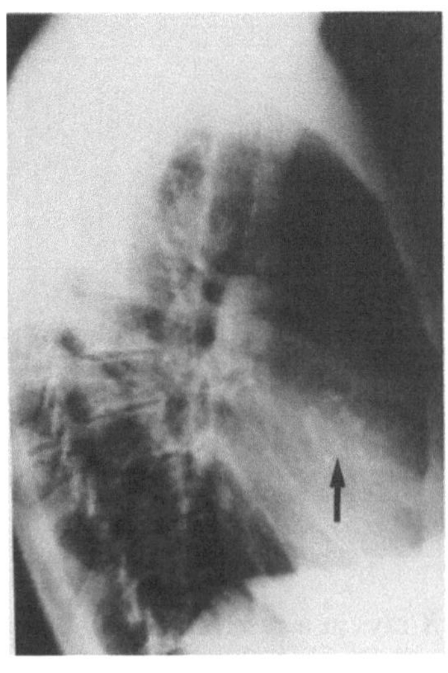

B

FIGURE 4.11. The X-rays in calcific aortic stenosis demonstrating enlargement of the ascending aorta and left ventricular hypertrophy in the frontal view (A) and calcification of the aortic valve (between arrows) (B).

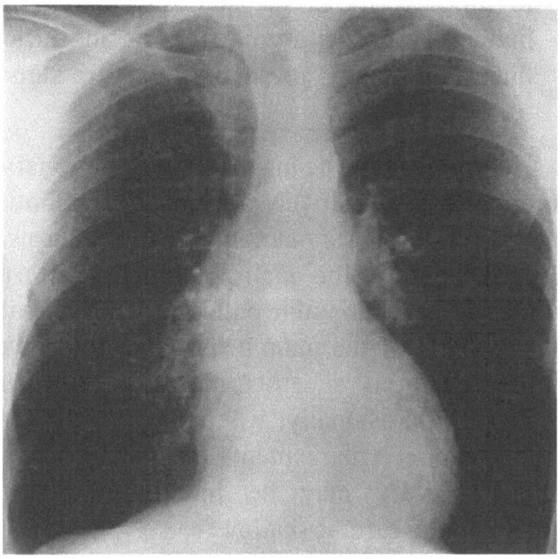

FIGURE 4.12. The X-ray in aortic insufficiency demonstrating enlargement of the ascending and descending thoracic portions of the aorta. There is also moderate left ventricular hypertrophy.

tinguished from enlargement of the ascending aorta as a result of aortic insufficiency. In the latter, both the ascending and the descending aorta are widened, whereas in aortic stenosis only the ascending aorta is dilated (Figs. 4.11 and 4.12).

A saccular aneurysm of the ascending aorta produces a sharply defined convex shadow, which has to be differentiated from other mediastinal space-occupying lesions. Aortic angiography or CT scan will differentiate an aneurysm from an extracardiac mass contiguous with the aorta. Calcification in the wall of such aneurysms is not uncommon. They are often a result of syphilis, dissecting aneurysm, or aortic arteritis (Fig. 4.13). Atherosclerosis usually produces a fusiform aneurysm, and rarely, if ever, a saccular aneurysm.

In congenital heart disease, a prominent aorta suggest Tetralogy of Fallot, patent ductus arteriosus, aortic stenosis, or coarctation. In coarctation, the aortic knuckle is replaced by a prominent left subclavian artery producing a double shadow resembling an Arabic 3. Obliteration of the space between the aorta and the pulmonary artery is highly suggestive of a patent ductus arteriosus. A right-sided aorta usually occurs in association with other defects, particularly Tetralogy of Fallot, and it is best recognized by a barium swallow.

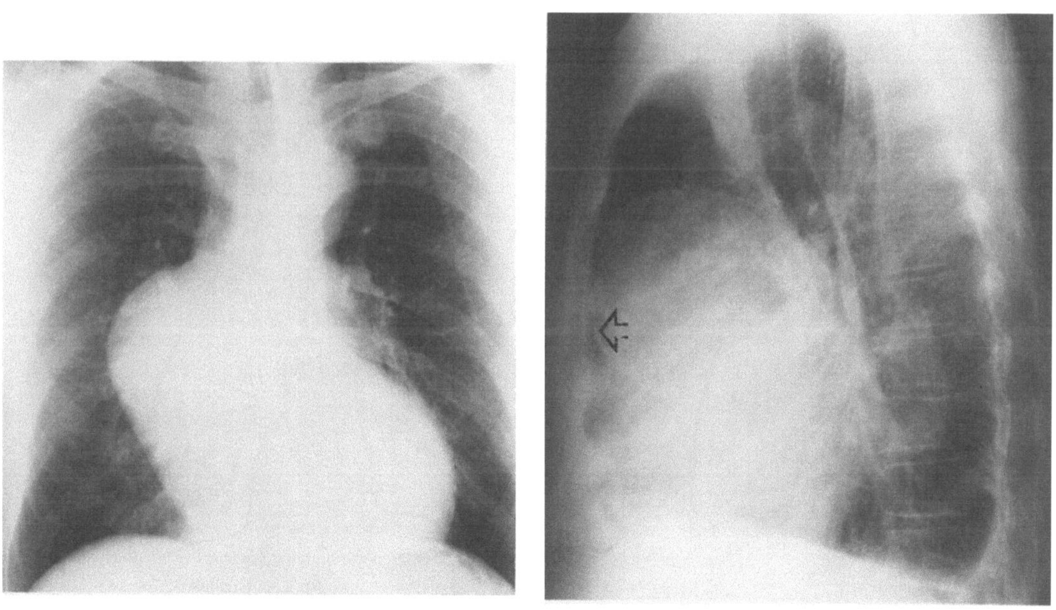

FIGURE 4.13. X-ray demonstrating a saccular aneurysm of the ascending aorta in Marfan syndrome. Calcification (arrow) is seen in the lateral view.

The Main Pulmonary Artery

This is best visualized in the PA projection and is normally separated from the aortic knuckle by a notch, unless a patent ductus is present. Enlargement of the main pulmonary artery may be a result of

1. Idiopathic pulmonary artery dilatation, which occurs as an isolated abnormality.
2. Increased pulmonary blood flow (e.g, atrial septal defect).
3. Increased pulmonary artery pressure (e.g., mitral stenosis).
4. Increased flow and pressure (e.g., ventricular septal defect).
5. Pulmonary valve stenosis. The size of the pulmonary arteries bears little relationship to the severity of the stenosis: dilatation may be severe with mild stenosis and little dilatation may be present with severe stenosis.

Enlargement of the main and left pulmonary arteries with a relatively normal right pulmonary artery suggests pulmonary valve stenosis. Enlargement of the main pulmonary artery alone suggests idiopathic pulmonary dilatation; enlargement of the main artery and both pulmonary arteries suggests increased flow of pressure. Occasionally, when there is associated chamber enlargement, an enlarged pulmonary artery may be incorporated and hidden in the cardiac shadow.

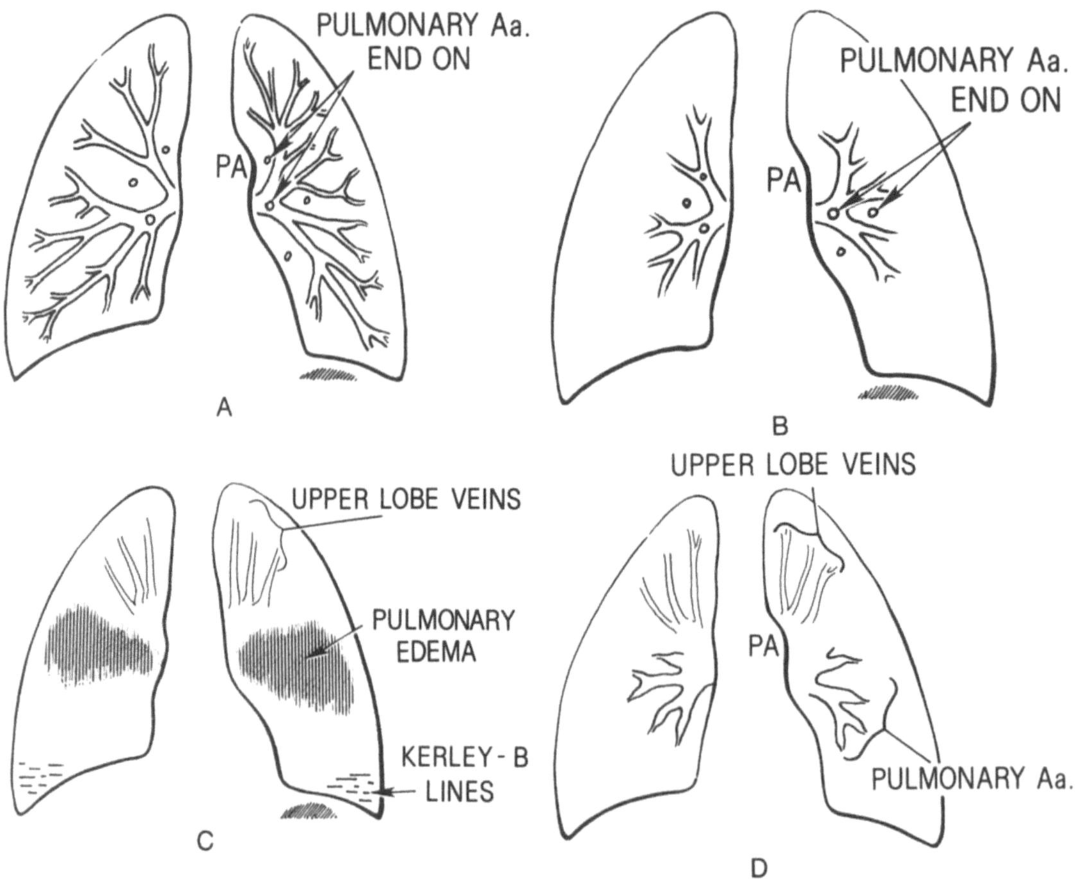

FIGURE 4.14. Diagrammatic representation of various changes in the pulmonary vasculature occurring with increased pulmonary blood flow (with and without pulmonary arterial hypertension) (A, B), pulmonary venous hypertension (C), and pulmonary venous and arterial hypertension (D).

An inconspicuous or absent main pulmonary artery is found in infundibular stenosis associated with Tetralogy of Fallot or pulmonary atresia with ventricular septal defect.

The Pulmonary Vasculature

Increased pulmonary arterial markings occur in left-to-right shunts (Fig. 4.14). This is best seen in the upper zones, but also involves the lower zones when the shunts are of greater magnitude (Fig. 4.15). Plethora leads to diminished translucency of the lung fields.

When the pulmonary vascular resistance rises, the degree of plethora diminishes, and when severely elevated, the pattern is modified. The pulmonary arteries remain enlarged proximally, but end abruptly (peripheral pruning), and this produces increased translucency of the peripheral lung fields (Fig. 4.16).

Thrombosis of the branches of the main pulmonary artery, and the site of the obstruction, can often be identified by oligemia distal to the enlarged proximal branch. It is most important therefore to compare the individual lung fields, because patchy loss of vascular markings, or localized plethora indicate regional impairment of flow resulting from obstruction, stenosis, or diversion of blood to an area of diminished resistance.

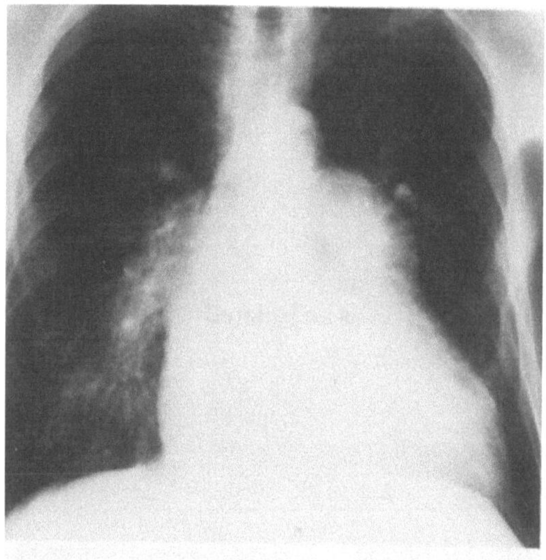

FIGURE 4.16. Secundum atrial septal defect with a predominant left-to-right shunt and elevated pulmonary vascular resistance. The main pulmonary artery is markedly enlarged. There is proximal prominence of the pulmonary arterial vasculature that diminishes peripherally ("peripheral pruning").

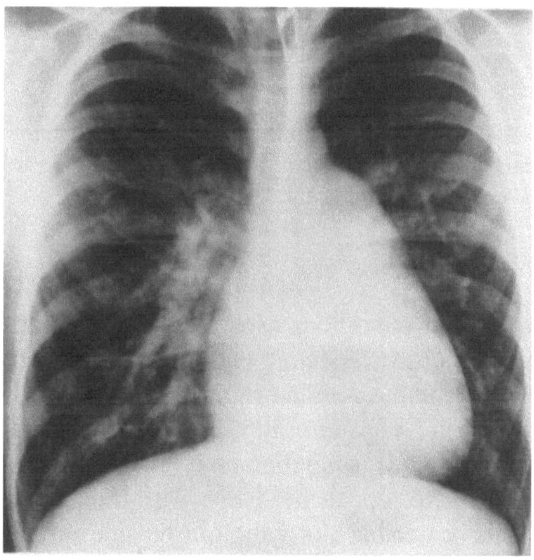

FIGURE 4.15. The X-ray in secundum atrial septal defect with large left-to-right shunt and low pulmonary vascular resistance. Pulmonary plethora is particularly evident in the right lung field and the arteries extend to the periphery.

Diminished pulmonary arterial markings are found in those congenital malformations where there is pulmonary oligemia resulting from obstruction to pulmonary blood flow and an associated right-to-left shunt. It is encountered occasionally in acquired heart disease such as emphysema and pericardial effusion.

Increased pulmonary venous markings occur in mitral valve disease and left ventricular failure. The redistribution of pulmonary blood flow associated with these conditions results in increased flow to the upper lobes leading to dilatation of the upper lobe veins. This disparity between the superior and inferior pulmonary venous shadows produces the characteristic "antler pattern" of mitral stenosis. There is also an increase in the hilar shadows resulting from both pulmonary arterial and pulmonary venous enlargement (Fig. 4.8). As

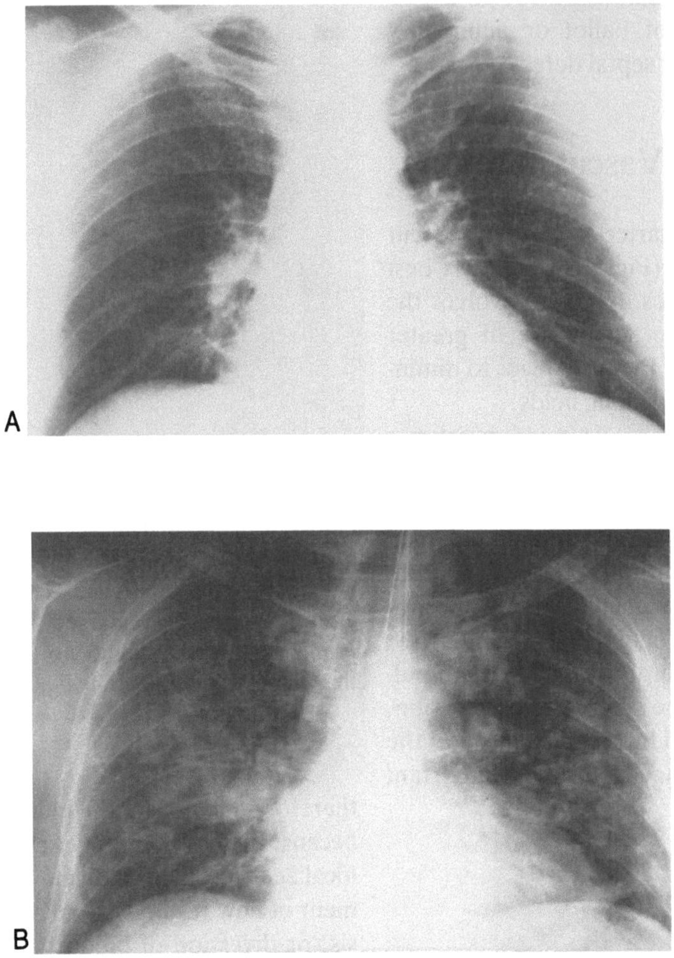

FIGURE 4.17. The radiological appearance of pulmonary edema (A) showing hilar flares and "solid" rounded opacities representative of pulmonary edema. This radiological appearance may simulate infective changes. In this patient with known ischemic heart disease there was a dramatic response to intravenous furosemide administration (B).

a result, the normal concave lateral border of the right hilum becomes straightened and even convex because of the dilated, laterally displaced, superior pulmonary veins.

With progressive increases in left atrial pressure pulmonary edema occurs producing fan-shaped hilar flares spreading peripherally, and when marked, giving rise to a "*butterfly*" appearance (Fig. 4.17). Pulmonary edema is characteristically central, sparing the bases and apices. Atypical manifestations such as unilateral edema (Fig. 4.18) or solid, rounded opacities ("phantom tumor") constantly give rise to problems in diagnosis. Pleural effusions develop in conditions associated with pulmonary venous or systemic venous hypertension, equally common on the right or left side. Less commonly, effusions may be interlobar, encapsulated, or subpulmonary. A useful maneuver is to repeat the X-rays with the patient on his or her back or lying on the side so that shifting of the fluid can be recognized radiologically.

Fine horizontal lines, best seen near the costophrenic angles (*Kerley's B-lines*), represent dilated lymphatic channels and are seen in conditions associated with a persistently high pulmonary venous pressure; this leads to exuda-

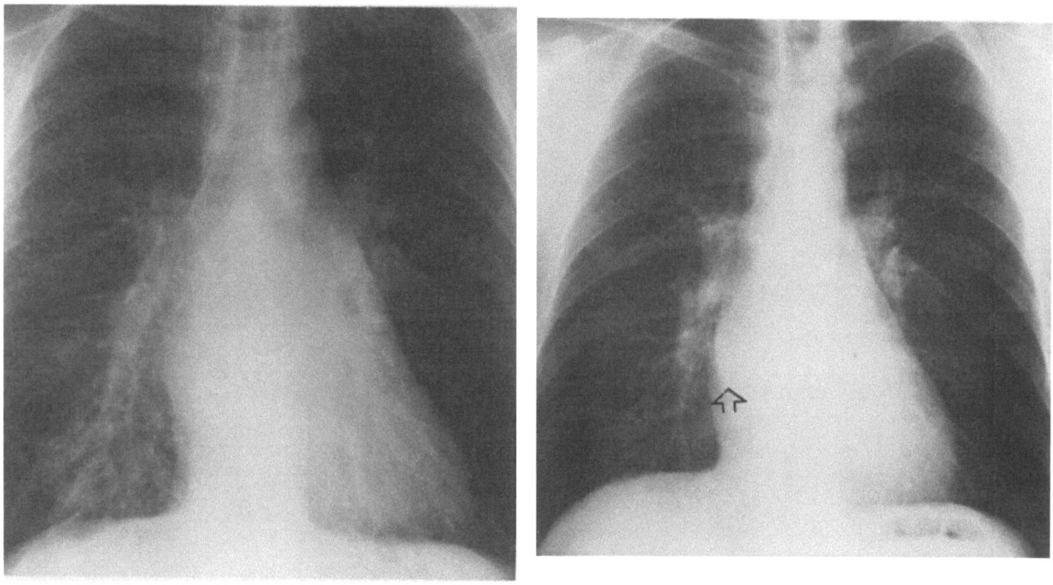

FIGURE 4.18. Unilateral pulmonary edema involving right lung. Following resolution a double density is evident (arrow).

tion of edema fluid into the lungs and promotes a voluminous lymphatic flow. Since mitral valve disease is the commonest cause of such a disturbance, these lymphatic lines are most regularly seen in this condition. They are occasionally encountered, however, in chronic left ventricular failure associated with other causes such as aortic valve disease. In chronic pulmonary venous congestion particularly secondary to mitral stenosis, a fine, diffuse reticular pattern is a result of hemosiderosis. Occasionally, the shadows are larger, dense, and more discrete because of calcification or even ossification.

In *anomalous pulmonary venous drainage*, the abnormal venous connection may be seen producing prominent superior medistinal shadows. When the enlargement is bilateral, total anomalous venous drainage should be suspected (Fig. 4.19).

Cardiac Calcification

This may involve the cardiac valves, pericardium, aorta, and coronary arteries. Calcification may be visible on a routine chest film, but more usually a specific search must be made using the image intensifier. Detection of calcification is of great diagnostic value.

Pericardial Calcification

This may be extensive, completely encasing the heart, or patchy. It is best seen in the anterior and diaphragmatic aspects of the heart and in the atrioventricular groove (Fig. 4.20). It is most commonly seen in association with constrictive pericarditis and is a useful confirmation of the diagnosis. Calcification does not, however, always imply that constrictive hemodynamics are present; the sign must be interpreted in relationship to the clinical and hemodynamic picture.

Valvular Calcification

Calcification of the pulmonary valve in pulmonary stenosis of Tetralogy of Fallot is extremely uncommon and when it does occur implies an episode of previous endocarditis. Calcification of the tricuspid valve, following rheumatic involvement, is extremely rare.

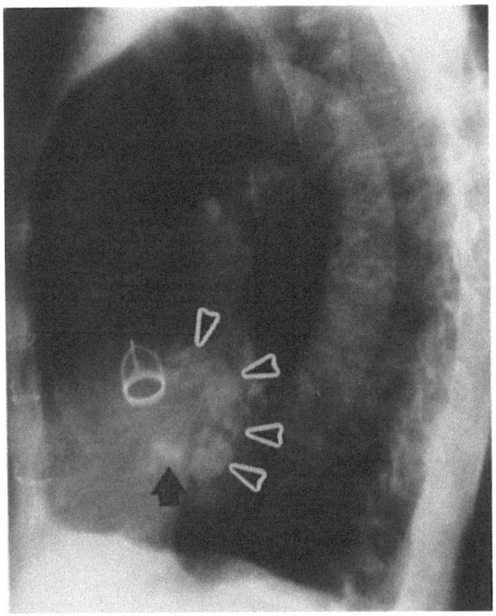

FIGURE 4.19. The characteristic enlargement of the superior mediastinum—the so-called "snowman" appearance in a case of total anomalous pulmonary venous drainage to the superior vena cava. The lung fields are plethoric.

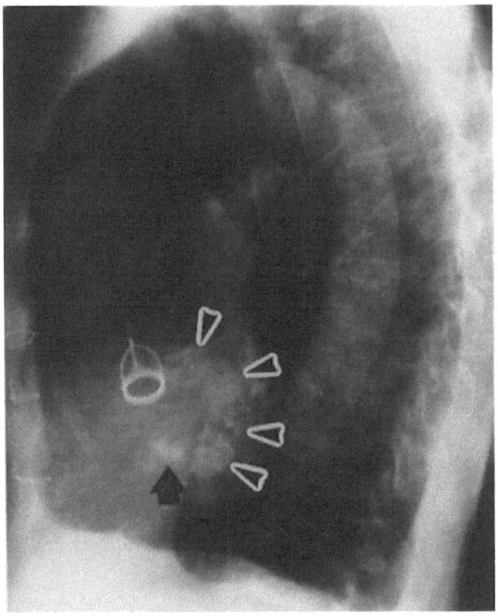

FIGURE 4.21. Lateral X-ray chest in a case of aortic stenosis following replacement with a Starr–Edwards valve, to illustrate position of various types of intracardiac calcification. There is heavy mitral annular calcification with characteristic C-shaped configuration (white arrows). Additionally, there is calcification of the mitral valve (black arrow). The aortic prosthesis indicates the anticipated site of aortic valve calcification.

Calcification of the mitral valve is almost invariably a result of previous rheumatic fever. It is usually irregular, clumped, and especially heavy at the commissures. In contrast, *mitral annular calcification* is the result of senile degeneration and has a characteristic U-shaped configuration occupying two-thirds of the mitral annulus (Fig. 4.21). Aortic valve calcification occurs following rheumatic involvement, on the basis of a congenital bicuspid valve or senile degeneration of the leaflet.

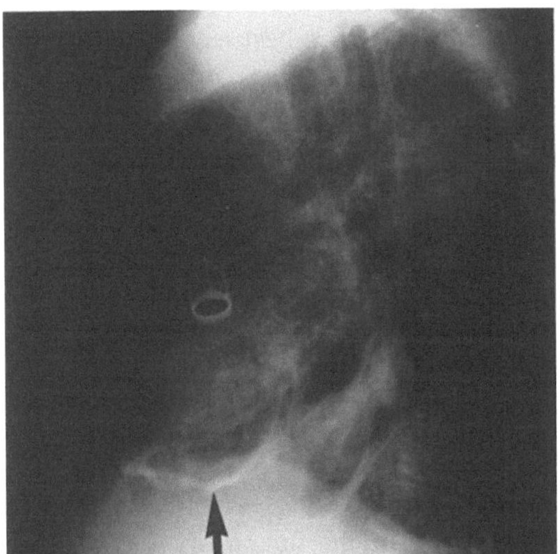

FIGURE 4.20. Lateral chest X-ray in postoperative constrictive pericarditis demonstrating pericardial calcification (arrow).

Valve calcification is best recognized by fluoroscopy in a position between the AP and RAO. The junction between the outwardly moving pulmonary artery and the inwardly moving right ventricle is selected and an imaginary angle of 45° is drawn toward the spine. The mitral valve is below and to the right and the aortic valve is above and to the left. The movement is distinct and rotatory.

Coronary Artery Calcification

This may be detected on a routine film when extensive, or by fluoroscopy. The presence of calcification does not necessarily imply critical atherosclerotic narrowing of the branches.

The Aorta

Calcification of the *ascending aorta* occurs in syphilis, aortitis, and atherosclerosis. Calcification of the aortic knuckle is common in the elderly and is a result of atherosclerosis.

Calcification of the *descending thoracic aorta* is frequently found in aortic arteritis, particularly in young women. In the elderly, diffuse calcification of the arch and the descending and ascending aorta is usually a result of atherosclerosis. In *coarctation* of aorta, the poststenotic segment may become calcified and appear as a calcified ring. In elderly patients, the *ductus arteriosus* and its connections with aorta and pulmonary arteries frequently calcify and can be seen as linear streaks between the aortic and pulmonary arch.

Myocardial Calcification

This is most commonly the result of calcified thrombus in an aneurysm; it is rarely a result of hydatid disease. Calcification may also involve cases of healed myocardial infarction without actual aneurysm formation.

Rib Notching

This occurs most commonly in coarctation of the aorta where it is bilateral, involving the fourth to ninth ribs. It is uncommon in aortic arteritis but when it occurs, involves the lower ribs. Unilateral notching occurs in coarctation when the narrowed segment is above, or includes the left subclavian artery. It is found in cyanotic heart disease after surgical intervention, particularly when the subclavian artery has been used for a palliative shunt. Occasionally, it is seen following pulmonary infections with pleural adhesions, neurofibromatosis, and superior vena cava occlusion.

Additional Reading

Edwards JE, Casey LS, Neufeld HN, Lester RG: "Congenital Heart Disease." W.B. Saunders, Philadelphia, 1965.

Kjellberg SH, Mannheimer E, Rudhe V, Jonsson B: "Diagnosis of Congenital Heart Disease," 2nd Ed. Year Book Publishers, Chicago, 1959.

Shanks SC, Kerley P: "A Text Book of X-ray Diagnosis," 4th Ed, Vol. 1. W.B. Saunders, Philadelphia, 1969.

5
Echocardiography

This is now widely used in the evaluation of cardiac disease and in some conditions is a critical part of the workup. In *acquired* heart disease these include

1. Pericardial effusion.
2. Idiopathic hypertrophic subaortic stenosis.
3. All forms of valve disease (rheumatic, myxomatous, and infective endocarditis).
4. Restrictive and infiltrative cardiomyopathies.
5. Cardiac tumors and thrombi.
6. Measurement of left ventricular chamber size, wall thickness, and detection of wall motion abnormalities.

The advent of Doppler echocardiography has changed the approach to the diagnoses of aortic valve stenosis. In the elderly, this is a common and difficult diagnostic problem, usually resolved by invasive catheterization. There is little place today for transseptal or transthoracic left ventricular puncture when the Doppler and two-dimensional echo show severe aortic stenosis.

It should be remembered that there are limitations to the usefulness of this technique. Good examinations are difficult in large patients, particularly when there is emphysema. Under these circumstances measurement and estimates of left ventricular ejection fraction may be grossly misleading because of failure to visualize and record a clear endocardial target.

In *congenital* heart disease echocardiography is a strong competitor to angiography and may in fact be superior in demonstrating complex malformations and malpositions.

Principles and Technique of M-Mode Echocardiography

Ultrasound refers to sound waves whose frequency lies above the audible range, that is above 20,000 cycles per second. They have no harmful effect on body tissue. Traversing a homogeneous medium such as fluid, these waves travel in a straight line, but on impact with an interface between two media of differing densities they are reflected like light waves. Ultrasound waves have a constant transit time through most types of soft tissue and the time between transmission and reception of the returning signal allows measurement of the transducer–interface distance. Ultrasound waves are produced by mechanical vibration of a piezoelectric (barium titanate) crystal stimulated by a high-frequency alternating current. For adult work a 2.25-MHz transducer is used but for pediatrics a frequency of 9 MHz is used to provide greater resolution.

Since the piezoelectric crystal is also capable of converting ultrasonic mechanical energy into electrical voltge, the transducer acts as a receiver in addition; returning echoes can therefore be made to appear on an oscilloscopic screen. The apparatus transmits intermittent passes of ultrasound at the rate of

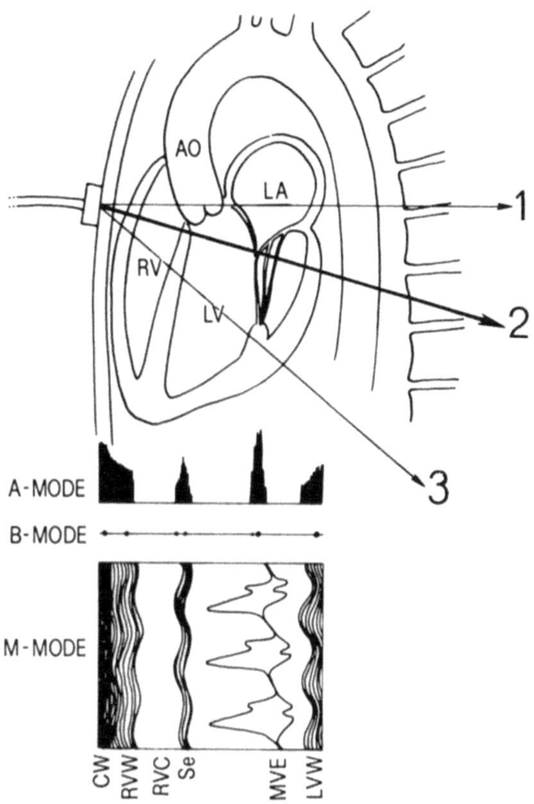

FIGURE 5.1. Diagrammatic representation of an echo beam as it serially traverses the intracardiac structures and displayed in various modes. In position (1) the beam traverses the right ventricular wall, right ventricular outflow tract, root of the aorta, and left atrium. In position (2) the beam passes through the right ventricular wall and cavity, ventricular septum, tip of the mitral leaflet, and posterior left ventricular wall. In position (3) the beam passes through the right ventricular wall and cavity, ventricular septum, cavity of the left ventricle, papillary muscles, and posterior left ventricular wall. The incoming signals from the various intracardiac structures are represented corresponsingly in the amplitude mode (A-mode), bright dots (B-mode), and in the time motion mode (M-mode). CW, chest wall; RVW, right ventricular wall; RVC, right ventricular cavity; SE, septum; MVE, mitral valve echo; LVW, left ventricular wall.

1000 per second and the crystal is free to receive echoes of each impulse before electrical stimulation generates the next impulse. Echoes may be displayed on the oscilloscopic screen in one of three forms (Fig. 5.1):

1. In the A-mode (amplitude modulation), echoes are displayed as vertical signals on a calibrated horizontal baseline showing the transducer–interface distance; movement occurs in a horizontal direction.
2. In the B-mode (brightness modulation), the vertical signals of the A-mode are turned on end electronically, so that the signals appear as moving dots.
3. M-mode recordings are obtained by passing a light-sensitive paper across the B-mode dots, thus obtaining a permanent record that may be incorporated with other noninvasive parameters such as a phonocardiogram, carotid pulse, and electrocardiogram. The M-mode recording contains a calibration scale represented by a series of dots, recorded each half second vertically and spaced 1 cm apart horizontally.

The Mitral Valve

The anterior leaflet of the mitral valve is located with the transducer placed in the left third to fifth intercostal space, pointing posteriorly (Fig. 5.2). In early ventricular systole, the tracing moves sharply in a posterior direction (A to C). During the rest of ventricular systole the mitral echo moves gradually anteriorly (C to D). In early diastole, the echo shows another abrupt, anterior opening movement to point E. There follows a steep backward movement to point F as the valve floats back toward the left atrium; normally the E–F slope velocity is 85–200 mm/sec in adults. In late diastole, when the left atrium contracts, the valve reopens to another anterior peak, point A (Fig. 5.3). The posterior leaflet of the mitral valve is recorded by slight lateral rotation of the transducer. The movement of the posterior mitral leaflet is in mirror image relationship to that of the anterior mitral leaflet. The left ventricular outflow tract lies between the anterior mitral leaflet and the left side of the ventricular septum. Between the right side of the septum and the anteriorly situated right ventricular wall, which moves inward during systole, is the echo-free space of the right ventricular cavity. Posterior to the mitral valve, the beam may locate the left atrial

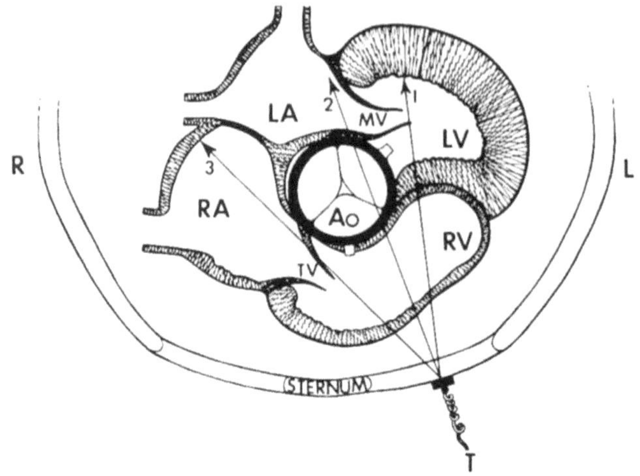

FIGURE 5.2. Diagrammatic representation of a transverse section of the heart at the level of the aortic root to illustrate location of the various intracardiac structures by the transducer (T). Positions 1, 2, and 3 indicate location of the mitral valve (MV), aortic root (AO), and tricuspid valve (TV), respectively. Reprinted, with permission, from Chesler et al. Ped Clin N Am 18:1163, 1971.

wall, which is recognized by its posterior movement in systole, or the left ventricular wall, recognized by its anterior movement in systole.

The Aortic Root

Medial and cephalic angulation of the transducer from the mitral valve recording position moves the echo beam up the outflow tract of the left ventricle (Figs. 5.1 and 5.2). The septal echo changes into that of the anterior margin of the aortic root. Aortic root echoes are parallel and move together in the same direction (anteriorly in systole and posteriorly in diastole). Between the two signals of the aortic root, echoes of the aortic valve leaflets are recorded. These have a characteristic "box-like" configuration (Fig. 5.4). The base of the aorta is in anatomical fibrous continuity with the anterior leaflet of the mitral valve. Recognition of this finding is important in the diagnosis of congenital heart disease. Behind the aortic root lies the left atrium (Fig. 5.5).

The Tricuspid Valve

This is located by angulating the transducer inferiorly and to the right from the aortic root. Its pattern of movement is identical to that of the mitral valve but the leaflets close later (at the time of the tricuspid component of the first heart sound).

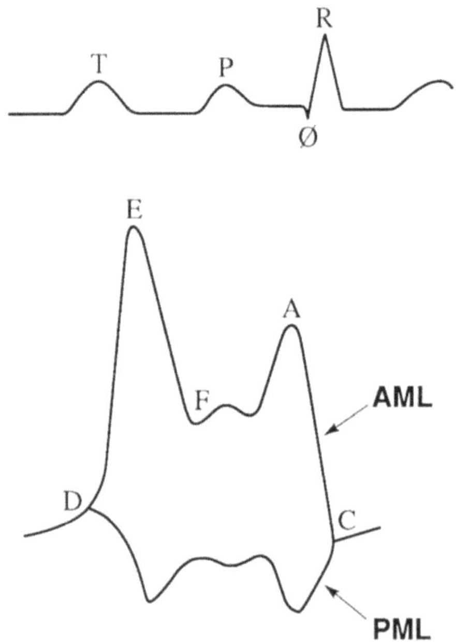

FIGURE 5.3. Diagram illustrating typical pattern of motion of the anterior and posterior mitral leaflets (AML and PML).

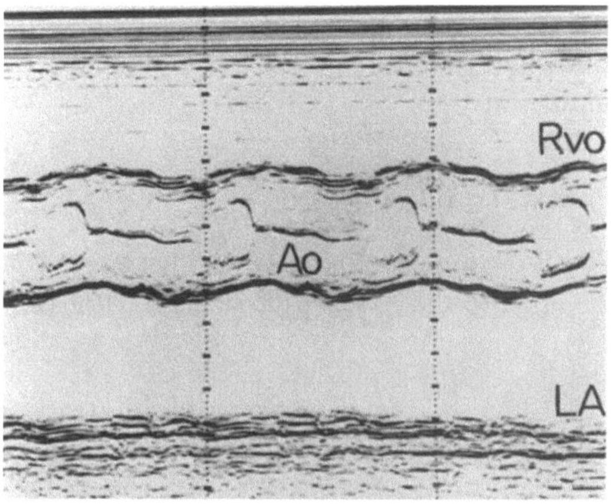

FIGURE 5.4. Echocardiogram of the aortic root. The right ventricular outflow tract (RVO) lies anteriorly and the left atrium (LA) posteriorly. Between the anterior aortic wall (AAW) and the posterior wall (PAW), the typical "box-like" opening movements of the right and noncoronary cusps of the aortic valve are demonstrated.

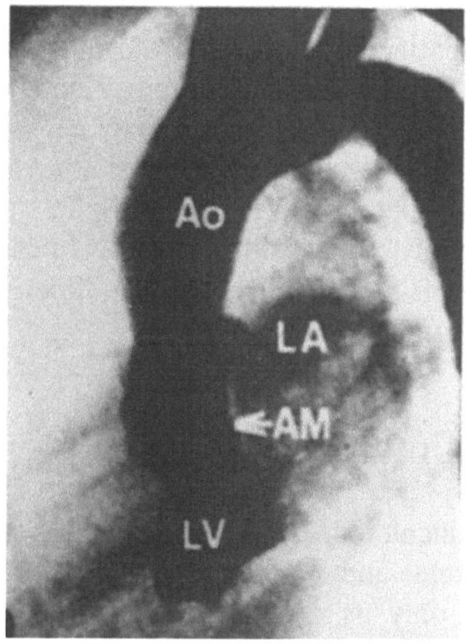

FIGURE 5.5. Left ventricular angiogram in the lateral view demonstrating continuity between the anterior mitral leaflet (AM) and the posterior wall of the aorta (AO). The cavity of the left atrium (LA) is immediately posterior to the aorta. LV, left ventricle. Reprinted, with permission, from Chesler et al. Ped Clin N Am 18:1163, 1971.

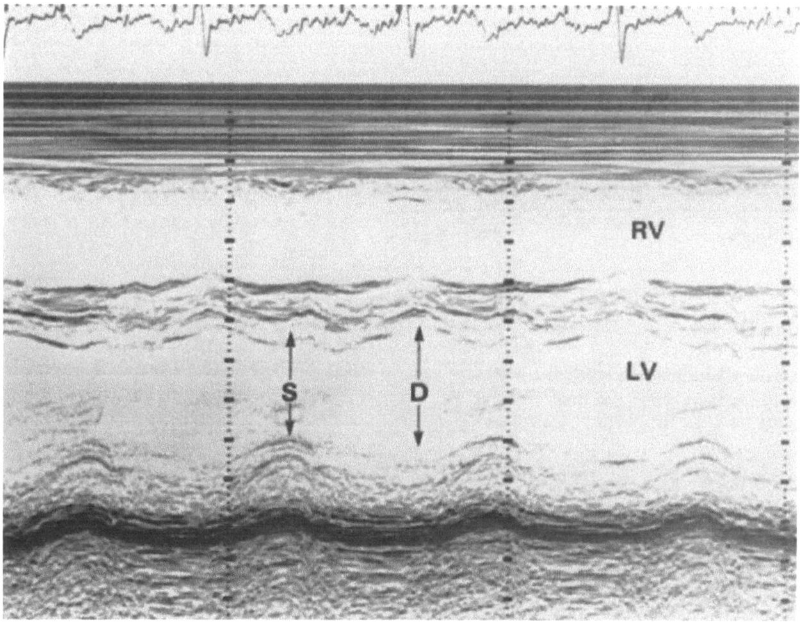

FIGURE 5.6. Echocardiogram from a normal patient demonstrating measurement of the left ventricular internal dimension in systole (S) and diastole (D), thereby permitting calculation of the ejection fraction. RV, right ventricle; LV, left ventricle.

The Ventricular Septum

This is identified by "sweeping" down from the aortic valve on to the anterior mitral leaflet and then into the left ventricular cavity below the chordae and papillary muscles of the mitral valve. The septum moves posteriorly in systole and anteriorly in diastole. It is in this position that the left and right ventricular dimensions are measured (Fig. 5.6).

The Pulmonary Valve

This is difficult to locate in the adult. It is found anterolateral and superior to the aortic root. Usually, only its posterior cusp is identified (Fig. 5.7).

Two-Dimensional (2D) Echocardiography

2D echocardiography uses one crystal rotated mechanically through a sector as a series of crystals in a transducer (phased array). A fan or pie-shaped slice, or tomographic cut, is obtained. Although the heart can be examined in an infinite number of tomographic slices, the following views are part of the standard examination:

Parasternal Long Axis

This is a composite of the M-mode sweep from the apex to the base of the left ventricle (Fig. 5.8).

Parasternal Short Axis

Views from this position may be recorded at multiple levels (Figs. 5.9, 5.10, and 5.11). They are ideal for demonstrating abnormalities of wall motion from the apex to the base. Also included are the papillary muscles, mitral valve leaflets, aortic valve, and crescentic-shaped right ventricle.

Apical Four Chamber View

This is probably the most informative of all views (Fig. 5.12). It magnificently displays all four chambers and the A–V valves in real time.

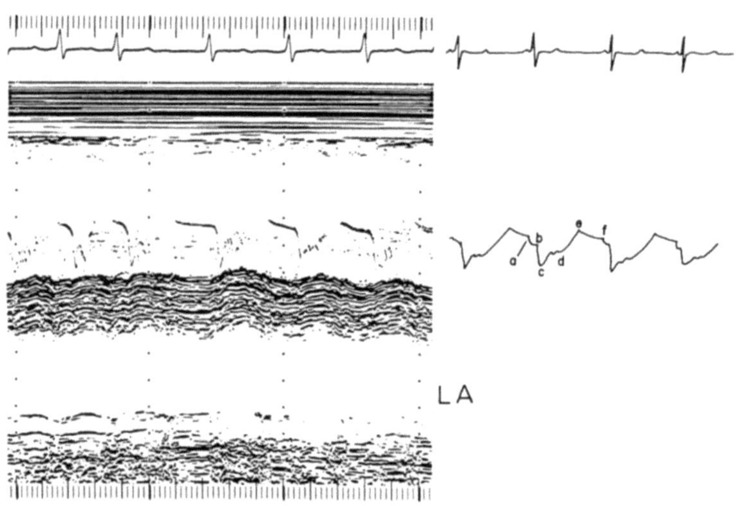

FIGURE 5.7. Echocardiogram of a normal pulmonary valve cusp (with a line diagram to the right) indicating reference points for cusp movement during the various phases of the cardiac cycle. LA, left atrium.

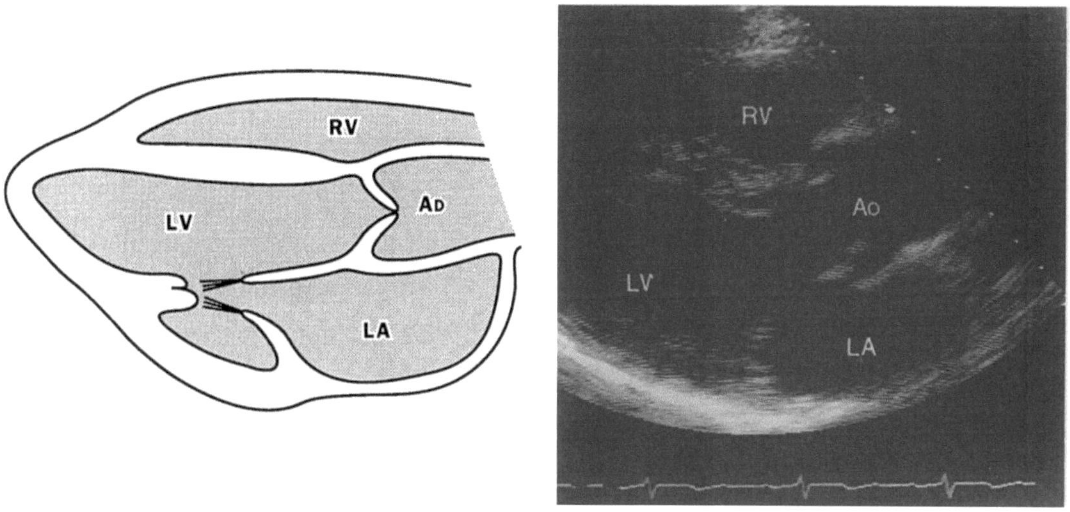

FIGURE 5.8. 2D Echocardiogram: Long axis parasternal view.

Subcostal Four Chamber View

This is similar to the apical four chamber view with the ventricle situated bottom left and the atria situated top right (Fig. 5.13). It has an advantage over the apical four chamber view in being able to scan the entire atrial septum.

Doppler Examination

This technique records the velocity of intracardiac blood flow and allows measurement of stenotic and regurgitant lesions.

The Doppler principle is that an apparent shift in transmitted frequency of sound will

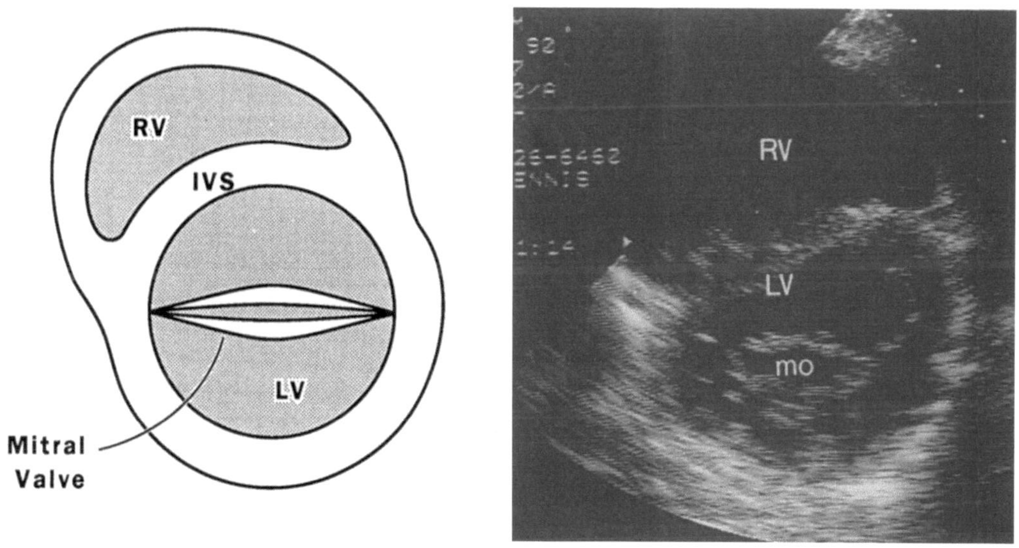

FIGURE 5.9. 2D Echocardiogram: Short axis view—mitral valve level.

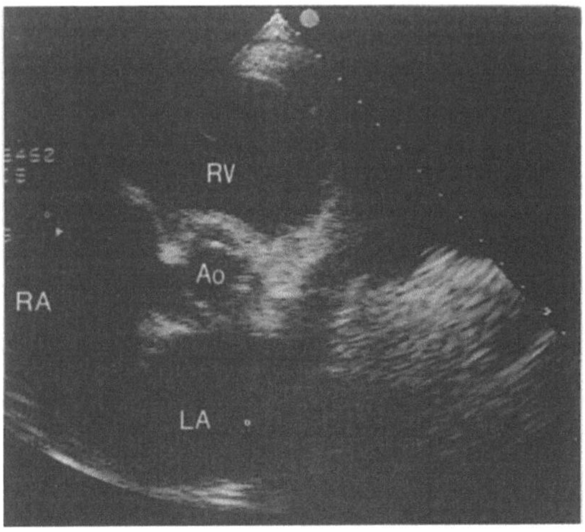

FIGURE 5.10. 2D Echocardiogram: Short axis view of aortic valve showing three leaflets in open position.

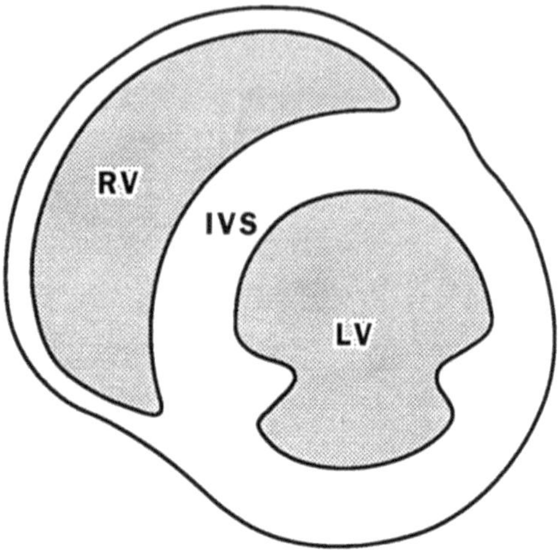

FIGURE 5.11. Diagram of 2D echo. Short axis level of papillary muscle.

occur when there is motion of either the source or the target. For example, when a stationary individual is approached by an automobile sounding its horn the frequency *appears* to increase (higher pitch), and when the vehicle moves away, the frequency *appears* to decrease (lower pitch). The change in frequency (Doppler shift) is proportional to the speed of the vehicle. In cardiology, the transducer is stationary and red blood cells are the moving target. Once the blood flow velocity is known, pressure gradients and valve orifice size can be measured by modifying the Bernoulli equation.

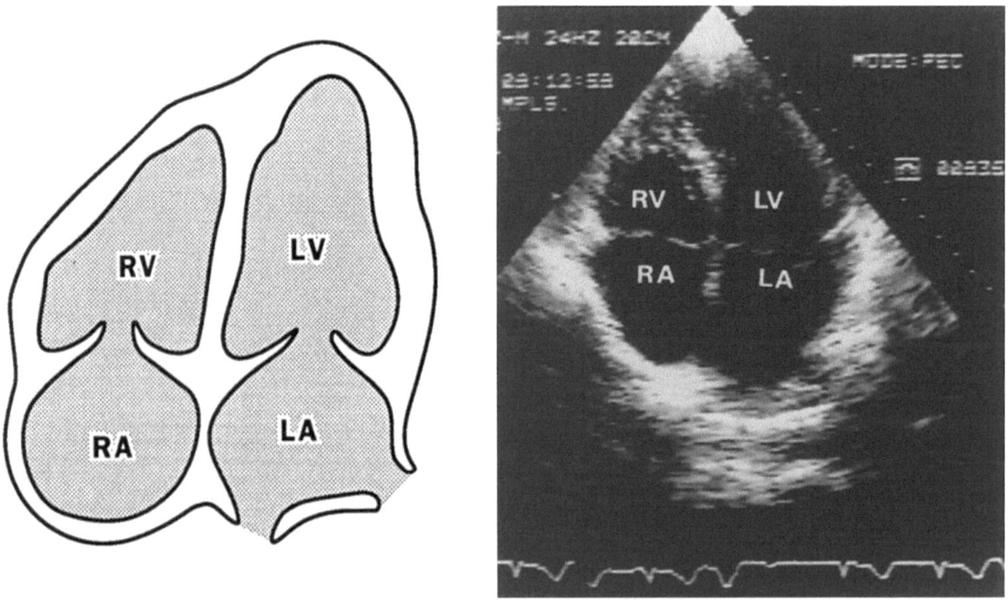

FIGURE 5.12. 2D Echocardiogram: Apical four chamber view.

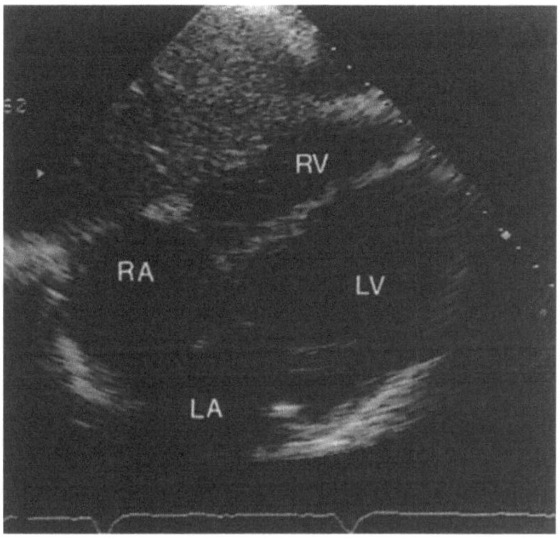

FIGURE 5.13. 2D Echocardiogram: Subcostal four chamber view.

Doppler instruments employ the usual piezoelectric ultrasound transducer, which emits ultrasonic energy at a constant frequency. When the reflected waves are detected by the same transducer it is called *pulsed* Doppler; when the waves are detected by an adjacent transducer it is called *continuous wave* Doppler. The combination of pulsed Doppler with a 2D image is called *duplex Doppler*.

Pulsed Doppler has an advantage over continuous wave in allowing precise depth resolution and is combined with imaging. Continuous-wave Doppler is a nonimaging technique that can measure the highest velocities of blood flow.

Color Flow Mapping

This is a sophisticated pulsed Doppler system that produces dramatic images. Flow toward and away from the transducer (blue or red) allows rapid identification of abnormal flow patterns. It makes detection of intracardiac shunts and valvular regurgitation much easier.

Transesophageal Echocardiography

All the preceeding techniques may be recorded through an esophageal probe. This is particularly useful (1) when transthoracic echograms are technically poor in large patients (2) for detection of valvular vegetations (3) intra- and post-operatively in myotomy for hypertrophic cardiomyopathy and annuloplasty for mitral valve prolapse.

Acquired Heart Disease

Mitral Stenosis

M-mode

In mitral stenosis the valve moves normally during systole, but in diastole the leaflets remain open and move posteriorly very slowly (Fig. 5.14). The slow diastolic closure rate is not only indicative of the presence of mitral stenosis but also correlates fairly well with its severity. With a mitral valve area of less then 1 cm^2 the E to F slope is usually less than 20 mm per second. The persistent pressure gradient between the left atrium and the left ventricle holds the mitral valve open and is responsible for this echocardiographic pattern. Additionally, the amplitude of valve movement is used as a measure of the mobility of the valve. Calcified valves produce wide, reduplicated echoes with restricted range of movement. Preoperative echograms are of considerable assistance in the assessment of patient for surgical treatment since calcification cannot always be seen radiographically. A slow E to F slope does not always indicate mitral stenosis. Since the E to F slope is indicative of the rate of flow across the mitral valve, the E to F slope may also be slow when left ventricular compliance is diminished or the cardiac output low.

2D

Doming of the leaflets in any view is the characteristic finding and a result of fusion of the tips of the leaflets (Figs. 5.15 and 5.16). Poor leaflet motion is also observed with low cardiac output, but doming is absent. 2D echocardiography provides detailed information about valvar and subvalvar anatomy (mobility, fibrosis, and calcification), which is helpful in deciding between commissurotomy (surgical or

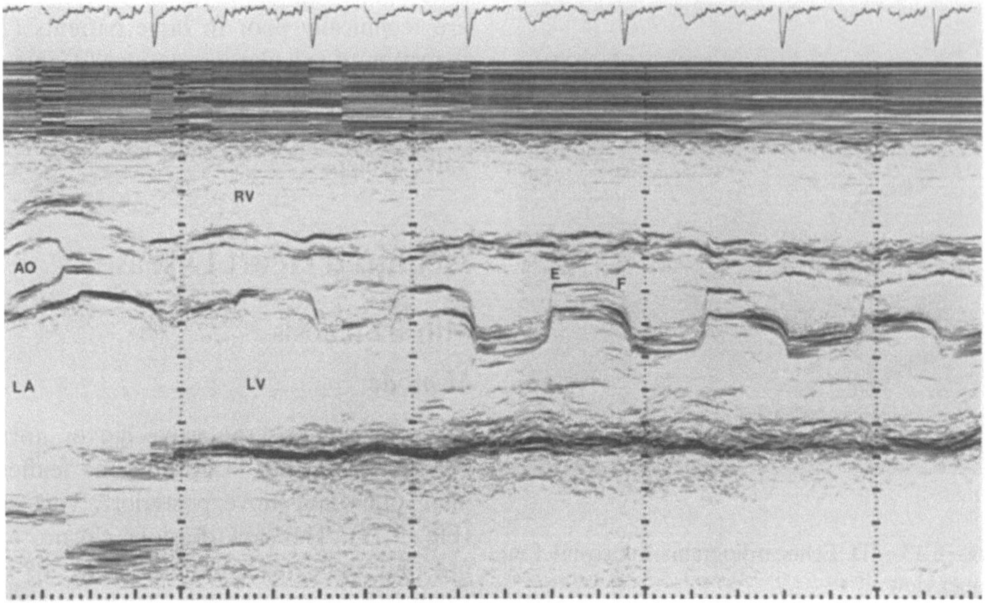

FIGURE 5.14. M-Mode echocardiogram showing enlarged left atrium, thickened anterior mitral leaflet with reduced E–F slope.

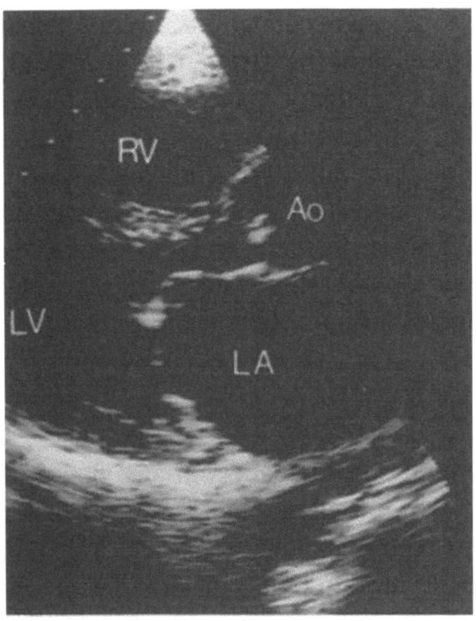

FIGURE 5.15. 2D Echocardiogram: Long axis parasternal view; mitral stenosis, showing doming of thickened leaflets and enlarged left atrium.

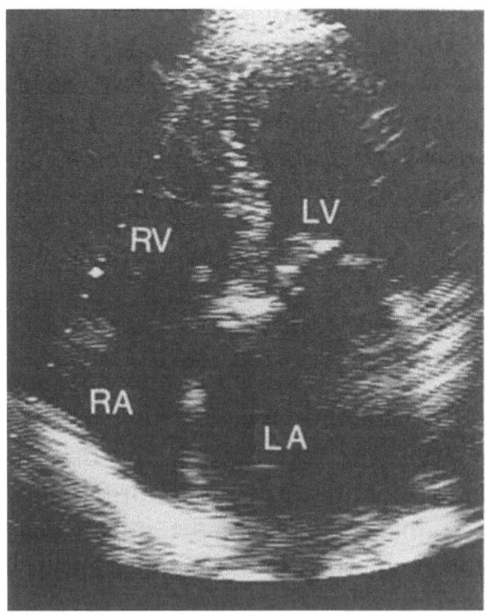

FIGURE 5.16. 2D Echocardiogram: Apical four chamber view; mitral stenosis, showing doming of thickened leaflets and enlarged left atrium.

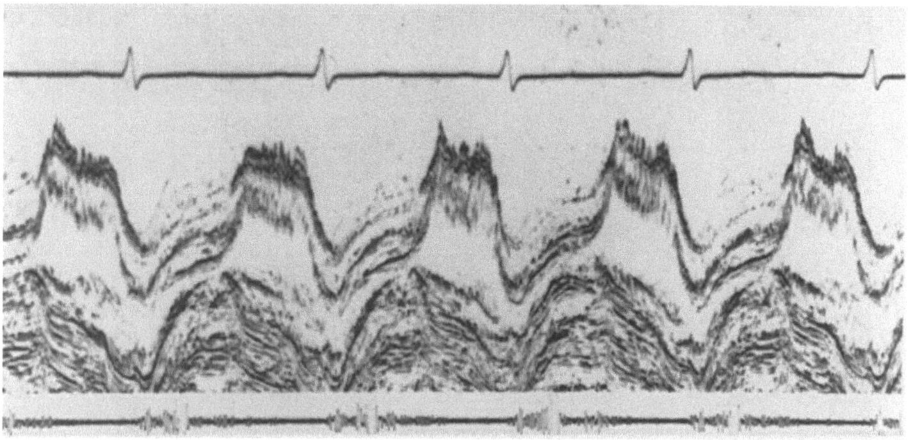

FIGURE 5.17. M-Mode echocardiogram showing fluttering of mitral valve leaflets in aortic regurgitation.

balloon) or valve replacement. Quantification of the severity of stenosis may be made by measuring the rate of decline of flow obtained by CV Doppler. The recording looks much like the pattern of an M-mode recording except that the atrial velocity is increased on the Doppler and decreased on the M-mode.

Aortic Insufficiency

M-Mode

Echocardiography can readily distinguish the Austin–Flint murmur from that of mitral stenosis. The regurgitant jet of aortic insufficiency striking the mitral valve produces a high frequency diastolic oscillation or flutter of the leaflets and the E to F slope is normal (Fig. 5.17). In patients with acute, severe aortic insufficiency premature closure of the mitral valve may be observed. Leaflet closure occurs before the onset of systole (before the R wave of the ECG) because the high diastolic pressure in the left ventricle rapidly exceeds that of the left atrium, thus closing the mitral valve before the onset of systole. This echocardiographic finding is extremely useful because in severe aortic insufficiency the diastolic pressures in the aorta and the left ventricle may be equal and there may not be an early diastolic murmur.

2D

Doppler echocardiography is the more sensitive and specific method for detecting aortic regurgitation. Tracking the depth of the diastolic signal into the left ventricular cavity produces a semiquantitative estimate of severity (Fig. 5.18).

Valvular Aortic Stenosis

M-Mode

Rheumatic aortic stenosis is characterized by thick multiple leaflet echoes enclosed within the aortic root (Fig. 5.19). However, there are no reliable criteria for predicting the severity of the gradient. These findings are particularly unreliable in an elderly patient with senile degeneration of cusps because the same findings may be evident in the absence of obstruction.

In a negative sense, an echocardiogram showing thin cusp echoes opening to the periphery of aortic root precludes the diagnosis of rheumatic aortic stenosis. It does not, however, rule out an uncalcified bicuspid valve that may dome up above the echo beam producing an apparently normal opening movement. An eccentric position of the aortic leaflets at the onset of diastole is suggestive of a

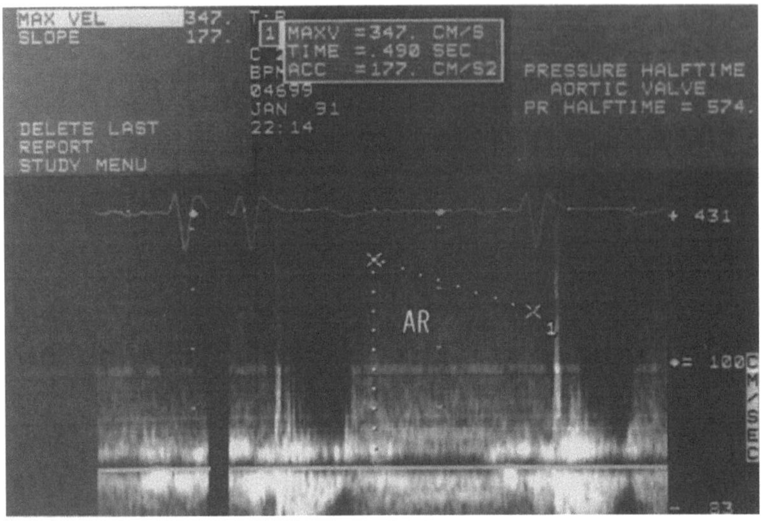

FIGURE 5.18. Continuous-wave Doppler recording in aortic regurgitation. The pressure half-time is slow and exists throughout diastole. In severe regurgitation aortic and left ventricular pressure equalize early in diastole.

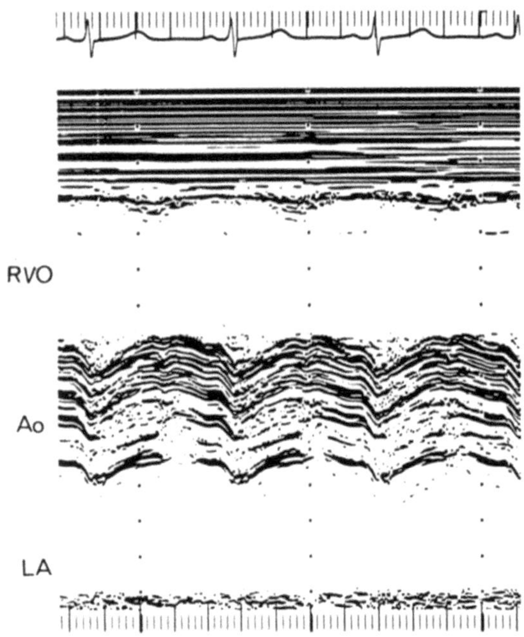

FIGURE 5.19. M-Mode echocardiogram in aortic stenosis showing multiple echoes from thickened leaflets.

congenital bicuspid valve, but this is not a reliable sign.

2D

Doppler echocardiography is the technique of choice. Continuous-wave recordings show a progressive increase in peak velocity across the valve with increasing degrees of stenosis. There is an excellent correlation between the mean gradient obtained this way and obtained in the catheterization laboratory (Fig. 5.20).

Mitral Regurgitation

Doppler echocardiography is the best technique for confirming mitral regurgitation and 2D echocardiography is the procedure of choice for determining the cause.

Rheumatic Mitral Regurgitation

Rheumatic valvular disease is characterized by thickening and calcification of the valve and subvalvular apparatus. The Doppler will show some degree of mitral stenosis.

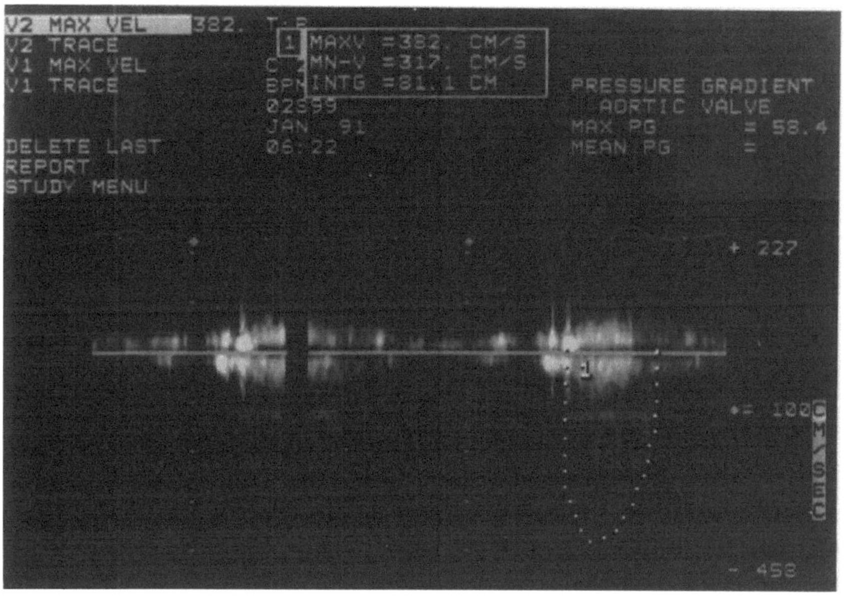

FIGURE 5.20. Continuous-wave Doppler recording in aortic stenosis. The aortic valve peak instantaneous gradient (p) is 58 mm Hg according to the simplified Bernoulli equation. ($p = V^2$).

Mitral Valve Prolapse

M-Mode

The characteristic finding is a midsystolic posterior bulge of one or both mitral leaflets so that they become separated during late systole (Fig. 5.21). Occasionally, there may be pansystolic posterior bulging and separation of both leaflets. In rupture of the chordae, whether spontaneous or the result of infective

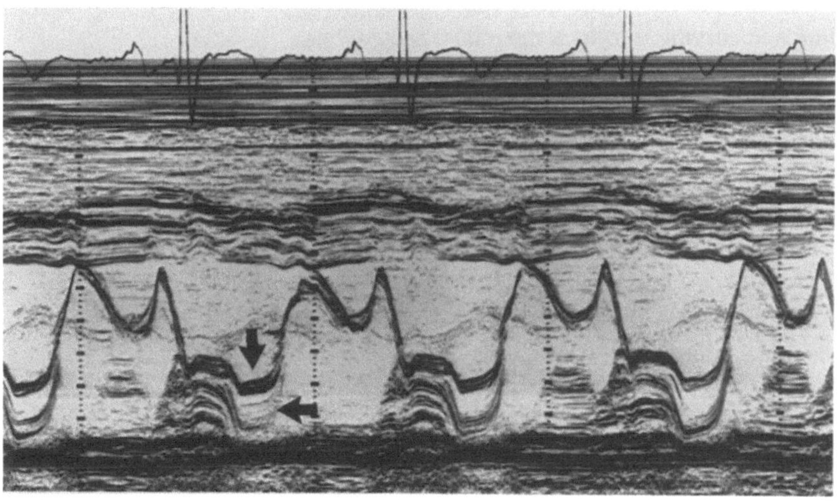

FIGURE 5.21. M-Mode echocardiogram of myxomatous mitral valve showing thickening and prolapse at both leaflets (arrows).

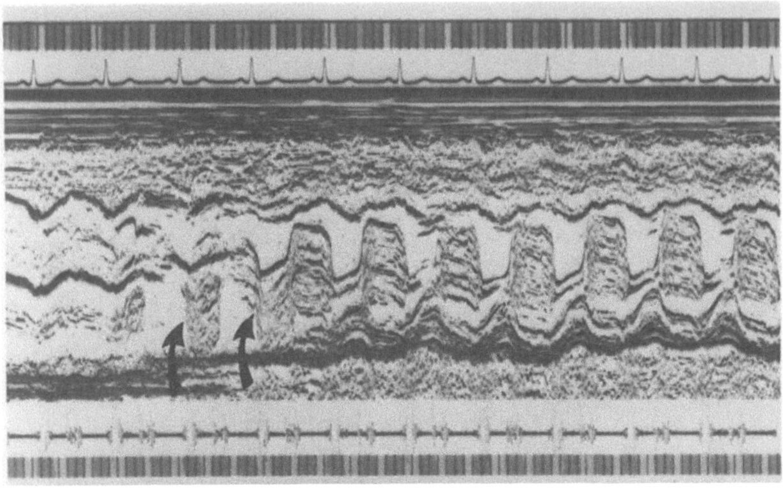

FIGURE 5.22. M-Mode echocardiogram in left atrial myxoma. There is a mass of echoes behind the anterior mitral leaflet: The tumor prolapses into the left atrium (arrows).

endocarditis, the mitral valve echo exhibits coarse chaotic diastolic fluttering movements produced by the flail leaflet; in systole the flail leaflets may prolapse into the left atrium.

2D

This demonstrates thickening of the leaflets that protrude into the left atrium beyond the plane of the mitral annulus. When the chordae rupture, the 2D shows the tip of the involved leaflet protruding and curving into face the left atrium. (When the chordae are intact, but there is marked prolapse, the tip of the leaflet points to the cavity of the left ventricle.)

Left Atrial Myxoma

M-Mode

Because a myxoma prolapses through the mitral valve orifice during diastole, a characteristic finding is a slow E to F slope with a mass of echoes observed behind the anterior mitral leaflet (Fig. 5.22). The absence of these findings does not, however, exclude a left atrial myxoma, since the pedunculated tumor may not prolapse through the mitral valve orifice and therefore be beyond the reach of the echo beam.

2D

This has made the diagnosis easy. Even small tumors attached to the atrial septum are demonstrable and distinguishable from thrombus layered against the atrial wall. The same applies to masses in the right atrium (Fig. 5.23).

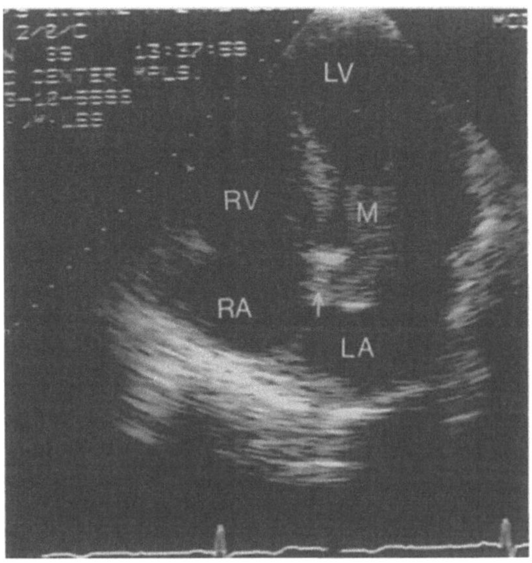

FIGURE 5.23. 2D echocardiogram, left atrial myxoma (M) prolapsing into the left ventricle. The tumor is attached to the atrial septum (arrow).

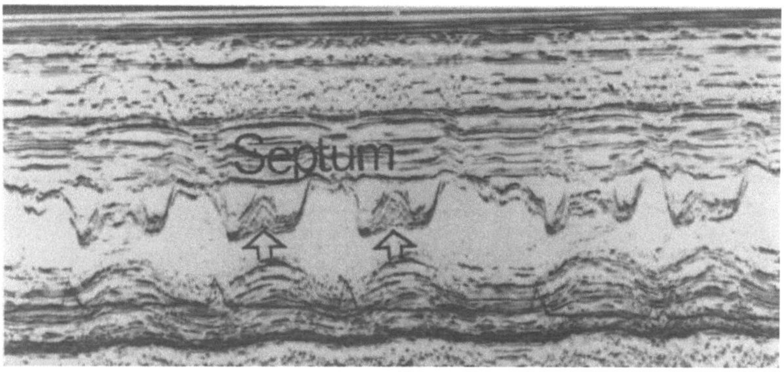

FIGURE 5.24. M-Mode echocardiogram in hypertrophic cardiomyopathy showing disproportionate septal hypertrophy and SAM (arrows).

Hypertrophic Subaortic Stenosis (IHSS)

Echocardiography is an extremely valuable noninvasive means of investigating symptomatic patients with this disease and their asymptomatic relatives.

M-Mode

During diastole, the pattern of the mitral valve motion is usually normal, but in midsystole the mitral valve echo exhibits an abrupt systolic anterior motion (SAM) (Fig. 5.24). This abnormal SAM moves abruptly back to its normal position just before the onset of ventricular diastole. The onset of SAM coincides with the occurrence of the pressure gradient between the left ventricle and aorta in mid- to late systole, with partial systolic closure of the aortic valve, and the onset of the characteristic murmur. This abnormal mitral valve movement correlates with all provocative tests known to obliterate or enhance the obstruction. The abnormal movement is the result of septal hypertrophy and distortion of the papillary muscles of the mitral valve. In addition to SAM, patients with hypertrophic cardiomyopathy may have a reduced mitral diastolic closure rate because of diminished ventricular compliance. Disproportionate septal thickening is the other characteristic finding and a septal/posterior wall thickness ratio of 1.3 : 1 or more is a characteristic finding.

2D

This is more sensitive and specific in identifying the size and extent of obstruction than the M-mode (Fig. 5.25). The normal septum is not always straight. A sigmoid (S-shaped) septum is an anatomic variant that becomes more frequent with advancing age. An oblique image of an M-mode beam through such a septum may

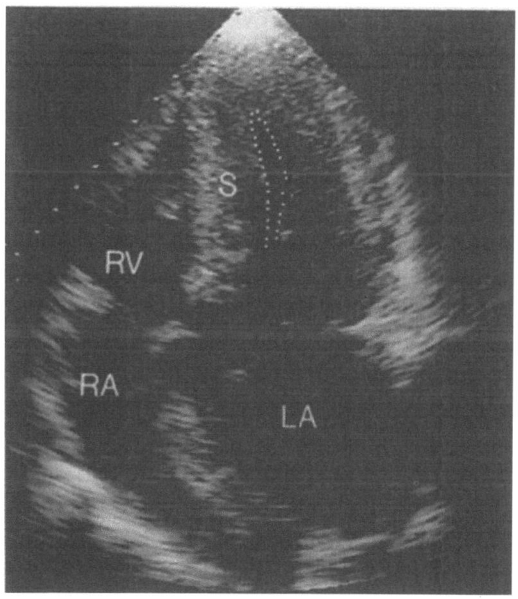

FIGURE 5.25. 2D echocardiogram in hypertrophic cardiomyopathy showing thickening of ventricular septum (S) and cavity obliteration (white dots).

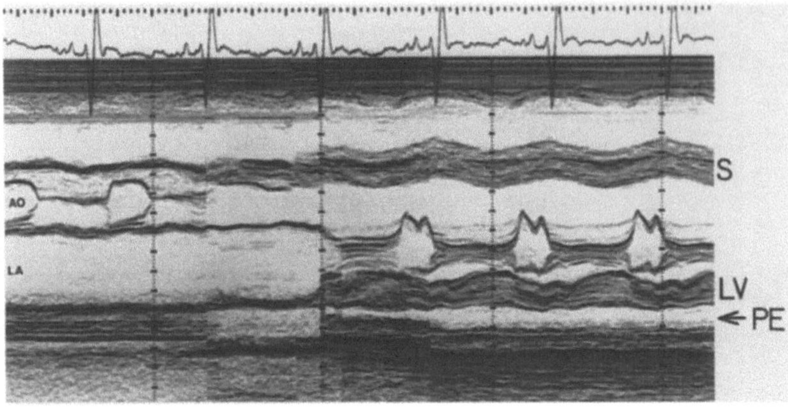

FIGURE 5.26. M-Mode echocardiogram in posterior pericardial effusion (PE), which disappears behind the left atrium.

falsely suggest IHSS. 2D may also detect the *apical* variety of this IHSS.

Pericardial Effusion

Echocardiography is the most accurate, and certainly the safest way to make a diagnosis of pericardial effusion.

M-Mode

The posterior wall of the left ventricle is made up of the endocardium, myocardium, and epicardium. Immediately behind the epicardium is the pericardium and behind this are the pleura and the lungs. A potential space exists between the epicardium and the pericardium, which when filled with fluid may be identified as an echo-free space. Pericardial effusions may be identified anteriorly between the right ventricular wall and the chest wall. An effusion is usually identified behind the posterior left ventricular wall and this disappears as the ultrasonic beam moves toward the left atrium where the pericardial space is much smaller (Fig. 5.26). This feature usually, but not invariably, serves to distinguish a pericardial from a pleural effusion. When a large effusion is present, the heart may be highly mobile in the pericardial sac, producing excessive movement of both anterior and posterior walls. The latter may distort the mitral valve echo and result in a false diagnosis of SAM, or midsystolic prolapse. With proper technique, echocardiography can detect 20 ml of pericardial fluid. However, if the gain settings of the machine are incorrectly adjusted, large effusions may be obscured. A calcified mitral annulus is another source of error since this produces an echo-free space behind the mitral valve (Fig. 5.27).

2-D

This plays an important role in detecting loculated effusions and in diagnosing cardiac tamponade features, which make the technique particularly useful after open heart surgery (Figs. 5.28 and 5.29). Diastolic collapse of the free walls of the right atrium and right ventricle is highly sensitive in the diagnosis of tamponade. The collapse may be timed by noting the position of the atrioventricular or semilunar valves on the 2D echocardiogram or by a simultaneous M-mode with ECG recording.

Evaluation of Left Ventricular Function

M-Mode

The size of the left ventricular cavity can be measured echocardiographically and the systolic and diastolic internal dimension compared, thereby permitting calculation of the ejection fraction (Fig. 5.6). This is useful clinically in

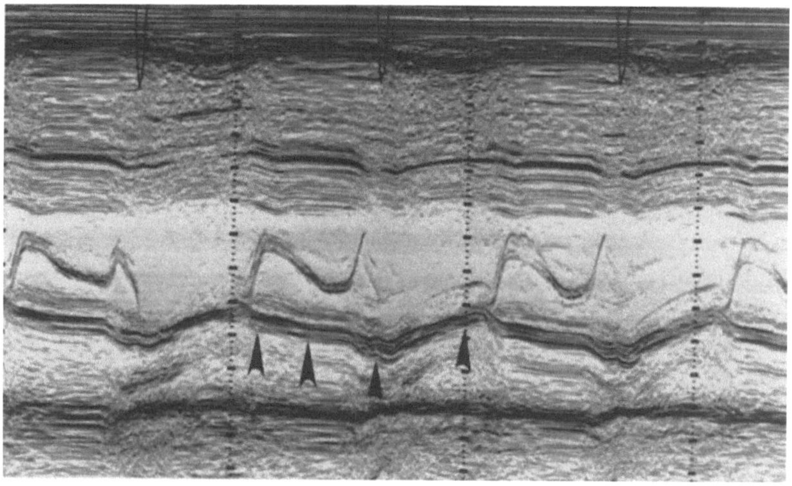

FIGURE 5.27. M-Mode echocardiogram showing mitral annular calcification (arrows) with space behind this resembling pericardial effusion.

the long-term follow-up and progression of heart disease, both naturally and with the effects of drug intervention. It should be remembered, however, that the ultrasonic beam provides only a limited view of the left ventricular cavity and dyskinetic segments may escape detection.

2D

This provides better visualization of the left ventricle and many machines incorporate computerized systems to calculate the ejection fraction. Its reliability depends on accurate tracing of the endocardial target, which is not always

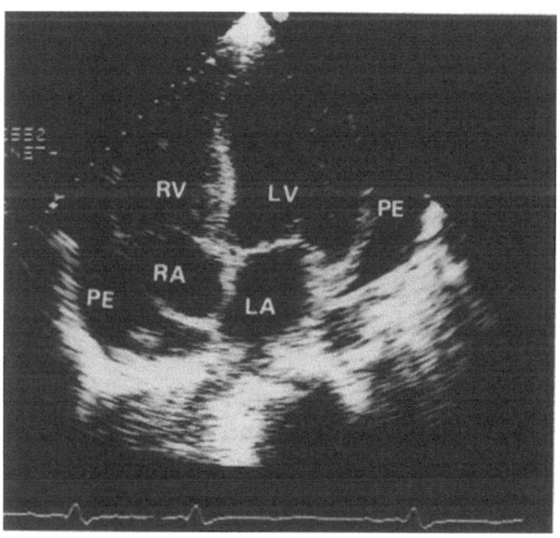

FIGURE 5.28. 2D Echocardiogram (four chamber view) in percardial effusion (PE).

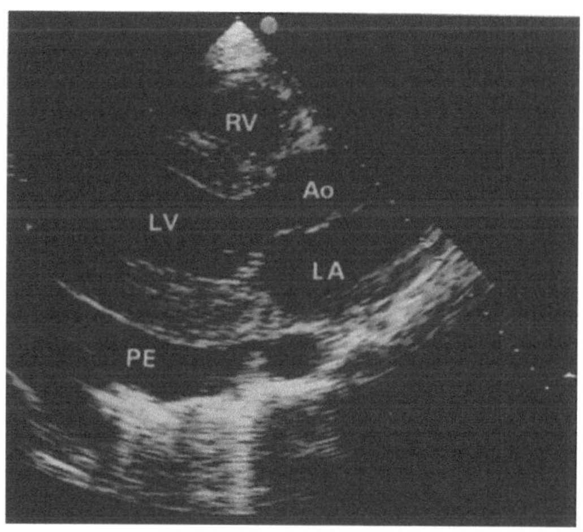

FIGURE 5.29. 2D echocardiogram (parasternal long axis view) showing pericardial effusion (PE) behind the left atrium (LA).

possible. A more practical approach is a visual estimate of the ejection fraction from all possible views made by an experienced echocardiographer. This allows simultaneous detection of abnormalities of wall motion (dyskinesis, hypokinesis, or akinesis), which is invaluable in ischemic heart disease.

Dissecting Aneurysm of the Ascending Aorta

Dissection of the root of the aorta produces an intimal flap. This can be recognized by 2D echocardiography fairly readily when the ascending and descending thoracic aorta is involved.

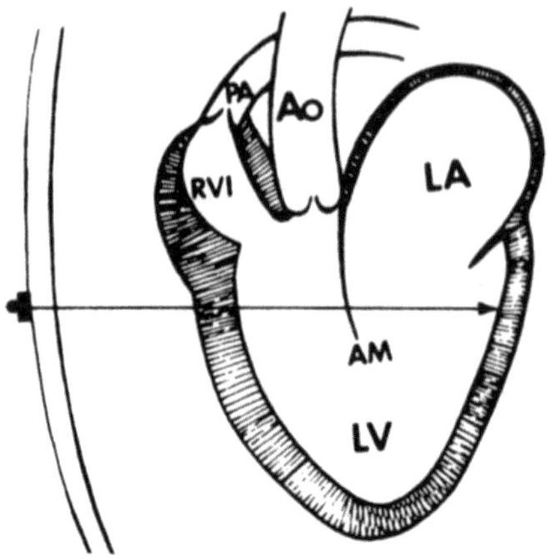

FIGURE 5.30. Diagrammatic representation of a functional single ventricle produced by tricuspid atresia with a single atrioventricular valve, absence of a septal echo, and a rudimentary outflow tract, features which may be identified by echocardiography. Reprinted, with permission, from Chesler et al. Ped Clin N Am 18:1163, 1971.

Congenital Heart Disease

Echocardiography is now firmly established as a valuable investigation, used in conjunction with electrocardiography and the chest X-ray in the initial assessment of infants with congenital heart disease. The technique is particularly easy to perform in the neonate because of the small chest and the uncalcified sternum. The 2D technique has proved to be particularly valuable in delineating the finer anatomic details of complex malformations and malpositions.

The pathological alterations that may be identified by echocardiography in the field of congenital heart disease may be approached, depending on whether it is possible to identify two atrioventricular valves, two ventricular chambers, and the ventricular septum. When the technique elicits the absence of a septal echo and a single atrioventricular valve (or occasionally two atrioventricular valves not separated by a ventricular septum), the anatomical counterpart is a *true* single ventricle or a *functional* single ventricle resulting from severe hypoplasia of the left or right sides of the heart (Fig. 5.30).

The clinical, electrocardiographic, and radiological diagnosis of the cause of heart failure in infancy may be difficult. Thus, many neonates who are hypoxic, for whatever cause, may exhibit a shock-like picture with poor peripheral perfusion, hepatomegaly, and cardiomegaly. It is essential to differentiate cardiac and noncardiac causes of this presentation. The differential diagnosis of the hypoplastic left heart syndrome in the neonate includes coarctation of the aorta, endocardial fibroelastosis, myocardial ischemia, large left-to-right shunts, truncus arteriosus, infradiaphragmatic total anomalous pulmonary venous drainage, and viral myocarditis. The hypoplastic right syndrome usually presents with more cyanosis and must be differentiated from transposition of the great vessels, pulmonary stenosis and atresia with an intact ventricular septum, and the Tetralogy of Fallot.

Ultrasonic recognition of a true or functional single ventricle narrows the differential diagnosis considerably and excludes all of the above-mentioned conditions in which two atrioventricular valves and two ventricles are present. Thus, in the neonate who presents with this picture, echocardiographic recognition of a diminutive aortic root and absent mitral valve echo would clearly indicate a diagnosis of aortic atresia. Or when the tricuspid valve echo is absent and a normal mitral valve is continuous with the aortic root echo, the diagnosis could be either a true single ventricle or tricuspid atresia. The identification of a hypoplastic right ventricular cavity in the less severe forms of tricuspid atresia would clinch the diagnosis, since a septal echo is not found in a true single ventricle.

Among patients in whom transposition of the great vessels is identified angiographically, the question of a single ventricle must always arise. Echocardiography may be of particular assistance by demonstrating the presence of the ventricular septum when the angiographic findings are inconclusive.

Single Functioning Ventricle

True Single Ventricle

A single ventricle receives both the tricuspid and mitral valves, or a common atrioventricular valve, and the ventricular septum is absent. Echocardiography demonstrates absence of the septum and a single leaflet moving to a markedly anterior position. Occasionally, two separate A–V valves are identified, but again the ventricular septal echo is absent.

Functional Single Ventricle (Hypoplasia of the Right Heart)

A single A–V valve (mitral) is identified moving abnormally far anteriorly. Continuity between the mitral valve and aortic valve is present. The ventricular septal echo is absent, but a small rudimentry right ventricular outflow tract may be identified and this is diagnostic.

The Hypoplastic Left Heart Syndrome

This malformation is characterized by a slit-like left ventricular cavity, atresia of the aortic or mitral valves, or both, and severe underdevelopment of the ascending aorta. The right ventricle functions as a single ventricle supplying not only the pulmonary circulation, but also the systemic circuit through a patent ductus arteriosus. The diagnostic echocardiographic criteria are the absence of a normal mitral valve echo, a small or absent aortic root echo, a small posterior ventricle, and a large anterior ventricle.

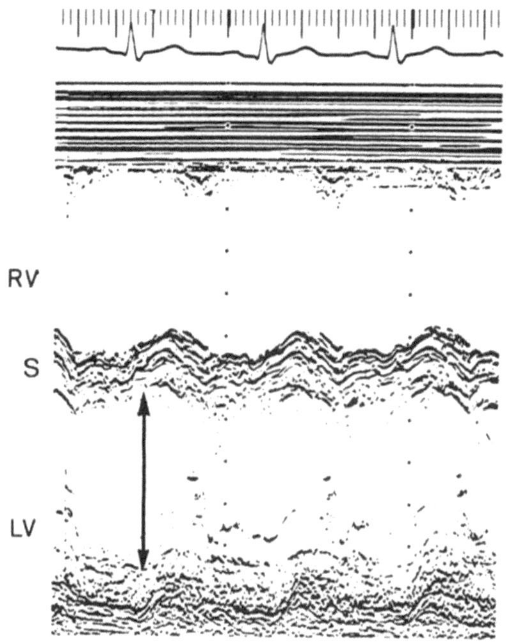

FIGURE 5.31. Echocardiogram in atrial septal defect demonstarting an enlarged right ventricular dimension and paradoxical motion of the septum (S).

Two Functioning Ventricles

Atrial Septal Defect

The M-mode echocardiographic findings in this condition are nonspecific and are a reflection of right ventricular volume overload. The findings are paradoxical septal motion and an increased right ventricular end-diastolic dimension (Fig. 5.31). Normally, the ventricular septum moves posteriorly toward the left ventricular wall during systole, and anteriorly or away from the posterior wall during diastole. Paradoxical movement consists of a systolic forward movement and a diastolic backward movement. Both paradoxical motion and an enlarged right ventricular dimension may result from other causes of right ventricular volume overload such as tricuspid insufficiency, pulmonary insufficiency, and partial or total anomalous pulmonary venous drainage. Paradoxical septal motion may also be a result of constrictive pericarditis, intraventricular conduction defects, and septal infarction.

In atrial septal defect, paradoxical motion disappears when the pulmonary vascular resistance or the right ventricular pressure is elevated.

2D echocardiography may directly demonstrate the actual defect or confirm its presence by a bubble study. When saline is injected into a peripheral vein the bubbles outline the right atrium. A negative jet demonstrates the left-to-right shunt and bubbles in the left atrium demonstrate a right-to-left shunt.

Total Anomalous Pulmonary Venous Drainage

The obstructive type of this anomaly may mimic the hypoplastic left heart syndrome, which may be excluded by the following features:

1. A normal mitral valve echo.
2. A left ventricle that, though small, generally exceeds the echo dimensions associated with aortic atresia.
3. An aortic root echo whose dimensions are normal.

When total anomalous pulmonary venous drainage is of the unobstructed variety and the clinical presentation is one of cyanotic congenital heart disease, the echocardiographic findings are paradoxical septal motion, increased right ventricular internal dimension, and an increased velocity of tricuspid valve movement. Similar findings, however, will be found in a common atrium.

Congenital Mitral Valve Disease

Congenital mitral valve stenosis is indistinguishable pathologically from rheumatic involvement and it is not suprising therefore that the echocardiographic features are the same. Echocardiography is useful in excluding other causes of left ventricular inflow obstruction such as a left atrial myxoma, supravalvular stenosing ring, and cor triatriatum. The mitral valve echo is normal but an abnormal band of echoes may be detected in the left atrium, separated from the posterior left atrial wall in cor triatriatum. Similarly, a supreavalvular stenosing ring may produce an abnormal echo just posterior to the mitral valve leaflet.

Ebstein's Disease

Echocardiography yields diagnostic information in this anomaly. The findings consist of (1) an enlarged right ventricle and (2) an easily recorded tricuspid valve echo lateral to its usual situation, demonstrating a retarded E to F slope, and a delayed closure. The delay in tricuspid valve closure is frequently in excess of 50 msec after mitral valve closure. Characteristically, the excursion of the tricuspid leaflet is of large amplitude, and when tricuspid insufficiency is present there may be paradoxical septal motion. Since Ebstein disease occurs with varying degrees of severity, the absence of these findings does not exclude a mild malformation.

Tetralogy of Fallot

The typical echocardiographic findings consist of right ventricular enlargement and a lack of continuity of echoes between the upper portion of the ventricular septum and the anterior aortic wall. Although the anterior aortic wall is abnormally displaced anteriorly, thus overriding the ventricular septal defect, the posterior wall is in normal continuity with the anterior mitral leaflet. These findings are very helpful in excluding double outlet right ventricle, which may mimic Tetralogy of Fallot in all respects. The presence of continuity between the anterior mitral valve leaflet and the posterior wall of the aorta excludes double outlet right ventricle but is compatible with the diagnosis of Tetralogy of Fallot or transposition of the great arteries and truncus arteriosus.

Endocardial Cushion Defect

An endocardial cushion defect may be suspected when the usual findings of an atrial septal defect (paradoxical septal motion and an enlarged right ventricular cavity) are associated with anterior displacement of the mitral valve, which approximates ventricular septum in diastole and the anterior tricuspid leaflet during systole. The anterior displacement of the mitral valve produces apparent narrowing of the left ventricular outflow tract. Additionally, the anterior mitral leaflet appears to cross the plane of the ventricular septum and to be continuous with the tricuspid valve.

Additional Reading

Chesler E, et al: Echocardiography in congenital heart disease. Ped Clin N Am 18:1163, 1971.

Clark RD: "Case Studies in Echocardiography." W.B. Saunders, Philadelphia, 1977.

Feigenbaum H: "Echocardiography," 4th Ed. Lea & Feibiger, Philadelphia, 1986.

Gramiak R: Echocardiography in acquired heart disease. In King DL (ed): "Diagnostic Ultrasound." CV Mosby, St. Louis, 1974.

Gutgesell HP, Huhta JC, Latson LA, Huffines D, McNamara DB: Accuracy of two-dimensional echocardiography in the diagnosis of congenital heart disease. Am J Cardiol 55:514, 1985.

Meyer RA: Noninvasive techniques in pediatric cardiovascular disease. Prog Cardiovasc Dis 4:341, 1973.

Popp RL.: Echocardiography (2 parts). N Engl J Med 323:2:101, 1990.

6 Electrocardiography

The electrocardiogram is a graphic representation of the electrical forces produced by the heart. Muscular contraction is preceded by depolarization of the cell membranes, during which the electrical charges on the surface of the muscle fibers change from positive to negative. Depolarization is followed by repolarization, whereby the cell membrane is restored to the resting state and the charge becomes positive once again. These processes depend on the movement of ions, particularly potassium, across the cell membranes.

Electrophysiologically, the atria function as one unit and the ventricle as another. Complete coordination and synchronization of atrial and ventricular contraction are achieved by the presence of two specialized tissues: the SA node, which spontaneously discharges at a high rate, and the AV node, which conducts impulses less rapidly.

The Conduction System

The sinoatrial (SA) node lies in the right atrium near the mouth of the superior vena cava. Impulses arising from this structure depolarize the atrium from fiber to fiber, but also through specialized intraatrial conducting pathways (Fig. 6.1). The AV node is also situated in the right atrium near the mouth of the coronary sinus and is a larger structure than the sinus node. It consists of a lattice-work of fibers that communicate with the bundle of His. The function of the AV node is to transmit atrial impulses to the ventricles in such a way that impulses are delayed. That this is due to decelerated conduction in the fibers seems unlikely. Most probably, the anatomical arrangement of the fibers results in a devious conducting pathway, with ample opportunity for impulses to cancel each other out, thus slowing the final arrival at the His bundle. Whatever the mechanism, the rate of transmission through the AV node is far slower than anywhere else in the heart. In addition to this remarkable property of conducting prograde impulses slowly, the AV node may conduct retrograde impulse even more slowly, or not at all.

From the AV node, a bundle of conducting fibers (bundle of His) runs through the ventricular septum and divides into the right and left bundle branches. Almost immediately on leaving the bundle of His the left bundle branch divides into the anterosuperior and the posteroinferior divisions (or fasicles), which lie in the subendocardium of the left ventricle. Peripherally, there is anastomosis between the fibers of the two divisions forming a syncytium that has rapid conduction characteristics. The anterosuperior division is long and thin and does not have as extensive a blood supply as the posteroinferior division. The anterosuperior division is in close proximity to the aortic valve. These factors combine to make it vulnerable to damage in aortic valve disease, ischemic injury, and diffuse subendocardial fibrosis.

The right bundle traverses the muscular

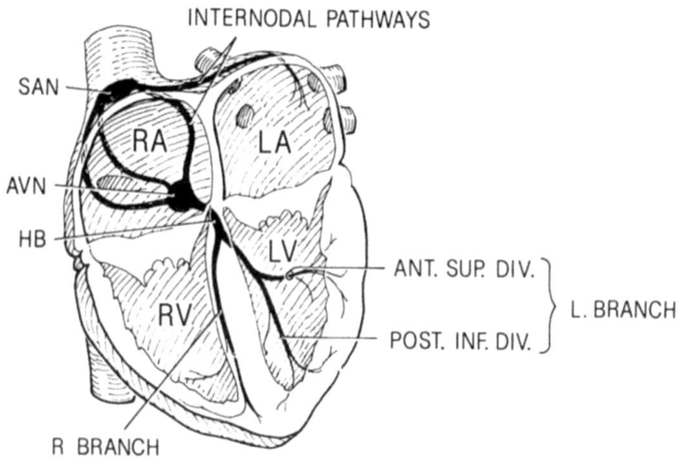

FIGURE 6.1. Diagrammatic representation of the normal conducting system (see text). SAN, SA node; AVN, AV node; HB, His bundle.

portion of the interventricular septum and emerges from the cavity of the right ventricle near the moderator band. From here it activates the right ventricle through the Purkinje system. Unlike the divisions of the left bundle, which lie diffusely in the subendocardium, the right bundle, because of its length and its discrete configuration, is readily damaged by a focal lesion.

Both AV and SA nodes are under humoral influence, particularly catecholamines and acetylcholine, either circulating in the bloodstream or released by the sympathetic or parasympathetic fibers. The left vagus nerve is distributed to the AV node and the right to the SA node.

Depolarization

Depolarization of the atria is represented electrocardiographically by the P wave. The QRS complex represents depolarization of the ventricles. The interval between the P and QRS represents the sum of the intraatrial, AV nodal, His bundle, and Purkinje fiber conduction times. The technique of His bundle electrocardiography demonstrates the following conduction times: (1) a P–A interval of 24–45 msec, measured from the onset of P to the low right atrium; (2) an A–H interval of 60–130 msec, measured from the low right atrium to the His bundle deflection representing the conduction time through the AV node; and (3) an H–V interval of 30–55 msec, measured from the His bundle deflection to the first portion of the QRS, representing His–Purkinje conduction.

Depolarization of the atria occurs from the right to the left atrium, the impulse reaching the AV node while the left atrium is still being traversed. Thus, when the left atrium is enlarged, the interval between the end of P and the beginning of the Q wave is short, whereas in right atrial hypertrophy this is not the case. There has been considerable dispute in the past as to whether atrial depolarization is achieved through specialized conducting pathways; however, recent studies have confirmed that several fairly well-defined conducting bundles traverse the atria and some pass directly from the sinus to the AV node. (The intraatrial tracts are named the anterior internodal pathway, middle internodal pathway, and posterior internodal pathway).

Depolarization of the ventricles is more complicated. The initial forces move from left to right through the ventricular septum followed by simultaneous activation of both ventricles. Since the left ventricle is bulkier than the right, right ventricular forces are outbalanced and the result is a single force moving

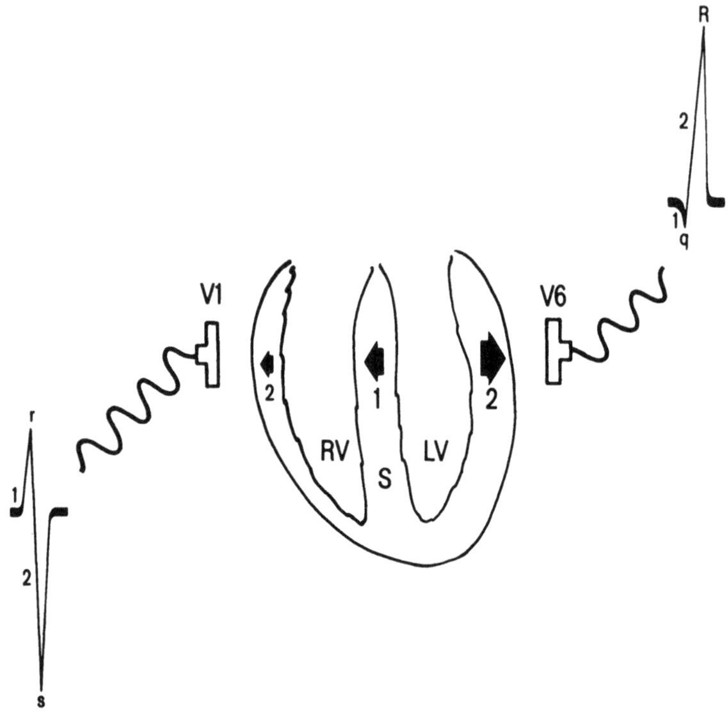

FIGURE 6.2. The mechanism of formation of the QRS complexes following ventricular depolarization in right precordial lead V_1 and left precordial lead V_6.

from right to left. Therefore electrodes facing the left ventricle demonstrate an initial small negative deflection produced by the left-to-right spread of the stimulus away from the electrode through the septum, followed by a large upward deflection caused by the spread of the stimulus toward the electrode through the left ventricle. Leads facing the right ventricle display the opposite pattern. The movement of these forces therefore inscribes a QRS over the left precordial leads and an RS complex over the right precordial leads (Fig. 6.2).

Repolarization

The T wave is produced by repolarization of the ventricle. In a simple muscle strip and in the atria, repolarization produces a negative deflection equal in area to the positive deflection of depolarization. The T wave, however, has the same polarity as the QRS complex and the mechanism for this is not understood. The T wave is usually followed by a small U wave, which has the same polarity as the T wave.

QRS Terminology

Q wave: the initial defection of QR—downward.
R wave: the initial deflection of the QRS—upward.
S wave: the initial deflection after R wave—downward.
R^1: the second upward deflection following S.
S^1: the second deflection of S following R^1.
QS: the entire QRS complex is negative.

Another convention is a lower case letter for a small deflection and a capital letter for a large deflection (e.g., RSr as opposed to rSR) (Fig. 6.3).

The Standard Leads

The Einthoven Triangle

A considerable amount of empiric knowledge has been gained from the three standard limb

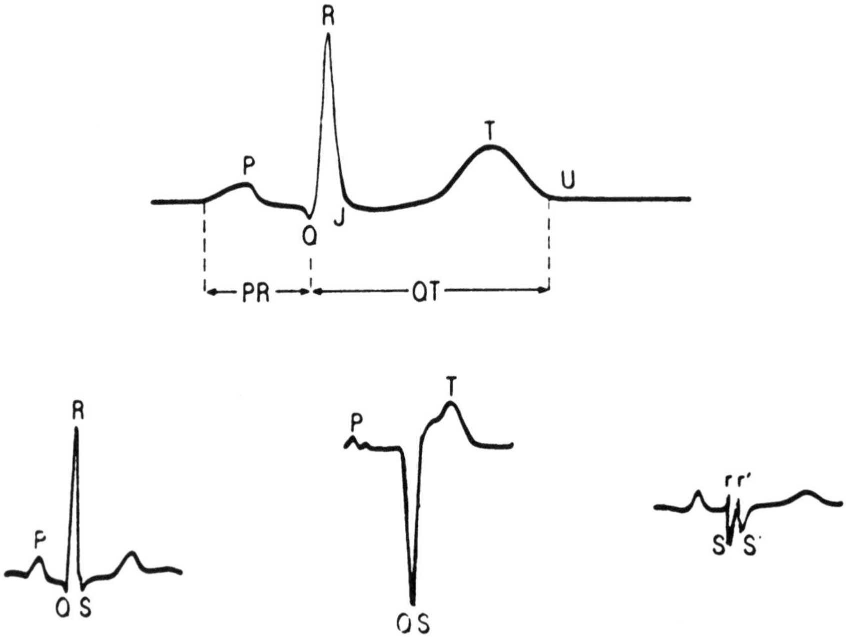

FIGURE 6.3. Nomenclature for the various types of electrocardiographic patterns.

leads since their introduction by Einthoven, and their use for more than 50 years. At present they still provide more valuable and reliable information than any other limb lead. Most abnormalities can be detected from them and they are useful in determining the frontal plane axis.

Einthoven used the combination of leads from both arms and left leg to obtain a triangle. The limbs should be regarded as convenient terminals, recording electrical forces generated by the heart, which is in the center of this triangle. The electrodes on the limbs are electrically equidistant from the heart. By using two limbs only the difference in potential between these two terminals can be obtained. It is conventional in physics to rèpresent a positive potential by a galvanometer deflection above the isoelectric line and a negative potential below the line. Standard lead I is obtained from electrodes on the right arm (negative terminal) and left arm (positive terminal). Standard lead II is obtained from electrodes on the right arm (negative terminal) and left leg (positive terminal). Standard lead III is obtained from the electrodes on the left leg (positive terminal) and the left arm (negative terminal). The Einthoven triangle is made up of each lead axis forming an equilateral triangle with the heart at the center.

Augmented Unipolar Limb Leads

It can be readily appreciated that information obtained from the bipolar limb leads, which measure difference of potential between two terminals, is mainly empirical. If some lead could be designed whereby the negative electrode could be attached to some terminal with zero potential, a unipolar lead would be possible. Wilson almost achieved this, by taking a lead with a resistance from all three limbs and joining them together to form a single terminal, which was connected to the negative pole of the galvanometer. The positive or exploring electrode was attached to the right arm (VR), left arm (VL), or left leg (VF). Deflections produced by this system were, however, small. Using the above technique, Goldberger augmented the voltage by omitting the connection from the central terminal to the extremity explored. Thus leads AVR, AVL, and AVF were obtained, the exploring leads being on the right arm, left arm, and left leg, respec-

tively. The letter A is used to designate that the lead has been augmented.

Precordial Leads

Limb leads have the disadvantage that they are derived from points distant from the heart and they are all in the same plane. Other leads can be obtained by placing the exploring electrode on the chest wall close to the heart. By general agreement the points chosen are as follows:

Lead V_1: just to the right of the sternum in the fourth interspace.
Lead V_2: just to the left of the sternum in the fourth interspace.
Lead V_4: in the midclavicular line in the fifth interspace.
Lead V_3: half-way between V_2 and V_4.

V_5, V_6, V_7: in the same plane as V_4, but in the anterior, mid, and posterior axillary lines, respectively. Leads to the right of the sternum correspond to the left, but are designated V_4R, etc.

Hexaxial Reference System

Without disturbing the polarity of the lead axis, the three leads of the Einthoven triangle may be represented as passing through the same zero point. This forms a triaxial reference system with each lead situated a 60° intervals. Similarly, a triaxial reference system may be constructed for the augmented unipolar limb leads. Combining the two results in a hexaxial reference system with leads separated at intervals of 30°. All portions of the upper hemisphere of the system are conventionally labeled negative and those in the lower hemisphere are labeled positive (Fig. 6.4).

Frontal Plane QRS Axis

Using the hexaxial reference system, the mean frontal plane QRS axis may be readily plotted. When the direction of a force is *toward* the *positive* pole of a lead, the deflection is *positive*; when the direction of a force is *toward* the *negative* pole, the deflection is *negative*. The

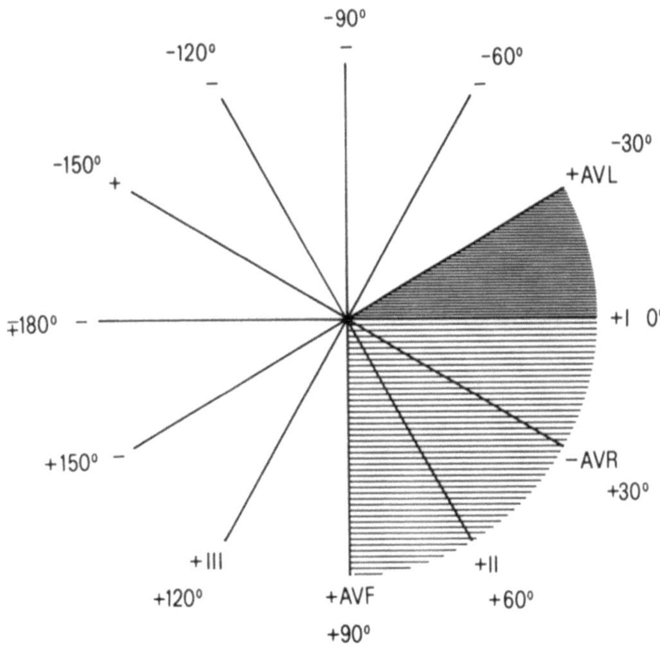

FIGURE 6.4. The hexaxial reference system and polarity of the various leads. The normal frontal plant QRS axis usually lies between O and +90°.

Deviation beyond −30° is compatible with left anterior hemiblock.

magnitude and direction of a force is known as a *vector*.

The mean frontal plane axis may be plotted on the hexaxial reference system as foilows. When an impulse travels parallel to a lead, the deflection is maximal (either positive or negative). However, when the impulse moves at right angles to a lead, the deflection is equiphasic. The vector therefore lies at right angles to the lead with an equiphasic deflection:

Equiphasic lead	Lead at right angles	QRS axis
Standard I	AVF positive	+90°
Standard I	AVF negative	−90°
Standard II	AVL positive	−30°
Standard II	AVL negative	+150°
Standard III	AVR negative	+30°
Standard III	AVR positive	+120°

In the case of bundle branch block the vectors for each 4-msec interval may be calculated for the initial, mid, and terminal portions of the QRS complex.

The following features should be examined in every lead in all electrocardiograms:

1. Rate.
2. Rhythm.
3. The voltage, timing, and shape of the PQRST complexes and measurement of various intervals.

Changes in the PQRST Complexes

P Wave

The P wave is produced by depolarization of the atria, initiated by an impulse from the SA node, which then radiates through the right and left atria. The direction of the P wave vector is thus oblique, from right arm to left leg, with an axis between +30 and +60° on the hexaxial frontal plane system. In cor pulmonale, the P wave vector is frequently directed to the right, between +60° and +90°.

Inversion of the P wave when it should be positive (superiorly directed P wave axis from −80° to 100°) implies that the sinus node is suppressed and the atria are activated from the AV node or low right atrium; there is therefore retrograde atrial activation (*inferior atrial rhythm*) (Fig. 6.5). In the setting of congenital heart disease inferior atrial rhythm is a strong indicator that there is *polysplenia* with interruption of the inferior vena cava. Retrograde atrial activation may also occur with ectopic AV nodal impulses.

In *dextrocardia with situs inversus*, the P wave axis is directed to the right and the P waves are inverted in standard I and AVL and upright in AVR. The same findings may be observed, however, when the right and left arm electrodes are inadvertently reversed. When the V leads have been placed in the usual position over the left chest, dextrocardia may be excluded by observing that the P waves are upright in V_6. In true mirror-image dextrocardia leads placed on the left side of the chest will demonstrate inverted P waves in leads V_4–V_6 because the cardiac apex points to the right (Fig. 10.1).

The normal duration of the P wave is 0.08 to 0.11 seconds measured in the lead where P is broadest, usually lead II. There is, however, a considerable degree of overlap, but a P wave duration of 0.14 seconds is certainly abnormal. Changes in the P wave may be due to hypertrophy of the atrial wall, dilatation, changes in intraatrial pressure, or disturbances in the intraatrial conducting pathways. The last factor is probably the most important and is referred to as intraatrial block.

Atrial Enlargement

The right atrium is situated anteriorly in the thorax whereas the left artium is situated more posteriorly (Fig. 6.6). In lead V_1 the right atrial forces are directed toward lead V_1 and inscribe the first component of the P wave, which is upright in this lead. The left atrial component is delayed and directed away from lead V_1 resulting in a P wave that is mainly negative or diphasic in lead V_1. Notching of the P wave is often present, and the first peak, which is sharp, arises from the right atrium and the second, which is broader and of lower voltage,

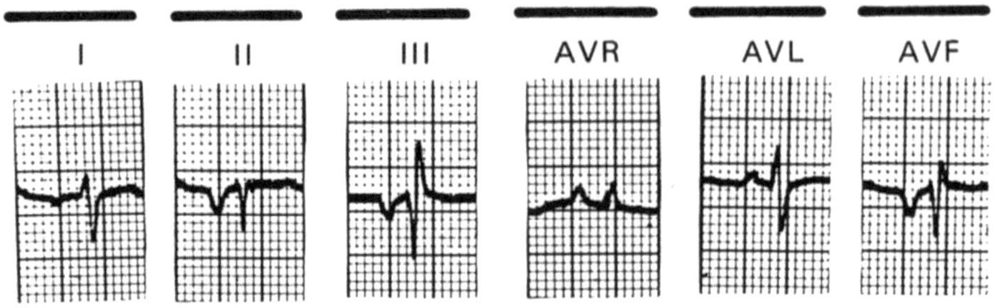

FIGURE 6.5. Inferior atrial rhythm showing left axis deviation of the P wave which is negative in II, III, and AF.

arises from the left atrium. An interval of 0.04 seconds or more between peaks is abnormal.

Left Atrial Enlargement

P "mitrale" is a broad, notched P wave in which the second peak represents left atrial enlargement (Fig. 6.7). It is classically observed in mitral stenosis and is best seen in leads I and II.

The best evidence for left atrial enlargement is found in lead V_1 when the P wave is diphasic and the terminal negative phase measures 0.03 seconds or more. Alternatively, the negative area may be measured and if the deflection is one square wide (0.04 seconds) and 1 mm deep a value of 0.04 is obtained. Any P wave negativity of this size or larger is abnormal.

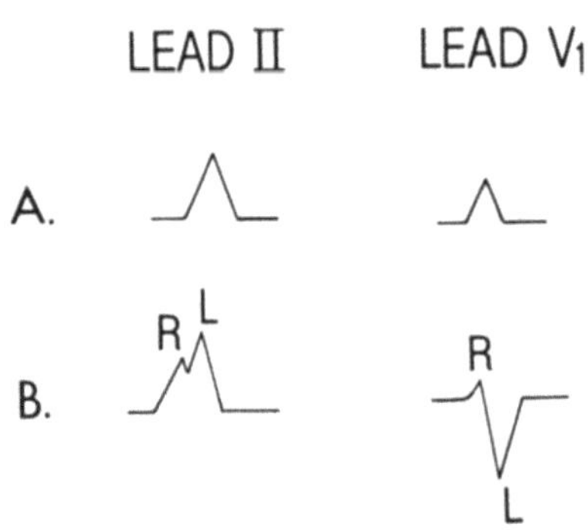

FIGURE 6.6. Diagrammatic representation of P wave abnormality in right (A) and left atrial enlargement (B).

Right Atrial Enlargement

This produces tall and peaked (gothic) P waves, also known as P pulmonale, and is best seen in leads II, III, and AVF (Fig. 6.7).

Electrocardiographically, left or right atrial enlargement may occur as a transitory phenomenon. Thus it may be encountered in acute left atrial overloading such as occurs in pulmonary edema, congestive cardiac failure, acute myocardial infarction, acute cor pulmonale, and during paroxysmal tachycardia. The P wave amplitude can also be altered by exercise and the Valsalva maneuver.

The PR Interval

The longest interval in any of the six limb leads, measured from the beginning of the P wave to the beginning of the QRS, represents the PR interval. The normal range is from 12 to 20 msec. The faster the heart rate, the shorter the PR interval. In infants, the PR interval is normally less than 0.12 seconds. Occasionally, a short PR interval is found in healthy normal adults, in whom paroxysmal atrial tachycardia may be associated (the Lown–Ganong–Levine syndrome). An abnormally short PR interval is also associated with the Wolff–Parkinson–White syndrome.

Prolongation of the PR interval beyond 0.20 seconds is regarded as evidence of AV block. It may occur, however, in healthy young people as a result of increased vagal tone because the PR interval shortens with upright posture. A long PR interval occurs in ischemic heart dis-

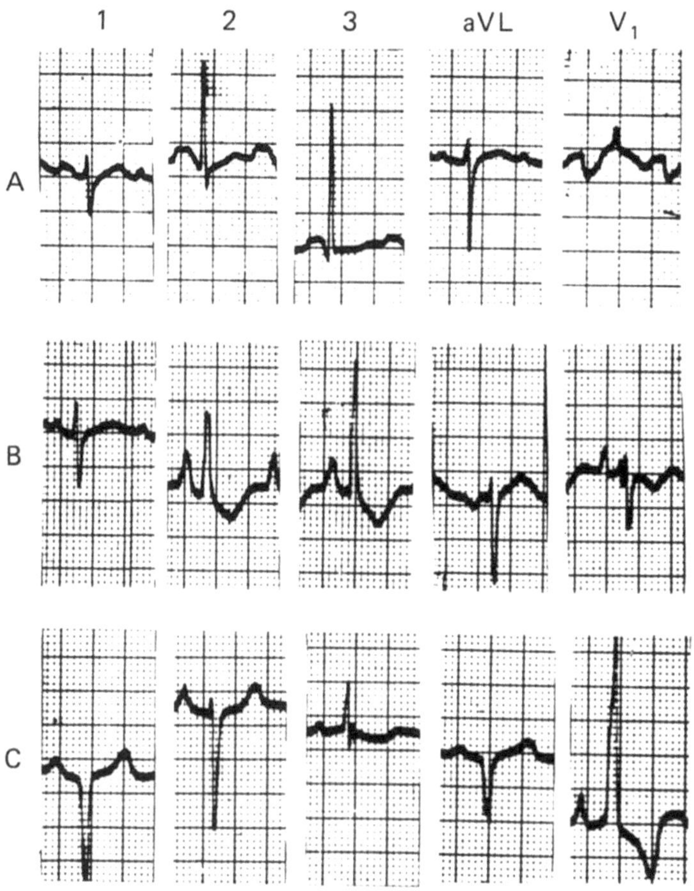

FIGURE 6.7. In left atrial overload (A) the P waves are large in I and II and bifid in lead II, with a large terminal negative reflection in V_1 (P mitrale). In right atrial overload (B) the P waves are peaked in II and III (P pulmonale) and negative in AVL because of right axis deviation of the P wave vector. In V_1 the P wave is peaked. In congenital heart disease with pulmonary hypertension (C) the P wave is usually upright in AVL in contrast to (B) because the P wave vector is usually less deviated to the right.

ease, hypertension, and rheumatic heart disease and is frequently induced by digitalis.

The QRS Complex

The QRS complex normally does not exceed 11 msec in duration in any lead. Prolongation of the QRS occurs chiefly in bundle branch block. Q waves are rarely deep in leads that face the left ventricle and in health do not exceed 0.04 seconds. The voltage of the QRS may be decreased or increased. Low voltage (sum of the R and S waves in any of the limb leads not exceeding 5 mm) may be normal in thick chests, but also occurs in emphysema, pericardial effusion, myxedema, and myocardial disease. Increased voltage occurs in healthy subjects with thin chest walls and in ventricular hypertrophy. The major changes in the QRS complex are discussed later.

The ST Segment

The ST segment is that part of the tracing between the end of the QRS complex and the beginning of the T wave. There are two im-

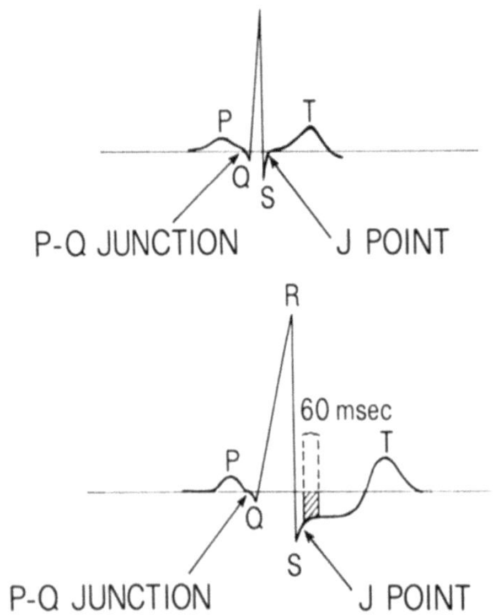

FIGURE 6.8. Diagram illustrating measurement of ST segment depression (see text).

portant observations to be made: the level of the ST segment compared with the baseline and the shape of the segment. This is of particular significance in the assessment of the exercise elecrocardiogram.

In determining ST-segment abnormalities, the baseline is taken at the PQ or PR junction and in normal individuals the ST segment during and after exercise is steeply upsloping, returning to the baseline within 80 msec after the J point. The J point is the junction between the S wave and the ST segment (Fig. 6.8). ST-segment depression of 1 mm or more, 80 msec after the J point, is indicative of myocardial ischemia.

Elevation of the ST segment, as much as 2 mm in the standard leads and 4 mm in the chest leads, is a normal variant encountered particularly in black subjects (so-called "junctional elevation") (Fig. 6.9). Usually, however, ST-segment elevation is a result of epicardial injury produced by myocardial infarction or pericarditis. The ST segments are elevated in those leads facing the damaged tissues and reciprocally depressed in leads facing normal tissue.

T Wave

In leads where the QRS complex is mainly positive, the T wave should also be positive and where the QRS is mainly negative, the T waves are usually negative. Thus, in leads I and

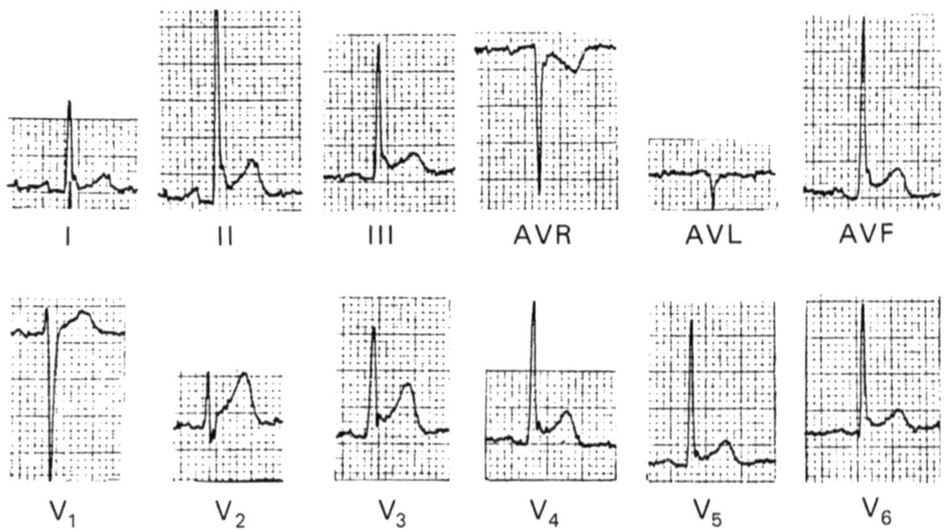

FIGURE 6.9. Junctional ST segment elevation particularly evident in the leads with the tall R wave, encountered frequently as a racial variant in blacks. This may be mistaken for the pattern seen in hyperacute myocardial infarction, but the latter is associated with a straight upward slope of ST segment to the T wave and reciprocal leads usually show marked ST segment depression.

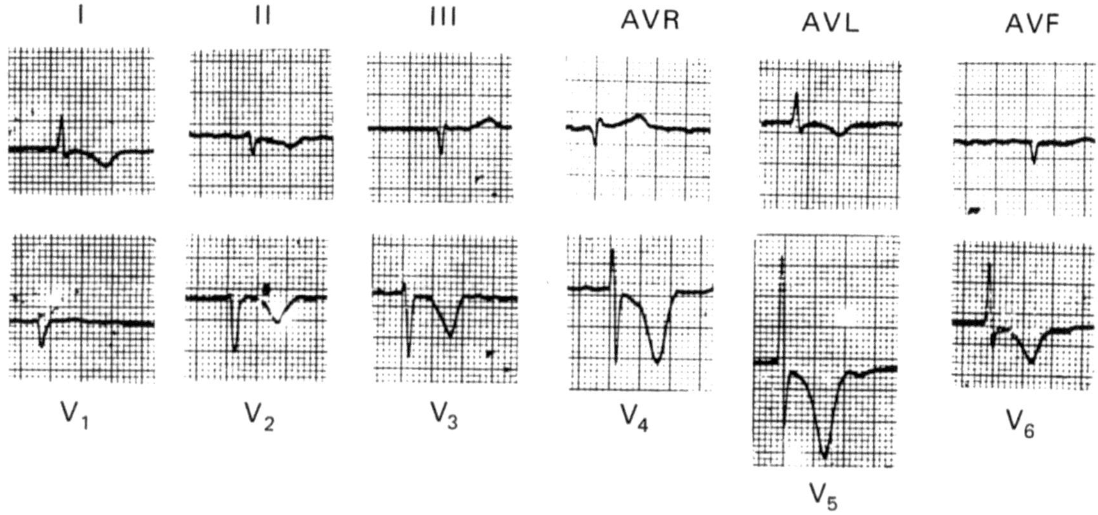

FIGURE 6.10. Marked inversion of the T waves encountered following subarachnoid hemorrhage.

II, and V_3–V_6, T is positive, and in AVR T is negative. In other leads it is variable. In the horizontal plane the QRS and T wave forces are directed toward lead V_6 and away from lead I. Therefore, V_6 is characterized by upright QRS complexes and T waves, whereas these are negative in lead V_1.

Myocardial ischemia results in an abnormal deviation of the T wave forces away from those of the QRS (wide QRS–T angle); therefore the T wave in lead V_1 is taller than the T wave in V_6. T waves are normally not greater than 5 mm Hg in the limb leads and 10 mm in the chest leads. In conditions associated with diastolic overload of the left ventricle, such as mitral or aortic regugitation, tall peaked T waves are often encountered.

The normal T wave is asymmetric. Tall symmetric T waves may be encountered in myocardial infarction, ischemia, and hypercalcemia. Massive, bizzare, "giant" negative T waves appear most commonly in cerebral disease, especially cerebrovascular accidents and head injuries, and in complete heart block following a Stokes–Adams attack. Leads V_1–V_4 are particularly affected (Fig. 6.10).

Flat T waves (1 mm or less) in leads I and V_6 are usually abnormal. The T waves are usually upright in leads V_1–V_6 in adult men. In infants and children the T waves are often inverted from V_1 to V_3 and less commonly inverted in V_4; this has been called the *juvenile precordial pattern*. In women and black men this may be a normal variant, and in the latter it is frequently labile. Isolated T wave inversion in one or two of the precordial leads (e.g., V_3 and V_4) with upright T waves in the other leads is a normal variant and this has been called the *null zone*.

The T waves are altered by a large number of factors, both physiologic and pathologic. Among these are conditions such as exercise, changes in posture, eating a meal, catecholamines, reflex response to pain or fright, and smoking. Cerebral disease, toxic and infectious agents, changes in acid–base balance, ischemia, trauma, and myocarditis may all produce T wave flattening or inversion. Positive T waves in V_1 in the neonatal period have been regarded as a sign of right ventricular hypertrophy. The T wave in this period of life is very unstable and this sign is therefore not very specific.

The U Wave

The U wave should have the same polarity as the T wave. When the U wave has a reversed polarity and is inverted this is usually a result of coronary artery or hypertensive heart disease. Prominent U waves in the right precordial leads are usually a manifestation of hypokalemia.

Junctional ST–T Changes

The junction of the QRS complex in the ST segment is referred to as the J segment. It is characteristically deformed by digitalis, which produces a distinctive sag at this site (like a mirror-image correction mark). The segment is frequently depressed following tachycardia induced by effort. The most bizarre and profound changes occur in hypothermia where the J deflection becomes broad and elevated well above the baseline and may be followed by T wave inversion.

The QT Interval

The QT interval may be a difficult interval to measure because it is difficult to determine where the T wave ends and the U wave begins. It has thus erroneously been regarded as increased in hypokalemia. The interval is best corrected for heart rate using Bazett's formula:

$$QT_c = \frac{QT}{\text{cycle length}}.$$

It is normally not more than 0.42 sec. A shortened QT interval may be a result of digitalis effect or hypercalcemia. It is prolonged in hypocalcemia, myocardial infarction, and acute rheumatic myocarditis, and is a result of Type I antidysrhythmic drugs such as quinidine and procainamide.

Conduction Disturbances

Because of the trifascicular nature of the conducting system, several types of disturbances are possible. Blocks may occur (1) in the right bundle branch, (2) in the anterosuperior division of the left bundle branch, (3) in the inferoposterior division of the left bundle branch, (4) in the entire left bundle branch, or (5) in the

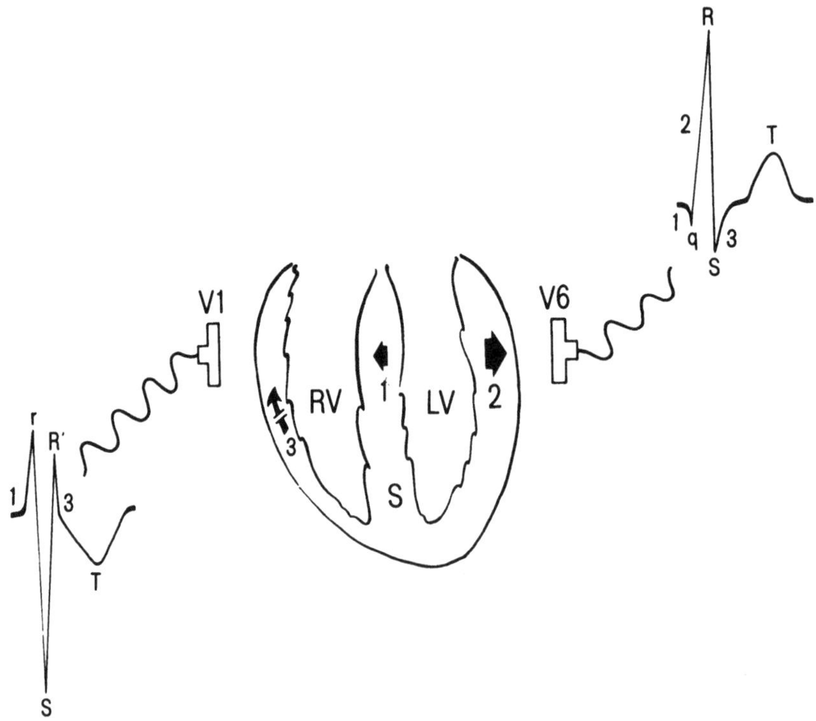

FIGURE 6.11. Diagrammatic representation of the conduction abnormality in right bundle branch block (see text).

right bundle and in one or both divisions of the left bundle.

Right Bundle Branch Block

The principal abnormality in right bundle branch block is a delay in the terminal vector of right ventricular depolarization because right ventricular activation is late (Fig. 6.11).

The initial vector produced by septal depolarization remains normal (from left to right) and therefore right ventricular surface leads show a small R wave and left ventricular surface leads show a Q wave. Depolarization of the left ventricle then occurs producing an S wave in the right ventricular surface leads and an R wave in the left ventricular surface leads. Late unopposed depolarization of the free wall of the right ventricle is produced by an impulse moving from left to right and anteriorly; this produces a wide terminal S wave in standard lead I and lead V_6.

The diagnosis is made more easily from the precordial, than from the limb leads, lead V_1 showing an rSR and V_6 a qRS pattern. The QRS complex becomes wide (by definition 0.12 sec or more) and notched, producing an M-shaped complex in leads facing the right ventricle. The ST segment and T wave in leads V_4–V_6 are opposite in direction to the terminal portion of the QRS deflection, are a result of the abnormal pattern of conduction, and do not indicate any primary abnormality of the ST segment or T wave (Fig. 6.12).

Since right bundle branch block does not affect the initial vector of the QRS complex, abnormalities that characteristically alter this deflection, such as the Q wave of a myocardial infarction, will still occur (Fig. 6.13). This is in contrast to left bundle branch block where the initial QRS forces are grossly changed and the Q waves of myocardial infarction are therefore obscured. Similarly, the occurrence of left anterior and posterior hemiblock, which produces left and right axis deviation, respectively, will be manifest in the presence of right bundle branch block (Figs. 6.12, 6.13, and 6.14).

The pattern of incomplete right bundle branch block is essentially the same, but the QRS duration is 0.11 msec or less and seldom less than 8 msec. This type of pattern is often a

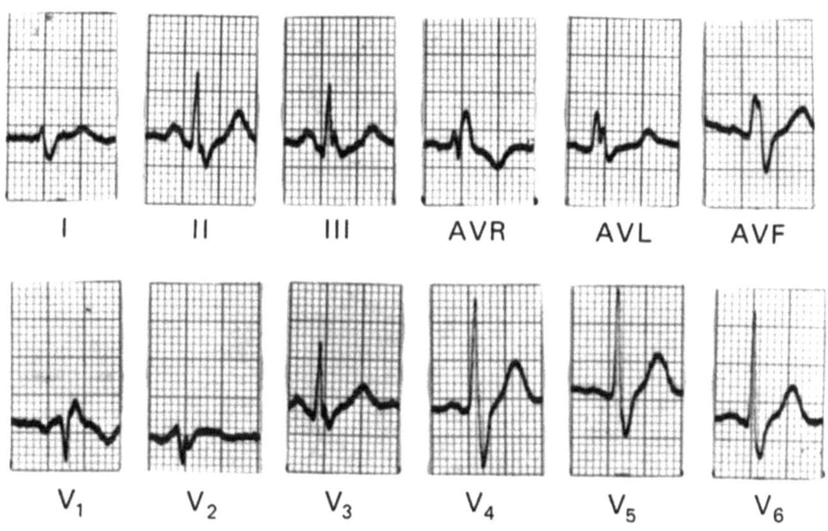

FIGURE 6.12. The electrocardiogram in complete right bundle branch block, old anterior myocardial infarction, and left posterior hemiblock (right axis deviation).

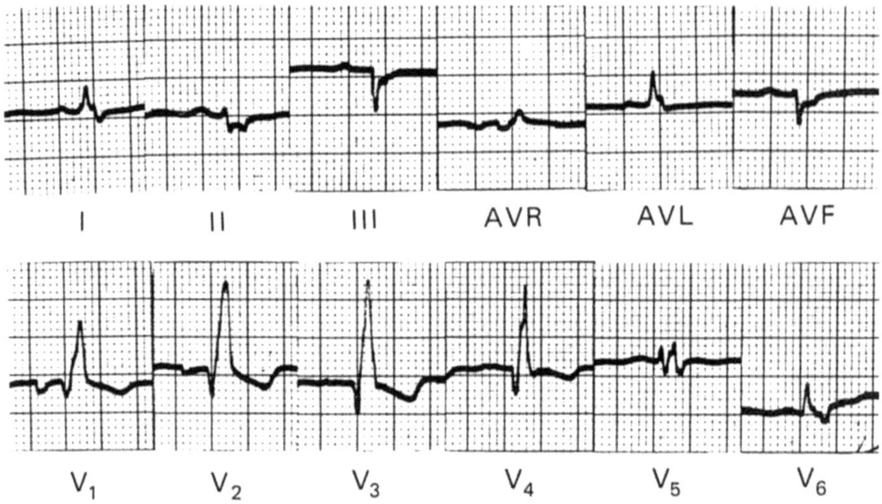

FIGURE 6.13. Electrocardiogram in old myocardial infarction complicated by complete right bundle branch block and left anterior hemiblock. The conduction abnormality does not obscure the pathological Q waves of anterior myocardial infarction in leads V_1–V_4. Left atrial enlargement in present (V_1).

normal variant, especially when the terminal deflection is small. The pattern may not be due to any disturbance in the right bundle, but rather to delayed activation of the right ventricular outflow tract or to right ventricular hypertrophy because the crista supraventricularis is the last part of the heart to be depolarized. This pattern has been referred to as diastolic overload of the right ventricle, since it occurs so frequently in conditions such as atrial septal defect.

Significance of Right Bundle Branch Block

Occasionally, right bundle branch block is encountered in apparently normal individuals and the prognosis in these circumstances is probably no different from that of the normal population of the same age, race, and sex.

Most commonly however, the disturbance is a result of myocardial damage produced by coronary atherosclerosis, virus myocarditis, or

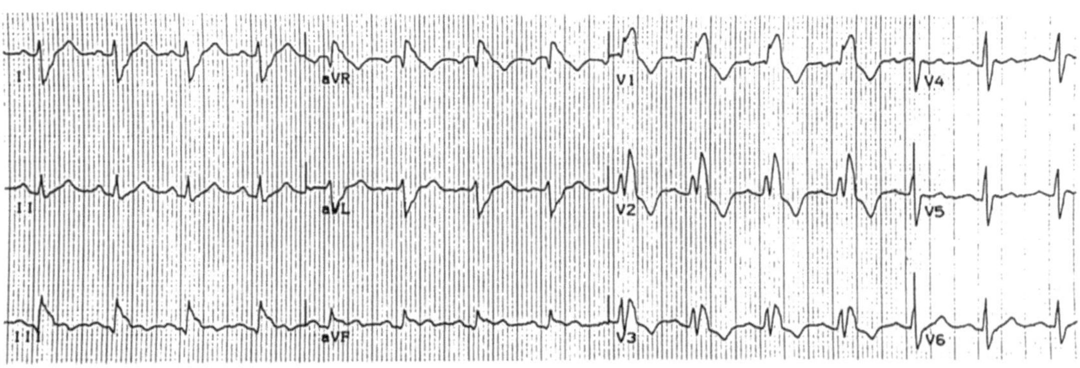

FIGURE 6.14. Electrocardiogram in complete right bundle branch block and left posterior hemiblock.

trypanosomiasis. It occurs in 95% of cases of atrial septal defect where it is a result of diastolic overload of the right ventricle—the abnormality disappears following closure of the defect. Surgical damage to the right bundle is common following repair of Tetralogy of Fallot or ventricular septal defect. It is commonly a result of aging and degeneration of the entire conducting system (Lev and Lenegre disease) where complete heart block is often the end result.

Intermittent right bundle branch block is often critically rate dependent. For example, it may appear only when the heart rate is increased above a certain level as during supraventricular tachycardia. Rarely, it appears with a very slow heart rate.

Left Bundle Branch Block

Here septal depolarization is reversed, the left ventricle being activated by impulses from the right bundle branch, which move from right to left to be followed by activation of the free wall of the left ventricle.

Conduction is such that right ventricular surface (V_1 and V_2) leads reflect a major movement away from the right ventricle producing a QS or rS type complex, whereas left ventricular surface leads show a broad notched R pattern (V_5 and V_6). M-shaped QRS complexes are present in standards lead I, AVL, V_5, and V_6. The duration of the QRS complex is prolonged to 12 msec or more, largely because of the delayed activation of the left side of the septum and the free wall of the left ventricle (Fig. 6.15). The ST segment and T waves are distorted secondarily to the abnormal pattern of intraventricular conduction and are opposite in direction to the terminal QRS deflection. Therefore, in leads V_5 and V_6 the ST segment is depressed and the T wave inverted. In leads V_1 and V_2 the ST segment is elevated and the T wave is upright (Fig. 6.16).

When a similar pattern occurs with a QRS duration of less than 12 msec, incomplete left bundle branch block is said to be present. Whether the block is complete or incomplete, the mean frontal plane QRS axis may be normally directed, or show left or right axis deviation. The mechanism of left axis deviation is not understood, but it may be a result of left anterior hemiblock with high grade, but incom-

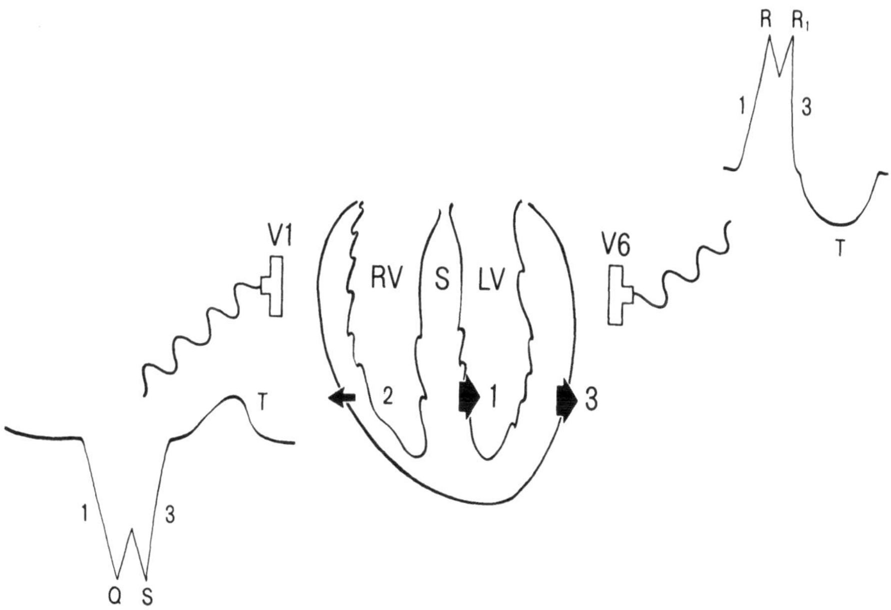

FIGURE 6.15. Diagrammatic representation of the conduction abnormality in left bundle branch block (see text).

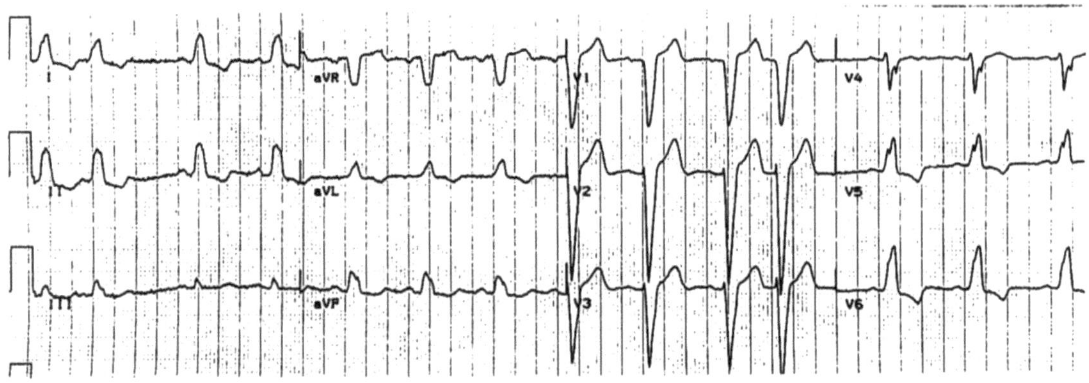

FIGURE 6.16. Electrocardiogram in complete left bundle branch block. The mean frontal plane axis is also deviated to the left at $-60°$.

plete block of the left posterior division. The result is that QRS duration is widened and when the impulse finally emerges through the left posterior division, the axis is swung to the left. Left axis deviation associated with left bundle branch block is purported to have a worse prognosis than left bundle branch block with a normal frontal plane axis.

Significance of Left Bundle Branch Block

The left bundle branch block nearly always connotes the presence of organic heart disease and there is no evidence that it ever occurs as an isolated congenital defect. Usually it is a result of coronary atherosclerosis, hypertension,

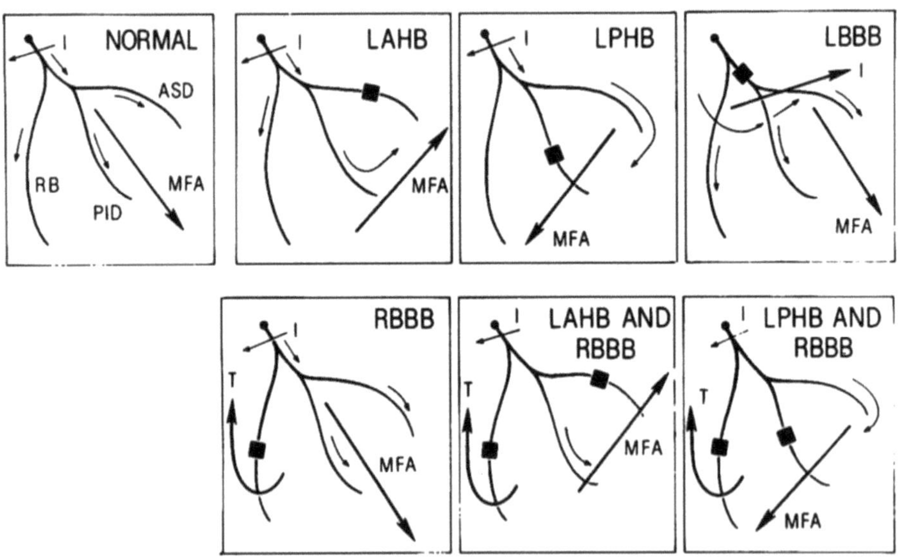

FIGURE 6.17: The patterns of intraventricular conduction in the normal, left bundle branch block (LBBB), right bundle branch block (RBBB), and (iv) left anterior and posterior hemiblock (LAHB, LPHB) with and without right bundle branch block (see text). MFA, mean frontal plane axis.

cardiomyopathy, myocarditis, senile degeneration of the conducting system, aortic stenosis with calcific extension into the conducting system, and rheumatic heart disease.

Left bundle branch block that occurs during myocardial infarction usually implies extensive myocardial damage and therefore carries a poor prognosis. Like right bundle branch block, it may be rate dependent, but this is less common.

Indeterminate Types of Intraventricular Conduction Defect

In some instances, conduction defects cannot be classified as typical left or right bundle branch block. Usually, there is a wide terminal S wave in leads I, III, and III and the chest leads have QRS complexes 120 sec or more wide. Frequently they are the result of ischemic heart disease or cardiomyopathy and are probably a result of extensive damage to the three fasicles of the conducting system.

The Hemiblocks

Normally, conduction through the posteroinferior division of the left bundle is in an upward and leftward direction, whereas conduction in the anterosuperior division is downward and to the right. When conduction occurs simultaneously through both divisions the mean axis is directed downward and to the left (+30 to +90°).

Interruption of both fascicles produces complete left bundle branch block, whereas interruption of one fascicle produces either left anterior or left posterior hemiblock with appropriate alterations in the direction of the frontal plane axis (Fig. 6.17).

When there is right bundle branch block in addition, a bifascicular block (left anterior or left posterior hemiblock) is present.

When both divisions of the left bundle branch are blocked and there is right bundle branch block, a trifascicular block (complete heart block) is present.

Left Anterior Hemiblock

Here, conduction occurs through the posteroinferior division resulting in the spread of the impulse through the left ventricle in an upward and leftward direction producing left axis deviation (Fig. 6.13).

Changes also occur in the precordial leads because the activation front also moves in a posterior direction in the horizontal plane (away from V_1). Therefore, common pattern in left anterior hemiblock is one of rS patterns in leads V_1–V_6. This may mimic anteroseptal myocardial infarction or so-called "clockwise rotation." Indeed, with leads placed in the usual precordial position, QS patterns may be present in leads V_1–V_4. However, when these leads are placed one interspace lower, a small r wave becomes evident; it should be appreciated that this is part of the hemiblock pattern and not a result of infarction.

Left anterior hemiblock is commonly a result of myocardial infarction, fibrous or calcific involvement of the bundle by cardiomyopathy or aortic valve disease, left ventricular decompensation with endocardial fibrosis, or congenital abnormalities such as tricuspid atresia and endocardial cushion defect.

Left Posterior Hemiblock

Activation occurs through the fibers of the anterosuperior division in a downward and rightward direction resulting in right axis deviation. This pattern results in an axis of +120°, and because the portions of the left ventricle that are located to the right are less significant than those located superiorly, the axis shift in posterior hemiblock is of lesser magnitude than that of left anterior hemiblock (Fig. 6.14).

It is important to appreciate that the same pattern of ventricular activation occurs in right ventricular hypertrophy, pulmonary hypertension of any cause, and a vertical heart position associated with a slender physique or chest wall

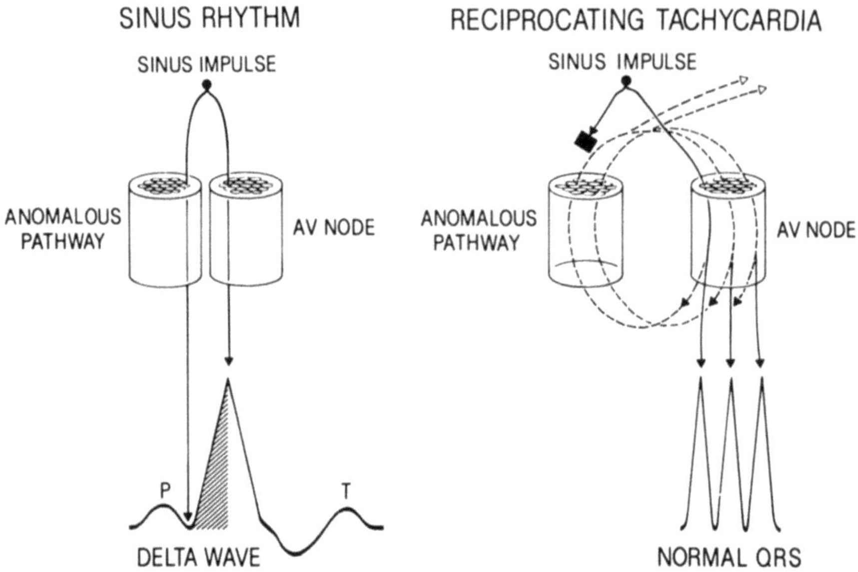

FIGURE 6.18. The mechanism of preexcitation and reciprocating tachycardia in the Wolff–Parkinsons–White syndrome (see text).

deformity. Therefore, the diagnosis of posterior hemiblock cannot be made from the electrocardiogram alone and the aforementioned conditions must be excluded clinically.

The Wolff–Parkinson–White (WPW) Syndrome

This syndrome is characterized by a short PR interval of 0.12 sec or less, prolongation of the QRS complex to 0.11 sec or more, and notching and slurring of the QRS, with a prominent slur on the upstroke of the R wave (the delta wave). The P waves are normal. This abnormality of AV conduction is a result of an anomalous pathway between the atria and the ventricle situated along the AV ring.

Atrial impulse travel down the normal and the anomalous pathway simultaneously, but the anomalous pathway has the facility for more rapid conduction. Therefore, the PR interval is shortened. However, subsequent conduction occurs through myocardium at the point of insertion of the anomalous pathway and not through specialized conducting tissues. Therefore, conduction is slower than normal, resulting in the slurred delta wave. Normal conduction through the AV node occurs at a slower rate, but when it reaches the ventricle subsequent conduction is through the specialized tissues of the bundle branches and the Purkinje system. This records the rest of the QRS complex, which is normal (Fig. 6.18).

The typical pattern of the WPW syndrome may be looked on as a form of fusion beat with the initial delta wave representing conduction through the anomalous pathway, and the normal portion of the QRS representing conduction through the AV node. When most of the ventricular depolarization is derived from the aberrant bundle, the QRS is bizarre and the PR interval is very short. However, the longer the PR interval the more normal the QRS (Fig. 6.19).

The WPW syndrome is associated fairly frequently with Ebstein disease. Usually, however, this conduction abnormality is an isolated finding of no importance and may be intermittent or persistent. On occasion it may be responsible for attacks of paroxysmal

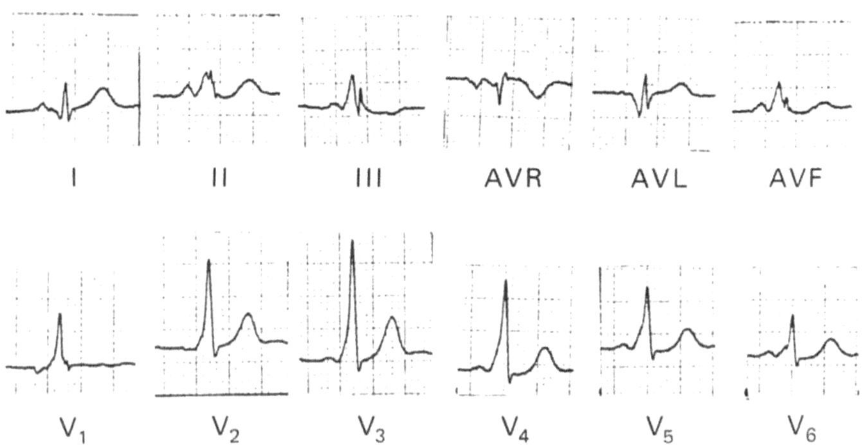

FIGURE 6.19. Electrocardiogram in Wolff–Parkinsons–White syndrome showing prominent R waves, leads V_1–V_3. This must be differentiated from true posterior myocardial infarction and right ventricular hypertrophy.

tachycardia, especially in infants. Fortunately, most infants with the syndrome display less tendency to develop tachyarrhythmias in childhood and adolesence. The tachyarrhythmias may be of two varieties: (1) reciprocating tachycardia and (2) paroxysmal atrial flutter or fibrillation.

In the presence of the WPW pattern, effort tests are of little diagnostic value since the ST segment may be strikingly depressed in the absence of coronary artery disease. The same phenomenon applies in left bundle branch block (Fig. 6.20).

Aberrant Ventricular Conduction

A wide QRS complex with a "bundle branch block" pattern does not necessarily mean permanent damage to the conducting system. Bundle branch block may be transient or intermittent, due to toxic or ischemic causes, or functional when it is a result of abnormal intraventricular conduction of a supraventricular impulse; this is known as aberrant ventricular conduction.

Fundamental to the occurrence of aberration is the presence of unequal refractory periods of the left and right bundle branches. A premature impulse is thus likely to find one bundle recovered and the other refractory. Usually, the left bundle recovers first, and aberration results in a right bundle branch block pattern. Possibly, because the right bundle is longer than the left, it is more subject to fatigue than the left. Normally, the refractory period shortens with tachycardia and lengthens with bradycardia. The same applies when the refractory periods are unequal. Therefore, when the preceding RR interval is long, the disparity between the refractory periods of the two bundles is accentuated and aberration is facilitated (the Ashman phenomenon) (Fig. 6.21).

The diagnosis of aberrant ventricular conduction has important therapeutic implications because it is usually mistaken for ventricular tachycardia. When P waves can be identified preceding the bizarre QRS complexes then the arrhythmia is supraventricular tachycardia with aberration; when the P waves are unrelated, or dissociated from the QRS complexes, the diagnosis is ventricular tachycardia. However, ventricular tachycardia may be accompanied by retrograde conduction to the atria and it is thus impossible to determine whether the P wave precedes or follows the QRS complex.

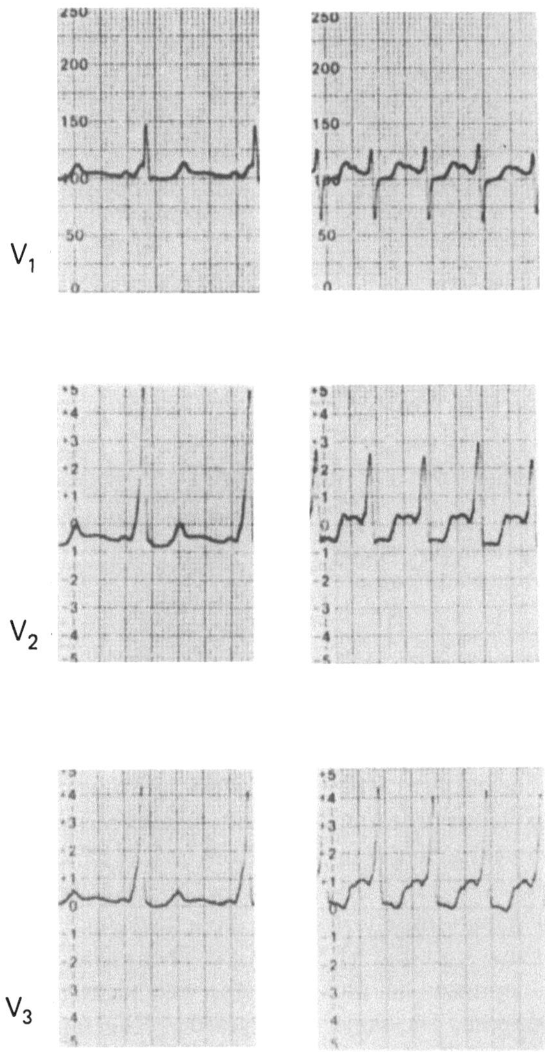

FIGURE 6.20. False-positive stress test in Wolff–Parkinsons–White syndrome. (A) The typical short PR interval and slurring of the QRS complex produced by the delta wave. (B) Progressive striking depression of the ST segment during exercise suggestive of ischemia; coronary angiograms were normal.

The configuration of the QRS complex itself may aid in the diagnosis: since most cases of aberrant ventricular conduction are the result of a partial right bundle branch block, the initial QRS vector will be the same during normal conduction and during aberration, whereas in ventricular tachycardia the initial vectors are grossly distorted. A certain diagnosis of ventricular tachycardia may be made when a fusion beat is identified. A fusion beat is produced by simultaneous activation of the ventricles by a supraventricular and ventricular impulse; the configuration of the QRS complex of a fusion beat thus has components of a normally conducted supraventricular beat and that of a pure ectopic beat.

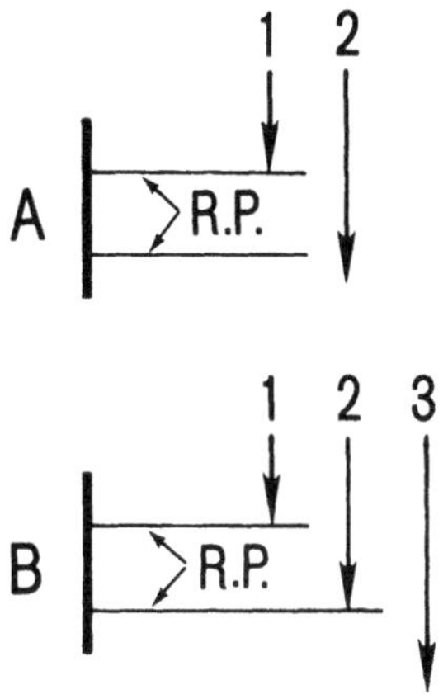

FIGURE 6.21. The mechanism of phasic aberrant ventricular conduction. (A) When the refractory periods of both bundles are equal impulse 1 is premature and blocked, whereas 2 is conducted normally. (B) Where the refractory periods are unequal, impulse 1 is premature and blocked whereas impulse 2 finds one bundle refractory and the other recovered the impulse is therefore conducted with a bundle branch block pattern; impulse 3 is conducted normally. Modified, with permission, from L. Shamroth and E. Chesler, Br Heart J 2:219, 1963.

The S_1, S_2, S_3 Syndrome

Late depolarization of the crista supraventricularis in the right ventricle produces deep S waves in the three standard lead and a large R wave in lead AVR; this is known as the $S_1S_2S_3$ syndrome. The syndrome may be associated with right ventricular hypertrophy but is also seen in people without evidence of cardiac disease. Occasionally it is associated with myocardial infarction, but there will always be other evidence such as ST segment, T wave changes, and the presence of pathologic Q waves.

Left Ventricular Hypertrophy

As the left ventricular muscle mass increases, the time taken for depolarization to progress from the endocardium to the epicardium increases. This results in an increase in the QRS voltage, widening of the QRS complex, and delay in onset of the intrinsicoid deflection (the time taken from the onset of the Q wave to the peak of the R wave). Abnormalities of repolarization are also manifest in the ST segment and the T waves. The width of the QRS complex is usually 0.08 to 0.11 seconds and rarely longer in the absence of bundle branch block. The intrinsicoid deflection is delayed to greater than 0.05 seconds in leads V_5 and V_6.

The voltage changes are characterized by deep S waves in the right precordial leads and tall R waves in the left precordial leads (e.g., the sum of S in $V_1 + R$ in $V_5/V_6 = 35$ mm or more, RV_5 or V_6 greater than 26 mm, AVL more than 11 mm, and AVF more than 20 mm) (Fig. 6.22). These criteria, however, lose specificity as they increase in sensitivity (i.e., these changes will detect most, but not all, patients who have left ventricular hypertrophy).

The overlap between normal and abnormal is particularly evident in young people and patients with thin chests and chest wall deformity. However, emphysema and a large chest cage artificially reduce the QRS voltage. ST-segment depression commencing below the isoelectric line, proceeding in a convex upward direction, and associated with inversion of the T wave adds specificity to increased QRS voltage, but false positives may be a result of digitalis, ischemia, or myocardial damage. Prolongation of the intrinsicoid deflection beyond 5 msec is not of great practical help because these changes are not commonly observed in left ventricular hypertrophy without total lengthening of the QRS duration. Left axis deviation (left anterior hemiblock) cannot be used as a criteria for left ventricular hypertrophy. In the absence of subendocardial fibrosis, hypertrophy alone does not produce left anterior hemiblock. The presence of left atrial enlargement in association with voltage and ST–T changes suggestive of left ventricular hypertrophy is supportive evidence.

Right Ventricular Hypertrophy

In well-marked examples, the right ventricular surface leads show signs of right ventricular hypertrophy, producing changes in the QRS

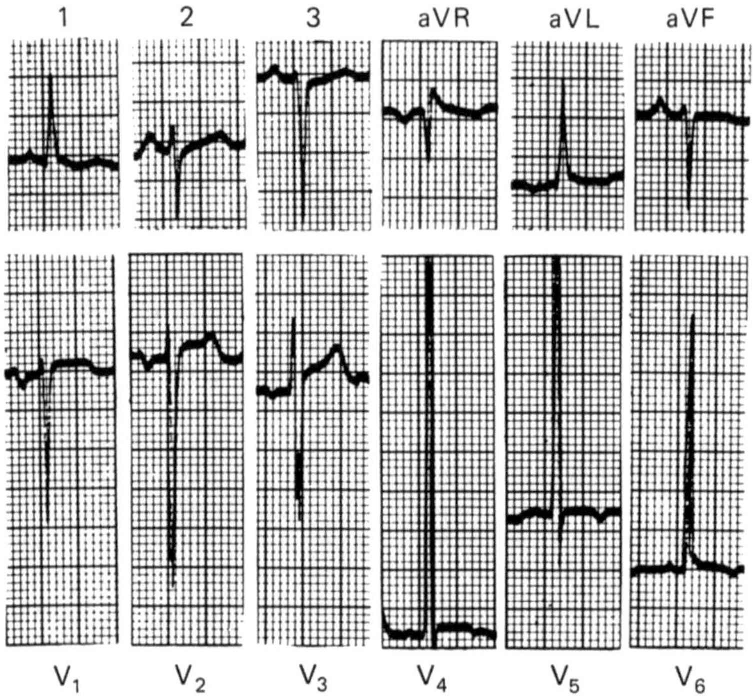

FIGURE 6.22. Electrocardiogram showing left ventricular hypertrophy, left atrial enlargement, and left anterior hemiblock (see text).

complex, the ST segments, and the T waves. The R/S ratio, which is normally 1/3, is reversed over the right precordial leads (Fig. 6.23). The following criteria are generally used:

1. Reversal of the ratio of R/S in V_1–V_6. In Vl the R wave is abnormally large relative to the S wave (R/S = more than 1) and is often slurred. The R/S ratio diminishes from V_1 to V_6, but the S wave remains dominant in V_6. A predominant R wave in AVR is confirmatory evidence. A small Q wave may be present in lead V_1 with severe right ventricular hypertrophy, particularly when there is tricuspid insufficiency.
2. ST-segment depression and T wave inversion in leads V_1 to V_3, or rarely further to the left.
3. Right axis deviation beyond +110°.
4. Incomplete or even complete right bundle branch block may be due to right ventricular hypertrophy, particularly with diastolic overload and hypertrophy of the cristus supraventricularis.
5. Right atrial enlargement may provide ancillary evidence.

The electrocardiographic diagnosis of right ventricular hypertrophy in childhood has good specificity and sensitivity. In adults, however, with similar degrees of right ventricular hypertrophy, these patterns are not as commonly observed.

Biventricular Hypertrophy

In children with congenital heart disease the presence of left and right ventricular hypertrophy may be recognized electrocardiographically when the features demonstrating hypertrophy of each ventricle are present. Equiphasic complexes over the midprecordial lead (R wave = S wave) is a common finding. The recognition of biventricular hypertrophy is more difficult in the adult where the changes of right ventricular hypertrophy are frequently overshadowed by those of left ventricular hypertrophy.

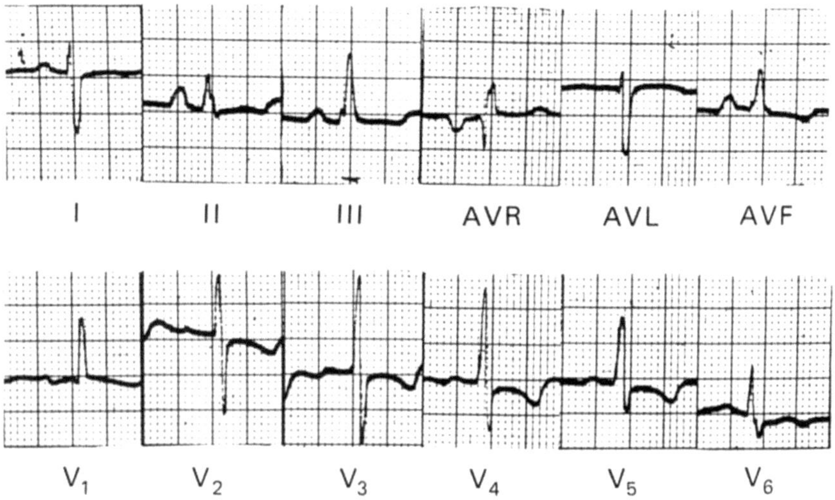

FIGURE 6.23. The electrocardiogram in right ventricular hypertrophy showing a dominant R wave in lead V_1. There is also right axis deviation and P pulmonale (lead II).

The Electrocardiogram in Ischemic Heart Disease

The electrocardiogram has its greatest use in the detection of ischemic heart disease. Alterations in the QRS, ST, and T waves provide evidence of transient or permanent myocardial damage, the degree of damage, and the extent of muscle involved. These changes may be localized, and for this reason at least 12 leads are routinely used. For example, the standard leads may be completely normal, but changes appear in the anterior chest leads only.

Myocardial Infarction

The electrocardiographic hallmark is the pathologic Q wave, which is a result of myocardial necrosis. Electrodes facing such an area detect forces moving away the from necrotic area.

Myocardial Injury

This is represented electrocardiographically by ST-segment elevation in leads facing such an area, and ST-segment depression in leads facing the adjacent uninjured area. Myocardial injury usually involves the epicardium; therefore leads facing such an area show ST-segment elevation, whereas endocardial leads show ST-segment depression.

Myocardial Ischemia

When the subendocardial region is ischemic during an episode of angina pectoris or during an effort test, precordial leads facing the epicardium show ST-segment depression. Myocardial ischemia is manifested by T wave inversion in leads facing such an area.

The earliest electrocardiographic changes following myocardial infarction are observed within a few hours and consist of an upward sloping ST segment, which merges with the T wave. The T wave becomes tall and may even exceed the height of the R wave (Fig. 6.24). Such tall T waves may be the most impressive of the early changes observed in myocardial infarction. These early "hyperacute" changes of myocardial infarction are evanescent and thus are not frequently observed. Usually when the patient is first seen, more typical electrocardiographic changes are

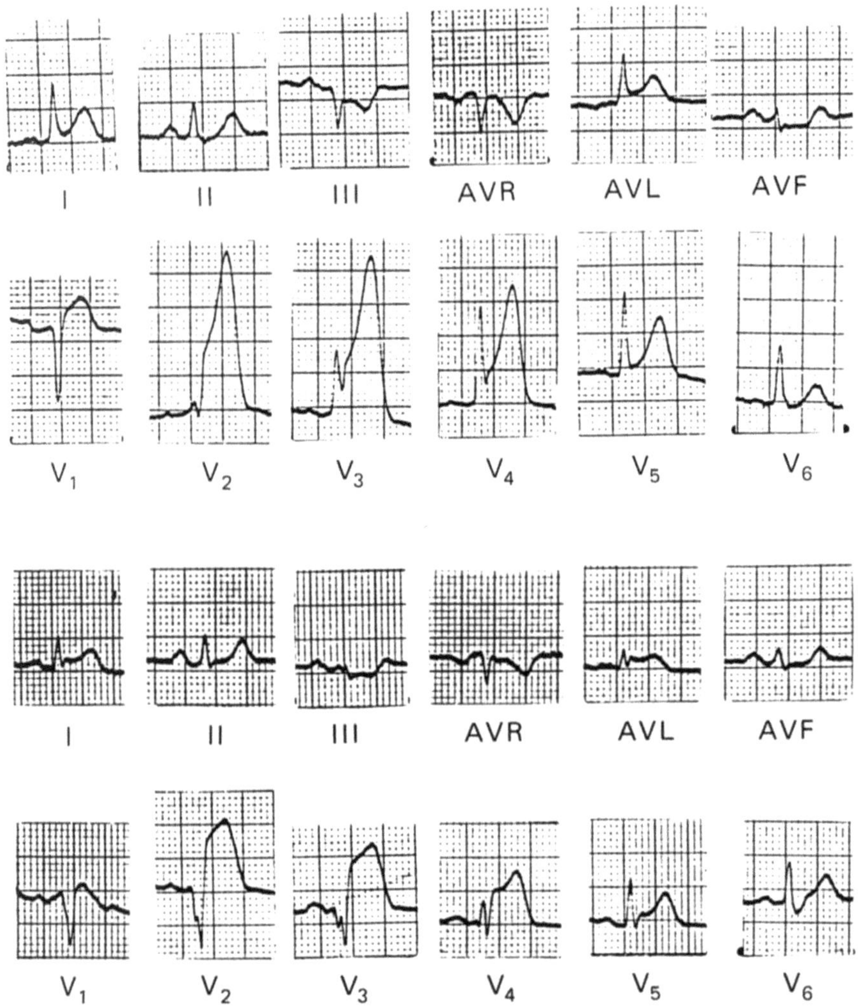

FIGURE 6.24. Electrocardiogram (top) of hyperacute myocardial infarction progressing to transmural myocardial infarction (bottom).

present. These include the presence of a pathologic Q wave and elevated ST segment, which persist for a few hours or days before returning to the isoelectric position. Later, the T waves become inverted and may persist in this way for a period of weeks or months before returning to normal. They may, however, remain abnormal indefinitely.

When the above sequence of changes as observed they are absolutely specific for the diagnosis of myocardial infarction. In the absence of Q waves, however, the ST–T changes are less specific because of the difficulty in distinguishing myocardial infarction from pericarditis and, less commonly, myocarditis.

Localization of the Infarction

Anterior Infarction

The infarction can be localized as follows (Figs. 6.25–6.29): Diagnostic QRST changes are seen

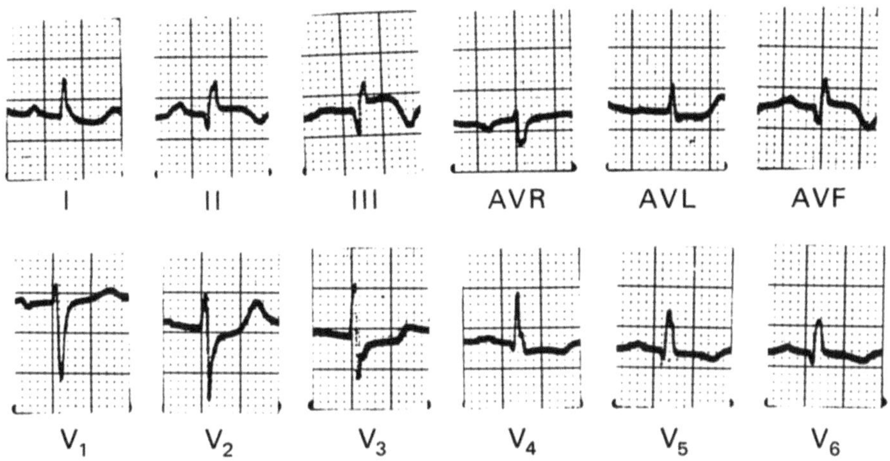

FIGURE 6.25. Electrocardiogram in inferolateral myocardial infarction showing pathological Q waves in leads II, III, AVF, and V_5 and V_6.

in the precordial leads, AVL, and standard lead I. The changes may be extensive, involving almost all of these leads, or may be more restricted. In the latter event the infarct may be *anteroseptal*—leads V_1–V_4, AVL, and lead I; *anterolateral*—leads V_4–V_6, AVL, and standard I; or *strictly anterior*—leads V_1–V_4 with normal limb leads.

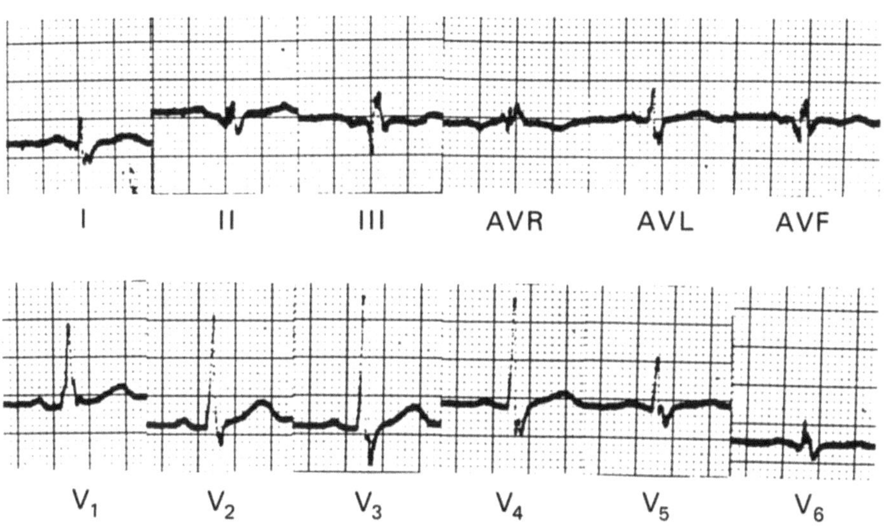

FIGURE 6.26. Electrocardiogram in inferolateral and true posterior myocardial infarction; evidence for the latter is the dominant R wave in lead V_1.

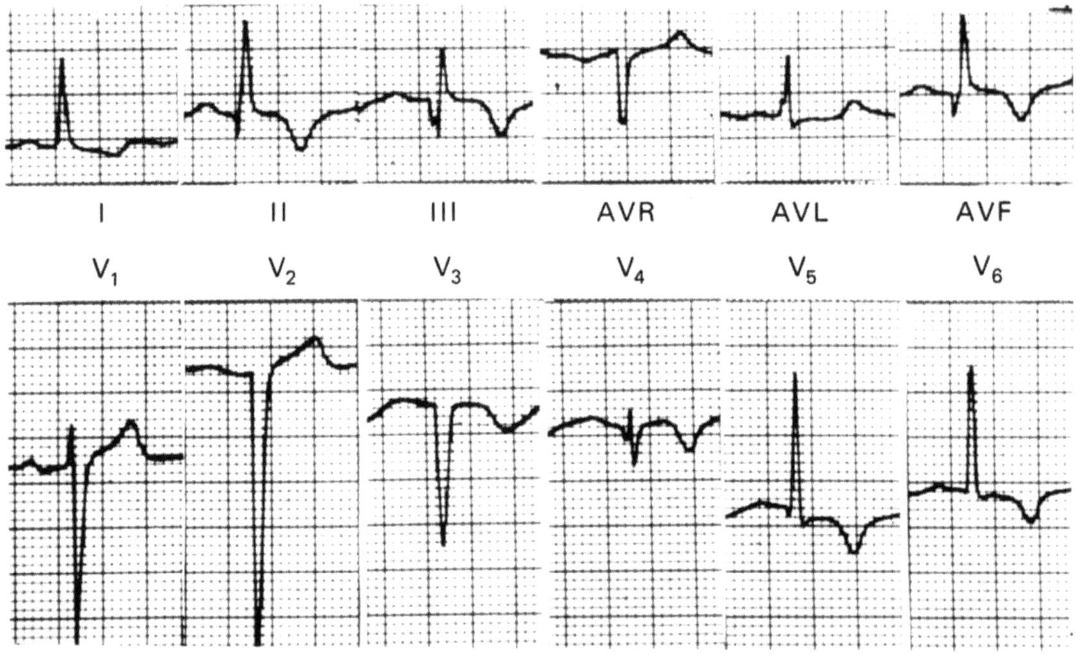

FIGURE 6.27. Electrocardiogram in old anterior myocardial infarction showing QS waves in lead V_2 and V_3 and a pathololgical Q wave in lead V_4. There is also evidence of old inferior infarction with pathological Q waves in leads II, III, and AVF. QRS axis is normal.

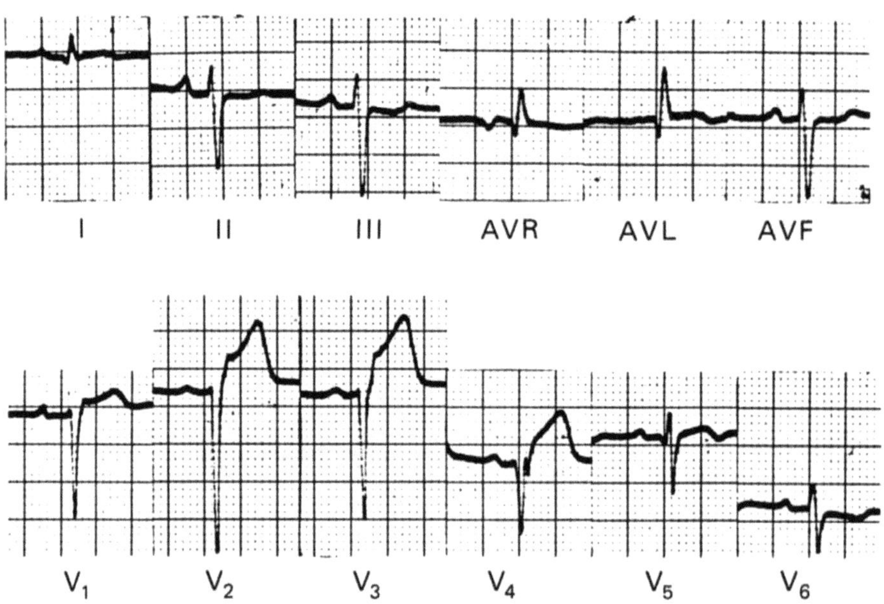

FIGURE 6.28. Electrocardiogram in old anterior myocardial infarction and left anterior hemiblock (QRS axis −60°).

Lateral Infarction

This is characterized by abnormal Q waves in leads I, AVL, V_5, and V_6.

Diaphragmatic (Inferior) Infarction

Changes are in standard leads II and III and AVF. When leads V_5 and V_6 are additionally affected the infarct is *inferolateral*.

True Posterior Infarction

Tall slurred waves in V_1 and V_2, similar to that of right ventricular hypertrophy, are seen. The R wave in V_1 is usually 40 msec wide and is a result of unopposed anteriorly directed vectors.

Right Ventricular Infarction

Among patients with inferior myocardial infarction, the electrocardiogram may provide evidence of right ventricular involvement. Elevation of the ST segments in the right precordial leads is a highly sensitive and specific sign (Fig. 6.29).

Pathologic Q Waves

These waves are at least 40 msec in duration, and their depth should exceed 25% of the height of the associated R wave.

Fully developed Q waves disappear in at least 20% of cases of myocardial infarction, or become smaller with the passage of time. Additional difficulty may arise in interpretation of Q waves in the presence of left ventricular hypertrophy, and incomplete left bundle branch block, which may produce QS waves in leads V_1–V_4. Similar changes may be seen in the Wolff–Parkinson–White syndrome and in idiopathic hypertrophic subaortic stenosis.

In the presence of right bundle branch block a pathologic Q wave is significant because this conduction abnormality interferes with the terminal vectors. However, when there is left bundle branch block the diagnosis of myocardial infarction is extremely difficult since QS waves are frequently present in the leads V_1–V_3. Persistent ST-segment elevation for months or years following myocardial infarction suggests the diagnosis of cardiac aneurysm.

Pericarditis

In the acute form, epicardial injury produces upward displacement of the ST segment in all three limb leads. This contrasts with the current of injury of infarction where lead III is the reciprocal of lead I. Similarly, upward ST-segment displacement is present in V_2–V_6 but rarely exceeds 4 or 5 mm. The T waves remain upright since myocardial ischemia is absent. Lead AVR, which faces the cavity of the heart, records reciprocal depression of the ST segment. Depression of the P–R interval is an early finding (Fig. 6.30).

In pericardial effusion and constrictive pericarditis, low voltage is commonly found in the limb leads and there is also reduction in voltage in the precordial leads. The P waves are normal. The T waves are flat or inverted in all surface leads and are a result of pericardial thickening or surrounding fluid. The same findings may be observed in myxedema (Fig. 6.31).

Effects of Drugs and Electrolyte Disturbances

The effects of the antidysrhythmic drugs are described in Chapter 8.

Digitalis

One of the first signs of digitalis activity is its effect on the T wave, which becomes flattened and then inverted as the dosage increases. ST-segment depression need not accompany T wave flattening but nearly always accompanies T wave inversion.

Characteristically, the effect of digitalis is to produce a gradual downward slope of the ST segment from the J point with a sharp terminal rise producing an appearance of a mirror-image correction mark; digitalis shortens the QT interval. Patients with underlying cardiac disease show a greater effect from digitalis

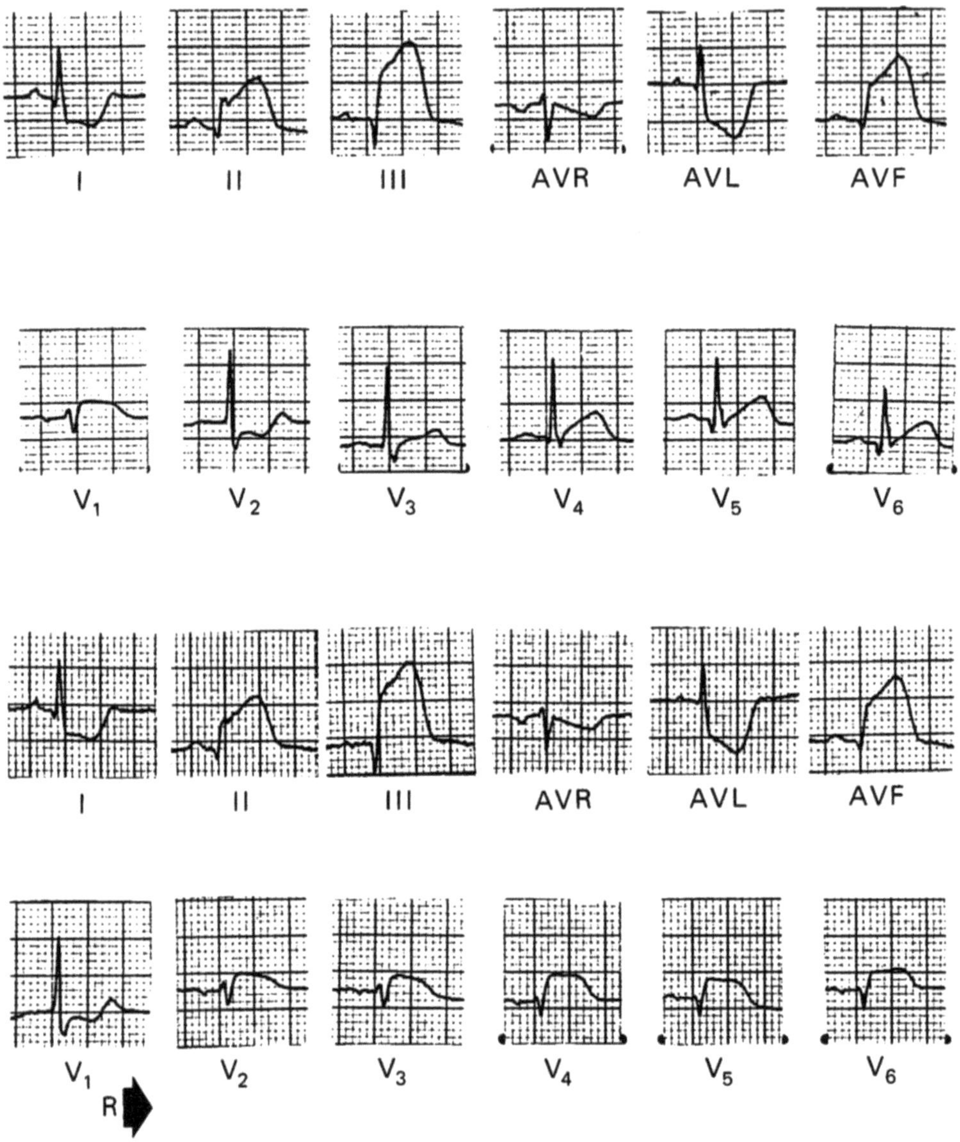

FIGURE 6.29. (Top) Electrocardiogram in acute inferior and right ventricular infarction—precordial leads in usual position. (Bottom) Precordial leads recorded to right of sternum showing ST segment elevation highly suggestive of RV infarction.

than normals, but the changes cannot be quantitated with the dosage. Toxicity may be associated with a normal tracing, whereas marked digitalis effect may occur with subtherapeutic doses. The effect of digitalis on the ST segment is usually best observed in those leads exhibiting the tallest R wave.

Hypokalemia

Hypokalemia produces increased amplitude and prolongation of the U wave (Fig. 6.32). The T waves are flattened or inverted. In severe hypokalemia the electrocardiogram superficially resembles a very long QT inter-

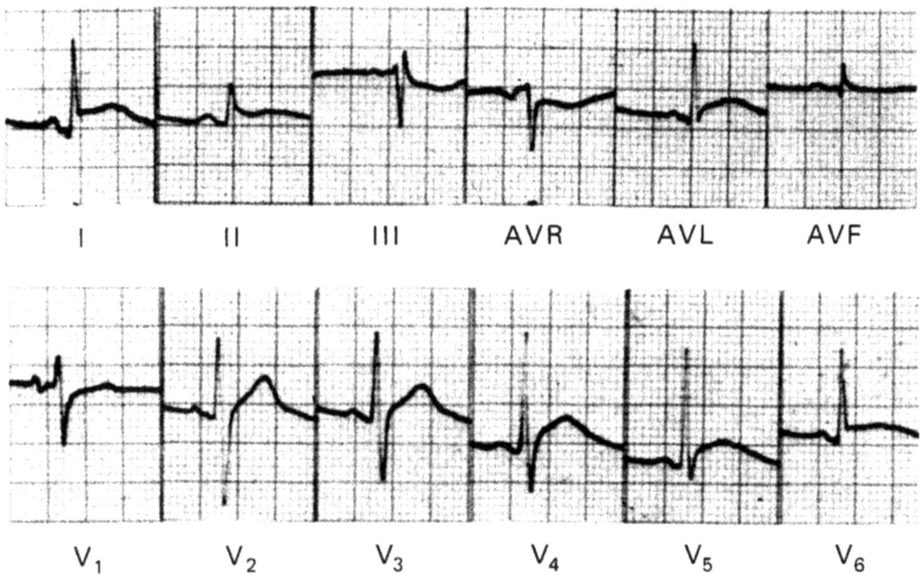

FIGURE 6.30. The electrocardiogram in acute pericarditis showing ST segment elevation in all the leads except lead AVR, which shows reciprocal depression (see text).

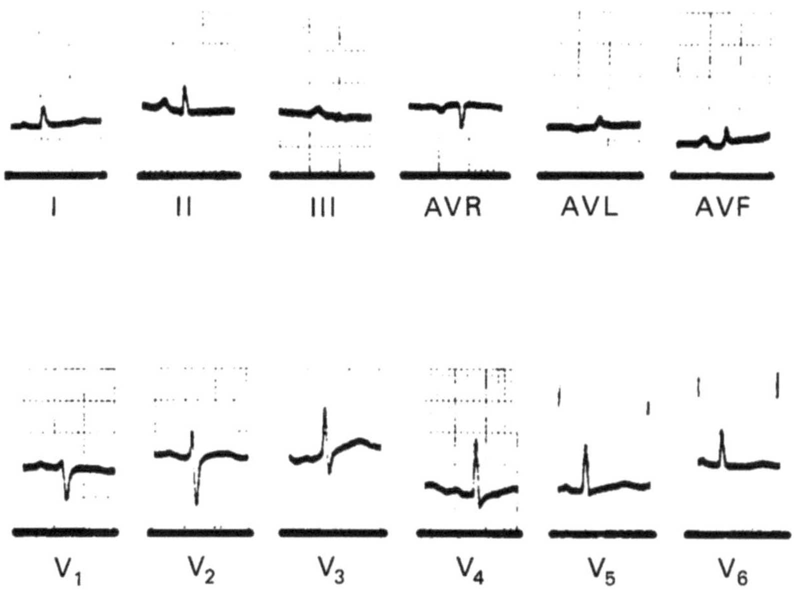

FIGURE 6.31. The electrocardiogram in constrictive pericarditis showing generalized low voltage and T wave flattening.

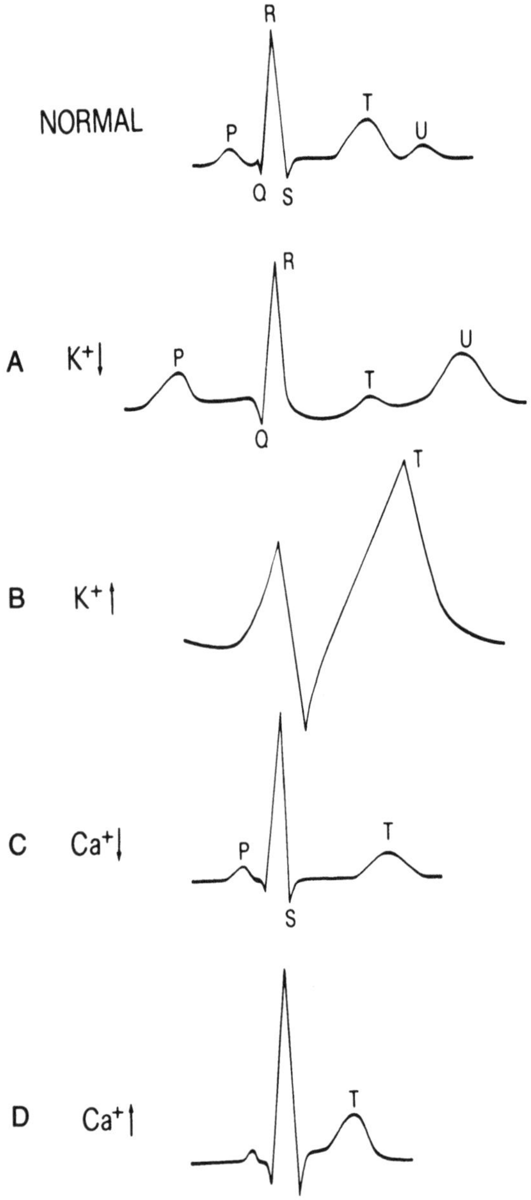

FIGURE 6.32. The electrocardiographic abnormalities in hypokalemia (A), hyperkalemia (B), hypocalcemia (C), and hypercalcemia (D).

val. The latter is, in fact, normal, and the appearance is due to the prominent U wave that is mistaken for a T wave. Additionally, flattening of the ST segment of 0.5 mm or more is not infrequently encountered. The appearance of electrocardiographic evidence of hypokalemia may be the forerunner of serious ventricular arrhythmias, particularly in patients who are receiving digitalis.

Hyperkalemia

One of the first manifestations of hyperkalemia is peaking or tenting of the T waves. In leads with positive T waves these become more positive and in those in which the T waves are inverted these become less inverted or even positive. As the serum potassium rises, the P waves decrease in voltage and widen, and the heart rate slows. The QRS widens gradually and blends with the tall peaked T waves.

Hypocalcemia

Hypocalcemia produces a long QT interval with small T waves and the tracing must be carefully distinguished from hypokalemia (Fig. 6.33).

Hypercalcemia

Hypercalcemia shortens the QT interval but does not disturb the T wave. The PR interval may be prolonged.

The electrocardiographic diagnosis of electrolyte disturbances is made difficult by the occurrence of similar changes in other conditions. QRS widening similar to that of hyperkalemia occurs in quinidine and procainamide toxicity. Also QT abnormalities may occur in patients with cerebral vascular disease and mimic those of hypocalcemia. Peaked T waves resembling hyperkalemia may be observed as a normal variant.

Exercise Electrocardiography in the Diagnosis of Coronary Artery Disease

This subject is also discussed in relation to the management of patients with ischemic heart disease (Chapter 17). The usual indications for exercise stress testing are to (1) diagnose the presence of coronary artery disease, (2) determine prognosis, (3) assess functional capacity, and (4) assess affects of treatment (medical, surgical or PTCA).

For many years stress testing was performed as the two-step test of Master. This test does

A

B

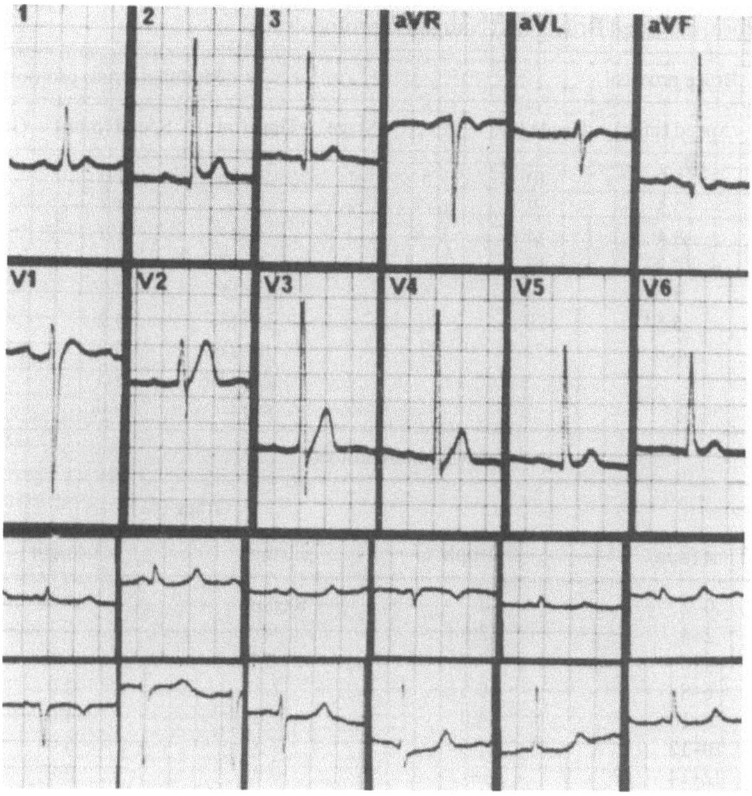

FIGURE 6.33. (A) The electrocardiogram in hypercalcemia showing a short QT interval and (B) in hypocalcemia showing a long QT interval.

not provide monitoring during the exercise period and therefore many of the important changes might have disappeared before recording of the ECG during the recovery stage. The Master's two-step exercise test has now been replaced in most institutions by the motorized treadmill. Additional advantages of the treadmill are the ability to adjust the speed and grade of walking to cater to individual subjects. The safety of the procedure is related to the experience of the physician supervising the test rather than the maintenance of rigid goals aimed at the patient reaching 85 or 100% of the predicted maximum heart rate. In experienced hands, the mortality is less than 0.01% and the morbidity less than 0.2%.

Technique

The procedure for stress testing includes continuous ECG monitoring, and facility to record the ECG and monitor the blood pressure during the test. A defibrillator and full resuscitative equipment should be available.

At least three EKG leads should be continuously monitored before, during each stage, and after the test until the heart rate and blood pressure have returned to normal. The most frequently used combination consists of leads V_2, V_5, and AVF. However, a 12-lead system is preferable since it not only increases the sensitivity of the test but also provides information about severity when ischemic chances are recorded in many leads.

Tracings should be recorded supine, standing, before and after hyperventilation to detect artifact related to these maneuvers.

Most protocols on a motorized treadmill follow a standardized test. For general testing, the Bruce Test in the most popular. Following myocardial infarction or cardiac surgery or to test deconditioned individuals, the modified

TABLE 6.1. The Bruce, modified Bruce, and Naughton protocols.

Bruce protocol					Modified Bruce protocol				
Stage	Time (min)	Speed (mph)	Grade (%)	mets	Stage	Time (min)	Speed (mph)	Grade (%)	mets
1	0–3	1.7	10	5	1	0–3	1.7	0	<5
2	3–6	2.5	12	6–7	2	3–6	1.7	5	<5
3	6–9	3.4	14	8–9	3	6–9	1.7	10	5
4	9–12	4.2	16	12–13	4	9–12	2.5	12	6–7
5	12–15	5.0	18	16	5	12–15	3.4	14	8–9
6	15–18	5.5	20	20	6	15–18	4.2	16	12–13
7	18–21	6.0	22	23	7	18–21	5.0	18	16
					8	21–24	5.5	20	20
					9	24–27	6.0	22	23

Naughton protocol					
		Grade (%)			
Stage	Time (min)	2.0 mph	3.0 mph	3.4 mph	mets
1	0–2	0	Resting	—	1
2	2–4	3.5	—	—	2
3	4–6	7.0	0	—	3
4	6–8	10.5	2.5	2.0	4
5	8–10	14.0	5.0	4.0	5
6	10–12	17.5	7.5	6.0	6
7	12–14	—	10.0	8.0	7
8	14–16	—	12.5	10.0	8
9	16–18	—	15.0	12.0	9
10	18–20	—	17.5	14.0	10
11	20–22	—	20.0	16.0	11
12	22–24	—	22.5	18.0	12

Bruce or Naughton protocols are preferred (Table 6.1).

Contraindications to Testing

1. Absolute (because of risk to patient).
   a. Unstable angina.
   b. Second- or third-degree heart block.
   c. Uncontrolled tachyarrhythmias.
   d. Severe aortic stenosis.
   e. Congestive cardiac failure.
   f. Uncontrolled hypertension.
2. Relative (difficulty in interpretation because of false positives).
   a. Digitalis administration.
   b. Hypokalemia.
   c. WPW syndrome.
   d. Left bundle branch block
   e. Left ventricular hypertrophy with or without baseline ST–T segment abnormalities.

Discontinuation of the Test

The patient is observed closely as exercise proceeds and constantly questioned about chest pain. The test should be discontinued (1) with the onset of arrhythmias such as atrial tachycardia, atrial fibrillation, heart block, salvoes of premature ventricular contractions, or ventricular tachycardia, (2) with a fall in the systolic blood pressure and pulse rate while exercise is in progress, (3) with the onset of severe dyspnea, fatigue, sweating, pallor, or faintness and (4) with the attainment by the subject of the maximum predicted heart rate.

Interpretation of the Test

As exercise proceeds a number of normal electrocardiographic changes occur: (1) the PR interval becomes shorter; (2) the wave of atrial repolarization increases, thus depressing the PR junction; and this may extend through the QRS complex causing factitious ST-segment depression; (3) the P wave becomes taller; (4) the total amplitude of the QRST complex becomes smaller; and (5) the QT interval shortens.

Evaluating a Positive Test

Depression of the ST segment is measured from the PQ segment, which is regarded as the baseline. J point (junction between the S wave and the ST segment) depression is frequently present in normal subjects. When the ST segment is depressed 1.0 mm or more below the baseline PQ level at a point 80 msec after the J point, the test is considered to be positive. The degree of depression considered to be normal is moot, but most observers would accept a figure of 1.0 mm or more. When figures in excess of this are used, the sensitivity drops but the specificity rises sharply.

Evaluating Severity and Prognosis of Coronary Artery Disease

The presence of severe disease and a poor prognosis is correlated with an "early" positive test. "Early" refers both to the duration of exercise and the double product attained at the time the test is stopped. Of these, the double product is the more reliable. (The double product is the multiple of heart rate and peak systolic blood pressure and is an index of myocardial oxygen consumption.) A positive test at a double product of less than 14,000 indicates severe disease, provided the chronotropic response to exercise has not been blocked by drugs (beta and calcium channel blockers).

Generally, this will correspond to 5 to 6 mets or less of exercise, provided the patient is not severely deconditioned. (A met unit is equivalent to an oxygen uptake of 3.5 ml O_2 kg/min.) Physically active men may have capacities of 12 mets and athletes more than 15 mets.

The predictive value of the test for severe disease is strongest when (1) it is positive at a low double product, (2) the ST-segment depression is more than 2 mm, (3) the ST-segment depression presents well into the recovery period, (4) ST-segment depression occurs in several leads, (5) exercise is accompanied by angina, pallor, sweating, or weakness, (6) blood pressure drops 20 mm Hg or more, and (7) there are salvoes of ventricular ectopic beats or runs of ventricular tachycardia.

Correlation Between Exercise Tests and Presence or Absence of Coronary Artery Disease

The ability of this test to identify patients with angiographically proven disease is not perfect. The correlations are expressed by the following epidemiological terms:

$$\text{Sensitivity (\%)} = \frac{\text{True positives}}{\text{Total with disease}}$$

$$\text{Specificity (\%)} = \frac{\text{True negatives}}{\text{Total without disease}}$$

$$\text{Predictive value (\%)} = \frac{\text{True positives}}{\text{True positives and false positives}}$$

$$\text{Predictive value (\%)} = \frac{\text{True negatives}}{\text{True negatives and false negatives}}$$

Sensitivity expresses the reliability of a test to identify patients with disease, whereas *specificity* expresses the reliability of a test to identify patients who do not have disease.

Sensitivity increases when the standard for a positive test is relaxed (1 mm rather than 3 mm ST-segment depression), but the specificity decreases. One of the major determinants of the predictive accuracy in the prevalence of disease in a test population. This is referred to as Bayes theorem, which states that the likelihood of disease after a diagnostic test must take into account the pretest risk for the population group being tested.

Because of these factors, exercise testing for coronary disease has marked limitations in diagnosis under certain conditions. In apparently healthy people the test has a sensitivity of approximately 50% and a specificity of 90%. Therefore, the test is of least value in testing population in which the prevalence is low. In young, asymptomatic people without coronary disease the yield of true positives will be outnumbered by the large number of false positives (i.e., the predictive value is low). The predictive value will also be low when there is atypical chest pain, so there is little value in testing under these circumstances. This is important in avoiding iatrogenic anxiety in healthy people. Also, ordering exercise tests in asymptomatic people as a "screening test" before surgery may have similar implications.

Additional Reading

Beckwith JR: "Grant's Clinical Electrocardiography." McGraw-Hill, New York, 1971.

Ellestad MH: "Stress Testing. Principles and Practice." Davis, Philadelphia, 1979.

Grant RP: "Clinical Electrocardiography." McGraw-Hill, New York, 1957.

Marriott HJL: "Practical Electrocardiography." Williams & Wilkins, Baltimore, 1952.

Rosenbaum MB, Elizari MV, Lazzari JO: "The Hemiblocks." Tampa Tracings, Oldsmar, 1970.

Schamroth L: "An Introduction to Electrocardiography." Blackwell Scientific, Oxford, 1976.

Schamroth L: "The 12-Lead Electrocardiogram." Blackwell Scientific, Oxford, 1989.

7
Other Methods of Investigation

Cardiac Catheterization and Angiography

In a text of this kind, mention can only be made of the indications, risks, and basic information to be obtained from these highly complicated techniques. Even in the most adequately equipped laboratory, staffed by highly trained operators, the basic question to be satisfied is that the information to be obtained from a contemplated procedure justifies the risks.

Indications

In the field of congenital heart disease, catheterization is indicated as an emergency procedure in all cyanotic neonates and those suffering from congestive cardiac failure. In older patients with congenital heart disease, catheterization is necessary for the precise delineation of the anatomy and hemodynamics of complicated malformations. For example, the selection of patients for closure of a ventricular septal defect complicated by pulmonary hypertension will be determined by measurement of shunt flows and measurement of the pulmonary vascular resistance. Catheterization is also indicated when clinical examination supported by all available noninvasive techniques has failed to resolve the question of whether a murmur is of pathological significance.

In many instances of valve disease surgery may be undertaken on the basis of clinical findings alone. For example, many surgeons justifiably perform mitral valvulotomy when clinical examination, fluoroscopy, and echocardiography indicate tight pliable mitral stenosis. Catheterization is indicated, however, when the patient's symptoms do not match the clinical assessment of severity of any valve lesion, and particularly when multivalvular disease is present. Under the latter circumstances, clinical evaluation of the severity of individual valve involvement and assessment of left ventricular function may be extremely difficult.

Selective *coronary angiography* is indicated in patients with angina pectoris intractable to adequate medical therapy and in those patients with an early markedly positive exercise test that suggests the possibility of critical left main stem disease. Coronary angiography plays an important role in delineating the problem of atypical chest pain and an abnormal electrocardiogram, when the patient's livelihood, psychological status, and insurability are at stake.

Risks

The risks are greatest in the *neonate* and are directly proportional to the skill of the operating team. In the best possible hands, the risk of mortality is 3 per 2000 procedures, but this will rise progressively with inexperience of the operators. For coronary angiography the risk should be less than 0.2%. The factors responsible for mortality include perforation of the heart or great vessels, arrhythmias, and myocardial infarction; other events resulting in mortality include arterial thrombosis, systemic embolism, knotting of catheters, and allergic reactions to iodine containing contrast material.

Right Heart Catheterization

Access to the *right side of the heart* is usually by cutdown on an arm vein or percutaneously from the leg using the femoral vein. In babies, the saphenous vein is used. Under fluoroscopy, pressures and oxygen saturations are recorded successively in the right atrium, right ventricle, and pulmonary arteries. The "wedge" pressure is recorded when the catheter is advanced firmly into a distal branch of the pulmonary artery; it then records the indirect left atrial pressure (PCWP). The normal pressures and saturations on the right side of the heart are as follows:

Site	Pressure (range) (mm Hg)	Oxygen saturation (%) (average)
Right atrium	−1 to +8 (mean)	75
Right ventricle	15–30/0–8	75
Pulmonary artery	15–30/5–16 (mean 10–22)	75
Wedge (PCWP)	6–15 (mean)	95
Left ventricle	90–140/4–15	95

Right heart catheterization detects the presence of a left-to-right shunt by a "step up" (more than 5%) in oxygen saturation in one of the chambers. It also documents the presence or absence of right heart failure, pulmonary hypertension, and gradients across the tricuspid or pulmonary valves (via pullback), and indirectly measures the left ventricular filling pressure.

Cardiac Output

While the catheter is in the pulmonary artery, the systemic pressure and saturation are obtained by needle puncture of an artery, or if left heart catheterization is to be performed, from a catheter introduced into the aorta by cutdown from the brachial artery, or percutaneously from the femoral artery. The oxygen content of mixed venous blood in the pulmonary artery and that of systemic blood is measured by the Van Slyke technique while the oxygen consumption is being measured. The cardiac output is then calculated by the Fick principle:

$$\text{Cardiac output (liters/min)} = \frac{\text{Oxygen consumption (ml/min)}}{\text{Arteriovenous oxygen difference (ml/liter)}}$$

cardiac output may also be measured by the indicator dye dilution technique.

Calculations of Resistance

$$\text{Pulmonary vascular resistance} = \frac{\text{Mean PA pressure} - \text{Mean LA pressure}}{\text{Pulmonary blood flow (Liters/min)}}$$

$$\text{Systemic vascular resistance} = \frac{\text{Mean arterial pressure} - \text{Mean RA pressure}}{\text{Systemic blood flow (Liters/min)}}$$

The pulmonary and systemic vascular resistance may be expressed in simple units (Wood) or in dyn/cm^2 by multiplying by 80. The normal cardiac output is 4–6 liters/min. When corrected for body surface area, the cardiac index is obtained, and this is normally 2.5–3.5 liters/min/m^2. The normal pulmonary vascular resistance is 1 unit and the systemic vascular resistance is 20 units.

Calculation of Shunts

A *left-to-right shunt* is calculated as the difference between pulmonary and systemic blood flow where

$$\text{Pulmonary blood flow} = \frac{\text{Oxygen consumption}}{\text{Systemic oxygen content} - \text{pulmonary artery oxygen content}}$$

and

Systemic blood flow

$$= \frac{\text{Oxygen consumption}}{\text{Systemic oxygen content} - \text{mixed venous oxygen content}}$$

A *right-to-left shunt* is calculated as the difference between systemic and pulmonary blood flow where

Pulmonary blood flow

$$= \frac{\text{Oxygen consumption}}{\text{Pulmonary vein oxygen content} - \text{Pulmonary arterial content}}$$

Systemic blood flow

$$= \frac{\text{Oxygen consumption}}{\text{Systemic oxygen content} - \text{Pulmonary arterial oxygen content}}$$

Measurement of the pulmonary blood flow and pulmonary vascular resistance is crucial in deciding whether to operate on patients with malformations associated with severe pulmonary arterial hypertension.

In general, for a favorable operative result the pulmonary to systemic blood flow should be at least 1.5 to 1 and the pulmonary vascular resistance less than 10 units/m^2. Lesser degrees of left-to-right shunting and a higher pulmonary vascular resistance are contraindicatations to operation.

Valve Areas

In the presence of semilunar or atrioventricular valve stenosis valve areas are calculated by the hydraulic formula of Gorlin where

Valve area

$$= \frac{\text{Cardiac output (ml/sec)}}{K \times \sqrt{\text{pressure gradient (mm Hg)}}}$$

It will be seen that calculations of valve area are critically related to measurement of the cardiac output, but much less so to the gradient. This is because the square root of a small variation between two measurements of a gradient will make an inconsequential difference. For example, a gradient of 20 mm across the aortic valve with a cardiac output of 6 liters/min is associated with mild aortic stenosis, whereas a similar gradient and a cardiac output of 2 liters/min indicates critical aortic stenosis.

Left Heart Catheterization

Access to the left heart is (1) retrograde across the aortic valve, (2) transseptal puncture of the atrial septum with a Brockenborough needle, (3) by transthoracic "stick" using a thin gauge needle, and (4) by crossing a foramen ovale from the right to the left atrium.

Left ventricular angiography is almost always selective (i.e., dye is injected directly into the chamber being studied). It may be performed using a large cut film that provides good anatomical detail, but at slow speed, or by cineangiography at much higher speeds. The technique provides details of the opacified chamber, and when performed biplane, demonstrates the relationship to other anatomical structures.

Left ventricular ejection fraction may be estimated as the

$$\frac{\text{end-systolic volume}}{\text{end-diastolic volume} - \text{end-systolic volume}}$$

and is normally 65% or more. In valvular heart disease angiograpy is used to establish the presence of regurgitation and grade its severity.

Coronary angiography is performed percutaneously from the leg (Judkins technique) or from the arm using a cutdown (Sones technique). Multiple injection in various views are made in both coronary arteries and for convenience a rotating cradle or rotating X-ray tube is used so that the patient is stationary.

Apexcardiography

The recording of precordial impulses may be performed by measuring *absolute* displacement at a point on the chest wall in relationship to a fixed reference point above the patient (*kinetocardiography*) or *relative* movement (*apexcardiography*) when the transducer is placed directly on the chest wall. The kinetocardiogram corresponds more closely to what is felt by the clinician.

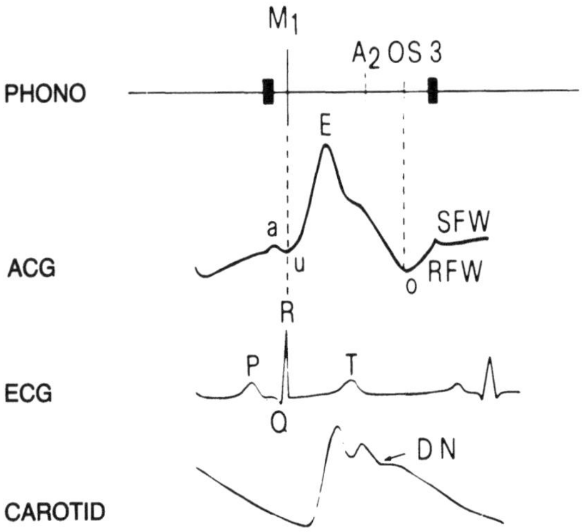

FIGURE 7.1. The normal apexcardiogram (ACG) with simultaneous phonocardiogram (phono) and carotid pulse tracing. SFW and RFW, slow and rapid filling waves respectively (see text).

These techniques provide useful corroboration of abnormal precordial impulses occurring with left and right ventricular pressure and flow overloads, and ischemic heart disease. Additionally, the apexcardiogram accurately reflects left-sided events of the cardiac cycle. As with phonocardiography, the technique requires meticulous attention to detail on the part of the operator and requires excellent equipment.

The *apexcardiogram* (Fig. 7.1) has the following features. The first upward deflection is the A wave produced by atrial contraction, which is normally less than 15% of the total apical displacement. It is accentuated in IHSS, hypertension, and aortic stenosis and corresponds to a loud fourth heart sound. Following descent of the A wave the first forward movement occurs at the U point, which signals very precisely the onset of isovolumic systole, corresponding with the initial low-frequency component of the first heart sound. The E point represents the maximum systolic peak, which is followed by a midsystolic descent reaching the O point, which signals the opening of the mitral valve (and opening snap). The O point is followed by the rapid filling wave and the slow filling wave; the angle between the latter two occurs at the time of the third heart sound. When diastolic flow is increased, as in aortic and mitral insufficiency, the rapid filling wave is peaked.

Phonocardiography

This technique finds its chief use in the elucidation of difficult auscultatory findings. Sounds should always be recorded with two microphones simultaneously with one placed at the base (to time A_2 and P_2) and the other at the apex. When recorded with a simultaneous electrocardiogram, apexcardiogram, and carotid pulse, accurate timing of sounds is possible.

The basal microphone should have a frequency around 300 cycles/sec to record the high-frequency sounds and the microphone at the apex should have the option of low-frequency sounds for middiastolic murmurs (40 cycles/sec) and high frequency range of 300 cycles/sec for high-pitched heart sounds and opening snaps.

Systolic Time Intervals

With phonocardiography and carotid pulse tracings the systolic time intervals may be recorded (Fig. 7.2). The intervals may also be recorded with the EKG and M-mode echocardiography of the aortic valve leaflets. These provide an assessment of left ventricular function.

The systolic time intervals consist of the left ventricular ejection time (LVET) and the preejection period (PEP). The LVET is the time between the upstroke and the dicrotic notch of the externally derived carotid pulse. The PEP is the time between the beginning of electrical activation of the heart and the opening of the aortic valve. Its length is mainly dependent on the isovolumic contraction time of the left ventricle. The PEP is obtained by measuring the Q to A_2 interval (electromechanical systole) and subtracting the LVET measured from the carotid pulse. This avoids the delay in pulse transmission when recording the external carotid pulse. The ratio of PEP/LVET

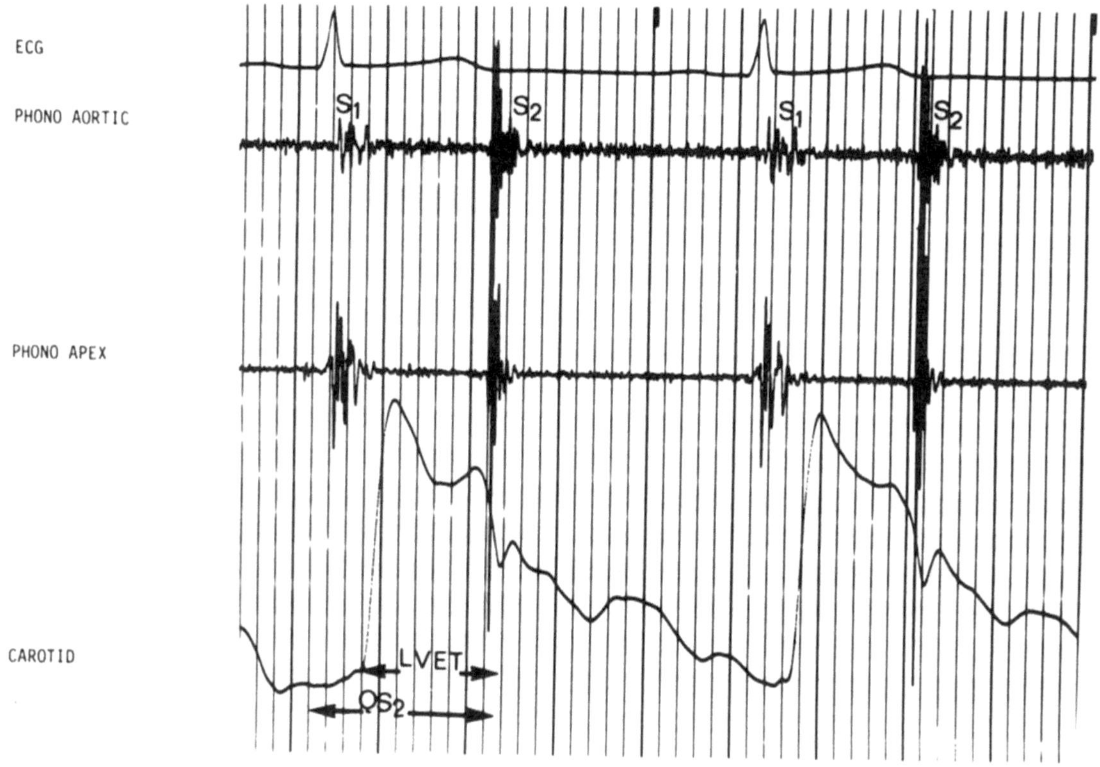

FIGURE 7.2. Technique for measuring systolic time intervals from the simultaneous ECG, phonocardiogram, and carotid pulse. The preejection period (PEP) is obtained by subtracting the measured left ventricular ejection time (LVET) from the Q to S_2 interval.

is affected by heart failure because the PEP is lengthened and the LVET is shortened. The lengthening of PEP is almost entirely a result of the diminished rate of rise of left ventricular pressure during isovolumic systole. The ratio of PEP/LVET is independent of the heart rate and the upper limit of normal is 0.38. The advantage of using the ratio PEP/LVET is that it can be used in a regression equation for estimating the ejection fraction in the formula E Fraction = 1.25 − (1.25 × PEP/LVET).

Measurement of the left ventricular ejection fraction by this technique correlates very well with the angiographically derived ejection fraction and is very simply obtained. They may be useful in the distinction between constrictive pericarditis and cardiomyopathy, where the ejection fraction is normal in the former and depressed in the latter. However, the correlation with angiography is weak when the ejection fraction is markedly depressed (less than 20%). The STIs may be useful for serial follow-up of individual patients to evaluate the effect of treatment on left ventricular function.

Radioisotopes

Radionucleotide Angiography

This is a much simpler technique than contrast angiography for visualization of the cardiac chambers, but does not provide nearly as much detail. Unfortunately the equipment is extremely expensive, but when available in a large hospital may provide useful information.

Following injection of technetium-99m, evaluation of left ventricular function is achieved by means of a gated cardiac study (Fig. 7.3). Emission of radioactivity is detected by a scin-

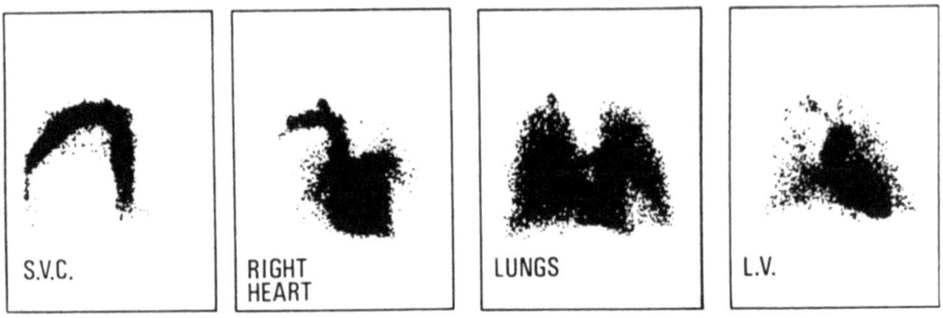

FIGURE 7.3. Gated blood pool scan obtained following injection of technetium-99m outlining the right and left sides of the heart (see text).

tilation camera and the amount of radioactivity is interfaced to a computer, which stores the data and makes it possible to calculate the left ventricular ejection fraction. This exhibits a high degree of correlation with the angiographic left ventricular ejection fraction. The advantage of the technique is that it permits single or repeated evaluation of left ventricular dynamics including information pertinent to regional abnormalities of contraction. It is applicable to ill patients in the Coronary Care Unit or in the postoperative period following saphenous vein bypass grafting. It is commonly used to differentiate diffuse left ventricular hypokinesis from left ventricular aneurysm when revascularization surgery is contemplated.

The exercise-gated cardiac study has been found to be highly sensitive and specific in detecting ischemic heart disease. Normal individuals respond by increasing their resting left ventricular ejection fraction, whereas patients with ischemic heart disease exhibit a decrease in the left ventricular ejection fraction and the appearance of left ventricular wall motion abnormalities such as dyskinesis. This technique provides more sensitive information than treadmill stress testing (Chapter 17).

The technique is useful in identifying enlargement of various cardiac chambers and is fairly sensitive in detecting a pericardial effusion by demonstrating a difference between the outline of the total cardiac shadow and the heart blood pool.

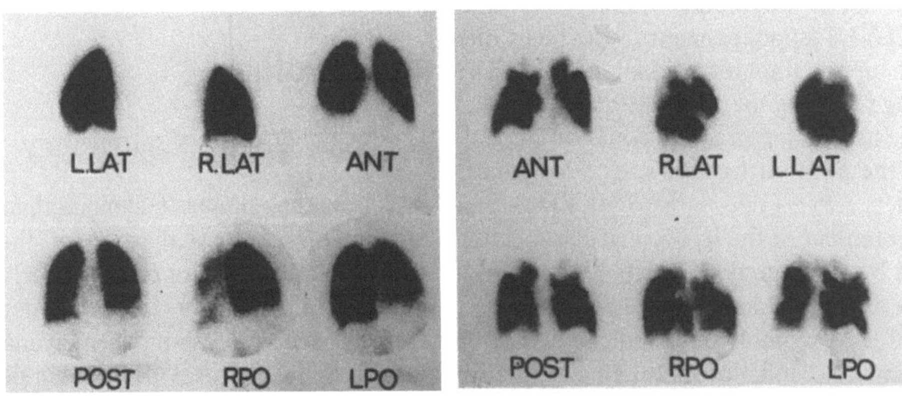

FIGURE 7.4. Lung scans. Left panel shows normal perfusion in a patient with deep vein thrombosis. One week later pulmonary embolism occurred. The right panel shows multiple perfusion defects. RPO and LPO, right and left posterior oblique views, respectively.

Lung Scan

Using technetium-macroaggregated albumin, this is a safe technique even in critically ill patients and takes only 10 to 20 minutes. Provided the chest X-ray is normal, pulmonary embolism can be detected with a high degree of accuracy (Fig. 7.4).

Thallium-201 Perfusion Scintigraphy

The use of this technique in the clinical management of ischemic heart disease is discussed in Chapter 17.

Additional Reading

Bancroft WH Jr, Eddleman EE, Larkin LN: Methods and physical characteristics of the vectorcardiographic and apexcardiographic systems for recording low frequency precordial motion. Am Heart J 73:756, 1967.

Gorlin R, Gorlin SG: Hydraulic formula for calculation of the area of the stenotic mitral valve, other cardiac valves and central circulatory shunts. Am Heart J 41:1, 1951.

Grossman W: "Cardiac Catheterization and Angiography." Lea & Feibiger, Philadelphia, 1980.

Lewis RP, Rittgers SE, Forester WF, Boudoulas H: A critical review of the systolic time intervals. Circulation 56:146, 1977.

Pitt HB, Strauss HW: Myocardial perfusion imaging and gated cardiac blood pool scanning: Clinical application. Am J Cardiol 38:739, 1973.

Rudolph AM: "Congenital Diseases of the Heart." Year Book Medical Publishers, Chicago, 1974.

Tavel ME: "Clinical Phonocardiography and External Pulse Recordings." Year Book Medical Publishers, Chicago, 1985.

Zimmerman HA: "Intravascular Catheterization." Charles C Thomas. Springfield, IL, 1972.

8
The Arrhythmias

Arrhythmias are a common problem in clinical practice. Their mode of presentation varies from a catastrophic event requiring immediate attention to an abnormality detected by routine clinical examination and electrocardiography in an asymptomatic patient. By common acceptance the term "arrhythmia" includes not only fast and slow irregularities of the heart beat, but also defects of conduction.

The approach to the patient with a cardiac arrhythmia should never be purely electrocardiographic. The cause of the arrhythmia, the identification of any predisposing factors, and, most importantly, the effects of an arrhythmia on the individual patient are critical assessments.

For example, an attack of supraventricular tachycardia in a young healthy athlete is frequently a benign, transitory event. Even when prolonged, the lack of hemodynamic embarrassment in such a case will dictate the most benign therapeutic measures. Yet, the identical arrhythmia in a patient with critically tight mitral stenosis may precipitate a life-threatening emergency complicated by acute pulmonary edema and hypotension necessitating immediate, aggressive medical treatment. Therefore, a careful clinical assessment must be made of the nature of the underlying heart disease, predisposing factors, and hemodynamic effects in the individual patient.

Circulatory Effects of Arrhythmias

Within the range of 40 to 160 beats/min, compensatory alterations in stroke volume will maintain cardiac output in a normal heart. Tachycardias beyond this range seriously impair ventricular filling and result in a fall in cardiac output. The wide range of heart rate at which the heart is able to maintain an adequate cardiac output does not apply when there is myocardial or valvular disease. The sudden development of a tachycardia or bradycardia will seriously depress cardiac output in patients with heart disease. In patients with mitral stenosis, the onset of tachycardia, whether regular or irregular, seriously abbreviates the diastolic filling period, producing not only a drop in cardiac output, but also pulmonary congestion. The bradycardia associated with complete heart block, even in the elderly, may be tolerated for long periods of time, provided the myocardium is normal. However, the cardiac output will fail to rise adequately and symptoms may occur when additional demands, such as the stress of infection or exercise, are superimposed.

Tachycardia increases myocardial oxygen consumption, whereas bradycardia reduces it. Since coronary blood flow is largely diastolic, tachycardia may precipitate angina or left ventricular failure because of increased oxygen demand and decreased coronary blood flow. The effect of atrial contraction is of great importance in the tachycardias and the bradycardias. When atrial systole is appropriately timed in relation to the QRS complex, this booster-pump effect increases ventricular filling by the Starling mechanism and increases cardiac output. When myocardial function is impaired, the onset of arrhythmias such as atrial fibrillation, A-V block, and ventricular tachycardia will deprive the patient of the atrial booster-pump and the cardiac output may drop as much as 40%. Loss of the atrial booster-pump is particulary important in patients with noncompliant left ventricles (valvular aortic stenosis, hypertrophic cardiomyopathy, and systemic hypertension) where there is impaired ventricular filling.

Etiology of Arrhythmias

The presence of an arrhythmia does not necessarily imply that heart disease may be detected by clinical or specialized forms of cardiac investigation. Such arrhythmias include supraventricular tachycardias, atrial and ventricular ectopic beats, sinus arrhythmia, sinus bradycardia, and sinus tachycardia.

Certain rhythms are particularly prone to occur with certain types of underlying pathological processes. Atrial fibrillation is most commonly encountered with mitral valve disease, any cause of left atrial enlargement, and thyrotoxicosis. Ventricular tachycardia is most commonly associated with ischemic heart disease.

Precipitating Factors

Hypoxia and Hypercapnia

These are important causes of arrhythmias, particularly when the abnormality of blood gases occurs suddenly, such as in the postoperative period following cardiopulmonary bypass or any other major surgical procedure. The usual factors are hypoventilation and severe pulmonary atelectasis.

Acidosis and Alkalosis

These are particularly important in the neonate.

Drug Toxicity

By far the commonest offender is digitalis, but catecholamines and other antiarrhythmic drugs such as quinidine and procainamide may also be responsible.

Thyrotoxicosis and Pheochromocytoma

Atrial ectopic beats and supraventricular tachycardia occur in both conditions and are thought to be a result of the chronotropic effect of catecholamines. Atrial fibrillation is the characteristic dysrhythmia of the elderly thyrotoxic patient.

Hypokalemia

This is important in the pathogenesis of digitalis toxicity. Severe hypokalemia may produce multifocal ventricular ectopic beats, eventually deteriorating to ventricular fibrillation.

Hyperkalemia

This produces varying degrees of A-V block and impaired intraatrial and intraventricular conduction with ventricular fibrillation as a terminal event.

Systemic Infections

Lobar or bronchopneumonia in the elderly is a potent cause of arrhythmias, which may disappear when the infection is successfully treated. Infective endocarditis may be a precipitating cause at any age.

Pulmonary Embolism and/or Infarction

This is a common cause for sudden onset of atrial fibrillation.

Myocardial Damage

An arrhythmia may be the presenting feature of so-called "silent" or overt myocardial infarction. Myocarditis (viral or rheumatic) is a recognized cause of ventricular irritability.

Hypotension

Blood loss from the gastrointenstinal tract or from a leaking abdominal aortic aneurysm may produce hypotension, myocardial ischemia, and ventricular arrhythmias.

Myocardial Metastases

The presenting feature of carcinoma of the bronchus may be the onset of atrial fibrillation. Lymphomas may present in a similar manner.

Failure to identify and correct these predisposing factors may lead to unsuccessful management of a cardiac arrhythmia.

Mechanisms of the Arrhythmias

As described in Chapter 6, the SA node is the dominant pacemaker, and the sequential subsidiary pacemakers (the A-V node and the conducting tissues below it) have lesser degrees of automaticity and are normally suppressed.

When the normal process of impulse *formation* or *conduction* is disturbed, various abnormalities of rate or rhythm occur. When a pacemaker other than the SA node assumes dominance, the ensuing arrhythmia is therefore by *escape* of a normally suppressed subsidiary focus. Alternatively, such a focus may assume dominance because of an increase in its inherent automaticity. In both circumstances impulse formation is from an *ectopic* focus that arises, therefore, by *default* of the higher pacemaker or by *usurpation* by the lower one. The ectopic focus may control the whole heart, the atria only, the ventricles only, or both.

Disorders of Impulse Formation

Normal Automaticity

The heart contains both pacemaking and nonpacemaking cells. Pacemaking cells differ fundamentally from nonpacemaking cells in that they have the property of spontaneous diastolic depolarization. The rate of spontaneous diastolic depolarization influences the activity of the pacemaker.

The action potential of a nonpacemaking cell is divided into four phases (Fig. 8.1). Phase 4 represents the resting negative potential, which rises slowly until an impulse depolarizes the cell and results in an abrupt positivity. Phase 0

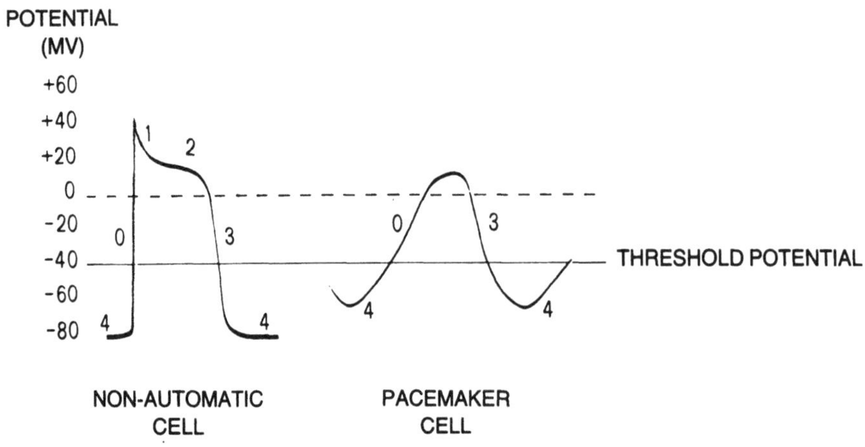

FIGURE 8.1. Action potentials of a nonautomatic and pacemaker cell. The latter exhibits spontaneous diastolic depolarization in phase 4 (see text).

represents initial rapid depolarization; it is followed by Phase 1, which represents early and rapid repolarization: Phase 2, which represents slow repolarization; and Phase 3, which represents relatively rapid repolarization. The action potential of a pacemaking cell has a shallower resting potential, a slower velocity of Phase 0, and a more rapid decline in Phase 2. The most striking difference, however, is the more rapidly upward slope of the resting potential during Phase 4 resulting in spontaneous depolarization. The effect of this is to automatically reach threshold potential so that there is regular spontaneous discharge. Inherent automaticity is dependent to a large extent by the slope and rate of Phase 4 depolarization. The slope and rate of depolarization in Phase 4 are influenced by cardiac medications, hypoxia, acid–base shifts, and autonomic function.

The configuration and duration of the action potential are important in the development of arrhythmias, which depend on *automaticity* (Phase 4, sodium and potassium dependent), or *reentry*, which depends on the fast response (Phase 0, sodium dependent), duration of the action potential, and slow response (Phase 2, calcium dependent).

Abnormal Automaticity

Atrial and ventricular muscles do not normally exhibit spontaneous diastolic depolarization and impulse formation. When diseased, however, these cells have reduced resting membrane potential, and spontaneous depolarization and abnormal automaticity may occur.

Abnormal Impulse Conduction

Arrhythmias resulting from *reentry* are more common than those arising from increased automaticity. Reentry may involve the SA node, the atria, the A-V node (dual A-V nodal pathways), and the ventricles. The reentry loop may be large (macroreentrant), as seen in the Wolff–Parkinson–White (WPW) syndrome and atrioventricular reentrant tachycardia, or small (microreentrant) when the ventricular muscle is involved. For reentry to occur there must be (1) two functionally distinct conducting pathways, (2) undirectional block in one pathway, and (3) slow conduction down the other pathway. A group of fibers, not activated by unidirectional block during the initial depolarization, may thus recover excitability and then reexcite areas that have just recovered. This becomes continuous and a tachycardia results (Figs. 8.2 and 8.3).

Approach to the Diagnosis of Cardiac Arrhythmias

History taking and clinical examination precede interpretation of the electrocardiogram and more sophisticated tests for the diagnosis of cardiac arrhythmias. It is helpful to have a rough clinical classification.

Rapid Regular Tachycardia

1. Sinus tachycardia
2. Supraventricular tachycardia:
   a. Atrial flutter
   b. Atrial tachycardias (reentrant or automatic)
3. Ventricular tachycardia

Rapid Irregular Tachycardia

1. Atrial fibrillation
2. Atrial flutter with varying block
3. Supraventricular tachycardia with varying A-V block
4. Multifocal atrial tachycardia

The Bradycardias

1. Sinus bradycardia
2. Various grades of A-V block
3. Atrial fibrillation of flutter with high degree A-V block
4. Junctional or ventricular escape rhythms

The History

Many patients are able to provide valuable information by imitating the arrhythmia. A simple technique is to request patients to reproduce the arrhythmia by tapping their finger on the physi-

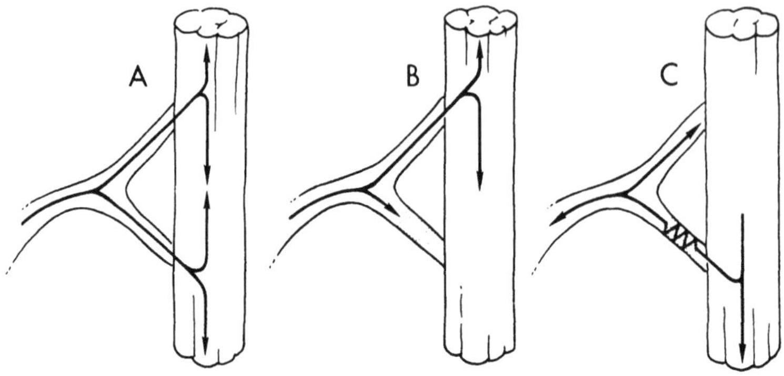

FIGURE 8.2. The reentry phenomenon. In (A) impulses are conducted uniformly from Purkinje fibers to cardiac muscle. In (B) antegrade conduction is impaired in a zone (shaded area) partially depolarized because of ischemia. The impulse can reenter the circuit retrogradely after a delay that permits normal tissue proximal to the depressed area to recover excitability (C). Thus, a second impulse is propagated as a premature beat that if repetitive may produce ventricular tachycardia.

cians desk. This is particularly helpful when a patient presents in regular rhythm, and episodes of tachycardia or bradycardia are infrequent. Regular supraventricular tachycardias are of dramatic onset and offset, and will be reduplicated with a regular tap of the finger. Sinus tachycardia accelerates and decelerates in gradual fashion, whereas the rhythm in atrial fibrillation and atrial flutter with variable A-V block may be entirely irregular.

The Intensity of the First Heart Sound

In arrhythmias in which the P wave is normally related to the QRS complex, the intensity of the first heart sound remains constant beat by beat. When there is dissociation between atrial and ventricular activity (complete A-V block, ventricular tachycardia) the first heart sound varies in intensity.

Atrial Sounds

When these are heard independently of the heart sounds, this signifies complete A-V block.

The Systolic Blood Pressure

Variation in the peak systolic blood pressure of more than 10 mm Hg in the presence of a tachycardia indicates a ventricular origin. This is because of the dissociation between atrial

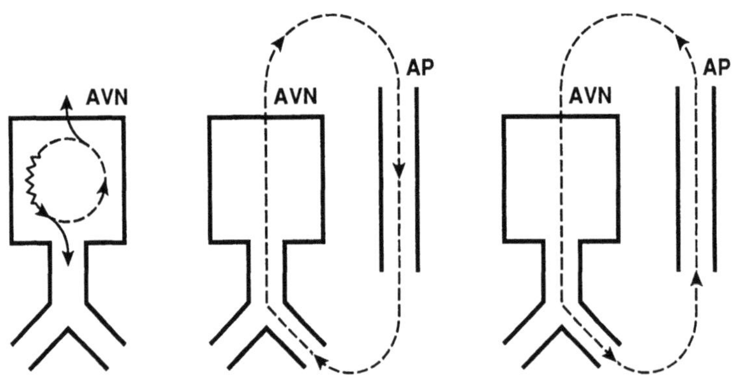

FIGURE 8.3. Types of reentrant junctional tachycardia. AVNRT, A-V nodal reentrant tachycardia; AVRT, atrioventricular reentrant tachycardia; AVN, A-V node; AP, accessory pathway.

and ventricular systole. In ventricular tachycardia, when atrial contraction fortuitously precedes ventricular systole, the output of the ventricle for that beat is augmented and the systolic blood pressure is correspondingly higher.

Splitting of the Heart Sounds

This implies asynchronous ventricular contraction and is either the result of ventricular tachycardia, supraventricular tachycardia with bundle branch block, or aberrant ventricular conduction. Wide splitting of both heart sounds excludes supraventricular tachycardia with normal intraventricular conduction.

The Jugular Venous Pulse

The appearance of irregular "cannon A waves" signifies dissociation between atrial and ventricular activity, and in the presence of a rapid tachycardia, is highly suggestive of ventricular tachycardia. In bradyarrhythmias, dissociation between the a, c, and v waves of the jugular venous pulse and the slower carotid pulse is diagnostic of complete heart block.

Vagal Stimulation

Carotid sinus massage and the Valsalva maneuver have no effect on ventricular tachycardia, may terminate an attack of supraventricular tachycardia, and may produce temporary slowing of the ventricular response to atrial flutter.

The Electrocardiogram

Usually, the only necessary form of investigation required for evaluation of an arrhythmia or conduction disturbance is the standard 12-lead electrocardiogram. A rhythm strip should be obtained from leads that best demonstrate P wave morphology (usually lead Vl and standard lead II).

If the atrial activity cannot be detected, an esophageal electrocardiogram may be helpful. Alternatively inducing temporary A-V block with i.v. adenosine may solve the problem.

Two Golden Rules

1. *Always Look for the P Waves*. Determine whether their morphology is normal, and analyze the relationship between the P waves and the QRS complexes.

2. *Always Examine the QRS Complex*. A QRS complex with normal configuration signifies activation of the ventricles through physiological pathways. Widened QRS complexes indicate bundle branch block or an intraventricular conduction defect that may be present before the onset of the arrhythmia or a manifestation of aberrant ventricular conduction, produced by the arrhythmia. Alternatively, broad QRS complexes represent arrhythmias whose substrate is below the bundle of His.

Ambulatory Electrocardiography (Holter Monitoring)

These portable recorders use two channels to record the electrocardiogram for up to 48 hours. Indications for its use are (1) patients with syncope or near syncope, (2) recording of symptomatic and asymptomatic dysrhythmias in conjunction with a diary, and (3) evaluation of the effect of antidysrhythmic drugs.

This technique is extremely useful in documenting transitory dysrhythmias such as occur in the sick sinus syndrome and complete heart block. Interpretation of the results, however, must take into account the wide range of findings among normal subjects, spontaneous variability in symptoms, and the infrequency of the rhythm disturbances.

In "normal" subjects, sinus bradycardia (less than 40 beats/min during sleep), sinus pauses, and transient second degree A-V block are frequent. Asymptomatic supraventricular and ventricular dysrhythmias increase with age and the presence of heart disease.

Event Recorders

These ambulatory monitors use transtelephonic transmission to document symptomatic episodes of rhythm disturbances that are too infrequent to be documented by 24 Holter recording. The advantage is that the tracing is recorded during the symptomatic period. Since the system contains a memory loop, 30 seconds of tracing prior to activation of the system by the patient will be recorded.

The test is also useful in a negative sense when tracings recorded during a typical "spell" show normal sinus rhythm.

Exercise Testing

Apart from its place in the evaluation of palpitation and other symptoms suggestive of a rhythm disturbance specifically induced by exercise, stress testing plays a limited role in diagnosis of dysrhythmia. Exercise-induced ventricular ectopy is common in asymptomatic patients and control subjects. It is expensive and not as sensitive as Holter monitoring.

Electrophysiologic Testing

This compliments the noninvasive techniques described above. The procedure is surprisingly safe despite the number of catheters used, and the deliberate, repeated provocation of dysrhythmias. Complications (deep venous thrombosis, infection, etc.) occur in less than 1% of procedures and the mortality is extremely low. The chief uses are as follows.

Wolff–Parkinson–White Syndrome

Patients with accessory pathways may have recurrent supraventricular tachycardia resistent to medical treatment. Rarely, patients may be at risk for sudden death because of a rapid ventricular response to spontaneous atrial fibrillation. Electrophysiologic studies assist in accurate diagnosis, location of accessory pathways, and determination of the conduction characteristics of the pathway.

Ventricular Tachycardia

The selection of drugs by trial and error in attempts to prevent recurrent sustained ventricular tachycardia has been replaced by programmed ventricular stimulation. Provocation of the dysrhythmia by critically timed premature stimuli, followed by serial drug testing until an effective agent is found, is much more reliable. The same technique is used to treat survivors of out-of-hospital cardiac arrest. Endocardial mapping is used to locate the site of origin of ventricular tachycardia prior to transcatheter or surgical ablation. Electrophysiological mapping can accurately locate the source of ventricular ectopy prior to aneurysmectomy.

Disturbances of Impulse Formation

Disturbances of the SA Node

Sinus Arrhythmia

This is produced by irregularity of impulse formation in the SA node resulting from changes in vagal tone. The commonest form of sinus arrhythmia is "phasic" and is related to respiration, the rate increases with inspiration and slows with expiration. It can be abolished by holding the breath, exercise, or atropine. "Nonphasic" sinus arrhythmia is unrelated to the phases of respiration. Both varieties are considered to be normal variants, which may be precipitated or made more obvious by increases in vagal tone. It is a common normal finding in children, but tends to disappear with advancing age.

Sinus Tachycardia

The sinus rate is over 100/min at rest in adults and over 140/min in infants. In adults, sinus tachycardia seldom exceeds 180/min, whereas in infants the rate may be well over 200/min. Sinus tachycardia is a normal response to exercise, hypotension, thyrotoxicosis, anemia, and other high output states.

The jugular venous pulse and heart sounds are normal. The electrocardiogram shows a normal P wave preceding each QRS complex, which is also of normal configuration. The importance of sinus tachycardia is to identify and treat the precipitating cause. When sinus tachycardia is the result of anxiety or automatic imbalance it may be effectively treated with propranolol.

Sinus Bradycardia

Impulses originate in the SA node at less than 60/min in the adult and less than 100/min in the infant. Physiological sinus bradycardia is encountered frequently among athletes, particularly marathon runners. Sinus bradycardia occurs with raised intracranial pressure, obstructive jaundice, and myxedema. It may follow the administration of β-receptor-blocking drugs, digitalis, reserpine, and quinidine. It not infrequently complicates the early phases of acute myocardial infarction, particularly the inferior variety. Under the latter circumstances it does not connote an adverse prognosis and will usually respond to the administration of atropine.

Electrocardiographically, it is recognized by a normal P-QRS-T relationship, recorded in slow sequence.

Sinoatrial (SA) Block

Here the sinus impulse is blocked between the node and the surrounding atrium. This results in the failure of atrial and ventricular activation and neither the P wave nor the QRS complex is inscribed. Sinoatrial block may occur irregularly, or occasionally a 2:1 sequence may be established. A period of SA block may be followed by a normal sinus beat or escape beat arising in either the A-V node or the ventricle.

Sinoatrial block is frequently the result of the administration of digitalis, but quinidine may also be responsible. In sensitive subjects vagal stimulation may produce episodes of sinoatrial block.

Electrocardiographically, SA block is diagnosed by failure of the P-QRS-T sequence to occur; the resulting pause equals two sinus cycles.

Usually SA block is not responsible for significant symptoms unless the condition is a component of the sick sinus syndrome as discussed below.

Sick Sinus Syndrome (Tachycardia–Bradycardia Syndrome)

In its typical form this manifests as various types of sinus node dysfunction including sinus bradycardia and periods of SA block. Additionally, there are episodes of atrial tachyarrhythmias and atrial fibrillation alternating with the periods of sinus node dysfunction.

The syndrome usually occurs in the fifth and sixth decades, but occasionally may affect younger age groups. Symptoms consist of syncope and dizziness and may follow a period of asymptomatic sinus bradycardia over many years. In those patients prone to tachyarrhythmias, palpitation is a troublesome symptom. The diagnosis of sick sinus syndrome is clinical and cannot be made until other conditions effecting the sinus node (e.g., digitalis, β-blocking drugs, inferior myocardial infarction) have been excluded. The electrocardiogram may be quite normal when a patient is seen for the first time but suggestive evidence may be present in the form of sinus bradycardia, periods of sinus arrest, and intervening episodes of atrial flutter or tachycardia. Failure to develop an adequate tachycardia following the intravenous administration of atropine or after exercise suggests the diagnosis. A prolonged sinus node recovery time following atrial pacing is evidence of sinus node dysfunction, but a normal recovery time does not exclude the syndrome. The diagnosis is therefore largely clinical assisted by Holter monitoring.

The treatment of the sick sinus syndrome involves permanent artificial pacemaking. Those patients whose symptoms are a result of sinus arrest and bradycardia are managed by pacemaking alone. When there are complicating episodes of tachyarrhythmia, digitalis or β-blockers will safely suppress these ectopic rhythms and in many instances the patient becomes completely pacemaker dependent. When A-V conduction is normal and atrial fibrillation is absent, atrial pacing with an activity mode may be used. Most commonly used is a DDD, a universal pacing system.

Atrial Arrhythmias

Supraventricular Ectopic Beats

This is a manifestation of increased automaticity. An ectopic focus (or foci), outside the SA node, located anywhere in the atrial mus-

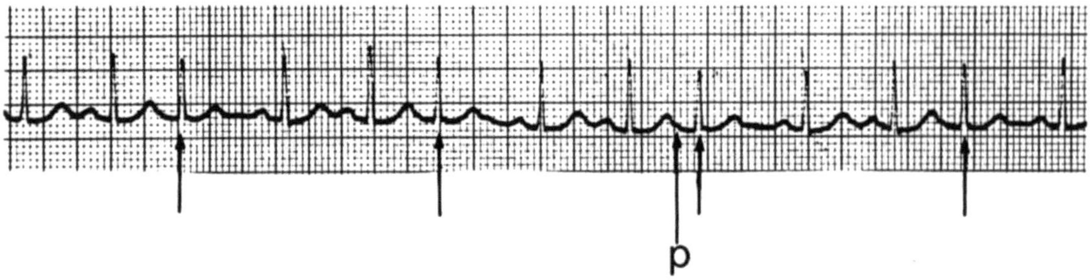

FIGURE 8.4. Atrial ectopic beats (arrow) with a normal QRS morphology and incomplete compensatory pace. A premature P wave deforms the descending limb of one T wave (arrowed P wave).

cle or in the junctional tissue, may discharge prematurely. Since the mode of activation of the ventricles is by the usual physiological pathways, the QRS configuration is normal. Both atrial and junctional foci may discharge as a single beat or in continuous ectopic rhythm. Repetitive successive premature beats constitute a paroxysm of automatic supraventricular tachycardia, the duration of which depends on the number of ectopic beats.

Supraventricular ectopics from any site may produce cannon A waves in the neck, provided atrial contraction occurs during ventricular systole. The first heart sound is generally accentuated in all premature beats, since filling of the ventricles is interrupted and the valves are still widely open. Splitting of the second heart sound is normal in contrast to the wide splitting produced by a ventricular ectopic beat.

In an *atrial ectopic* beat the P wave is always present and since the atria are usually activated differently, the P wave morphology is abnormal. If, however, the ectopic beat arises near the sinus node, the P wave will not differ greatly from the sinus P wave and will have the same frontal plane axis as those of the sinus beats. Since the ectopic impulse depolarizes the sinus node prematurely, a compensatory pause is present (i.e., the sum of the pre- and postectopic periods is less than the sum of two consecutive normal intervals) (Fig. 8.4). Depending on whether the A-V node is refractory or not, and on the degree of prematurity of the ectopic beat, they may or may not be conducted to the ventricles, in which case they are referred to as "blocked."

Atrial ectopic beats are common in healthy people of all ages and they may be precipitated by emotion, tobacco, alcohol, or coffee. They may be a result of digitalis intoxication, in which case they may precede atrial tachycardia with 2:1 A-V block. They are common during the course of myocardial infarction, and in any form of atrial distension (classically mitral stenosis) where they precede the onset of atrial fibrillation.

AV Junctional Ectopic Beats

These spread simultaneously upward toward the atria and downward toward the ventricles. Depending on the rate of conduction, the atria may be activated at the same time, simultaneously, or after the ventricle. The characteristic electrocardiographic features are "retrograde" P waves that are inverted in leads II, III, and AVF. (Their frontal plane axis is leftward and close to $-90°$.) When this is continuous, it is also known as "inferior atrial rhythm" (Fig. 6.5). The P waves may coincide with, precede, or follow the QRS. Usually the QRS complex is normal in configuration unless aberrant ventricular conduction is present.

The physical signs associated with junctional ectopy are much the same as with atrial ectopy.

Treatment of supraventricular ectopic beats, whether atrial or junctional, is generally not required. Avoidance of precipitating factors such as alcohol and tobacco may be helpful. Withdrawal of digitalis is indicated when toxicity is suspected.

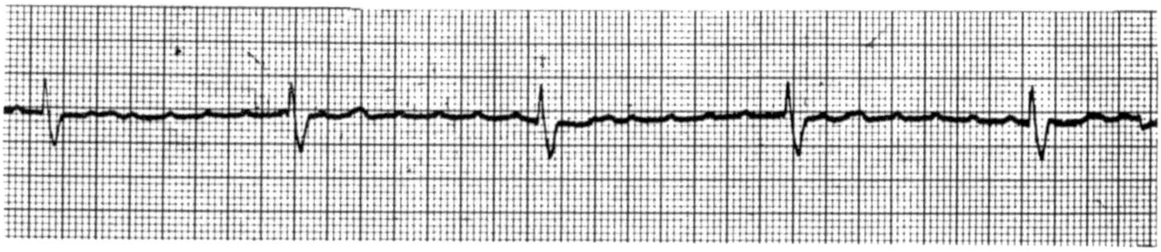

FIGURE 8.5. Electrocardiogram demonstrating atrial flutter and complete A-V block with a regular, nodal response of 40/min. Note the characteristic flutter waves.

Atrial Flutter

Atrial flutter, unlike atrial fibrillation, is characterized by extremely rapid atrial contractions, which may at least produce a partially effective atrial contraction. It is the result of rapid regular atrial excitation and, therefore, in many respects is highly similar to atrial tachycardia. Atrial flutter is rarely encountered among normal subjects. It responds to vagal stimulation, adenosine, calcium channel blockers, and digitalization by an increase in the degree of A-V block rather than by termination of the attack. Clinically, it tends to be associated with the same conditions as atrial fibrillation (mitral valve disease, thyrotoxicosis, atrial septal defect, myocardial infarction, following operations on the heart and lung, and pericardial metastases). It is an unusual manifestation of digitalis intoxication but commonly occurs during the course of treatment of atrial fibrillation with quinidine.

Electrocardiographically, it is characterized by irregular flutter or "f" waves at a rate of 250

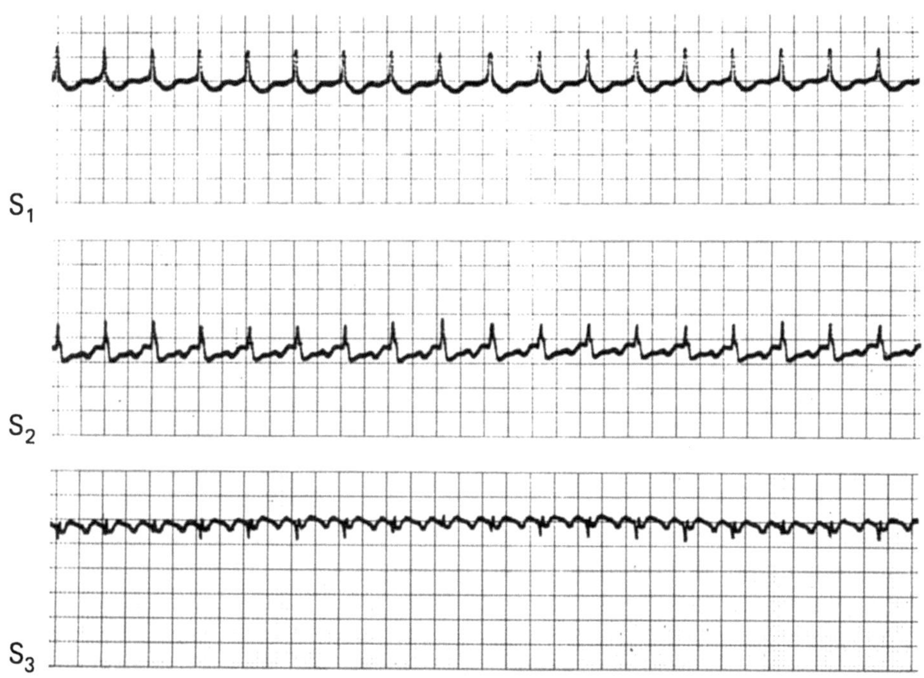

FIGURE 8.6. Electrocardiogram in atrial flutter simulating supraventricular tachycardia with a "P wave" preceding each QRS complex in standard II. Close inspection of standard III, however, demonstrates the characteristic "saw-tooth" appearance.

to 300/min producing a "saw-tooth" appearance without an isoelectric line between the individual flutter waves. Some degree of A-V block is usual and this is frequently 2:1. One-to-one conduction may result in an extremely rapid tachycardia with rates up to 300/min. When 2:1 A-V block is present, alternate flutter waves merge with the QRS complex and their appearance may simulate sinus rhythm. However, carotid sinus stimulation or adenosine-induced transient A-V block may demonstrate the underlying "saw-tooth" pattern (Figs. 8.5 and 8.6).

Atrial flutter, like atrial fibrillation, may occur in paroxysms. In the absence of valvular disease or cardiomyopathy and in the presence of a high degree of A-V block (4:1) a patient may be quite asymptomatic. On the other hand, with lesser degrees of A-V block and underlying heart disease, the rapid ventricular response may produce hemodynamic deterioration, angina, and congestive heart failure.

The commonest finding on physical examination is regular tachycardia in the region of 150/min, which may be difficult to distinguish from other forms of supraventricular tachycardia. When the ventricular response is regular at a normal rate, the arrhythmia may not be obvious clinically. A helpful physical sign is observation of flutter waves in the jugular venous pulse, which are particularly evident with higher grades of A-V block. Auscultation frequently detects variations in intensity of the first heart sound because of varying relationship between ventricular contraction and the preceding atrial contraction. The response to carotid sinus pressure is diagnostically helpful and the rate may drop by 50% during the procedure.

Treatment

When the general condition of the patient dictates urgent resolution of the arrhythmia, cardioversion is effective in low-energy doses of 25–100 J in approximately 90% of patients. When the situation is less critical, digitalis is highly effective and rapidly increases the degree of A-V block until a satisfactory ventricular rate is achieved. Although the A-V blocking effect of digitalis is predictable, the effect on the atrial arrhythmia is variable. Frequently it will convert flutter to fibrillation, but occasionally there may be a direct conversion to sinus rhythm. When digitalis converts flutter to fibrillation, digitalis should then be discontinued since there is a distinct possibility that conversion to sinus rhythm will take place spontaneously. If this does not occur, digitalis should be introduced and quinidine should be used in an attempt to restore sinus rhythm. Quinidine should *never* be used to convert flutter to sinus rhythm without prior digitalization, since quinidine may induce a dangerous degree of acceleration of the ventricular response. Atrial overdrive pacing is a useful alternative when there digitalis toxicity is a possibility and when sedation for cardioversion is undesirable as in emphysema.

Atrial Fibrillation

This is the commonest atrial tachyarrhythmia and may occur in paroxysmal or chronic form. Atrial fibrillation may occur in otherwise healthy subjects ("lone fibrillation") but usually is associated with organic heart disease. Rheumatic heart disease, especially mitral stenosis, essential hypertension, and coronary artery disease account for over 90% of the cases. Thyrotoxicosis is the next commonest cause and should always be considered, especially when there is no obvious heart disease in an elderly subject. Other toxic causes such as pneumonia and infection become more important with advancing age. In fact, age is important in the pathogenesis, and the majority of cases of atrial fibrillation occur after the age of 40. Less common associations are constrictive pericarditis, atrial septal defect, infective endocarditis, cor pulmonale, and hemochromatosis. Atrial fibrillation occurs commonly after any operation on the thorax, particularly following mitral and aortic valve procedures. Paroxysmal attacks occur frequently before the arrhythmia becomes permanently established. Episodes may vary in duration from a few seconds to a few days and usually the onset and offset are sudden.

Lone atrial fibrillation occurs most commonly after the age of 40 and, as the name indicates, evidence of underlying heart disease or precipitating factors is absent. Heart failure may occur and may resolve when sinus rhythm is restored.

Atrial fibrillation is characterized by ineffective atrial contraction, and a rapid and irregular bombardment of the A-V node by supraventricular impulses. Most of these impulses are blocked within the A-V node but enough are conducted to make the ventricular contractions rapid and irregularly irregular. The combination of these effects depends on the duration of the arrhythmia and the state of myocardial function. The irregular tachycardia and lack of effective atrial contraction may produce a precipitous drop in cardiac output resulting in congestive cardiac failure or pulmonary edema. Furthermore, there is a predisposition to the development of static thrombus in the atria, which may result in systemic and pulmonary emboli.

Physical Signs

The arrhythmia is suspected when an irregularly irregular pulse is found, independent of the rate. When the rate is rapid there are mole cycles audible at the apex than are palpable at the peripheral pulse, producing a "pulse deficit." The irregularity and the pulse deficit are not diagnostic of atrial fibrillation since the same findings may be detected in atrial tachycardia with varying degrees of block, multiple ectopic beats, and atrial flutter with varying degrees of A-V block.

The jugular venous pulse reflects the lack of atrial contraction and the "a" wave and the "x" descent are replaced by positive CV waves, which may be very prominent when tricuspid insufficiency is associated. The magnitude of the arterial pulse varies in relationship to the cycle length. The first heart sound varies in intensity, being loud after short diastolic cycles and softer after longer cycles. These changes depend the position of the A-V valves at the onset of ventricular systole. The long cycles allow the valves to refloat almost completely to the closure position and the sounds are therefore soft.

The Electrocardiogram

Atrial fibrillatory waves or "f" waves are present at a rate between 300 and 700/min and are best seen in V1. Usually these "f" waves are irregular and vary in size and shape. Large "f" waves are usually encountered in rheumatic heart disease, particularly mitral valve disease, whereas small "f" waves tend to be associated with ischemic heart disease (Fig. 8.7).

The ventricular response is totally irregular. If the rhythm suddenly becomes regular in atrial fibrillation, digitalis toxicity should be suspected since it represents an idioventricular rhythm. The ventricular rate will also be regular when there is associated complete heart block, and when ventricular tachycar-

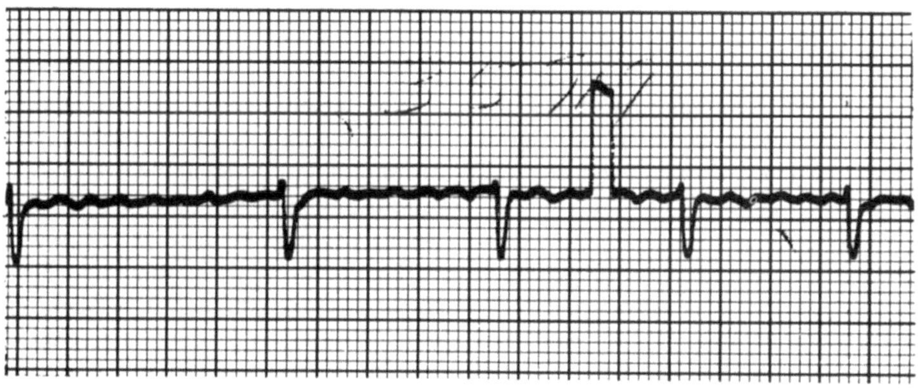

FIGURE 8.7. Electrocardiogram of lead V1 showing the fine high-speed atrial fibrillatory waves in a case of ischemic heart disease. The ventricular response is irregular.

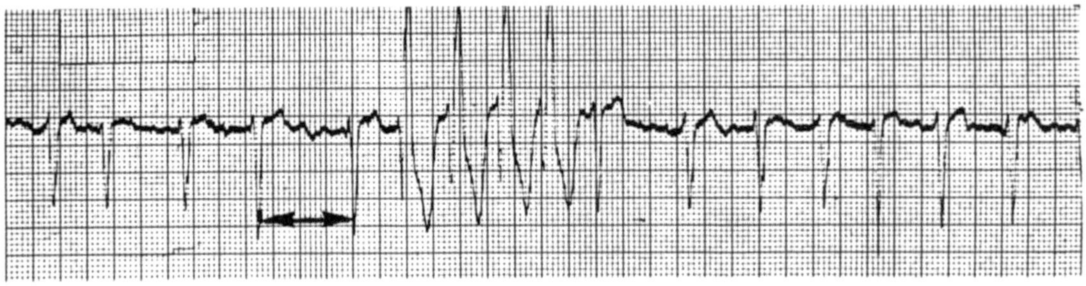

FIGURE 8.8. Electrocardiogram demonstrating atrial fibrillation with an irregular ventricular response complicated by a run of five aberrantly conducted beats. The latter are preceded by spontaneous lengthening of the RR interval, which predisposes to aberration (the Ashman phenomenon).

dia is associated with atrial fibrillation. The QRS complex is usually normal but with rapid rates it may be widened because of aberrant ventricular conduction. However, the marked irregularity differentiates this from true ventricular tachycardia. Aberration is particularly prone to occur when a long ventricular cycle is followed by a short one: the beat terminating the short cycle may show ventricular aberration. This sequence is conducive to aberration and has been called "Ashman's phenomenon" (Fig. 8.8).

The diagnosis of aberration may be difficult when the rate is extremely rapid and regular, and P waves are not available for assistance. The distinction is important because atrial fibrillation with a rapid ventricular response, complicated by aberrant ventricular conduction, is best treated by adequate digitalization. Generally, aberrant beats have a right bundle branch block pattern and the initial vector is the same as that of normally conducted beats. Also, there is no compensatory pause and the abnormal beat is not constantly related to the previous complex with a fixed coupling interval.

Treatment

Before a decision is made to convert atrial fibrillation to sinus rhythm it should be understood that the chances of sinus rhythm being permanently maintained are inversely proportional to (1) the duration of atrial fibrillation, and (2) the age of the patient. Therefore, the best chance of success is the young patient with recent onset of atrial fibrillation and a small or normal size left atrium. The least likelihood of success is the elderly patient with long-standing atrial fibrillation, who, in addition, has cardiomegaly. Naturally, patients do not always separate readily into these two groups and individual decisions must be made. In addition, the clinical condition of the patient at the time will be a stong modifier of the therapeutic regime. For example, the young patient who presents in acute heart failure or pulmonary edema because of rheumatic mitral valve disease is best treated with immediate intravenous digitalization to control the ventricular response. Following successful cardiac surgery in such a case, there is a good chance that electrical or drug-induced conversion to sinus rhythm will be maintained for a considerable time, provided the patient is young and the left atrium is not unduly enlarged.

Elderly patients should be treated to control the ventricular response with digitalis and/or propranolol or verapamil when there is a large left atrium and long-standing atrial fibrillation, whether successful cardiac surgery has been performed or not. The same approach applies to the elderly patient with ischemic heart disease. When atrial fibrillation complicates acute myocardial infarction, the objective again should be to slow the ventricular response with digitalis.

Reversion to sinus rhythm with electrical

countershock or quinidine or other antidysrhythmic drugs is likely to be successful and should be used in young patients with mild rheumatic heart disease with recent onset fibrillation, and young patients who have undergone successful operation for mitral valve disease. Electroshock therapy is the treatment of choice for the restoration of sinus rhythm unless small doses of quinidine (given with digitalis to control the ventricular response) is promptly effective. Embolism immediately following cardioversion is rare. It may also follow quinidine conversion and can occur days after restoration of normal rhythm and is associated with the return of mechanical atrial function. The role of anticoagulant therapy is controversial. Whether cardioversion is successful electrically or pharmacologically, many patients will revert to atrial fibrillation within 1 year. Long-acting quinidine or procainamide may be effective, however, in maintaining sinus rhythm. Approximately one-third of patients with atrial fibrillation remain in sinus rhythm 6 to 12 months after conversion. The procedure is nevertheless worthwhile in most patients and can be repeated when the arrhythmia recurs.

Restoration of atrial fibrillation to sinus rhythm does not necessarily mean that atrial function is restored. This is an example of electromechanical dissociation (i.e., the electrocardiogram shows normal P waves but hemodynamically there is no evidence of left atrial contraction). It may take several days for mechanical function to be restored. Furthermore, right atrial function may return sooner than left and this may be the explanation for the development of pulmonary edema in rare cases after cardioversion, particularly when mitral stenosis is present.

Among patients with long-standing atrial fibrillation in whom a decision has been made to control the ventricular response pharmacologically, digitalis and/or propranolol may not always be completely effective. There are the occasional instances where adequate digitalization is complicated by too rapid a ventricular response during exercise. Under these circumstances verapamil is an extremely useful drug for regularizing the ventricular response.

Atrial Tachycardias

These may be reentrant or a result of increased automaticity. Automatic tachycardias are much less frequent than reentrant junctional tachycardias and occur in patients with serious underlying heart disease. Also, they do not respond to calcium channel blockers like junctional tachycardias.

Sinus Node Reentrant Tachycardia

This is an uncommon form of atrial tachycardia, usually occurring in elderly patients with heart disease. Since the reentry is in the SA node itself atrial activation is normal. The tachycardia ranges from 100 to 140 beats/min and the P waves are normal. It starts and stops suddenly and may respond to vagal stimulation, features that may help distinguish it from sinus tachycardia. The attacks may be terminated by digoxin, quinidine, and β-blockers.

Multifocal Atrial Tachycardia (MAT)

Also called chaotic atrial tachycardia, this is an irregularly, irregular rhythm with P waves of at least three different morphologies (Fig. 8.9). The atrial rate is between 100 and 130 beats/min. This dysrhythmia is usually encountered in elderly patients with severe lung disease. Aminophylline toxicity and hypokalemia may be precipitating factors.

The treatment of MAT is that of the underlying disease since it is not responsive to antidysrhythmic drugs.

Automatic (Ectopic) Atrial Tachycardia

This dysrhythmia is a result of enhanced automaticity of an atrial focus. Characteristically, it has a "warm-up" phase with the rate accelerating to reach 125 to 200 beats/min. The P wave of the ectopic focus is different from that of sinus rhythm and precedes the QRS complex. Automatic atrial tachycardia is usually a result of digitalis toxicity, chronic lung disease, and ischemic heart disease. It should be treated by withholding digoxin and replacing potassium

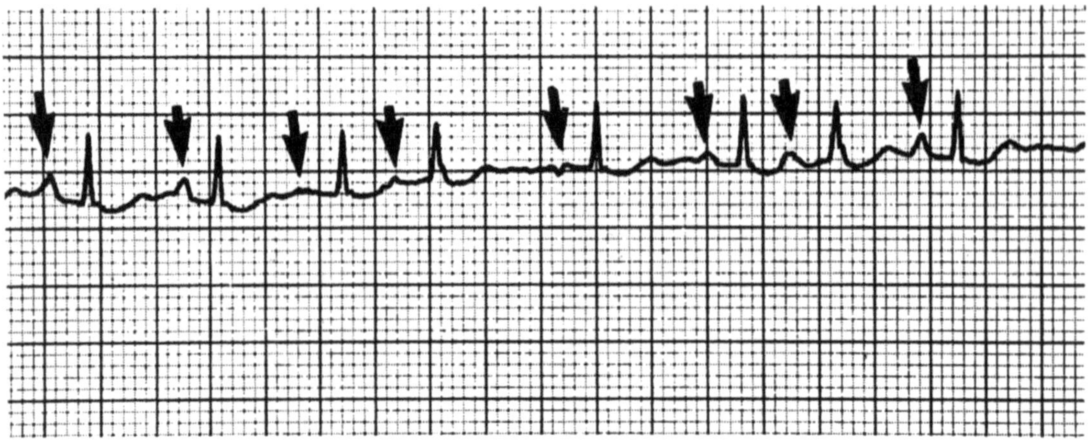

FIGURE 8.9. Electrocardiogram showing multifocal atrial tachycardia (MAT). The P waves "arrows" are of differing morphology.

when necessary. Type Ia antidysrythmic drugs are effective.

Atrial tachycardia with A-V block (frequently 2:1) has a strong association with digitalis toxicity in patients with severe heart disease. It is frequently accompanied by ventricular ectopy and is frequently mistaken clinically for atrial fibrillation.

The electrocardiogram demonstrates an atrial rate varying from 150–250/min and a ventricular rate generally over 100. A-V block is present, but is variable and this is responsible for irregularity. The P waves are abnormal in shape, differing from sinus P waves, and are frequently very small, unlike flutter waves. The baseline is isolectric between the P waves and this contrasts with the "saw-tooth" effect of atrial flutter.

When the arrhythmia is purely a result of digitalis intoxication, the drug should be withheld. When digitalis-toxic dysrhythmias are life threatening, digoxin-specific Fab fragments (antibodies to digoxin) should be given intravenously.

Atrial tachycardia with 2:1 A-V block may also occur among patients with cor pulmonale in the absence of digitalis administration. It usually responds poorly to digitalization and since the arrhythmia is dangerous in patients with chronic obstructive airway disease and right ventricular failure, cardioversion may be life-saving.

Junctional Reentrant Tachycardias and the Preexcitation Syndromes

Prior to the advent of electrophysiological studies, all narrow complex tachycardias were loosely classified under the generic term "paroxysmal atrial tachycardia." It is known that when atrial flutter and atrial fibrillation are excluded, the majority of such tachycardias (80%) are a result of reentry within the A-V node (A-V nodal reentrant tachycardia) or, less frequently, via an accessory pathway (atrioventricular reentrant tachycardia).

A-V Nodal Reentrant Tachycardia

This usually occurs in the absence of heart disease and the electrocardiogram between attacks is normal. The reentry circuit is within the A-V node and is a functional, not an anatomical entity. The A-V node is said to be "longitudinally dissociated," having two, or dual, pathways that are functionally different. The pathways have different conduction velocities (a slow pathway and a fast pathway) and different refractory periods (short or long) (Fig. 8.3).

The common form of A-V nodal reentry uses a slow pathway with a short refractory period and a fast pathway with a long refractory period. An atrial premature beat will therefore be conducted down the slow pathway (short refractory period) by which time the fast

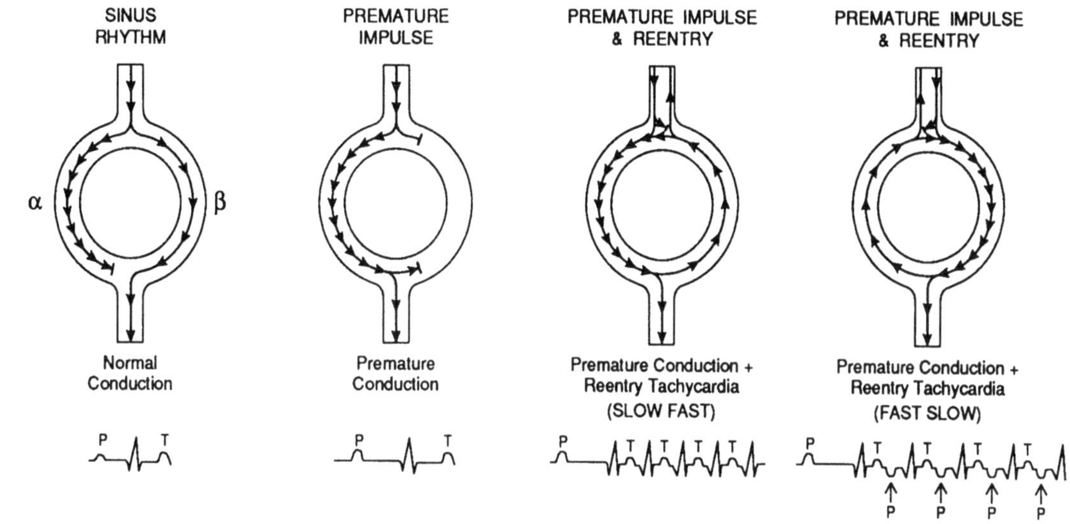

FIGURE 8.10. Mechanism of reentrant tachycardia. Proximal and distal pathways within the A-V node (or myocardium) are linked by a pathway with slow conduction and a short refractory period and a pathway with fast conduction and a long refractory period. In sinus rhythm impulses traverse the rapid pathway producing a single QRS complex. A premature impulse finds the fast pathway refractory in both directions and is blocked; a single premature beat results. When retrograde conduction is possible, reentry tachycardia may occur and may be slow antegrade and fast retrograde (P waves invisible) or fast antegrade and slow retrograde (inverted P waves follow T waves).

pathway (long refractory period) has recovered to conduct retrogradely, thus initiating the circus movement and a tachycardia (Fig. 8.10). Because the atria and the ventricles are depolarized simultaneously the P waves are hidden in the QRS complex. Uncommonly there is a fast–slow mechanism: the P waves then occur well after the QRS complex.

Clinical Features. The dysrhythmia frequently affects normal young people and is recurrent. Attacks start and stop suddenly and the duration is variable; they may be precipitated by anxiety and alcohol ingestion. Usually the tachycardia is absolutely regular and in the range of 140–200 beats/min. Clinical examination will detect a constant intensity of the first heart sound, since the normal sequence of atrial and ventricular contraction is maintained, unlike ventricular tachycardia where the first heart sound varies in intensity because of A-V dissociation.

Electrocardiographic Features. The findings are those that suggest reentrant supraventricular tachycardia whether A-V nodal or atrioventricular: (1) initiation and termination by an appropriately timed premature beat; (2) the initial ectopic P wave that starts the tachycardia has a different shape from succeeding P waves; and (3) absence of "warm-up," or tachycardia accentuation, as occurs in an automatic tachycardia.

Treatment. Frequently an attack will respond to vagal stimulation (carotid sinus massage or Valsalva maneuver). The drugs of choice are i.v. verapamil or adenosine. Should these fail digoxin may be given i.v. Because of its negative inotropic effect, verapamil should not be used if there is any suggestion of heart failure—electrocardioversion is safer.

Atrioventricular Reentrant Tachycardia

Unlike A-V nodal reentry, atrioventricular reentry has an identifiable anatomic pathway. This is the characteristic finding in the WPW syndrome. These "reciprocating" or "circus movement" tachycardias account for 30% of supraventricular tachycardias. One limb of the circuit is the A-V node and the other is the accessory connection. In most cases, conduction is "orthodromic," that is, in the normal antegrade direction through the A-V node and "retrograde" through the accessory connection—the QRS complex is therefore normal (Fig. 8.3). When conduction is antidromic or retrograde through the A-V node and antegrade through the connection, the QRS complex is widened, as in the "delta wave" of the WPW syndrome. In both instances the retrograde P wave is seen well after (more than 0.07 seconds) the QRS complex.

Compared to the A-V node, the accessory pathway has faster conduction and a longer refractory period. A premature beat can then block the pathway (because of its long refractory period), traverse the A-V node, and return to the atria by the accessory connection. If the pathway conducts only retrogradely, the QRS complex in sinus rhythm is normal and the pathway is "concealed." If the pathway allows antegrade conduction, the electrocardiogram snows preexcitation (delta wave) with a WPW type complex.

Diagnosis. During tachycardia the retrograde P wave is seen after the QRS complex. These retrograde P waves are later than in A-V nodal reentrant tachycardia (more than 0.07 seconds) because atrial activation follows ventricular activation. In A-V nodal tachycardia the atria and ventricles are activated simultaneously. When preexcitation is absent ("concealed") in sinus rhythm, the pathway may be revealed by delaying A-V nodal conduction (vagal stimulation or i.v. adenosine), which permits antegrade conduction through the accessory pathway; When identified, these patients should have electrophysiologic studies to assess the risk of rapid preexcited tachycardia—they may be candidates for surgical ablation of the pathway.

Treatment. Termination of the acute attack may be achieved with vagotonic maneuvers, or i.v. verapamil or adenosine. Long-term control is by suppressing premature beats and modifying the reentry circuit. The A-V node may be made more refractory by β-blockers or calcium channel antagonists and the accessory pathway made more refractory by procainamide, disopyramide, or quinidine. Refractory tachycardias are candidates for catheter or surgical ablation.

Preexcitation Syndromes

Early activation of the ventricles by a stimulus conducted through an accessory pathway that bypasses the A-V node is referred to as "preexcitation" or "accelerated A-V conduction" (Figs. 6.18 and 6.19). The phenomenon is typical of, but not exclusive to the WPW syndrome. The characteristics of the WPW syndrome are as follows:

1. P-R interval less than 0.12 seconds.
2. QRS wider than 0.12 seconds.
3. Initial slurring of the QRS by the delta wave of preexcitation.
4. Susceptibility to paroxysmal tachycardias:
   a. Atrioventricular reentry tachycardia.
   b. Atrial fibrillation or flutter with anomalous A-V conduction.

Preexcitation and the delta wave are not always manifest depending on the location and conduction time through the accessory pathway and the effect of drugs and autonomic tone. This differs from a "concealed bypass" tract that can conduct retrograde only from ventricle to atrium, so that the 12-lead EKG is unaffected.

WPW—Tachyarrhythmias

Narrow QRS—A-V Reciprocating Tachycardia. The QRS complex is narrow because the conduction is orthodromic through the A-V node and retrograde through the anomalous pathway. The tachycardia is in the range of 150 to 240 beats/min. When P waves are visible, they usually follow the QRS and are superimposed on the ST segment or T wave. The QRS is always narrow unless rate-related aberrant ventricular conduction supervenes.

Wide QRS—A-V Reciprocating Tachycardia. This is due either to (1) aberrant ventricular conduction complicating an orthodromic tachycardia as described above or (2) an antidromic tachycardia with antegrade conduction through the anomalous pathway resulting in continuous preexcitation of the ventricles with

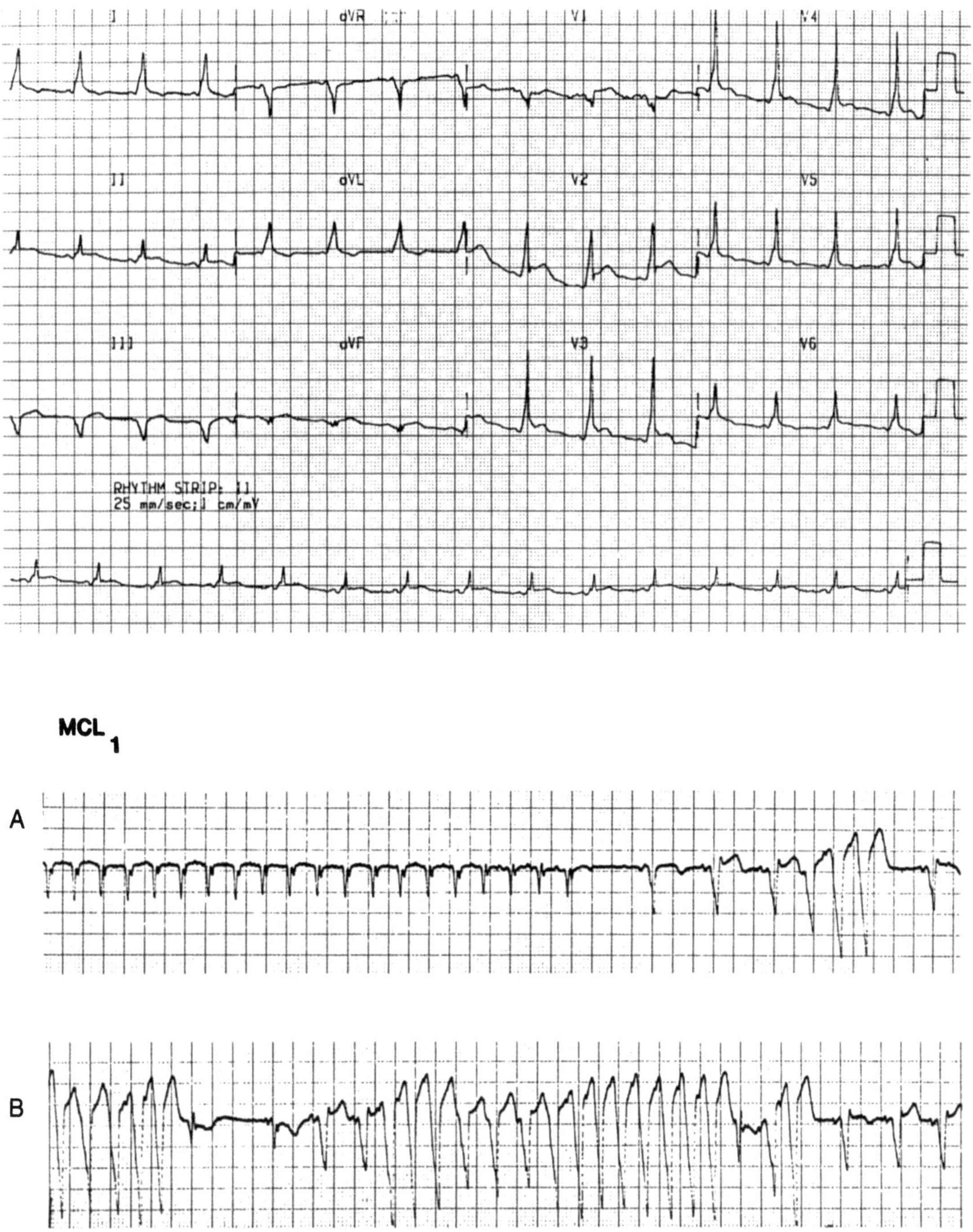

FIGURE 8.11. Top: EKG showing typical morphology of WPW syndrome. Bottom: Rhythm strips (A & B) showing narrow QRS—A-V reciprocating tachycardia followed by bursts of atrial fibrillation with irregular wide QRS complex tachycardia because of antegrade conduction through the anomalous pathway; rate 300/min.

delta waves and wide QRS complex. In both situations the tracings may be impossible to distinguish from ventricular tachycardia.

Atrial Fibrillation. This is a dangerous dysrhythmia among patients whose bypass tract can conduct at rapid rates. The resultant wide complex QRS tachycardia may be indistinguishable from ventricular tachycardia—except that the rhythm is irregular (Fig. 8.11). This dysrhythmia may lead to hemodynamic collapse and in some cases to ventricular fibrillation. Ventricular fibrillation may be precipitated by the use of verapamil or digoxin in an irregular wide complex tachycardia when the mechanism is atrial fibrillation and preexcitation.

Treatment. The typical WPW electrocardiographic findings occur in one to three EKGs per thousand of nonselected individuals. There is a miniscule risk for sudden death from ventricular fibrillation in an asymptomatic individual without heart disease and no further evaluation is necessary.

Among patients known to have WPW the use of digoxin or verapamil is absolutely contraindicated in the presence of an irregular wide complex tachycardia; electrical cardioversion is the treatment of choice. Acute termination of reentrant, narrow complex tachycardias is by vagotonic maneuvers or i.v. verapamil or adenosine. Long-term control is aimed at suppressing premature beats or altering conduction through the reentry circuit. The A-V node may be made more refractory with β-blockers, digoxin, or calcium antagonists. The accessory pathway may be made more refractory with disopyramide, procainamide, or quinidine. Surgical ablation of the pathway is reserved for patients with resistant tachycardias, and in particular for those who have a rapid ventricular response to atrial fibrillation; the mortality and morbidity are negligible and it is effective in more than 95% of cases.

The Lown–Ganong–Levine Syndrome. This consists of a short P-R interval, a normal QRS complex, and paroxysmal tachycardia. It is a result of bypass tracts preexciting the A-V node or bundle of His. It is much less frequent than the WPW syndrome.

Other Junctional Dysrhythmias

Junctional Extrasystoles

These have already been referred to as a form of supraventricular ectopic beats. When there is retrograde conduction to the atria from the junctional tissues, the premature P wave is inverted in leads II, III, and AVF. The sinus node is prematurely discharged and, therefore, the compensatory pause is incomplete. When there is retrograde block of the junctional impulse, the sinus discharge is uninterupted and there is a complete compensatory pause; there is, however, no P wave representative of atrial depolarization. When beats originate at distal sites in the bundle of His, or when there is marked delay in retrograde conduction to the atrium, the P wave follows the QRS complex. The QRS complexes of junctional ectopic beats are usually normal in configuration and duration, unless there is aberrant ventricular conduction. The significance is the same as for atrial extrasystoles.

Junctional Escape Beats

If for any reason there is a failure of discharge of the normally dominant SA node, a slower pacemaker in the atria, A-V node, or ventricles may discharge spontaneously after an interval longer than the cycle set up by the more rapid sinus node. This is known as an escape beat. Long pauses may be provoked by sinus arrhythmia, SA block, or extrasystoles and may therefore result in escape beats. Continuous firing of such a focus produces an *escape rhythm.* Escape beats are characterized by the late occurrence of a junctional beat and the P wave may or may not be visible. The significance of escape beats is related to the cause of sinus bradycardia, sinoatrial block, and so on.

A-V Junctional (Nodal) Rhythm

In junctional rhythm the A-V node is in control of both the atria and the ventricles. It may follow any cause of default of the sinus node (sinus bradycardia, SA block, sinus bradycardia) and the rate is usually between 30 and 60 beats/min (Fig. 8.12).

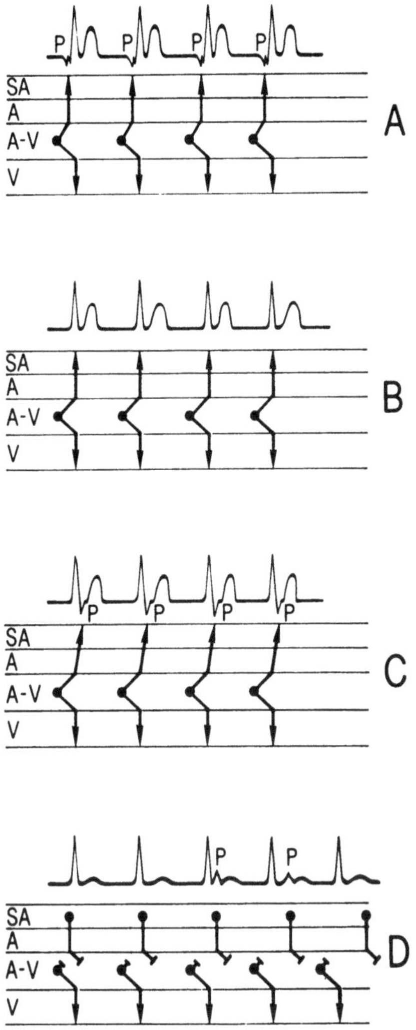

FIGURE 8.12. Junctional rhythm. In (A) retrograde P waves precede each QRS and the PR interval is short. In (B) retrograde P waves are obscured. In (C) retrograde P waves deform the ST segment. In (D) there is complete A-V dissociation; none of the P waves is conducted to the ventricles. The atria and the ventricles beat independently and the P waves "march through the QRS complex."

Electrocardiographically, retrograde P waves may occur before, following, or within a normal QRS complex. When the P waves are inscribed they are narrow and inverted in leads II, III, and AVF.

This rhythm may be recognized clinically by its slow rate and a loud first heart sound produced by the early relationship between atrial contraction and ventricular contraction. When atrial contraction coincides with that of the ventricle, cannon A waves may be present in the jugular venous pulse.

Idionodal Tachycardia

When A-V nodal automaticity is sufficiently enhanced to produce a rate between 70 and 100 beats/min, "idionodal" or "nonparoxysmal" A-V nodal tachycardia" is present. Should the sinus node speed up, idionodal tachycardia will be abolished. The significance of idionodal tachycardia, like that of idioventricular tachycardia to be discussed later, is one of nonspecific increase in automaticity of the A-V node, produced by myocardial infarction, administration of digitalis, or fever. Because of its rate, it does not produce hemodynamic embarrassment and does not require active specific treatment.

Paroxysmal Extrasystolic Junctional Tachycardia

This is a run of three or more junctional extrasystoles, usually with a normal QRS configuration, and has the same significance as paroxysmal atrial tachycardia discussed previously.

Wandering Pacemaker

When the pacemaking focus oscillates between the sinus and the A-V nodes, in the absence of premature beats, a "wandering pacemaker" is said to be present. Electrocardiographically, this is represented by P waves of different shape with a group of sinus P waves replaced by retrograde P waves originating in the A-V node. P waves of intermediate contour represent a fusion of sinus node and A-V node impulses. Wandering atrial pacemaker is produced by fluctuating vagal tone and, therefore, does not have any specific connotation.

Ventricular Dysrhythmias

Ventricular Extrasystoles

This is the commonest abnormality of cardiac rhythm. They have as their mechanism the reentry phenomenon with the following electrocardiographic features:

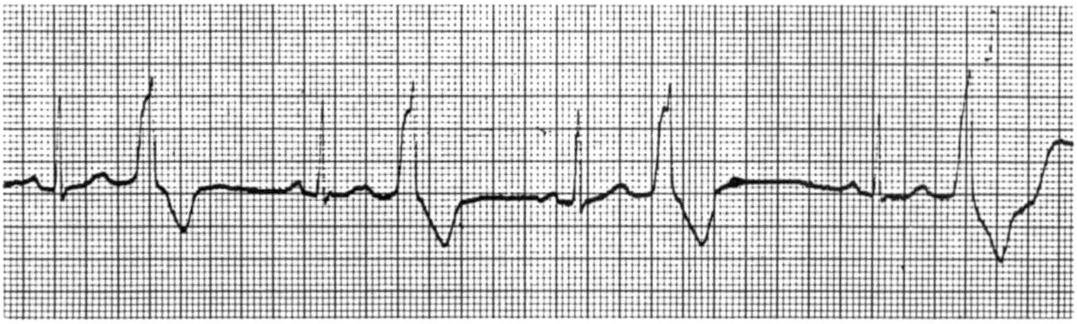

FIGURE 8.13. Electrocardiogram showing ventricular bigeminy. The interval between the sinus and ectopic beat is constant ("fixed coupling interval").

1. The QRS complex is premature and wide, with the ST segment and T wave inscribed in opposite direction to the terminal QRS complex.
2. The relationship between the preceding normal sinus beat and the extrasystole has a fixed relationship, called a "fixed coupling interval" (Fig. 8.13).
3. They often reset the sinus node so that the compensatory pause is complete (i.e., the pre- and postectopic periods equal two consecutive sinus intervals).
4. Occasionally, ventricular extrasystoles are perfectly interposed between two sinus beats without a compensatory pause; they are then said to be "interpolated."

Most premature beats are wide. Those that arise in the right ventricle have a left bundle branch block pattern, whereas those that arise in the left ventricle have a right bundle branch block pattern. Beats arising in a normal heart frequently have a right ventricular configuration.

Simple Premature Beats

These are isolated (i.e., no couplets or triplets), infrequent (less than 10/hours), not superimposed on the preceding T wave, and have the same shape (uniform).

Simple premature beats are common in healthy asymptomatic individuals, occurring at rest but sometimes precipitated by exercise. When they result in palpitation, patients should be reasurred as to their benign nature. Avoidance of alcohol, tobacco, and sympatheticomimetic drugs may help. When acompanied by vayue chest pain, fatigue, and anxiety, the symptoms are those of panic disorder and should be treated as such.

Complex Premature Beats

These occur as couplets, triplets, salvoes, or three or more and are multiform (two or more different shapes).

In the setting of acute myocardial infarction, complex premature beats are forerunners of ventricular fibrillation. This risk has been significantly reduced by treatment with lidocaine and procainamide.

Among the survivors of acute myocardial infarction, patients with hypertrophic and congestive cardiomyopathy, and those with chronic valvular disease, the presence of VPBs carries an adverse prognosis. Whether to treat such patients is controversial since the efficacy of antidysrhythmic therapy has not been established. Patients with significant symptoms should be treated for their relief. Many authorities also recommend treatment for high grade ventricular ectopy when there is severe underlying heart disease. Under both circumstances therapy should be carefully monitored with 24 hour Holter recordings and blood drug levels to detect aggravation of the arrhythmia (proarrhythmia) that may occur with any antidysrhythmic drugs.

Parasystole

Not all ventricular ectopic beats are characterized by a fixed coupling interval. In parasystole the ectopic beats are of similar morphology to the usual type of ventricular ectopic beats, but the coupling interval is not fixed. In parasystole there is an ectopic pacemaker that is *protected* from the impulses of the sinus node, which is normally the dominant pacemaker. Therefore, the ectopic pacemaker fires in undisturbed fashion at its own rate and will activate the ventricles when they are not refractory. Parasystole is characterized by (1) the absence of fixed coupling intervals, and (2) interectopic intervals that have as their common denominator the shortest interectopic interval; all other intervals are multiples of this. *Fusion beats* are commonly associated with parasystole because the two pacemakers fire at their own rates and eventually the ventricles will be activated by a combination of a pure sinus beat and a pure ventricular beat producing a fusion beat with intermediate configuration.

Parasystole is not a common arrhythmia and the principles of treatment of the condition are the same as those for ventricular ectopy. This usually occurs in the setting of acute myocardial infarction when a parasystolic tachycardia may be present.

Ventricular Tachycardia

By definition, this is a series of three or more ectopic ventricular complexes at a rate of 100 to 250/min.

Sustained ventricular tachycardia refers to episodes of 30 seconds or more that require drugs or cardioversion to terminate the attack. When the duration of the tachycardia is less than 30 seconds but longer than 3 beats and aborts spontaneously, it is said to be *nonsustained*.

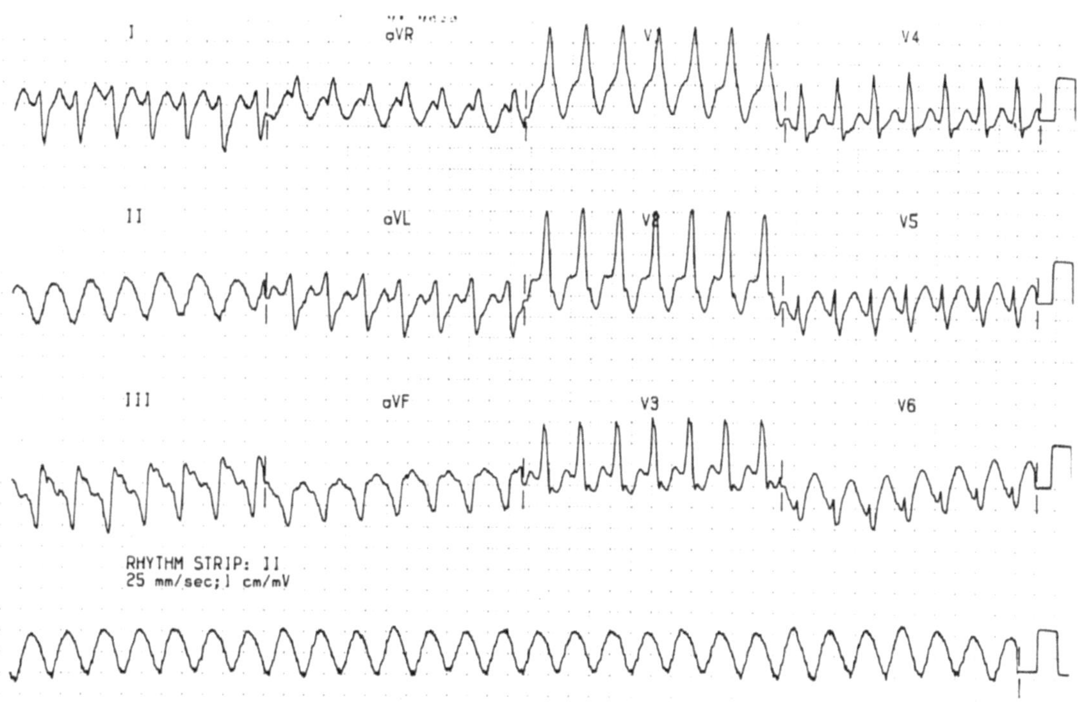

FIGURE 8.14. Ventricular tachycardia, 180 beats/min. The QRS axis is −150°, QRS duration is 0.18 seconds, and right bundle branch block configuration—features highly suggestive of ventricular tachycardia.

Electrocardiographic Features

The ventricular rate is usually in the range of 150 to 200/min and the QRS complexes have the characteristics of ventricular ectopic beats (Fig. 8.14). The QRS duration is wide: more than 140 m/sec with a right bundle branch block and more than 160 m/sec with a left bundle branch block pattern. Typically, the QRS complexes are of the same shape and position in all leads (positive concordance). The mean frontal plane QRS axis is deviated to the left of −90°. In 50% of cases there is A-V dissociation, so there is no relationship between the P waves and the QRS complexes. In the other 50% there is retrograde conduction to the atrium, so that P waves follow the QRS complexes. In many cases, however, it is impossible to discern the P waves. During the paroxysm, the A-V node is refractory to most supraventricular impulses, but occasionally a *capture beat* may occur. This is recognized by a P wave preceding a QRS complex, which differs in shape from that of the ectopic ventricular focus. *Fusion beats* represent partial capture of the ventricles and have a QRS shape intermediate between a sinus and an ectopic beat. The presence of *capture* and *fusion* beats is a pointer to the diagnosis of A-V dissociation and therefore ventricular tachycardia, rather than supraventricular tachycardia with aberrant ventricular conduction.

Bidirectional ventricular tachycardia refers to beat-by-beat variation in the direction of the QRS complexes. This type of ventricular tachycardia is almost invariably associated with digitalis toxicity and is probably a result of a supraventricular tachycardia with alternating left anterior and left posterior hemiblock as a result of aberrant conduction in these bundles.

Ventricular flutter is a variant of ventricular tachycardia at a faster rate, and an immediate precursor of ventricular fibrillation, is recognized by sine wave or zig-zag pattern making a clear separation of the QRS complexes and T waves difficult.

Idioventricular tachycardia is a manifestation of an accelerated idioventricular rhythm characterized by an idioventricular rate of 70 to 90 beats/min. Like idionodal tachycardia it represents acceleration of a subsidiary pacemaker overcoming the normally dominant SA node. It has the same nonspecific connotation as idionodal tachycardia and may occur with myocardial infarction, rheumatic fever, and digitalis administration.

The electrocardiogram demonstrates bizarre QRS complexes at a rate of approximately 70 to 80 beats/min. Capture beats and fusion beats are common because of the slow rate of the idioventricular focus, which provides adequate recovery time for capture by a sinus impulse.

Like idionodal tachycardia, this rhythm does not produce serious hemodynamic effects and treatment is not usually required. Occasionally, in myocardial infarction the loss of atrial contraction may be important and the ectopic ventricular rhythm can then be overdriven with the use of atropine, which accelerates the sinus node discharge rate.

Torsade de pointes means a "twisting of points". It refers to a form of polymorphic nonsustained ventricular tachycardia where the electrical polarity alters so that the peaks of the QRS complexes appear to twist around the isoelectric line (Fig. 8.15).

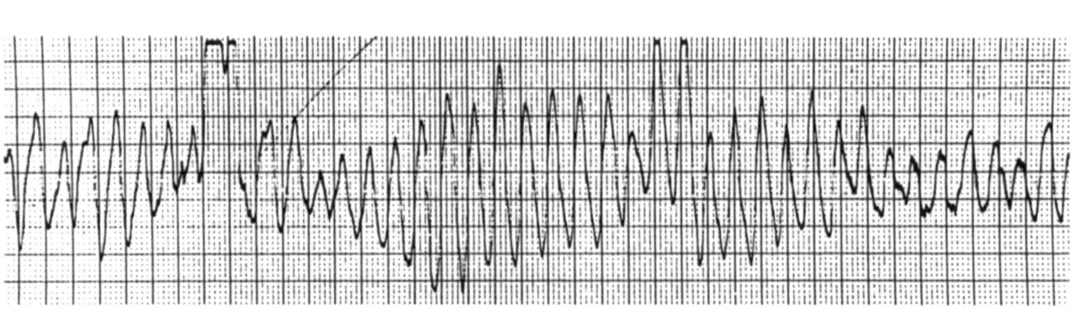

FIGURE 8.15. Electrocardiogram of "torsade de pointes" (see text).

This episodic dysrhythmia is frequently associated with a long QT interval and has been called the "long QT syndrome". The *congenital* variety of the syndrome is associated with a strong family history of syncope and sudden death (Romano syndrome) and there may also be associated deafness (Jervile–Lange–Nielsen syndrome). The *acquired* variety occurs as a result of electrolyte abnormalities, drug toxicity, ischemia, and myocarditis. The treatment is to remove any predisposing cause such as Class Ia and Ic drugs. When rapid control of the dysrhythmia is necessary, overdrive atrial pacing and infusion of isoprotenolol may be effective. The congenital examples are treated by β-blockade and stellate ganglion sympathectomy.

Electrocardiographic Distinction between Ventricular Tachycardia and Ventricular Tachycardia with Aberrant

Ventricular Conduction (Wide QRS Complex Tachycardia)

Abnormal intraventricular conduction of a supraventricular impulse may occur in temporary (phasic) or permanent (nonphasic) forms. In phasic aberrant ventricular conduction bizarre QRS complexes occur during rhythms with otherwise normal intraventricular conduction. When phasic aberrant ventricular conduction occurs the bizarre complexes characteristic of ventricular ectopic rhythms (ventricular tachycardia) are closely mimicked. The distinction between the two has important prognostic and therapeutic implications.

Any supraventricular rhythm may be complicated by aberrant ventricular conduction. Normally the refractory periods of the left and right bundle branches are equal. When the refractory periods are unequal early impulses may find the one bundle refractory and the other recovered; they will therefore be conducted with a pattern of bundle branch block. The preceding RR interval is highly critical in determining whether aberrant ventricular conduction will occur. Teleologically, the refractory period must shorten with tachycardia and lengthen with bradycardia. When the refractory periods are unequal this same effect pertains. When the preceding RR interval is long, the ensuing refractory period will be long and any disparity between the refractory periods of the two bundles will therefore be greater. Should an early impulse occur in the beat following a long preceding RR interval, the chances of finding one bundle refractory and the other recovered are much greater; this, therefore, predisposes to aberration of the conducted beats. This phenomenon may occur with isolated ectopic beats or with more sustained arrhythmias such as atrial fibrillation, atrial flutter, and supraventricular tachycardia (Fig. 8.8).

When a single beat, or a salvo of bizarre beats is inscribed, the possibility exists that either ventricular ectopy or aberrant ventricular conduction of a supraventricular impulse is present. The distinction between the two rests on (1) the relationship of the P wave to the QRS complex and (2) the morphology of the QRS complex.

To diagnose supraventricular tachycardia with aberrant ventricular conduction, it should be demonstrated that supraventricular impulses precede the abnormal QRS complexes; in ventricular tachycardia there is dissociation between the P waves and the QRS complexes. This is not always easy to detect because a rapid tachycardia may obscure the P waves, and they are absent in atrial fibrillation; even when they are detected it may be difficult to determine whether they are conducted antegrade, or retrograde from an etopic ventricular focus. Knowledge of a preexisting bundle branch block is valuable in making the distinction—in supraventricular tachycardia with bundle branch block, the "wide QRS" tachycardia is of the same morphology. However, with ventricular tachycardia and preexisting bundle branch block, the QRS morphology is quite different.

Fusion beats favor the diagnosis of ventricular tachycardia since they represent simultaneous activation of the ventricles by supraventricular and ventricular impulses. A fusion beat can be diagnosed only when a pure ectopic beat, a pure conducted supraventricular beat, and the intermediate configuration of the fusion beat itself are present. The presence of a considerably longer cycle following a run of anomalous beats favors ventricular ectopy because this represents a compensatory pause. This may be particularly helpful in the diagnosis of atrial fibrillation complicated by aberration since the QRS complexes are not usually followed by a compensatory pause.

Despite all these pointers, the diagnosis of a wide QRS complex tachycardia is difficult. Helpful practical clues are as follows:

1. Ventricular tachycardia is much more frequent than supraventricular tachycardia with aberrant conduction.
2. Ventricular tachycardia is much more likely when there is heart disease (particularly ischemic) and when the patient is elderly.
3. Ventricular tachycardia characteristically has
   a. atrioventricular dissociation,
   b. mean frontal QRS axis to the left of −90°,
   c. QRS duration more than 140 msec with right bundle and 160 msec with left bundle branch block,
   d. concordant upright complexes in the precordial leads, and
   e. tachycardia QRS complexes different to previous tracings in patients with bundle branch block.

Treatment

Ventricular tachycardia is usually a medical emergency since it commonly occurs in the setting of acute myocardial infarction. If there is hypotension with poor peripheral perfusion, the patient should be electrically cardioverted immediately. The same approach should be used when there is uncertainty as to whether the diagnosis is ventricular tachycardia or supraventricular tachycardia with aberrant conduction. The use of i.v. verapamil may lead to fatal hypotension in cases of ventricular tachycardia.

When the clinical situation is stable, drug treatment should be tried. Lidocaine 100 mg i.v. is given as a bolus over 1 minute followed by a second dose of 100 mg at 10 minutes. If this is successful a maintenance infusion of 1–5 mg/min is started. If lidocaine fails, procainamide may be given i.v. at a rate of 50 mg/min for a total dose of 500 mg. If successful it should be followed by an i.v. infusion at 1 to 4 mg/min, with close observation of the blood pressure and monitoring of the QRS complex for widening.

Burst pacing using a pervenous temporary pacing wire will terminate most attacks of ventricular tachycardia. The ventricle is paced at a rate of 50 beats/min faster than the tachycardia for a total of 50 beats.

In the absence of acute myocardial infarction or other acute precipitating factors, such as hypokalemia and drug toxicity, all patients with recurrent sustained ventricular tachycardia are candidates for electrophysiologic evaluation because of the risk for sudden death. Programmed stimulation induces and terminates ventricular tachycardia and allows sequential testing of various drugs for their efficacy in preventing induction of the dysrhythmia. One or two closely coupled paced beats are used to stimulate the apex of the right ventricle. These stimuli scan diastole to change a reentry circuit, blocking one limb and provoking a tachycardia. The technique is highly sensitive (80%) and almost completely specific. It can be made more sensitive by adding a third stimulus. Serial drug testing is then used to identify an effective agent that makes the tachycardia noninducible. When an effective agent is identified and then used orally, it is likely that the tachycardia will be clinically suppressed. These principles are valid for most drugs, except amiodarone and propafenone, where failure to suppress induction may not necessarily predict a poor clinical response. Repeat testing with amiodarone should be delayed for at least 2 weeks. Programmed stimulation is much more efficacious than Holter monitoring and exercise testing.

Surgery is the next option for the treatment of patients with drug-resistant tachycardia. Preoperative electrophysiological study will determine the type of tachycardia and also locate the reentry circuit. The site of origin of the tachycardia is confirmed by endocardial mapping at operation. The focus is then ablated by aneurysmectomy and endocardial resection when necessary.

Antidysrhythmic Drugs

The various antidysrhythmic drugs have been classified according to their physiologic effects on pacemaking and nonpacemaking cells. It is important to realize, however, that this classification does not help in the clinical selection of an appropriate agent—the choice is largely empirical.

When choosing an antidysrhythmic drug there are two important considerations apart from the action of a drug on a specific dysrhythmia.

1. *Negative Inotropic Effect.* Many antidysrhythmic drugs have this action but it is most significant with β-blockers, disopyramide, and verapamil. These drugs should not be used in the presence of congestive heart failure or when there is a markedly depressed left ventricular ejection fraction.

2. *Proarrhythmia.* Drug-induced arrhythmias occur in 5 to 10% of patients. Deaths occur in 1 to 3% of patients treated for serious ventricular dysrhythmias but much less commonly in those treated for less serious dysrhythmias (0.1%). This is a significant problem and patients starting treatment should be closely monitored for a few days. Ventricular tachycardia may be provoked with Class Ia drugs and this usually takes the form of *torsade de pointes*. This may occur in patients with no history of ventricular tachycardia and is independent of drug dosage and serum levels. Class Ic drugs (encainide and flecainide) may also provoke ventricular tachycardia, particularly among patients with left ventricular dysfunction and a history of ventricular tachycardia. The tachycardia usually has a sustained monomorphic configuration. The actions of the various drugs depend on their effect on the phases of the action potential.

Classification of Antidysrhythmic Drugs

Class I. Local anesthetic drugs
1. Quinidine, procainamide, disopyramide
2. Tocainide, mexiletine, lidocaine
3. Encainide, flecainide, propafenone

Class II. β-Blockers

Class III. Prolong repolarization amiodarone sotolol, bretyllium

Class IV. Calcium channel blockers

Class I

These agents act by depressing to varying degrees the fast inward sodium current (phase 0 upstroke velocity) or V_{max}, which is the maximum rate of change of voltage over time. The class is subdivided into subgroups Ia, Ib, and Ic depending on their effects on repolarization and resultant EKG changes.

Class Ia

These drugs reduce V_{max} and also prolong the action potential. They delay both conduction and repolarization, widening the QRS complex and prolonging the QT interval.

Quinidine

This is almost completely absorbed after oral administration, begins to act within 30 minutes, and has a peak effect in 2 to 3 hours. It is metabolized chiefly in the liver, resulting in loss of its antiarrhythmic effects. Its elimination is impaired in the presence of liver disease. However, elimination by the kidneys is not significantly impaired among patients with renal dysfunction or congestive cardiac failure. When used in combination with digoxin, blood levels of the latter are increased and toxicity may ensue.

Quinidine, like other group I drugs, depresses excitability and conductivity and also has an anticholinergic action. Indications for its use are as follows:

1. Paroxysmal atrial arrhythmias (flutter, fibrillation, and tachycardia).
2. Premature atrial and ventricular beats.
3. Ventricular tachycardia.
4. WPW syndrome.
5. Prevention of recurrences of the above arrhythmias.

Dosage. Following an initial 200 mg dose of quinidine sulfate to test for idiosyncrasy or hypersensitivity, the usual maintenance dose is 200–400 mg every six hours. Therapeutic blood levels range from 2 to 6 μg/ml. Since quinidine prolongs the refractory period of the atria it may be effective in converting atrial fibrillation or flutter to sinus rhythm. The drug should be used with caution in the treatment of atrial flutter since 1:1 conduction may result from slowing of the flutter rate. This may be prevented by prior digitalization.

EKG Effects. Because the drug slows conduction and repolarization it may prolong the PR, QRS, and QT intervals. Quinidine should not be used in patients with heart block or a tendency to develop heart block.

Adverse Reactions. Diarrhea, nausea, and vomiting are the commonest. Hypersensitivity reactions include hemolytic anemia, skin rashes, thrombocytopenia, and angioneurotic edema. An immune response may be responsible for thrombocytopenia and hepatic granulomatosis. The cardiotoxic effects are sinus arrest, atrioventricular block, torsades de point, ventricular tachycardia, ventricular fibrillation, and sudden death. These effects are usually observed with high doses, but occasionally with normal doses. Usually EKG changes (QRS widening, Q-T-U prolongation) precede cardiac toxicity and there is time to stop the drug. Rarely, ventricular fibrillation may occur with no warning. It may occur in paroxysms (*quinidine syncope*) and this presages a fatal outcome.

Idiosyncrasy may take the form of allergic bronchospasm, rash, shock, and thrombocytopenia. The most serious effect, however, is that of cardiotoxicity. Treatment is to withdraw the drug whereon toxic effects abate rapidly because of its short half-life.

Procainamide

The electrophysiological actions of pronestyl are much the same as those of quinidine, but clinically the drug is more efficacious in ventricular arrhythmias.

Pronestyl is virtually completely absorbed after oral administration and approximately 50% is excreted unchanged in the urine. The drug undergoes acetylation in the liver and therefore plasma levels should include estimation of both procainamide and *N*-acetylprocainamide. The effective blood level for procainamide is 4–8 μg/ml and when the acetylated product is included the effective level is double.

Procainamide may lengthen the PR and QRS intervals, but less commonly than quinidine.

Adverse Reactions. Like quinidine, procainamide may produce gastrointestinal symptoms such as nausea, anorexia, and diarrhea. Approximately three-quarters of patients who receive the drug long-term will develop a positive antinuclear-antibody test. In some instances this will be associated with all the signs and symptoms of disseminated lupus erythematosus (apart from renal involvement), which may disappear when the drug is discontinued. Like quinidine, conduction disturbances, asystole, ventricular tachycardia, and ventricular fibrillation may occur.

Dosage. Orally, the short acting preparation of the drug is given at 4–6 hour intervals in doses of 250 to 500 mg. The slow release form may be given every 6 or 8 hours. The drug must be used cautiously intravenously. The maximum dose is 100 mg given slowly every 5 minutes until a total dose of 1 g is reached. More rapid administration results in severe hypotension and myocardial depression.

Disopyramide

This is an effective agent for the treatment of both ventricular and supraventricular dysrhythmias. Its usefulness is limited by its side effects, which may be serious.

Electrophysiologically, its actions are similar to those of quinidine and procainamide, and it prolongs the PR, QRS, and QT intervals.

Disopyramide has a significant negative inotropic effect. It may precipitate heart failure in patients who have a history of heart failure or in those patients with a depressed left ventricular ejection fraction. It should never be used in patients who are actually in heart failure.

The vagolytic effect of the drug produces urinary retention, constipation, and dry eyes.

The dose is 100 to 200 mg three to four times daily.

Class IB

In this group are drugs that do not reduce V_{max} but shorten the duration of the action potential.

Lidocaine

In contrast to its lack of effect on the conduction velocity in normal fibers, lidocaine slows conduction in the ventricular myocardium and His–Purkinje system in the presence of acute ischemia. It has little effect on A-V conduction.

The chief clinical use of lidocaine is the prevention and treatment of ventricular arrhythmias. It has no place in the treatment of supraventricular arrhythmias. It is rapidly metabolized in the liver and lower doses should be used in the presence of liver disease to avoid toxicity. Important side-effects of lidocaine are produced by its action on the central nervous system. Toxic doses produce drowsiness, confusion, psychosis, and seizures. In normal doses the drug has little or no negative inotropic effect. Less than 10% is excreted unchanged in the urine and therefore renal failure produces little effect on blood levels.

The dosage of lidocaine consists of an initial loading dose of 1 to 1:5 mg/kg given intravenously followed by an infusion of 1–4 mg/min. Derivatives of lidocaine (tocainide and mexiletine) have similar effects but are effective orally and have a slower rate of hepatic metabolism.

Tocainide and Mexiletine

These are lidocaine cogeners administered orally. Both are effective in treating ventricular dysrhythmias and neither has a significant negative inotropic effect. Like lidocaine, these drugs do not significantly change the QRS intervals.

The side effects of these agents, like lidocaine, involve the central nervous system and gastrointestinal tract. These include dizziness, tremor, slurred speech, ataxia, nausea, vomiting, and diarrhea.

Dosage: Tocainide. The usual dose is 400–800 mg tid. The therapeutic plasma level is 4 to 10 mg/liter. It is largely metabolized by the liver but one-third is excreted unchanged by the kidney; therefore caution is necessary when there is renal failure.

Dosage: Mexiletine. The usual dose is 150–400 mg tid. It is largely metabolized in the liver but 115% is excreted unchanged in the urine.

Class Ic

In this group are drugs that reduce V_{max}, primarily slow conduction, and have little effect on refractoriness.

Encainide

This is an effective agent for the treatment of ventricular ectopy. It has a definite proarrhythmic effect, which seriously limits its use.

The usual dose is 25 to 50 mg three or four times daily. The drug produces significant lengthening of the PR and QRS intervals. Unfortunately, QRS widening does not predict the proarrhythmic effect and runs of ventricular tachycardia may occur without warning.

Flecainide

This is an agent that is effective in the treatment of supraventricular and ventricular dysrhythmias. Like encainide, it has a definite proarrhythmic effect and is therefore not available for general use. It produces significant prolongation of the PR and QRS intervals. The usual dose is 100 to 200 mg bid.

Propafenone

This is effective in the treatment of supraventricular and ventricular dysrhythmias and the WPW syndrome. The drug slows impulse conduction, lengthening the PR and QRS intervals. Side-effects are usually mild. The chief limitation to its use is its negative inotropic effect, therefore, it should not be used when there is heart failure or left ventricular dysfunction.

Class II: β-Adrenergic Blocking Agents

The drugs in this group are the β-receptor blockers whose antiarrhythmic action depends on their β-adrenergic blocking effect rather than any direct "membrane effect." β-Blockers slow the velocity of the upstroke of the action potential and suppress phase 4 depolarization.

β-Blockers are useful in the treatment of atrial and ventricular ectopic beats and in supraventricular and ventricular tachycardias of the automatic or reentry type. They are usually used in conjunction with a group I agent for the suppression of ventricular dysrhythmias. Through their action on the A-V node, the ventricular response is reduced in atrial flutter and atrial fibrillation. They are particularly useful in the treatment of tachyarrhythmias that are a result of digitalis toxicity or hyperthyroidism.

Propranolol, the prototypical β-blocker, is largely metabolized in the liver and the drug should be used with caution in liver disease. In high dosage, severe bradycardia and heart block may be precipitated. Its negative inotropic effect may produce heart failure by removing sympathetic stimulation from a failing left ventricle. Similarly, it may precipitate acute bronchospasm in asthmatics or among patients with chronic obstructive airways disease. The drug should be used with caution when there is evidence of peripheral vascular disease because unopposed α-adrenergic activity may reduce peripheral blood flow. Symptoms of hypoglycemia may be obscured in diabetic patients because of its effect in blocking the action of epinephrine.

The cardioselective β-blockers (atenolol and metropolol) may be more useful because they have fewer side effects.

Class III

In this class are drugs that block potassium channels and prolong repolarization.

Amiodarone

This is a Class III agent, but also has Classes I, II, and IV effects. Its major electrophysiologic action is to prolong the duration of the action potential of cardiac tissues. It exhibits mild α-receptor, β-receptor, and calcium channel blocking activities. Amiodarone is widely used and is a highly effective treatment for ventricular tachycardia. It also prevents atrial flutter, fibrillation, WPW arrhythmias, and other junctional tachycardias.

The drug has a negative inotropic effect but cardiac output is usually unaffected because of peripheral vasodilatation. The drug lengthens the PR and QT intervals and produces prominent U waves. The dosage is variable and requires weeks to months of loading to reach a steady state. The recommended dose is 800–1600 mg daily for 3 weeks, 600–800 mg for the next month, and thereafter 200–400 mg daily for maintenance.

Side effects are common and increase with duration of therapy. Corneal microdeposits occur in 90% of patients and may result in ulceration. Dermatitis and photosensitivity are less common. The most serious side effect is the occurrence of pulmonary infiltrates and irreversible pulmonary fibrosis. Therefore, the drug should be used with caution. Reasonable indications for its use are the WPW syndrome and atrial fibrillation when operation is not feasible and life-threatening ventricular dysrhythmias in hypertrophic and congestive cardiomyopathy.

Bretylium Tosylate

The use of bretylium is restricted to those patients with life-threatening ventricular dysrhythmias unresponsive to Class Ia drugs.

The drug acts on the sympathetic ganglia. Initially, there is a release of catecholamines followed by their suppression. The most important side effect is severe hypotension. The drug in available only in intravenous form.

Class IV

These are drugs that block the slow calcium channels.

Verapamil

The important antidysrhythmic effect of Verapamil and other calcium channel blockers is on nodal tissue. It is commonly used to terminate reentry tachycardia involving the A-V node, and whether an accessory pathway is present or not, it is successful in more than 90% of cases. The drug has a powerful negative inotropic effect when given intravenously and this is particularly dangerous when patients are receiving β-blockers: hypotension, bradycardia, A-V block, and asystole may occur. Intravenous verapamil should be used with great caution in hypertrophic cardiomyopathy.

Verapamil slows the response through the A-V node in atrial fibrillation but is rarely effective in converting the dysrhythmia to sinus rhythm. The drug is contraindicated in the WPW syndrome complicated by atrial fibrillation since dangerous acceleration of the ventricular response may result. It is highly effective, as noted earlier, in the treatment of reentrant tachycardias.

The dose of i.v. verapamil is 10 mg given by slow injection. A further 10 mg may be given 30 minutes later. The oral dose is 80 to 120 mg four times daily. Verapamil may decrease the excretion of digoxin by 30%.

Other Antidysrhythmic Drugs

Adenosine

Adenosine, like verapamil, has depressant effects on the SA and A-V nodes, but does not have a negative inotropic effect. After i.v. injection, it acts within 30 seconds and is eliminated from the bloodstream in seconds so that there are few side-effects. Many patients may react with facial flushing, chest discomfort, or dyspnea, all of which are transient. Sequential doses of 3, 9, and 12 mg will convert more than 90% of supraventricular tachycardias. The usual starting dose is 6 mg.

Adenosine is also useful in diagnosis. When it produces A-V block without terminating a tachycardia, an atrial tachycardia is much more likely than a junctional variety.

Digoxin

Digoxin is the mainstay in the control of the ventricular response in atrial fibrillation. This effect is largely through increasing vagal inhibition on the A-V node. Because this effect is re-

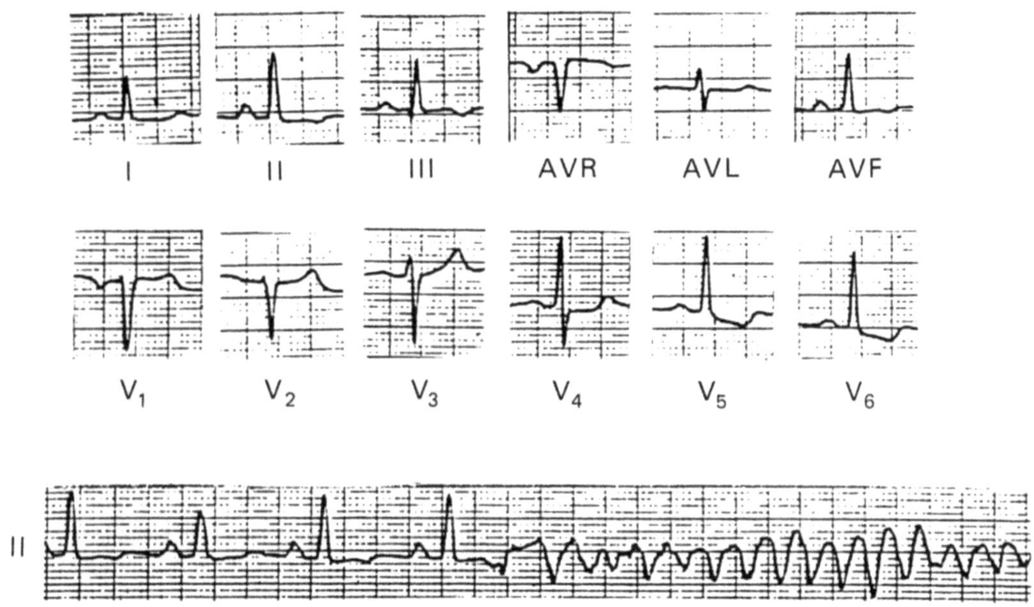

FIGURE 8.16. Electrocardiogram recorded during an episode of angina pectoris showing ST segment depression V4–V6. There is the sudden onset of ventricular fibrillation during recording of rhythm strip II.

duced during exercise, it may be advantageous to add a calcium channel or β-blocker.

Like verapamil, digoxin may produce a dangerous acceleration of the ventricular response to atrial fibrillation in the WPW syndrome.

Ventricular Fibrillation

Electrocardiographically, ventricular fibrillation is a totally irregular arrhythmia characterized by disorganized undulating deflections varying in height and width (Fig. 8.16).

Ventricular fibrillation is most commonly a result of ischemic heart disease and is usually seen in the setting of acute myocardial infarction. Following myocardial infarction, the recurrence rate is only 2%, presumably because of healing and much less ischemic myocardium at risk.

In the case of survivors of out of hospital cardiac arrest the prognosis is poor. These victims are often resuscitated promptly by paramedic teams and frequently do not have electrocardiographic and enzymatic evidence of myocar-

TABLE 8.1. Ventricular fibrillation (and pulseless ventricular tachycardia).[a,b]

Witnessed arrest	Unwitnessed arrest
↓	↓
Check pulse—If no pulse	Check pulse—If no pulse
↓	
Precordial thump	
↓	
Check pulse—If no pulse	
↓	

↓
CPR until a defibrillator is available
↓
Check monitor for rhythm—if VF or VT[c]
↓
Defibrillate, 200 J[d]
↓
Defibrillate, 200–300 J[d]
↓
Defibrillate with up to 360 J[d]
↓
CPR if no pulse
↓
Establish i.v. access
↓
Epinephrine. 1:10,000, 0.5–1.0 mg i.v. push[e]
↓
Intubate if possible[f]
↓
Defibrillate with up to 360 J[d]
↓
Lidocaine, 1 mg/kg i.v push
↓
Defibrillate with up to 360 J[d]
↓
Bretylium, 5 mg/kg i.v. push[g]
↓
(Consider bicarbonate)[h]
↓
Defibrillate with up to 360 J[d]
↓
Bretylium, 10 mg/kg i.v. push[g]
↓
Defibrillate with up to 360 J[d]
↓
Repeat lidocaine or bretylium
↓
Defibrillate with up to 360 J[d]

[a]Reprinted, by permission, from "Textbook of Advanced Cardiac Life Support," 1987, Copyright American Heart Association.

[b]This sequence was developed to assist in teaching how to treat a broad range of patients with ventricular fibrillation (VF) or pulseless ventricular tachycardia (VT). Some patients may require care not specificed herein. This algorithm should not be construed as prohibiting such flexibility. Flow of algorithm presumes that VF is continuing. CPR indicates cardiopulmonary resuscitation.

[c]Pulseless VT should be treated identically to VF.

[d]Check pulse and rhythm after each shock. If VF recurs after transiently converting (rather than persists without ever converting), use whatever energy level has previously been successful for defibrillation.

[e]Epinephrine should be repeated every 5 minutes.

[f]Intubation is preferable. If it can be accompanied simultaneously with other techniques, then the earlier the better. However, defibrillation and epinephrine are more important initially if the patient can be ventilated without intubation.

[g]Some may prefer repeated doses of lidocaine, which may be given in 0.5-mg/kg boluses every 8 minutes to a total dose of 3 mg/kg.

[h]Value of sodium bicarbonate is questionable during cardiac arrest, and it is not recommended for routine cardiac arrest sequence. Consideration of its use in a dose of 1 mEq/kg is appropriate at this point. Half of original dose may be repeated every 10 minutes if it is used.

dial infarction. Because there is myocardium at risk, the recurrence rate at 2 years is 40%.

Treatment

The treatment is immediate nonsynchronized dc shock using 200 to 400 J. Cardiopulmonary resuscitation should be employed only when a defibrillator is not available or when the circulation is inadequate after reversion to sinus rhythm. Time should not be wasted in attempting to determine whether cardiac arrest is a result of ventricular fibrillation or asystole. Dc shock may cause the asystolic heart to discharge as well as converting ventricular fibrillation. An algorithm for the treatment of ventricular fibrillation has been developed by the American Heart Association (Table 8.1).

Cardiac Asystole

This is usually a result of myocardial infarction but may also occur in other forms of severe heart disease. Depression of automaticity may be precipitated in these cases by hypoxia, electrolyte imbalance, and acidosis. Asystole may degenerate into ventricular fibrillation.

Cardiac asystole may be a manifestation of a syndrome of neurally mediated hypotension and bradycardia in the absence of heart disease. This is thought to be a result of stimulation of mechanoreceptors in the left ventricle by hypovolemia. Syncope and profound bradycardia may be reproduced by orthcstatic tilt, which decreases left ventricular volume. It is an important cause of syncope.

The algorithum for the management of asystole of the American Heart Association is given in Table 8.2.

Table 8.2. Asytole (cardiac standstill).[a,b]

If rhythm is unclear and possibly ventricular fibrillation, defibrillate as for VF, if asystole is present[c]

↓

Continue CPR

↓

Establish i.v. access

↓

Epinephrine, 1:10,000, 0.5–mg i.v. push[d]

↓

Intubate when possible[e]

↓

Atropine, 1.0 mg i.v. push (repeated in 5 min)

↓

(Consider bicarbonate)[f]

↓

Consider pacing

[a]Reprinted, by permission, from "Textbook of Advanced Cardiac Life Support," 1987, Copyright American Heart Association.

[b]This sequence was developed to assist in teaching how to treat a broad range of patients with asystole. Some patients may require care not specified herein. This algorithm should not be construed to prohibit such flexibility. Flow of algorithm presumes asystole is continuing. VF indicates ventricular fibrillation.

[c]Asystole should be confirmed in two leads.

[d]Epinephrine should be repeated every 5 minutes.

[e]Intubation is preferable; if it can be accomplished simultaneously with other techniques, then the earlier the better. However, cardiopulmonary resuscitation (CPR) and use of epinephrine are more important initially if patient can be ventilated without intubation. (Endotracheal epinephrine may be used.)

[f]Value of sodium bicarbonate is questionable during cardiac arrest, and it is not recommended for the routine cardiac arrest sequence. Consideration of its use in a dose of 1 mEq/kg is appropriate at this point. Half of original dose may be repeated every 10 minutes if it is used.

Disturbances of Impulse Conduction

Atrioventricular (A-V) Block

The specialized anatomy of the conducting system and its branches has already been described. Interruption or delay in conduction of supraventricular impulses through the A-V node is customarily classified into three degrees:

1. *First-degree A-V block*: a delay in conduction without dropped beats.
2. *Second-degree A-V block*: intermittent interruption of conduction.
3. *Third-degree A-V block*: complete interruption of conduction.

First- and second-degree A-V blocks are sometimes referred to as partial or incomplete degrees of A-V block.

First-Degree A-V Block

At normal heart rates in adults, a PR interval in excess of 21 msec is regarded as abnormal. At rates of over 100, 19 msec or less may be abnormal. The commonest causes are conduction system disease, vagal stimulation (carotid sinus pressure), digitalis, and hypoxia. If vagally mediated it can often be reversed by atropine. Occasionally, it is congenital, and may also occur as an isolated abnormality in apparently healthy people. In normal and diseased hearts prolonged PR interval may be shortened by atropine, exercise, or standing. Usually, the diagnosis is made electrocardiographically, although occasionally it be suspected by irregular cannon A waves in the neck, by a soft first heart sound, or by presystolic triple rhythm.

Second-Degree A-V Block

In this condition there is failure of conduction of sinus beats to the ventricle (Fig. 8.17). The atria are activated normally and the P wave is inscribed, but the impulse is blocked within the A-V conducting system. There are three varieties of second-degree A-V block.

Mobitz Type I A-V Block: (the Wenckebach Phenomenon)

This is the commonest type of second-degree A-V block and it is characterized by progressive lengthening of the PR interval until a beat is dropped. The sequence may begin with a PR interval that is normal or prolonged. Following the dropped beat the conducting system recovers so that the next sequence begins and ends in another dropped beat.

The commonest conduction ratio is three P waves to two ventricular complexes producing paired groups of ventricular complexes. The sequence of PR lengthening is usually maintained and although the lengthening of the PR interval is progressive, the amount by which it increases over the previous PR interval decreases. The first lengthening of the PR inter-

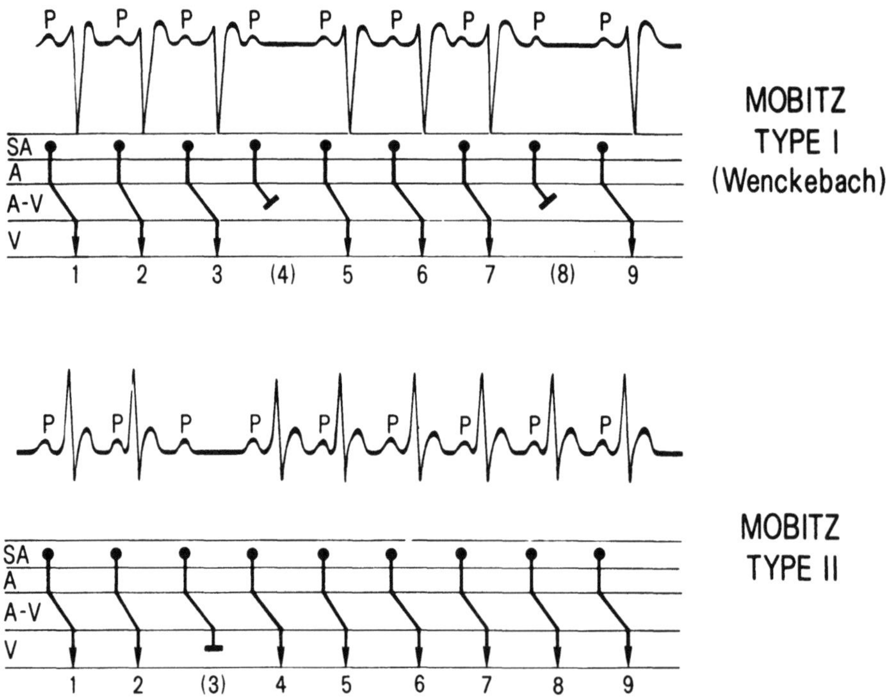

FIGURE 8.17. Second-degree A-V block. In Type I dropped beats follow progressive lengthening of the PR interval whereas in Type II dropped beats occur at a constant RR interval.

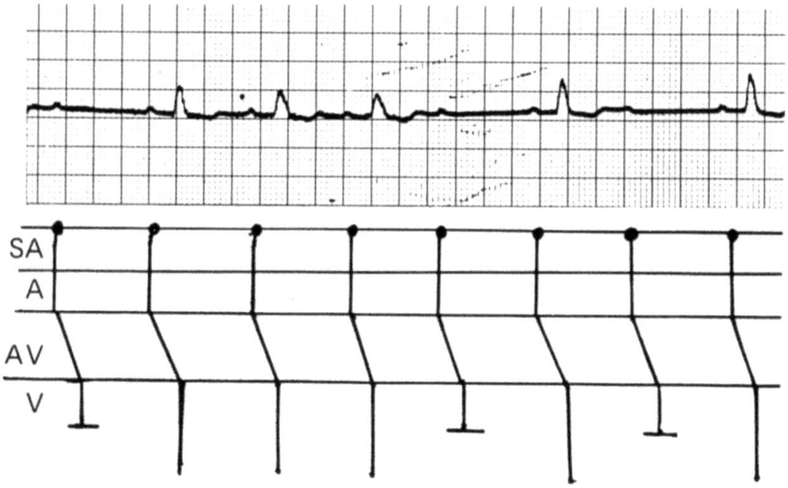

FIGURE 8.18. Rhythm strip showing Mobitz Type II A-V block. The PR interval is 0.20 seconds. Beats are dropped without progressive lengthening of the PR interval. The QRS is wide, compatible with block below the bundle of His.

val to occur is the longest. The effect on the ventricular cycle is therefore somewhat paradoxical, in that as the PR interval lengthens, the RR interval shortens. This is a highly characteristic feature of the Wenckebach type of abnormal conduction.

This type of A-V block is due to a conduction delay in the A-V node and like first-degree A-V block may occur with vagal stimulation in normal individuals, or may result from digitalis intoxication, rheumatic fever, or myocardial infarction (particularly inferior). The prognosis is good.

Mobitz Type II A-V Block

In this type of A-V block beats are dropped without a preceding lengthening of the PR interval (Fig. 8.18). The PR interval of the conducted beats may be either normal or prolonged. The delay in conduction occurs in or below the bundle of His and is usually a result of bilateral bundle branch disease. Therefore, the QRS complexes are frequently wide and aberrant. In the presence of 2:1 A-V block it is impossible to distinguish Mobitz Type II from Type I A-V block. There is a strong tendency for progression to complete A-V block with idioventricular rhythm, requiring permanent pacing.

Third-Degree A-V Block (Complete A-V Block)

In complete heart block the atria beat at a normal rate of 70 to 80/min, but none of these impulses is conducted to the ventricles, which are activated by an ectopic pacemaker below the level of block (Fig. 8.19). When the subsidiary pacemaker is located in the A-V node or the proximal bundle of His, the ventricles are activated through a near-normal pathway and the QRS complex may be normal in shape. However, when the ectopic pacemaker is located more distally in the fascicles the QRS complexes become broad. The rate of the ventricular pacemaker depends on its location. Pacemakers within the bundle of His or A-V node have rates of 35 to 50 beats/min, whereas pacemakers within the ventricular musculature have rates of 25 to 35 beats/min. Not uncommonly, the ventricles at different times may be under the control of pacemakers in different sites. Thus, the QRS complexes may vary in configuration as the pacemaker shifts from the one site to another.

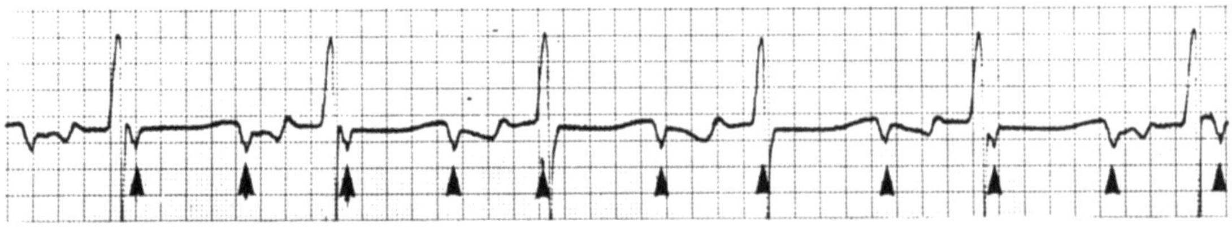

FIGURE 8.19. Monitor strip demonstrating complete heart block with a regular ventricular response of 34 beats/min. The P waves (arrows) are completely dissociated from the QRS complexes. The PP intervals enclosing a QRS complex are shorter than the other PP intervals, a phenomenon known as "ventriculophasic sinus arrhythmia."

Causes of Complete A-V Block

Congenital. This may occur as a sole abnormality without any associated malformations. There is a tendency, however, for congenital heart block to be associated with corrected transposition of the great vessels. In general, the subsidiary pacemaker in congenital A-V block is situated within the A-V node and the QRS complexes are relatively normal in shape and fire at a rate of 50 to 65 beats/min. The ventricular rate may increase with exercise or with atropine and although there is a definite tendency to Stokes–Adams attacks, this is less frequent than in the acquired forms of A-V block.

Lev's Disease and Lenegre's Disease

These conditions account for the great majority of cases of complete A-V block. Lev's disease is a fibrocalcific invasion of the conducting system from a calcific aortic valve, mitral annulus, and superior aspect of the muscular septum. Lenegre's disease is a sclerodegenerative process restricted to the conducting system, starting in one fascicle to involve the others successively, until trifascicular block produces complete A-V block. Commonly, the earliest finding is left anterior hemiblock, which after many years is complicated by right bundle branch block, and when the left posterior division is finally affected, trifascicular or complete A-V block is present.

Ischemic Heart Disease

Complete A-V block complicates approximately 5% of cases of myocardial infarction. Inferior infarction has a greater tendency to be complicated by A block than anterior infarction. In inferior infarction the block is usually transitory and there will be a reversion to sinus rhythm following the use of temporary electrical pacing. When complete A-V block complicates anterior myocardial infarction the prognosis is extremely poor even when pacing is employed, since most patients die of cardiogenic shock.

It should be emphasized that ischemic heart disease accounts for relatively few cases of chronic complete A-V block; the usual cause is Lev's or Lenegre's disease.

Traumatic A-V Block

Penetrating and nonpenetrating chest trauma may involve the conducting system, thereby causing complete A-V block. Operative trauma (closure of a VSD, repair of Tetralogy of Fallot or corrected transposition, and aortic and mitral valve replacement) may be complicated by traumatic heart block.

Unusual causes of complete heart block are involvement of the conducting system by secondary malignant tumors, ankylosing spondylitis, sarcoidosis, and amyloidosis. Thyrotoxicosis and myxedema are occasional causes. Diphtheritic myocarditis is now fortunately uncommon, but when heart block does complicate the disease it may be successfully managed by temporary pacing. The combination of aortic valve disease and complete heart block should immediately arouse a suspicion of rheumatoid arthritis, ankylosing spondilitis, Reiter syndrome, or bacterial endocarditis of the aortic valve with invasion of the conducting pathways. Calcific aortic stenosis may also be complicated by invasion of the conducting system. Digitalis intoxication commonly causes first- or second-degree A-V block but is a rare cause of complete A-V block. In the presence of bundle branch block, antidysrhythmic drugs may further depress intracardiac conduction and precipitate complete heart block.

Physical Signs. The jugular venous pressure is generally slightly elevated and irregular cannon A waves are present. Unless atrial fibrillation is present, there is marked variation in intensity of the first heart sound and independent atrial sounds may be audible. Occasionally, atrial systole is associated with a murmur, and when the ventricular rate is half the atrial rate a mitral diastolic murmur may be misdiagnosed as mitral valve disease. Cardiomegaly and a basal systolic ejection murmur are usually present and are simply a manifestation of increased stroke volume.

The electrocardiogram shows infrequent ventricular complexes (either with a normal QRS, or a left or right bundle branch block pattern), completely unrelated to the atrial complexes. Complete heart block may be confused with 2:1 block, when the atrial rate is coincidently twice the ventricular rate. Exercise or amyl nitrite can be used to solve this problem since the increase in atrial rate will unmask the essential independence of each pacemaker.

Occasionally, the PP intervals that enclose the QRS complexes are shorter than those that do not and this has been termed "ventriculophasic sinus arrhythmia." The early P wave following the QRS complex has been ascribed to mechanical stimulation of the sinus pacemaker to discharge slightly earlier (Fig. 8.19).

Symptoms. These depend on the heart rate and associated conditions. Patients with congenital complete heart block may be asymptomatic and the cardiac output well maintained. Heart block in the elderly is commonly associated with some reduction of effort tolerance and when underlying heart disease is fortuitously associated, the bradycardia may be responsible for heart failure.

Stokes–Adams attacks are transient episodes of unconsciousness complicating established complete heart block. They are particularly prone to occur when there is a sudden change from partial to complete heart block. Approximately one-half of Stokes–Adams attacks are a result of asystole and the other a result of transient ventricular fibrillation or ventricular tachycardia. Loss of consciousness is abrupt and the patient appears to be dead, since the circulation has ceased. After about 10 seconds if the circulation is not restored, twitching is followed by generalized convulsions. Usually, ventricular activity returns spontaneously and, with this, highly oxygenated pulmonary venous blood is delivered to the systemic circulation resulting in a bright flush, since pronounced peripheral vasodilatation follows the period of hypoxia. The return of consciousness is abrupt. The attacks vary considerably in frequency, from an isolated single episode to more or less continuous seizures. In elderly patients, recovery from an attack may be complicated by hemiplegia or by stupor, coma, and prolonged mental confusion. Remarkable return to normal mental function can be achieved by pacing.

Pacemakers

Permanent pacemakers are marvels of technology, but the decision to implant one is clinical and involves a consideration of the patients symptoms and associated cardiac and general medical disorders, which within themselves may shorten life expectancy.

Indications for Permanent Pacing

In general, permanent pacing is indicated in any symptomatic patient with persistent bradycardia (i.e., unrelated to myocardial infarction or drug toxicity). The most common causes are the sick sinus syndrome, complete A-V block, hypersensitive carotid sinus syndrome, and ventricular response to atrial fibrillation.

Sinus Node Dysfunction

Documented Symptomatic Bradycardia. This includes cases that are drug induced for the long-term treatment of tachyarrhythmias. Pacing is not indicated in asymptomatic patients or those with symptoms not clearly related to documented heart rates of less than 45 beats/min.

Acquired A-V Block

Complete Heart Block. Whether intermittent or permanent, pacing is indicated when associated with:

1. Congestive heart failure or marked exercise-intolerance.
2. Syncope, presyncope, dizziness, or lightheadedness.
3. Escape rate of less than 40 beats/min, whether symptomatic or not.

Second-Degree A-V Block. Pacing is indicated when symptomatic bradycardia is associated with second-degree A-V block. Pacing is probably also indicated when there is asymptomatic second-degree A-V block and a wide QRS complex, since there is a high incidence of progression to complete A-V block.

Pacing is not indicated when there is first-degree or second-degree A-V block with a normal QRS complex.

Myocardial Infarction

Permanent pacing plays a minor role in the survivors of acute myocardial infarction. Varying degrees of heart block commonly complicate inferior infarction and resolution is usually spontaneous, or follows a short period of temporary pacing. Acute anterior myocardial infarction complicated by complete heart block carries a very high mortality and it is doubtful whether temporary pacing makes a difference. Most cardiologists would agree that persistent Mobitz Type II and complete heart block should be paced. Again, however, it is by no means certain whether this improves life expectancy, since the fatal arrhythmia in these patients is ventricular fibrillation and not asystole.

Bifascicular Block

Asymptomatic patients with bifascicular block and without clinical evidence of heart disease are commonly encountered in the elderly. The rate of progression to complete heart block is slow and pacing is not required. Pacing is necessary when there is intermittent, complete, or Mobitz Type II heart block associated with symptoms such as syncope, dizziness, confusion, seizures, or congestive heart failure.

Carotid Sinus Hypersensitivity

Permanent pacing is effective when recurrent syncope is associated with a *cardioinhibitory* response (i.e., asystole for 3 seconds or more due to sinus arrest or A-V block). When syncope is a result of the *vasodepressor* response (i.e., severe hypotension due to withdrawl of sympathetic overactivity), pacing is ineffective. The relative contribution of each modality to the patients symptoms must be carefully assessed.

Types of Pacemakers

Pacemakers have two basic functions: (1) stimulation of the heart (*pacing*) and recognition of spontaneous cardiac electrical events (*sensing*). When a pacemaker does not sense an electrical stimulus at the appropriate time, it fires. Both sensing and pacing are usually accomplished with a bipolar lead in which both electrodes are in contact with the myocardium. Two varieties of pacemakers are available for permanent implantation:

1. *Single chamber*—used in either atrium or ventricle.
2. *Dual chamber*—used in both atrium and ventricle.

A letter code has been devised to identify various types of pacemakers used:

The first position indicates the chamber paced, the second, the chamber sensed, the third, the mode of response and the fourth, programmability. The most commonly used pacemakers are

1. *VVI*: Paces and senses the ventricle and is inhibited from discharging (I) by ventricular sensing.
2. *DDD*: Pacing and sensing of both chambers and inhibition of atrial or ventricular output.

Four-position pacemaker code.

I. Chamber paced	II. Chamber Sensed	III. Mode of response	IV. Programmability
V = Ventricle	V = Ventricle	I = Inhibited	P = Programmable rate and/or output
A = Atrium	A = Atrium	T = Triggered	M = Multiprogrammable
D = Atrium and ventricle	D = Atrium and ventricle	D = Atrial triggered and ventricle inhibited	O = None
	O = None	R = Reverse	
S = Single chamber	S = Single chamber	O = None	

3. *AAI*: Atrial pacing inhibited by sensed atrial activity.

The VVI pacemaker is used for any symptomatic bradycardia, particularly when there is no significant atrial contribution (flutter or fibrillation). The AAI pacemaker is used for symptomatic sinus node dysfunction with normal A-V conduction. The DDD, or universal pacemaker, preserves the best hemodynamic relationship between atrial and ventricular systole. This may be further enhanced by the rate-responsive variety, which increases its rate with physical activity.

Additional Reading

Akhtar M., Henasa M., et al.: Wide QRS complex tachycardia reappraisal of a common clinical problem. Am Int Med 109:11.1, 905, 1988.

Gornick CC, Almquist A, Benditt DG, Francis GS: A practical approach to diagnosis and initial management of cardiac dysrhythmias: Part I. Supraventricular tachycardia. Intern Med 8:217–230, 1987.

Gornick CC, Almquist A, Benditt DG, Francis GS: A practical approach to diagnosis and initial management of cardiac dysrhythmias: Part II. Ventricular tachycardia. Intern Med 9:224–232, 1987.

Kapoor WN, Hammill SC, Gersh BJ: Diagnosis and natural history of syncope and the role of invasive electrophysiologic testing. Am J Cardiol 63:730, 1989.

Kapoor WN, Karpf M, Levey G: Issues in evaluating patients with syncope. Ann Intern Med 100:755, 1984.

Schamroth L: "The Disorders of Cardiac Rhythm." Blackwell Scientific, Oxford, 1973.

9
Heart Failure

The epidemiology of heart failure in western countries has changed considerably over the last two decades. Rheumatic valvular disease has receded into the background and the leading causes of chronic congestive heart failure are now coronary artery disease and cardiomyopathy. Their principal deleterious effect is left ventricular damage or dysfunction.

The expansion of the geriatric population coupled with the fact that the incidence of heart failure increases with age has made this the most common hospital discharge diagnosis for people over the age of 65. There is also a considerable impact on mortality. It is not generally appreciated that the prognosis for congestive heart failure is worse than that for many types of cancer: only 40% of men and 55% of women will survive 5 years.

Heart failure is readily described and recognized as a clinical entity but a precise physiological definition is more difficult. For clinical purposes it may be defined as the state where the heart fails to maintain a cardiac output sufficient to supply tissue needs. In terms of the venous circulation it implies an inability of the right heart to eject the venous return through the pulmonary circulation.

Normally, the heart is capable of increasing its output several times to meet changing physiological needs such as strenuous exercise. The potential to increase the output is known as the *cardiac reserve* and any encroachment on this represents the first step toward heart failure.

Regulation of Cardiac Output

The following factors are responsible for the control of cardiac output and performance:

Preload

According to Starling's Law, the force of myocardial contraction is related to the end-diastolic length of the muscle fibers, and therefore to the end-diastolic ventricular volume. An increase in end-diastolic volume leads to an increase in end-diastolic length and a more forceful ensuing contraction. A major determinant of end-diastolic volume and therefore cardiac output is the venous return and any reduction in venous return produced by hemorrhage, dehydration, redistribution of blood volume by gravity or the Valsalva maneuver is soon reflected by a decrease in the cardiac output. The venous return is also affected by the intrathoracic and intrapericardial pressures, venous tone, and skeletal muscle activity. Atrial contraction, when appropriately timed, effectively augments end-diastolic volume and therefore increases cardiac output—the so-called "atrial booster pump." This effect is lost in atrial fibrillation and myocardial performance is appropriately diminished (Fig. 9.1).

Afterload

The afterload (or impedance) is the sum of all forces opposing ejection of blood from the left

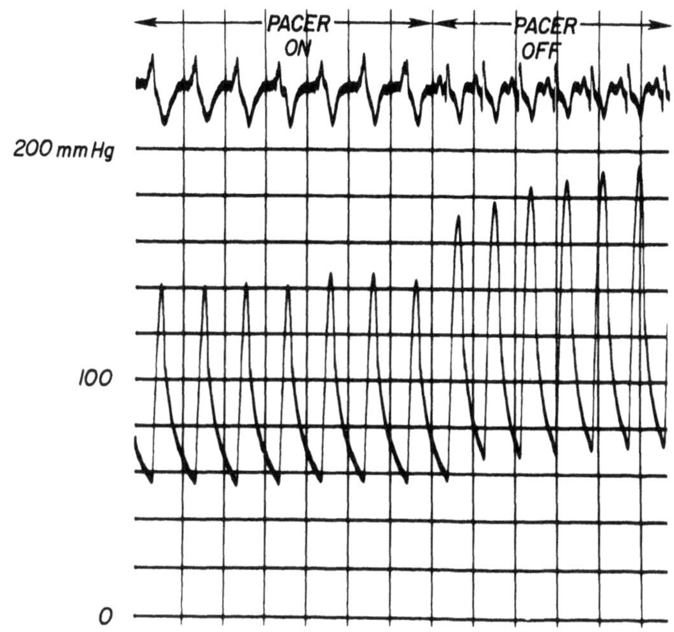

FIGURE 9.1. The effect of the atrial booster pump in a patient with a temporary pacemaker. When the pacemaker fires the booster effect is lost because of A-V dissociation. When the P wave precedes the QRS complex appropriately (pacemaker off) the booster pump comes into effect and raises the systolic pressure by 55 mm Hg.

ventricle during systole. The major components of impedance are the compliance of the large arteries and the resistance to flow of the smaller muscular arterioles. At any given end-diastolic volume and inotropic state, the left ventricular stroke volume depends on the afterload.

The Inotropic State

When preload and afterload are constant, the stroke volume depends on the state of myocardial contractility. Factors that increase contractility shift Starling's curve to the left. For example, sympathetic stimulation and norepinephrine increase the peak systolic pressure, diminish the end-diastolic pressure, produce more rapid myocardial shortening and ejection of blood, and increase the rate of rise and fall of ventricular pressure. This effect is of great importance in the response of the circulation to stress and exercise. Drugs that increase myocardial contractility (positive inotropic effect) include digitalis and β-stimulators such as isoprenaline. Drugs with a negative inotropic effect (such as propanolol) reduce the cardiac output and heart rate during exercise: they may induce heart failure when myocardial function is compromised and dependent on sympathetic stimulation to maintain a normal cardiac output.

Heart Rate

Tachycardia is important in maintaining the cardiac output when the venous return is suddenly reduced by hemorrhage or there is sudden severe myocardial damage because of infarction or myocarditis.

Compensatory Mechanisms

The aforementioned factors operate in the normal situation to maintain an appropriate cardiac output and cardiac reserve. When cardiac disease is present the important abnormality is that the Starling curve is shifted downward and to the right. The cardiac output at rest may be within normal limits but is maintained only by an elevated end-diastolic volume. When the left ventricle becomes markedly distended there may be a considerable rise in end-diastolic pressure that is transmitted to the left atrium and to the pulmonary vessels.

Dilatation of the ventricle is an important compensatory mechanism that utilizes the Starling mechanism as the first line of defense to maintain cardiac output when contractility declines because of left ventricular damage. Dilatation is also an important compensatory mechanism in cases of mitral and tricuspid insufficiency where the regurgitant volume leads to an increase in the diastolic volume of the affected ventricle. Up to a point dilatation is an effective way of increasing cardiac output but this occurs at the price of increased intramyocardial tension, and therefore oxygen demand, and this eventually leads to failure.

Sympathetic stimulation and increased concentration of circulating catecholamines act by augmenting contractility (shifting the Starling curve to the left) and producing tachycardia (Fig. 9.2).

Tachycardia is not as efficient a compensatory mechanism as dilatation or hypertrophy. Its value is limited by the shortening of diastole, which reduces ventricular filling and

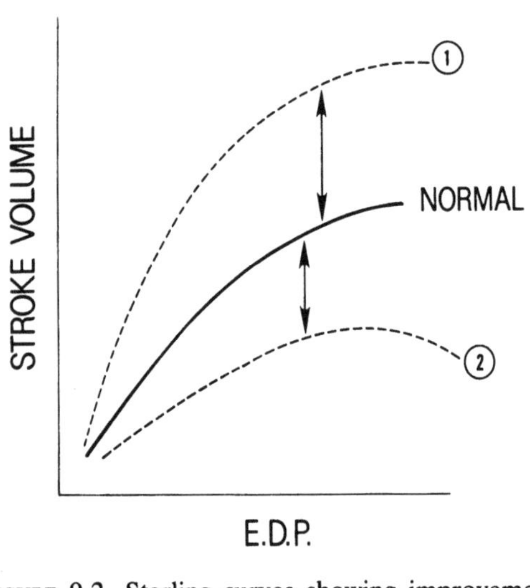

FIGURE 9.2. Starling curves showing improvement (1) and deterioration (2) in left ventricular function (See text).

coronary blood flow. The latter is particularly deleterious when there is coronary atherosclerosis.

Hypertrophy is a compensatory response to an increase in afterload. It adds more contractile units to the myocardium and up to a point is physiological. When, however, it becomes extreme, the thickened muscle outstrips its blood supply leading to subendocardial ischemia and fibrosis and eventually, heart failure.

The earliest evidence of heart failure is an encroachment on the cardiac reserve and an inability of the heart to increase cardiac output under conditions of stress such as exercise or pregnancy. With progressive impairment of ventricular function, the ventricle becomes distended and empties inadequately. The ventricular end-diastolic pressure, and therefore, the atrial, and the pulmonary and systemic venous pressures rise and produce pulmonary and systemic venous congestion ("backward failure").

Peripheral and neurohormonal factors are important compensatory mechanisms in response to a fall in cardiac output ("forward failure"). Activation of the sympathetic nervous system, the renin–angiotensin–aldosterone system, and secretion of arginine vasopressin produces volume expansion and vasoconstriction. This is certainly helpful when the heart is normal and the cardiac output decreased because of loss of blood volume. When myocardial performance is diminished, however, a vicious cycle may ensue where the increase in peripheral resistance and decrease in vascular distensibility further impairs left ventricular function (Fig. 9.3). Interruption of this vicious cycle forms the rationale for vasodilator therapy.

Sympathetic activity is increased in patients with congestive heart failure. The decreased stroke volume and cardiac output in heart failure produces a drop in arterial pressure, which is counteracted by baroreceptor-mediated increase in sympathetic tone. Also, increased sympathetic activity with secretion of catecholamines enhances myocardial contractility. Plasma norepinephrine levels are increased and plasma levels are generally higher in the more symptomatic patients.

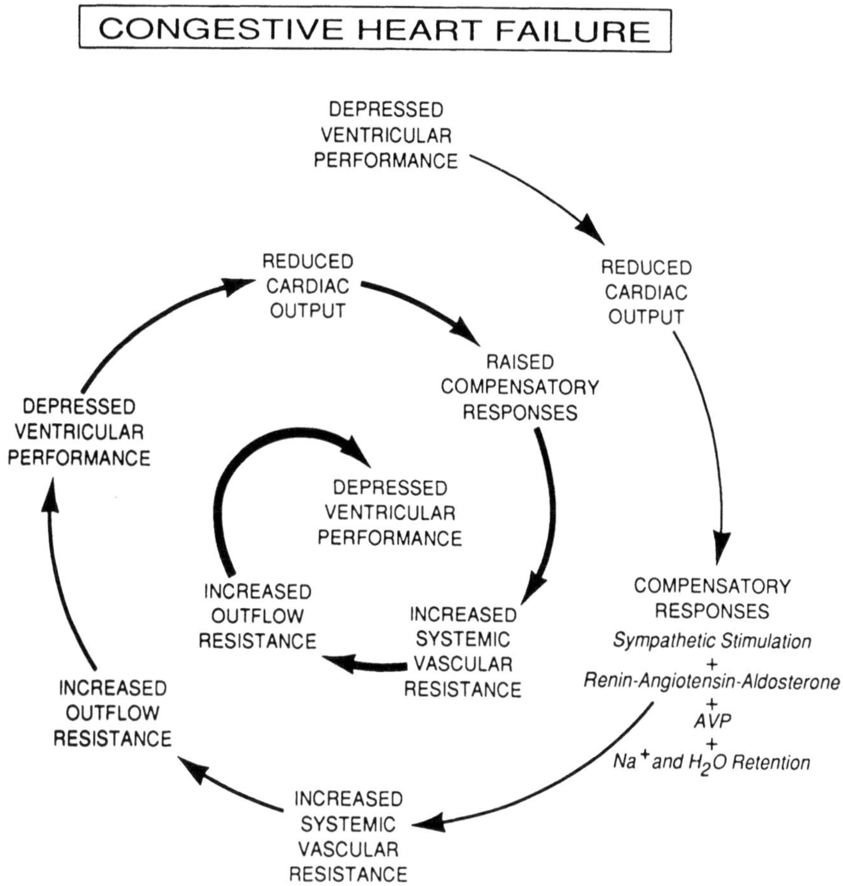

FIGURE 9.3. The vicious cycle whereby depressed left ventricular function activates compensatory respons which further aggravates left ventricular performance. Reprinted, permission, from Francis GS: Congestive heart failure. In Taylor B (ed): "Difficult Medical Management." W.B. Saunders, Philadelphia, 1990.

The *renin–angiotensin–aldosterone system* is activated by those factors usually operative in congestive heart failure (i.e., decreased renal perfusion, reduced serum sodium, and increased sympathetic tone). Secretion of renin converts angiotensinogen to angiotensin I, which is converted to angiotensin II by converting enzyme. Angiotensin II has powerful effects that may aggravate the vicious cycle referred to earlier: (1) it is a powerful vasoconstrictor, (2) there is a feedback to the adrenal glands, which release aldosterone and this further increases the salt retention associated with heart failure, (3) sympathetic outflow is enhanced and this may further elevate plasma norepinephrine levels. The degree of elevation of plasma norepinephrine correlates fairly well with prognosis: high levels are associated with a poor prognosis. Patients who have the highest mortality rates have the lowest serum sodium and the highest renin levels. They may respond well to angiotensin-converting enzyme (ACE) inhibitors, which should be used cautiously because of the risk of hypotension.

The arginine vasopressin system is activated in most patients with congestive heart failure. The antidiuretic hormone is a powerful vasoconstrictor and may aggravate heart failure.

Types of Heart Failure

Two forms of heart failure are recognized depending on the measured cardiac output:

Low-Output Failure

Here the demands of the tissues at rest are normal or reduced, but the heart is unable to deliver the required amount of oxygen. This is the type of heart failure that occurs in ischemic heart disease, hypertension, cardiomyopathy, and rheumatic heart disease.

High-Output Failure

Here the cardiac output may be close to the upper limit of normal even in the presence of severe heart failure, or may actually be above the upper limit of normal. Diseases that produce high cardiac output, such as thyrotoxicosis, anemia, Paget's disease, arteriovenous fistula, and beriberi are characteristically associated with this syndrome. Because of the underlying condition, the demands of the tissues, even at rest, are abnormally high, and this the heart cannot provide, so that failure occurs with the cardiac output above normal.

Systolic and Diastolic Dysfunction

This is an important concept in clinical practice. Most commonly heart failure is a result of failure of systolic pump function and the left ventricular ejection fraction (whether measured by cineangiography, radionuclide techniques, or echocardiography) is depressed. In systolic dysfunction, heart failure is of the low output, forward failure, type. The usual causes are coronary artery disease, cardiomyopathy, and end stage rheumatic valve disease.

Diastolic dysfunction (with a normal left ventricular ejection fraction) is much less common. Here the fault is impaired left ventricular filling. When sustained, it is usually associated with concentric left ventricular hypertrophy of any cause. It is routinely found in idiopathic hypertrophic subaortic stenosis and accounts for the high left ventricular filling pressure. Infiltrative diseases of the myocardium (amyloid disease or hemochromatosis) are not uncommon and importantly have to be distinguised from constrictive pericarditis, which is the classic, remediable cause of impaired left ventricular filling.

Diastolic dysfunction with impaired relaxation accounts for some of the symptoms in ischemic heart disease. Acute reversible ischemic episodes may manifest as attacks of dyspnea or even pulmonary edema in the face of a near-normal ejection fraction. Chronically, diastolic failure and reduced compliance are a result of fibrous replacement of zones of myocardial infarction. Among cases of ischemic heart disease there are instances where the signs and symptoms are a result of both systolic and diastolic dysfunction.

Left Heart Failure

Causes

Myocardial dysfunction:

1. Coronary atherosclerosis (the most common).
2. Cardiomyopathy.
3. Myocarditis.

Systolic overload of the left ventricle:

1. Hypertension.
2. Aortic valve stenosis.
3. Subvalvular aortic stenosis.
4. Coarctation of the aorta.

Diastolic overload of the left ventricle:

1. Mitral insufficiency.
2. Aortic insufficiency.
3. Congential defects with left-to-right shunt (VSD, PDA).

Systclic and diastolic overload:

1. Aortic stenosis and insufficiency.
2. Aortic stenosis and mitral insufficiency.

Left ventricular failure is the commonest and most important cause of congestive cardiac failure, commencing as isolated chamber failure and, unless it is of rapid onset, usually leading to biventricular failure.

Acute left ventricular failure with pulmonary edema is most commonly observed in acute myocardial infarction, or the catastrophic onset of aortic or mitral insufficiency because of leaflet perforation, rupture of chordae tendinae, or rupture of a papillary muscle. Pulmonary venous hypertension and engorged pulmonary capillaries lead to exudation of fluid into the alveoli. The lungs become heavy and noncompliant with thickened alveolar membranes and narrowed bronchi. This may be completely reversible, with normal lung function, before and after the attack. In chronic left ventricular failure, however, persistent left atrial hypertension leads to passive pulmonary arterial hypertension, right ventricular hypertrophy, and ultimately right heart failure.

With the development of right ventricular failure, episodes of acute pulmonary congestion may cease because of the reduced output of the right ventricle. Occasionally, the initial presentation of left ventricular failure is overshadowed by signs and symptoms of right-sided congestion and this has been called "Bernheim syndrome." It was originally attributed to bulging of the ventricular septem into the right ventricular cavity and this allegedly interfered with right ventricular filling and stroke output. The development of vasconstrictive pulmonary arterial hypertension is, however, a much more likely explanation.

Changes in afterload have a marked effect on left ventricular performance. As the afterload increases, left ventricular stroke volume decreases. Elevated afterload in left ventricular failure is a regular occurrence and dependent on the peripheral and neurohumoral mechanisms previously described.

Symptoms

The presenting symptom is nearly always effort dyspnea; eventually, effort tolerance becomes more and more reduced until dyspnea is present at rest.

Orthopnea is dyspnea in the recumbent position and is usually a symptom of more advanced heart failure. It results from a redistribution of blood from the extremities and splanchnic bed to the lungs on assuming the recumbent position. The increase in intrathoracic blood volume elevates the pulmonary venous and capillary pressures leading to interstitial pulmonary edema, stiffening of the lungs, and increased work of breathing. The Hering–Breuer reflex, which inhibits inspiration, is augmented and results in the shallow breathing of cardiac dyspnea.

Paroxysmal cardiac dyspnea is usually nocturnal and consists of sudden attacks of respiratory distress, with coughing, choking, and tightness in the chest. When wheezing is associated, the picture may closely resemble bronchial asthma. Usually, however, the respiratory difficulty is as marked during inspiration as it is during expiration, and the untreated attack lasts for no more than 10 to 20 minutes, points that are useful in differentiating paroxysmal cardiac dyspnea from bronchial asthma. Typically, paroxysmal cardiac dyspnea wakens the patient in the early hours of the morning. Like orthopnea, it is a result of redistribution of fluid in the recumbent position and the total blood volume is augmented at night because of reabsorption of edema from dependent portions of the body.

Pulmonary edema may develop in a severe attack of paroxysmal cardiac dyspnea. The dyspnea is more acute and severe and cough may be productive of copious, frothy, blood-stained sputum. Gas exchange is impaired, producing hypoxia and cyanosis in severe cases.

The usual progression of effort dyspnea to paroxysmal cardiac dyspnea and orthopnea does not always occur in left ventricular failure. Paroxysmal nocturnal dyspnea, or less commonly orthopnea, may be the presenting symptom, so that a patient may be able to continue work, apparently well, despite these ominous symptoms.

Cough is a frequent complaint and results from congestion and engorgement of the bronchial mucous membranes. Increased mucus secretion and reduction of resistance to infection result. Upper respiratory infections not only complicate, but may also precipitate failure.

Paroxysmal cough related to effort, is an occasional symptom of left heart failure and may be associated with the expectoration of small quantities of blood-stained sputum.

Fatigue is a common syptom of heart failure

and like weakness, results from reduction of blood flow to skeletal muscles.

Physical Signs

The Heart

Cardiomegaly is usually present with palpable evidence of left ventricular enlargement. Presystolic gallop rhythm occurs early in the course of left ventricular failure, particularly when a result of systolic overload. It is not as ominous a physical sign, however, as diastolic gallop rhythm. Murmurs are frequently audible and are a result of underlying organic aortic or mitral valve disease. Alternatively, mitral systolic murmurs may be functional when they result from dilatation of the valve ring.

The Pulse and Blood Pressure

Pulsus alternans is a particularly ominous prognostic sign; it is almost invariably associated with a loud diastolic gallop rhythm. The blood pressure is usually normal unless the underlying cause is systemic hypertension. Occasionally, hypertension may be present during an acute episode of heart failure, and is a result of excessive peripheral vasoconstriction in response to the low cardiac output. Conversely, a normal blood pressure may be encountered among patients with systemic hypertension when severe heart failure is a result of myocardial infarction.

Cheyne-Stokes Breathing

This is frequently encountered in the elderly patient with left ventricular failure. It is a result of depression of the respiratory center produced by low cardiac output and there is usually associated cerebral atherosclerosis. It is aggravated by respiratory center depressants such as morphine and relieved by stimulants such as CO_2 and aminophylline.

Fever

Although an intercurrent illness, pulmonary infection or pulmonary infarction must be excluded. It is not sufficiently appreciated that pulmonary congestion alone may be responsible. Usually, the temperature is only a degree or two above normal but occasionally may reach 104°F, lasting for a few hours, until diuresis occurs.

The Lungs

There are no physical signs of pulmonary venous hypertension, even in the presence of orthopnea and paroxysmal cardiac dyspnea, unless pulmonary edema is present. In the presence of pulmonary edema, rales are heard at both bases posteriorly since the patient is generally recumbent. The rales disappear with postural change, reappearing in the dependent areas of the lung. When there is complicating bronchospasm and bronchitis, rhonchi and wheezing are more diffuse, occurring both anteriorly and posteriorly and they are unaffected by change in posture. In acute pulmonary edema, rales become more extensive and, in severe attacks, the entire chest may be filled with bubbling noises. Pleural effusions are common in the later stages of heart failure and may be unilateral or bilateral, without particular predisposition for either side.

The Electrocardiogram

Tracings are always abnormal when symptoms are advanced. Left ventricular hypertrophy is the rule but this pattern may be obscured by bundle branch block or the changes of myocardial infarction. Electrocardiographic evidence of left atrial enlargement is usually present and this is a fairly sensitive indicator of sudden elevation of the left atrial pressure.

The X-Ray

The radiological appearance of the heart depends on the underlying disease but some degree of left atrial enlargement is usually present. When there is concentric left ventricular hypertrophy the left ventricular contour may show little or no abnormality (e.g., aortic stenosis). When there is eccentric hypertrophy, the chamber may be prominently enlarged (e.g., aortic insufficiency).

Dilatation of the upper lobe veins is the first sign of left ventricular failure. This is followed by hilar congestion manifested by an increase in density and width of the hilar shadows producing a fuzzy appearing "bats-wing" appearance. With more extensive edema, diffuse haziness of the lungs appears, but the periphery remains relatively clear. Sometimes the edema is more solid and isolated, involving one lung or only one lobe. Interlobar, or loculated pleural effusion produces a similar picture and both may be mistaken for solid tumors of the lung ("phantom tumor"). When there is prolonged elevation of the pulmonary venous pressure dilated lymphatic vessels (Kerley B-lines) are visible as thin horizontal lines at the bases of the lung fields. Occasionally, prolonged interstitial edema may produce nodular deposits as a result of pulmonary hemosiderosis. The diagnosis of left ventricular failure and pulmonary edema is usually readily made clinically. Occasionally, there may be difficulty in the presence of obstructive airways or pulmonary embolism.

Adult Respiratory Distress Syndrome (ARDS)

The clinical distinction between noncardiogenic pulmonary edema and cardiogenic pulmonary edema may be impossible. Noncardiogenic pulmonary edema is a result of disruption of the alveolar membrane leading to increased alveolar capillary permeability and pulmonary edema. There are a wide variety of initiating factors including infectious pneumonia, aspiration of gastric contents, shock lung, and hemorrhagic pancreatitis.

When the possibility of ARDS arises in patients in whom there is a strong background prevalence of ischemic heart disease and cardiomyopathy the easiest solution is to measure the indirect left atrial pressure with a Swan Ganz catheter. Physical signs such as cardiomegaly, gallop sounds, and rales are of little diagnostic help. The situation is made even more difficult because left ventricular failure may be superimposed on ARDS by the excessive use of intravenous fluids.

Right Heart Failure

Causes

Systolic Overload

Pulmonary hypertension:

1. Left heart failure.
2. Pulmonary embolism.
3. Congenital heart disease.

Diastolic overload of right ventricle:

1. Atrial septal defect.
2. Total anomalous pulmonary venous drainage.
3. Isolated tricuspid insufficiency.

Restriction to right ventricular filling:

1. Endomyocardial fibrosis.
2. Loeffler's parietal endocarditis.
3. Isolated tricuspid stenosis.
4. Right atrial myxoma.

Primary right ventricular myocardial failure (rare):

1. Myocarditis.
2. Cardiomyopathy.
3. High output states (especially beriberi), the right ventricle may bear the brunt.

Symptoms and Signs

The abdomen becomes distended and the liver tender. Pain in the right upper quadrant on effort (hepatic angina) is an occasional complaint. Chronic congestion of the liver gives rise to impaired function, jaundice, and ultimately cirrhosis. Congestion of the gastrointestinal tract produces loss of appetite and occasionally, vomiting. In some conditions, particularly constrictive pericarditis and chronic tricuspid valve disease, protein-losing enteropathy aggravates the cachexia.

Edema

This is at first latent, leading only to a gain in weight, but will become manifest after approximately 10 pounds have accumulated. Initially, it is dependent, appearing in the feet at the end of the day. During the night, the fluid is mobilized and nocturia results. In children, however, the face and abdomen are involved rather than the feet and, in fact, hepatic congestion is one of the earliest signs of heart failure. Later the edema becomes persistent and is orthostatic, tending to collect over the sacrum and back when the patient is confined to bed. When extensive, it may involve the penis and scrotum giving rise to difficulty in micturition. Swelling of the face and eyes is less common than in nephritis. Chronic edema of the skin leads to trophic changes and the lesions heal with difficulty. Unilateral leg edema suggests venous insufficiency or thrombosis of the deep veins on the affected side.

Dyspnea

This is usually present in right-sided failure, even in the absence of pulmonary congestion, hydrothorax, and pulmonary disease. The exact mechanism is obscure, but receptors in the great veins, the right heart, and pulmonary arteries may be involved. Weakness, fatigue, depression, oliguria, cyanosis, and peripheral circulatory symptoms are manifestations of advanced failure.

Jugular Venous Pressure

This is the most important physical sign and is best recognized with the patient lying at an angle of 45°, or sitting upright. Pulsation is always present. When cardiac reserve is markedly reduced, short of actual congestive failure, gentle pressure on the abdomen will produce elevation of the jugular venous pressure (hepatojugular reflux).

Hepatomegaly

This reflects the same process as above. Systolic pulsation of the liver is well appreciated in tricuspid incompetence but presystolic pulsation occurring in tricuspid stenosis is less easy to time. Liver distension is very helpful in the diagnosis of heart failure in infants and young children, in whom the jugular veins are difficult to see, bearing in mind that in this age group, the liver may be normally palpable. Tenderness of the liver is associated with failure of fairly recent onset. In acute heart failure hepatic pain and tenderness may be so severe that an acute abdominal condition such as cholecystitis may be suspected. In long-standing failure, the liver loses its tenderness, becomes very hard with a rounded edge, and in the course of time cirrhosis may develop. This is particularly common in chronic tricuspid valve diseae and constrictive pericarditis. Jaundice may develop and ascites is often a prominent feature. When congestive failure is controlled, the venous pressure drops but it may take time before the liver returns to normal size. Conversely, pulsating raised jugular veins with a normal sized or impalpable liver suggest the presence of cirrhosis.

Splenomegaly

This is the result of chronic passive congestion and is usally encountered in patients who have hepatomegaly. If sought for it can be frequently detected, but palpation is difficult because of edema of the abdominal wall and ascites. It is often palpable in chronic rheumatic heart disease with tricuspid incompetence. The presence of splenomegaly, therefore, does not automatically mean infective endocarditis.

Ascites

Usually this is less prominent than subcutaneous edema except in the presence of liver disease, which frequently complicates tricuspid disease and chronic constrictive pericarditis. In the latter two conditions, gross ascites may be present with little subcutaneous edema. Pleural effusions may develop because of the high azygos venous pressure and is almost a constant finding in severe chronic constrictive pericarditis. Pericardial effusion occurs occasionally and may be detected by echocardiography.

Peripheral Cyanosis

This is a result of sluggish peripheral circulation with excessive extraction of oxygen by the tissues. A cyanotic malar flush is common in tricuspid incompetence especially when it is associated with multivalvular rheumatic heart disease.

Exophthalmos

This may be pronounced when there is long-standing severe heart failure with increased intraorbital pressure and cardiac cachexia. It must be differentiated from the endocrine variety.

The Heart

The signs associated with the underlying disease are evident. Most commonly, therefore, there is evidence of left ventricular disease, mitral stenosis, obstructive airways disease, pulmonary-embolism, atrial septal defect, and so on.

Cardiomegaly, with signs of right ventricular, or combined ventricular enlargement is present. A left parasternal systolic lift produced by the enlarged right ventricle, and a palpable diastolic pulmonary closure sound may be detected. When there is severe tricuspid insufficiency, however, the major lift is diastolic and is produced by the marked influx of blood into the right ventricle from the overfilled right atrium. Ventricular gallop rhythm is best heard over the right ventricle, unless the signs of right-sided congestion are a result of tricuspid stenosis. In cases where the right ventricle enlarges toward the apex the gallop may be heard toward the "mitral" area. A presystolic gallop is frequently heard in patients with pulmonary hypertension and is a result of augmented atrial systole. It is frequently associated with a poorly compliant thick ventricle and is therefore not a specific indicator of congestive cardiac failure. In the second left interspace, the pulmonary component of the second heart sound increased in intensity and an ejection click may be present.

The Electrocardiogram

In pure right heart failure, the electrocardiogram is a fairly sensitive and specific indicator of right atrial and right ventricular enlargement and hypertrophy. Where left ventricular enlargement coexists, the pattern of left ventricular hypertrophy persists and there is evidence of biventricular hypertrophy. Occasionally, the changes are balanced out, producing a relatively nonspecific tracing.

The X-Ray

This frequently demonstrates left ventricular enlargement, which is commonly responsible for right-sided failure and the cardiac enlargement is therefore marked and generalized. Pure right-sided enlargement does, however, occur. In acute right heart failure dilatation produces a marked increase in heart size, which may reduce with treatment or resolution of the cause of heart failure (e.g., pulmonary embolism). Disproportionate right atrial enlargement is a valuable clue to the diagnosis of tricuspid stenosis. When pulmonary venous and arterial hypertension is responsible for right ventricular failure there are appropriate changes in the pulmonary vasculature, and the main pulmonary artery is enlarged. When chronic pulmonary disease is reponsible, the lung fields are hyperaerated, the diaphragms depressed, and bullae may be present.

Other Systems

Oliguria with proteinuria is present. Usually, the proteinuria is slight, but may be heavy even in the absence of renal disease. The specific gravity is high and the urinary sodium concentration reduced. Elevation of the blood urea is common in advanced heart failure and may reach levels encountered in primary renal disease.

Fluid and Electrolyte Disturbances in Heart Failure

In congestive cardiac failure there is a marked increase in total body water and when renal function is intact urinary sodium concentration may be reduced to virtually zero. Thus, patients may have the capacity to retain nearly all of the sodium taken in the diet. The result is hypervolemia and edema. The serum sodium concentration in the early stages of heart failure is usually normal, but later there is a tendency to develop hyponatremia. Total body sodium, however, is elevated and there is an increase in intracellular sodium. Retention of sodium results from the decreased glomerular filtration rate, increased output of aldosterone, and increased filtration fraction.

Hypokalemia

This is a common complication of congestive cardiac failure. It is provoked by inadequate food intake, nausea, anorexia, and diarrhea and is aggravated by intensive diuretic therapy and sodium restriction. It is particularly prone to occur when thiazide diuretics induce a rapid weight loss over a short period of time. Under the latter circumstances evidence of hypokalemia, and digitalis toxicity may he expected unless potassium supplements have been administered.

Hypokalemia is recognized by drowsiness, anorexia, and weakness, which progress to paralysis with loss of tendon reflexes. The electrocardiogram may show characteristic changes correctable by treatment with potassium. Contrariwise, hyperkalemia is liable to occur among those patients with severe congestive cardiac failure who are refractory to diuretics and are also receiving potassium supplements. The sudden appearance of sinus bradycardia, sinus arrest, complete heart block, and widening of the QRS complexes in an oliguric patient should immediately arouse suspicion of hyperkalemia.

Hypochloremic Alkalosis with Hypokalemia

This is not an uncommon complication of diuretics leading to a disproportionate excretion of chloride and potassium. It is encountered with the use of ethacrynic acid and furosemide. It is recognized clinically by diuretic "fastness" and is confirmed biochemically. It may be corrected by the administration of ammonium chloride and potassium supplements. Acetazolamide is also frequently effective since this drug produces a hyperchloremic acidosis.

Depletion Hyponatremia

Drastic diuretic therapy in the face of rigid sodium restriction produces this derangement. It is aggravated by aspiration of large effusions and excessive sweating. Characteristically, the syndrome presents with anorexia, weakness, muscle cramps, hypotension, and severe thirst. A state of prerenal uremia is present and confirmed by a marked increase in the ratio of blood urea to creatinine. The abnormality may be corrected by temporary cessation of diuretics and sodium supplementation if necessary.

Dilutional Hyponatremia

These patients are edematous and have all the signs of intractable cardiac failure. Serum sodium concentration is low because of inappropriate water retention. The mechanism responsible for the latter finding is not entirely clear but may be related to excessive secretion of antidiuretic hormone. Dilutional hyponatremia is usually a manifestation of intractable impairment of cardiac function. It is frequently precipitated by recurrent myocardial infarction, pulmonary infection, or pulmonary embolism. In the majority of such patients there are no clinical manifestations of this type of electrolyte disturbance and the symptoms are those of severe heart failure. Occasionally, a sudden drop in sodium concentration and osmolality may produce "hyponatremic encephalopathy," in which case small amounts of hypertonic saline solution may be effective therapy. In the remaining cases the electrolyte abormality is best treated by fluid restriction in the hope that the cardiac condition can be remedied or ameliorated.

Treatment of Congestive Heart Failure

The treatment of congestive cardiac failure falls under two headings: (1) treatment of, or removal of the cause, and precipitating factors, and (2) control of cardiac failure itself.

Cardiac failure occurs as part of the natural history of rheumatic valvular disease, systemic hypertension, and ischemic heart disease. Recognition of the underlying cause is obviously crucial, since surgical relief (e.g., mitral valvotomy or valve replacement) may cure cardiac failure. Frequently heart disease exists in well compensated form until a precipitating factor supervenes. Identification of these factors is crucially important, although they are not always readily evident clinically.

Thyrotoxicosis

Even with mild endocrine manifestations this may increase the cardiac output sufficiently, particularly in the elderly, to precipitate cardiac failure. The usual presentation is the onset of atrial fibrillation with minimal or no evidence of thyrotoxicosis such as exophthalmos, sweating and tremor—the diagnosis must be made by laboratory assessment of thyroid function.

Pregnancy, Anemia, Infection, and Arteriovenous Fistula

These cause high cardiac output, which may produce failure in an overloaded but otherwise compensated heart. Heart failure not infrequently occurs for the first time in pregnancy in women suffering from rheumatic heart disease. Arteriovenous fistula is not commonly thought of, but every so often is in fact the cause of profound heart failure. For example, operations for the removal of lumbar discs are not uncommon and occasionally these are complicated by a surgically induced fistula between the aorta and the inferior vena cava, which leads to progressive cardiomegaly and intractable cardiac failure. A careful search should always be made, therefore, for a continuous murmur among cases of obscure cardiac failure.

Pulmonary Embolism

Bed-ridden patients with low cardiac output are particularly susceptible. Embolism may precipitate or aggravate heart failure without dramatic signs. There is progressive elevation of pulmonary arterial pressure, which aggravates right ventricular failure.

Infective Endocarditis

Anemia, tachycardia, and fever increase the cardiac output. It is particularly liable to produce intensification of heart failure when there is rupture of chordae tendinae or perforation of the aortic or mitral valves.

Systemic Hypertension

Spontaneous aggravation of systemic hypertension or uncontrolled hypertension following withdrawal of effective therapy is a potent precipitator of heart failure.

Rheumatic Fever

Recurrence of acute rheumatic fever will precipitate heart failure in patients with established valve disease.

Arrhythmias

The onset of the arrhythmia may be new or may become uncontrolled by inadvised cessation of medication by the patient. Tachyarrhythmias shorten diastole, impair ventricular filling, and thereby reduce stroke volme by the Starling mechanism. The onset of atrial fibrillation produces heart failure by the latter mechanism, but additionally, there is loss of effective atrial contraction and the atrial booster pump. Ventricular tachycardia is associated with poor myocardial performance because of asynchronous ventricular contraction and shortened diastole. The bradycardia of complete heart block necessitates a markedly increased stroke volume to maintain a normal cardiac output, which a damaged myocardiuln may not be able to provide.

Reduction in Physical Activity

This remains the keystone of medical treatment and patients should be nursed in an upright position in a cardiac bed if available. Except in severe cases, both active and passive movements of the leg should be encouraged. An adequate amount of sleep is essential and sedatives may be required to allay anxiety and encourage relaxation. Adequate physical and emotional rest diminishes the cardiac output and the work of the respiration and slows the heart rate. The duration of bed rest depends on the response to treatment and on the underlying cause.

Diet

Salt restriction is essential in all but the mildest forms of heart failure. The normal diet contains approximately 8 g of sodium chloride. To be effective, the sodium intake should be reduced to between 500 and 1000 mg/day, but this is unpalatable. With the advent of powerful diuretics a diet containing 2 to 4 g of sodium chloride daily may be achieved by avoiding salty foods and omitting added salt for cooking and during the meal. There is no necessity to decrease water intake except in the advanced forms of congestive cardiac failure complicated by dilutional hyponatremia. The obese patient should have the demands on cardiac output lessened by undergoing a weight reduction program. In individuals with protracted severe heart failure, cardiac cachexia will supervene if adequate nutritional intake is not maintained. This is particularly important in patients with anorexia and vomiting.

Digitalis

This is the traditional drug used for the treatment of congestive cardiac failure. The drug is readily absorbed from the gastrointestinal tract and is rapidly cleared from the blood. Although dispersed throughout all the tissues of the body, its prime action is on the myocardial cells. The most important effects of digitalis are (1) enhancement of contractility and efficiency of the failing heart—the inotropic effect; (2) blocking of conduction through the A-V node—the dromotropic effect; (3) slowing of the heart by a direct action on the heart muscle, and reflexly through the vagus—the chronotropic effect.

Digitalis is used for three reasons: (3) to slow transmission of impulses through the A-V node, thereby controlling the ventricular response in atrial fibrillation and atrial flutter; (2) for its antiarrhythmic action where it is effective in controlling supraventricular tachycardia and atrial ectopic activity; and (3) for its enhancement of myocardial contractility.

The therapeutic value of the drug for the first two indications is established beyond doubt. Atrial fibrillation and atrial flutter with uncontrolled ventricular response (frequently complicated by severe heart failure) respond dramatically to the administration of digitalis glycosides. The chief effect under these circumstances, however, is related to control of the ventricular response, thereby allowing sufficient time for adequate ventricular filling. Similarly, the drug is highly effective in aborting an attack of paroxysmal supraventricular tachycardia and preventing further attacks of this, and other supraventricular arrhythmias. However, the positive inotropic effect of digitalis in heart failure associated with sinus rhythm is not so clearly demonstrated. Almost invariably, such patients receive concomitant powerful diuretics, bed rest, and restricted sodium intake.

Although there is ample experimental evidence supporting the inotropic effect of digitalis acutely, the long-term effect on cardiac output has been the subject of much debate. It has no place in the treatment of heart failure resulting from diastolic dysfunction. In the presence of impaired systolic dysfunction it may be useful in sinus rhythm, particularly when vasodilators may aggravate hypotension or renal failure. Although it is fairly easy to titrate the dose of digitalis required for adequate control of ventricular response in atrial fibrillation without risking toxicity, this is certainly not the case with heart failure and sinus rhythm and there is a serious potential for the development of digitalis toxicity. Indeed, digitalis toxicity is now a widespread problem among patients being treated in hospital and in those receiving the drug as outpatients.

Digoxin is the most widely used preparation. The drug is rapidly absorbed and excreted. Approximately 80% of the oral dose is absorbed and peak levels occur within 30 to 60 minutes. Intravenously, it is effective within 15 to 30 minutes. One-half of the dose is eliminated in 30 to 38 hours and almost all in 7 days. Ninety percent of the drug is excreted in the urine and 10% in the stool. In renal failure the half-life is prolonged to over 80 hours. The rapid excretion with normal renal function, though advantageous in some circumstances, often leads to problems in the state of digitalization in patients who take their therapy sporadically or erratically.

Generally, the digitalizing dose is 1.25 mg orally and the maintenance dose is 0.25 to 0.375 mg daily. Unless the clinical situation is urgent, Digoxin should be given orally. The digitalizing dose can be given orally over 24 hours: 0.5 mg stat and 0.25 mg 8 hourly for 3 doses. Intravenously over 24 hours it may be given as 0.5 mg stat and 0.125 mg 8 hourly for 3 doses. Elderly patients are frequently exquisitively sensitive to digitalis and the drug should be used with yreat caution, and in smaller dosage.

In contrast to the marked sensitivity to digitalis displayed by the elderly, infants and children are relatively resistant to the drug. The average digitalizing dose is 0.03 mg/pound given in four divided doses over 24 hours, with a maintenance dose of one-fourth of the digitalizing dose. When intravenous administration is required one-half of the digitalizing dose is given immediately. Since the margin between therapeutic and toxic doses is wider in infants and children than in adults, treatment is relatively safe and simple because it is assessed on body weight.

Digitoxin is completely absorbed in the gastrointestinal tract and half of the drug is excreted in 9 days. Ninety percent of the drug is metabolized in the liver and the metabolites are excreted in the urine. Because of its long duration of action the potential for toxicity is greater than with Digoxin. The oral and intravenous digitalizing dose is the same, and the average adult requires about 1.2 mg over a period of 24 to 48 hours. The effect of the drug may last for 14 to 21 days. It may be given as 0.6 mg initially followed by 0.3, 0.2, and 0.1 mg every six hours. Given intravenously, it has an effect in 30 minutes to 1.5 hours, with a peak effect at 6 hours. The maintenance dose is usually 0.1 mg daily.

Strophanthin. There are two main strophanthus preparations, Strophanthin-K and Strophanthin-G. Their effects are like those of digitalis but the drugs have to be given intravenously. They are probably the most rapid acting preparations available, having a maximum effect in 30 minutes, the drug being excreted within 24 hours. The usual dosage schedule is 0.5 mg followed by 0.1 mg every 30 minutes until digitalized, without exceeding 1 mg on the first day. Usually, strophanthin is discontinued when the emergency is over and oral Digoxin or Digitoxin is substituted.

The Use of Digitalis in Special Clinical Situations

1. *Renal Disease*. At least half of the administered dose of diyitalis glycoside is eliminated by the kidneys and therefore the toxic effects of the usual maintenance dose of digitalis is magnified. The dosage of digitalis must therefore be reduced in the presence of renal failure.
2. *Pulmonary Disease*. The primary defect here is pulmonary hypertension either because of pulmonary arterial obstruction or because of hypoxia with hypercapnea. Digitalis therapy plays only a minor role in treatment and the incidence of toxicity is definitely increased.
3. *Thyroid Disease*. The ventricular response in atrial fibrillation is characteristically difficult to slow with usual doses of digitalis and larger doses may result in toxicity. The addition of small doses of propranolol is preferable to increasing the dose of digitalis.
4. *Quinidine*. The administration of quinidine to a digitalized patient elevates the serum Digoxin level with a propensity for toxicity. When quinidine is given, the dose of Digoxin should be reduced and the Digoxin level should be assayed.

Toxic Effects of Digitalis

Digitalis therapy is made difficult by the great individual variation in tolerance to the drug. Normal subjects and the very young car tolerate the largest doses of the drug without toxicity. There is a large margin between the therapeutic and toxic dose in patients with relatively mild cardiac disease. However, in patients with severe heart disease, the glycoside is often so poorly tolerated that toxic manifestations appear before the therapeutic level has been reached. Occasionally, susceptibility is so extreme that even small doses cannot be tolerated.

Toxicity develops particularly in the elderly, in whom renal function is often impaired and body weight reduced. Elderly patients with atrial fibrillation are frequently readily controlled with doses as small as 0.125 mg/day. Toxicity readily occurs in patients with renal failure, and caution is required when there is hepatic dysfunction, myocarditis, or chronic cor pulmonale with hypoxia, and whenever depressed A-V nodal function is present. Most important are situations in which there is a disturbance of ionic equilibrium, especially hypokalemia.

Potassium plays a crucial role in digitalis intoxication. In congestive cardiac failure there is a decrease in intracellular potassium and a fall in the potassium gradient. Depletion of total body potassium occurs very readily with powerful diuretics, and is aggravated by inadequate potassium intake.

Extracardiac Toxicity

Gastrointestinal disturbances are characteristically anorexia followed by nausea and vomiting. Diarrhea is less common. Neuropsychiatric manifestations are not uncommon in the elderly and include vertigo, headache, restlessness, confusion, and psychosis. Ocular symptoms include blurring of vision, flashes of light and colored vision (especially yellow), flickering, and scotomata. Rarely, retrobulbar neuritis and ocular paralysis may occur. The latter are more likely to be a result of Wernicke's encephalopathy produced by digitalis-induced anorexia and vomiting and thiamine deficiency, rather than a direct effect of the drug itself. Allergic reactions such as urticaria or eosinophilia are extremely rare. Gynecomastia may occur after prolonged administration of digitalis, and this is related to its steroid structure.

Cardiac Disturbances

Any arrhythmia may occur, the commonest being ventricular ectopic beats. These may be isolated, unifocal, or multifocal, occur in salvoes, and may eventually lead to ventricular tachycardia and ventricular fibrillation. Occasionally, ventricular tachycardia is of the bidirectional type where the QRS complex alternates its direction from beat to beat: this arrhythmia is virtually diagnostic of digitalis toxicity.

A characteristic supraventricular arrhythmia is paroxysmal atrial tachycardia with 2:1 A-V block. However, this may also occur in the absence of digitalis administration (particularly in cor pulmonale). Great caution must be exercised before digitalis is used if it is uncertain whether the drug has been administered previously since ventricular fibrillation will certainly ensue.

Digitalis prolongs the refractory period of the junctional tissue and thus produces all grades of A-V block. First degree A-V block (long PR interval) is generally not a sign of digitalis toxicity. Digitalis toxicity should be suspected in atrial fibrillation or flutter whenever the rhythm becomes regular, whether the period of regularity is short or prolonged.

Depression of the ST segment is a characteristic electrocardiographic effect of digitalis and may occur with small doses. However, severe toxicity may be present without any ST segment change. In this respect therefore, the electrocardiogram is a poor guide to toxicity. Toxicity is recognized by the presence of atrial, nodal, or ventricular irritability, or by depression of A-V conduction.

Treatment of Digitalis Toxicity

The drug should be stopped when any of toxic manifestations are present. Ventricular ectopic beats, Wenckebach block, and A-V dissociation require no specific additional therapy other than correction of hypokalemia when this is present. More vigorous therapy is required for uni- and bidirectional ventricular tachycardia and paroxysmal atrial tachycardia with 2:1 A-V block. In urgent cases, complicated by hypokalemia, intravenous administration of potassium may be required in the form of a slow infusion of 20–40 mEq of potassium chloride in 1000 ml of 5% glucose water; continuous electrocardiographic monitoring is mandatory. Procaine amide, quinidine, magnesium lidocaine, dilantin, and propronolol have all been successful at times but it is difficult to document which agent is the most efficacious. Termination of these arrhythmias by cardioversion is hazardous and should be used only as a last resort.

When toxicity manifests with high grade A-V block, antiarrhythmic drugs and potassium should not be used since these drugs further impair A-V conduction and may induce ventricular fibrillation. When the patient is in severe cardiac failure and unable to tolerate bradycardia, temporary transvenous pacing may be necessary.

Drug-specific antibody fragments (FAB) is now available for the treatment of digitalis toxicity. Given intravenously this has proven to be rapidly effective with full recovery.

Digitalis Assays

Radioimmunoassay techniques are available for measuring Digoxin and Digitoxin levels in the blood. There is a considerable overlap between patients who have ineffective levels, those within the therapeutic range, and those within the toxic range. The test is useful, however, in the evaluation of arrhythmias that are compatible with digitalis toxicity. Levels in the low range makes it likely that the arrhythmias are unrelated to digitalis, whereas levels in the toxic range make it reasonable to assume that digitalis is responsible for the arrhythmia. Unfortunately, help is most often required when the clinical evidence of toxicity is equivocal and it is in this group that the serum Digoxin levels overlap considerably between toxic and nontoxic levels.

Diuretics

Therapy with various diuretic drugs is an effective way of controlling congestive cardiac failure. Diuretics produce dramatic relief of symptoms in acute pulmonary edema and are highly effective in preventing a recurrence of congestive cardiac failure in patients who have recovered from a previous episode. These are powerful drugs that must be used with caution in the smallest effective dose. Diuresis may be profound and there are several deleterious effects that may arise: (1) electrolyte depletion, particularly potassium, leading to serious cardiac arrhythmias and aggravation of digitalis toxicity; and (2) overdiuresis may result in hypovolemia and a decrease in left ventricular end-diastolic volume, which deprives the patient of one of the major compensatory mechanisms required to maintain an adequate stroke output. A high venous filling pressure is required, particularly in those conditions characterized by impaired diastolic filling (e.g., constrictive pericarditis, restrictive cardiomyopathy, and obstructive cardiomyopathy) and under these circumstances, overvigorous diuresis may be harmful. The use of powerful diuretics should be monitored by daily weighing and frequent measurement of the blood electrolytes. The commonly used diuretics fall into the following groups.

Distal Tubular Diuretics

Thiazide and Related Sulfonamide Diuretics

Chlorothiazide, hydrochlorothiazide, chlorthalidone, metolazone, and furosemide are all sulfonamide derivatives that act on the *distal* tubule to produce an increase in urinary excretion of sodium, potassium, chloride, and water. These drugs are moderately potent and there is little to choose between the various types. Chlorothiazide is given in doses of 50 to 150 mg twice daily. All thiazide diuretics may induce hyperuricemia and precipitate acute gout. Hyperglycemia is also a well-recognized complication but is usually not severe. The commonest side-effect is severe hypokalemia, which may be avoided by conscientious potassium supplementation.

Potassium Sparing Distal Tubular Diuretics

These include spironolactone and triamterene. They are less effective than other diuretics, but are useful in combination with the thiazides and furosemide. Spironolactone has an action commencing 24 to 48 hours after oral administration with a peak effect reached after 3 days. It antagonizes the effects of aldosterone, promoting sodium excretion and potassium retention. Triamterene acts independently of aldosterone, but also promotes potassium retention. Both drugs, particularly triamterene, may produce dangerous, and occasionally fatal hyperkalemia. Spironolactone may, like Digoxin, produce gynecomastia, because of its steroid structure.

Loop Diuretics

Ethacrynic acid and Furosemide are chemically unrelated to each other but have similar modes of action. Bumetanide is a more powerful cogener of furosemide. They are the most powerful diuretics available and may be administered both orally and intravenously. They exert their effect on the proximal renal tubule and the ascending limb of the loop of Henle. Furosemide is a sulfonamide derivative that has become the drug of choice in the severe forms of heart failure. It is rapidly absorbed from the gastrointestinal tract and the diuretic effect commences within an hour and lasts for 6 hours. Intravenously the effect begins within 15 minutes and is maximum within 3 hours. Some patients respond with massive diuresis when the drug is used for the first time. The commencing dose should be 40 mg and if this is ineffective the dose should be progressively doubled. It is not uncommon for patients to receive 1000 mg/day. The drug can be used in high dosage even in the presence of renal disease and uremia. Furosemide is effective when other diuretics fail, provided it is given in sufficient dosage: a combination of metolazone and lasix may be more effective than lasix alone. The dose of metolazone is 2.5 to 5 mg daily. It is diagnostically helpful in the oliguric patient when it is uncertain whether dehydration or renal tubular necrosis is present. Intravenous furosemide is followed by excretion of urine in the presence of dehydration but not when there is renal failure. Intravenous therapy is particularly useful in refractory cases of edema or in acute pulmonary edema. Direct toxic effects of the drug are rare but include skin rashes and hyperuricemia.

The action of ethacrynic acid is somewhat more unpredictable in that a gradual, or an overwhelming diuresis may result even after relatively small doses. Great care must be exercised in its use, for even a small dose in patients with heart failure refractory to all other diuretics may produce a drastic response. The average dose is 50 mg b.i.d., but it may be safer to commence with 25 mg. Side-effects are infrequent when the drug is used intermittently, but there is a high incidence of nausea, vomiting, and diarrhea, forcing discontinuation of the drug in patients on long-term therapy. Ethacrynic acid may induce hyperglycemia, hyperuricemia, and rarely acute hearing loss.

Bumetanide (Bumex) may be substituted for furosemide in allergic patients since cross-sensitivity is rare. One milligram of Bumex has an equivalent diuretic potency to 40 mg of furosemide.

NSAIDS

The diuretic effect of all loop diuretics may be offset by the effect of nonsteroidal anti-inflammatory drugs (NSAIDS). These drugs (indomethacin, sulindac, ibuprofen) and also aspirin limit the effect of prostaglandin, which increases renal blood flow as part of the natriuretic response to loop diuretics. These drugs may aggravate congestive heart failure and produce renal failure in some instances.

Proximal Tubular Diuretics

Carbonic Acid Anhydrase Inhibitors

Acetozolamide (Diamox) is a sulfonamide derivative that acts on the *proximal tubule*. This drug is occasionally useful in counteracting the hypochloremic metabolic alkalosis that complicates the use of loop diuretics. It produces an excretion of bicarbonate resulting in a hyperchloremic acidosis, which may restore diuretic potency. The usual dose is 250 to 500 mg daily or b.i.d.

Vasodilators

These drugs are now standard therapy for congestive heart failure. When used in combination with an inotropic agent or a diuretic the hemldynamic effects are additive.

In left ventricular failure there is a characteristic response to vasodilator drugs. They act by reducing the filling pressures and the systemic resistance thus breaking up the vicious cycle previously described (Fig. 9.3). Following reduction of the elevated systemic vascular resistance, the left ventricular filling pressure falls and the cardiac output increases significantly while the systemic arterial pressure is only modestly reduced; the heart rate remains the same. Unlike normal subjects who respond to vasodilators with tachycardia, this does not occur in the presence of heart failure—the reason for this is not known. The rise in cardiac output appears to be greatest in those patients with the highest initial left ventricular filling pressures and the lowest cardiac outputs.

The action of the various drugs is given in Table 9.1. Usually, a nitrate should be administered with an arteriolor dilator such as hydralazine, since the latter class of drugs is more effective is raising the cardiac output.

Sodium Nitroprusside

This relaxes smooth muscle of arteries and veins. Given intravenously, these effects are observed within 5 minutes and should be monitored by Swan Ganz catheterization and frequent measurement of the arterial pressure. It may produce severe hypotension. Fortunately, its effect wears off within 10 minutes after the infusion is stopped. It is extremely useful in the treatment of acute pulmonary edema and uncontrolled hypertension.

The initial infusion rate is 10 μg/min increasing by 5 μg/min to a maxium of 300 μg/min. Unwanted hypotension may be counteracted by intravenous phenylepherine or norepinepherine. Use of high doses, particularly in the presence of renal insufficiency, may produce thiocyanate intoxication.

Nitrates

Whether given orally, intravenously, or topically these agents are predominant venodilators with minimal effect on the arterioles. Their predominant effect is to reduce the filling pressures of both ventricles.

Isosorbide Dinitrate

This is given orally 20 to 60 mg t.i.d. The sublingual dose is 2.5 to 10 mg every 2 to 4 hours.

Intravenous Nitroglycerine

This preparation finds its chief use in the treatment of heart failure complicating myocardial infarction. The infusion is usually started at a rate 10 μg/min increasing by 10 μg/min every 10 minutes to a maximum of 100 μg/min until the systemic and pulmonary capillary pressures fall and there is a clinical response.

Topical Nitroglycerin (Ointment or Patch)

Tolerance may develop to these preparations; their efficacy in treating heart failure is being studied.

Hydralazine

A direct effect of this drug on the arterioles reduces the vascular resistance in the renal, splanchnic, and cerebral circulations more than in muscle and skin. The usual dose of 100 mg t.i.d. increases the cardiac output with little, if any change, in left ventricular filling pressure. The latter may be reduced when hydralazine is used in conjunction with a nitrate. Large doses of hydralazine may induce a lupus-like syndrome. *Minoxidil* has effects very similar to those of hydralazine. It has not gained much popularity in the treatment of chronic heart failure because of side-effects such as hirsutism and fluid retention.

Prazosin is an α-receptor blocker that dilates arterioles and veins. It produces the same hymodynamic effect as does a combination of hydralazine and isosorbide dinitrate. Prazosin was not effective in prolonging life in the V-Heft trial. This is undoubtedly related to hemodynamic tachyphylaxis, which occurs with prolonged use. Therefore, it has no place in the treatment of chronic heart failure.

Angiotension-Converting Enzyme (ACE) Inhibitors

Captopril, Enalapril, and Lisinopril

These drugs, are currently the vasodilators of choice. In comparative trials they have been

TABLE 9.1. Classification of vasodilators according to site and mechanism of action.

Agent	Action	Heart rate	Right atrial pressure	Pulmonary capillary pressure	Cardiac output	Blood pressure
			Venodilators			
Nitrates	Direct venodilator; direct arteriolar dilator (mild); direct coronary dilator (NTG)	No change	Marked decrease	Marked decrease	No change or slight increase	Slight decrease
			Arteriolar Dilators			
Hydralazine and minoxidil	Direct arteriolar dilators	No change or slight increase	No change	No change or slight decrease	Marked increase	Slight decrease or no change
Phentolamine	α_1- and α_2-Blocker	Increase	Decrease	Decrease	Increase	Slight decrease
			Combined Arteriolar Dilator and Venodilator			
Nitroprusside	Direct veno- and arteriolar dilator	No change	Decrease	Decrease	Increase	Slight decrease
Prazosin and trimazosin	α_1-Blockers	No change or slight decrease	Marked decrease	Marked decrease	Increase	Moderate decrease
Captopril and enalapril	Converting enzyme inhibitor	Slight decrease	Decrease	Marked decrease	Moderate increase	Moderate decrease

shown to improve life expectancy. They are efficacious in advanced heart failure with elevated levels of circulating angiotension IL. Diuretics and arteriolar vasodilators activate the renin–angiotension–aldosterone system paving the way for ACE inhibitors. In effective doses the cardiac output increases, the filling pressures fall, and the blood pressure is maintained without tachycardia.

To avoid hypotension, dosage should be gradual. The starting doses are captopril 12.5 mg t.i.d., enalapril 5 to 10 mg b.i.d., and lisinopril 10 to 20 mg daily. The dosage is then titrated until the maximum clinical effect is obtained. Their effects are markedly diminished in the presence of renal failure. They may decrease renal function and produce glomerulonephritis as a toxic effect.

TABLE 9.2. Comparison of hemodynamic effects of dopamine and dobutamine.

<table>
<tr><th></th><th>Dobutamine</th><th>Dopamine</th></tr>
<tr><td>Heart rate</td><td></td><td></td></tr>
<tr><td>Low dose</td><td colspan="2">No change</td></tr>
<tr><td>High dose</td><td colspan="2">Increase</td></tr>
<tr><td>Blood Pressure</td><td></td><td></td></tr>
<tr><td>Low dose</td><td colspan="2">No change</td></tr>
<tr><td>High dose</td><td colspan="2">Increase</td></tr>
<tr><td>Cardiac Output</td><td></td><td></td></tr>
<tr><td>Low dose</td><td colspan="2">Increase</td></tr>
<tr><td>High dose</td><td colspan="2">Increase</td></tr>
<tr><td>Left ventricular filling pressure</td><td></td><td></td></tr>
<tr><td>Low dose</td><td colspan="2">Variable</td></tr>
<tr><td>High dose</td><td>Decrease</td><td>Increase</td></tr>
<tr><td>Peripheral vascular resistance</td><td></td><td></td></tr>
<tr><td>Low dose</td><td colspan="2">Variable</td></tr>
<tr><td>High dose</td><td>Decrease</td><td>Increase</td></tr>
</table>

Inotropic Agents

Sympathomimetic Drugs

At the outset it should be made clear that these agents play a minor role in the management of patients with *chronic* congestive heart failure. Most importantly, there is no evidence to show that they improve life expectancy, even though a 72-hour infusion may improve the ejection fraction and duration of exercise for several weeks. Indeed, their inotropic effect may produce an increase in oxygen consumption and produce serious ventricular dysrhythmias. Even in cardiogenic shock, dopamine does not appear to favorably influence survival. Also, these drugs have to be given intravenously with Swan Ganz and arterial-line monitoring.

Among patients with chronic heart failure there seems little, if any, justification for a so called routine "tune up." When heart failure is precipitated by factors such as (1) withdrawal of medication, (2) infection, or (3) dysrhythmia in an otherewise stable patient they may have a place in management until the situation is stabilized.

Intravenous sympathomimetic amines stimulate β_1-receptors, thus enhancing myocardial contractility. Differences in their overall action are related to effects on peripheral β_2- and α_1-receptors. The actions of dopamine and dobutamine are compared in Table 9.2.

Dopamine

This catecholamine is the immediate precursor of norepinephrine. Although it has the inotropic effect of norepinephrine, it has less vasoconstrictor and chronotropic effects.

The vasodilation induced by dopamine follows activation of specific dopaminergic receptors in blood vessels and the central and peripheral nervous system. In low doses (less than 2 μg/kg/min) is direct effect is to dilate the coronary, renal, mesenteric, and cerebral vascular beds. In heart failure this dopamine-induced diuresis is a result of its positive inotropic effect and renal vasodilatation. With larger doses (2 to 5 μg/kg/min) the positive inotropic effect is still evident, but the peripheral effects are variable. When 5–10 μg/kg/min is given, there is significant vasoconstriction with a decline in renal blood flow. This dosage may raise the left ventricular filling pressure, producing tachycardia and dysrhythmias. Therefore, the dosage must be carefully titrated when treating congestive heart failure.

Dobutamine

This is a synthetic sympathomimetic amine with β_1-, β_2-, and α-adrenergic activity. The effect of dobutamine is to increase the cardiac output without changing the heart rate or blood pressure; there is not a selective renal vasodilator effect. Dobutamine has the advantage over dopamine in treating heart failure because it has little effect on heart rate and blood pressure and reduces ventricular filling pressure. The usual dose is 1 to 4 μg/kg/min.

Phosphodiesterase Inhibitors

Amrinone and *milrinone* are not available in the United States for oral use; amirinone is available in intravenous form. Although their mechanisms of action are quite different, the hemodynamic effects of amirinone are similar to those of dobutamine. Inhibition of phosphodiesterase increases cyclic adenosine monophosphate (AMP), which enhances calcium entry and improves contractility. There is a direct vasodilator action, an increase in cardiac output and a decrease in filling pressures, and an improvement in exercise tolerance. The long-term effect of these agents is uncertain and there are no studies to indicate an improvement in life expectancy.

Arrhythmias

Sudden death is a common event in heart failure and the presence of complex ventricular dysrhythmias is a predictor of this event. Unfortunately, antiarrhythmic drugs have not been shown to alter this. In the absence of symptoms, such treatment cannot be justified since these patients are at high risk for proarrhythmic effect; also virtually every antiarrhythmic drug has a negative inotropic action that may aggravate heart failure.

Treatment of Acute Pulmonary Edema

1. *Morphine*. This terminates most of the mild, and some of the severe attacks, given in a dose of 15 to 20 mg intramuscularly, or 10 mg intravenously slowly in a diluted solution. Respiratory depression and vomiting are the main side-effects associated with its use. Morphine acts by decreasing venous and arterial tone, producing venous pooling, and decreased venous return, in addition to its effect of decreasing arterial resistance. These factors improve ventricular function. Additionally, it is extremely valuable in relieving the anxiety which aggravates the attack.
2. *Sodium Nitroprusside*. This is the next step in treatment. Its effects are dramatic, particularly when left ventricular dysfunction is a result of hypertension. The initial dose is an infusion rate of 10 μg/m/min, increasing this every 5 minutes by 10 μg until the signs and symptoms are relieved and the wedge pressure returns to normal, or until the arterial pressure falls to limiting levels.
3. *Intravenous diuretics* such as furosemide (20 mg) or ethacrynic acid (50 mg) are rapidly effective. The effect of lasix is extremely rapid and precedes diuresis. The drug has a venodilator effect, thereby relieving pulmonary congestion.
4. *Aminophylline* also has a direct vasodilating effect on arteries and veins that is useful in the treatment of patients with acute heart failure. Also, it increases myocardial contractility through a positive inotropic effect, and relieves bronchospasm, which frequently accompanies cardiac dyspnea. It promotes diuresis by increasing renal blood flow and the glomerular filtration rate. It is given intravenously in a dose of 0.5 g in 20 ml of saline at a rate of 1 ml/min to avoid vomiting. A total daily dose of 1000 mg should not be exceeded because of the risk of toxic effects, which include hypotension, convulsions, and serious cardiac arrhythmias.
5. *Digoxin* is particularly valuable when acute pulmonary edema is precipitated by uncontrolled atrial fibrillation in patients with mitral stenosis.
6. *Oxygen* should be administered to correct the associated hypoxia and is best given by nasal mask. Occasionally, artificial positive pressure respiration is required and may be life saving, particularly after operations on the mitral valve, because these patients have noncompliant lungs and severe chronic pulmonary congestion.

Intractable Cardiac Failure

This is a common problem despite the use of modern treatment. When heart failure is truly refractory or intractable the question of cardiac transplantation arises in suitable patients. Before taking this step, the situation should be reviewed to identify subtle precipitating or aggravating factors.

Systolic Pump Function

The left ventricular ejection fraction (LVEF) should be determined by MUGA or by echocardiography. This is a powerful predictor of mortality in congestive heart failure and is usually depressed. A normal or mildly decreased ejection fraction would point to impaired diastolic filling and the possibility of constrictive pericarditis, which is remediable. Other causes of impaired diastolic filling include amyloid disease, endomyocardial fibrosis, and cardiac tumors, all of which may be detected by echocardiography.

High Output States

Anemia should be identified and the cause treated. The clinical diagnosis of mild *thyrotoxicosis* is extremely difficult or impossible. It should be searched for by routine biochemical testing, particularly when there is atrial fibrillation.

Pulmonary Thromboembolism

This commonly complicates protracted heart failure and may be occult. It should be identified by ventilation–perfusion scan and selective angiography if necessary.

Infective Endocarditis

This is particularly difficult to diagnose in the elderly among whom aortic ejection murmurs are so frequent. Echocardiography may not be so helpful in diagnosing vegetations because of the presence of heavy senile calcification of the aortic valve. Other infections (pulmonary, renal, etc.) aggravate heart failure by increasing cardiac output.

Electrolyte Abnormalities

These are frequently a result of overdiuresis and may be correctable (e.g., hypokalemia, hypochloremic alkalosis).

Digitalis

Toxicity. This may result in bradycardia (sinus, junctional, or A-V dissociation) or tachycardia (paroxysmal atrial tachycardia with A-V block, bidirectional tachycardia), both of which may aggravate heart failure. Toxicity is particularly likely when quinidine is administered and when hypokalemia complicates vigorous diuresis.

Resistance

Infections alter the gastrointestinal flora may produce resistance by inactivating digoxin. Absorption is decreased by aluminum hydroxide, kaopectate, and cholestyramine.

Compliance

This requires careful attention. Is the medication being taken regularly? Are other medications from another practitioner being taken? (Estrogens, steroids, and NSAIDs product salt retention). Vasodilators and dietary indiscretion also produce salt retention.

Alcohol

Abuse of alcohol may result in poor compliance. In large doses, alcohol may have a direct cardiotoxic effect or may aggravate heart failure through thiamine deficiency.

Myocarditis

Rheumatic myocarditis may produce heart failure in an otherwise stable patient with valvular disease.

Hypertension

Among patients with ischemic or valvular heart disease, uncontrolled hypertension will aggravate heart failure.

When these factors have received attention and heart failure remains intractable, transplantation should be considered.

Cardiac Transplantation

Candidates for this procedure should be less than 60 years of age, psychologically stable, and compliant with treatment. Contraindications are insulin-dependent diabetes, pulmonary hypertension (vascular resistance more than 8 units), coexisting liver or renal disease, and active peptic ulceration. With the advent of cyclosporine, the 5-year survival rate is 75%, which is as good as kidney transplantation with unmatched donor and recipient.

A shortage of donors and financial constraints inhibit the fullest use of this procedure.

Additional Reading

Cohn JN: Current therapy of the failing heart. Circulation 1099–1106, 1988.

Cohn JN, Archibald DG, Phil M, Ziesche S, et al.: Effect of vasodilator therapy on mortality in chronic congestive heart failure. N Engl J Med 1547–1552, 1986.

Franciosa JA, Wilen M, Ziesche S, et al.: Survival in men with severe chronic left ventricular failure due to either coronary heart disease or idiopathic dilated cardiomyopathy. Am J Cardiol 51:831–836, 1983.

Francis GS: Development of arrhythhmias in the patient with congestive heart failure: pathophysiology, prevalence, and prognosis. Am J Cardiol 57:3–7B, 1986.

Friedberg CK: Edema and pulmonary edema. Pathologic physiology and differential diagnosis. Prog Cardiovasc Dis 13:546, 1971.

McKee PA, Castelli WP, McNamara PM, et al.: The natural history of congestive heart failure: The Framingham study. N Engl J Med 285:1441–1446, 1971.

Parmley WW: Pathophysiology and current therapy of congestive heart failure. J Am Coll Cardiol 13:771, 1989.

Wood P: Heart failure: In "Diseases of the Heart and Circulation," 3rd ed. Eyre and, Spottiswoode, London, 1968, p. 291.

10
Congenital Heart Disease

The incidence of congenital heart disease is about 8 per 1000 live births. Of these cases, one-third have anomalies that if untreated result in death within the first year of life; two-thirds of these deaths occur in the neonatal period. With early recognition and prompt referral to a specialist center equipped for 24-hour emergency cardiac catheterzation and surgery, many of these infants can now be expected to survive.

Although there clearly is a need for aggressive early investigation of the neonate with heart disease, skilled clinical examination is nowhere more rewarding and challenging. With the additional corroborative information available from the chest X-ray, electrocardiogram, and echocardiogram, a fairly accurate clinical diagnosis may be made prior to cardiac catheterization, and in critically ill babies this helps in the planning of the procedure.

There should be no illusion, however, about the potential for serious diagnostic clinical errors. Therefore, in the neonatal period all infants with cyanotic congenital heart disease should be promptly investigated. Undue reliance on a clinical diagnosis may delay the procedure and result in fatality. Similarly, neonates in congestive cardiac failure should be catheterized following institution of appropriate medical treatment: when there is a rapid good response, the procedure may be delayed for a day or two but if the response is incomplete, catheterization should be undertaken without delay.

The value of clinical examination is more clearly evident in the management of older infants and children where the situation is less urgent. A firm diagnosis of a malformation (such as ventricular septal defect) and its hemodynamic significance can frequently be made, thus avoiding unnecessary invasive procedures. There is no justification for catheterizing children with vibratory or pulmonary ejection systolic murmurs, small ventricular septal defect, or mild pulmonary stenosis. However, when a complicated anomaly is considered to be hemodynamically significant and operation is contemplated, cardiac catheterization is necessary to confirm the diagnosis and also to exclude unsuspected associated lesions.

A good clinical approach to the diagnosis of congenital heart disease requires a knowledge of the pathology of the various malformations and the changing disturbances in physiology resultant therefrom. These, in turn, influence the clinical findings and the abnormalities found in the electrocardiogram, chest X-ray, is echocardiogram.

Many classifications have been proposed, but none is entirely satisfactory or provides an easy route to diagnosis. This is particularly evident in the neonate. Here, a helpful perspective is to know the following:

The leading causes of neonatal cyanotic heart disease:

1. Transposition of the great vessels
2. Tetralogy of Fallot
3. Tricuspid atresia

4. Total anomalous pulmonary venous drainage
5. Truncus arteriosus
6. Aortic atresia
7. Pulmonary atresia

The leading causes of neonatal heart failure:

1. Aortic atresia
2. Coarctation of the aorta
3. Transposition of the great vessels
4. Ventricular septal defect
5. Endocardial fibroelastosis

In the neonate therefore (and also in older children) the first decisions to be made relate to the presence or absence of (1) central cyanosis, (2) heart failure, and (3) central cyanosis and heart failure.

Central Cyanosis

In the assessment of the significance of central cyanosis in the neonate, the *respiratory distress syndrome* is a major source of difficulty. It occurs most frequently in premature infants, infants who are the product of diabetic mothers, or those delivered by cesarean section. Infants with the respiratory distress syndrome frequently have sternal retraction and grunting prior to the onset of cyanosis. At first the heart is not enlarged and there are no murmurs. Subsequently, hepatomegaly, rales, a systolic murmur, and cardiomegaly may develop. The presence of a significantly enlarged liver would tend to point away from the diagnosis of respiratory distress syndrome. Usually the chest roentgenogram shows characteristic reticulation of the lungs and an air bronchogram, which is evidence of hyperaeration. Occasionally, the clinical distinction between severe cardiac disease and the respiratory distress syndrome is impossible. Two-dimensional echocardiography and cardiac catheterization should be undertaken if necessary to elucidate the problem, although there is a higher than usual risk for the procedure.

When it has been established that central cyanosis is a result of cardiac disease, auscultation of an apical short rumbling middiastolic murmur indicates the presence of excessive mitral, and therefore pulmonary blood flow. This may be confirmed by the radiological finding of an increase in the pulmonary *arterial* vasculature. Likewise, cyanosis without an apical middiastolic murmur and with diminished pulmonary vasculature indicates decreased pulmonary blood flow. The same assessment may be made in the absence of cyanosis. When a radiological diagnosis of pulmonary *venous* obstruction is made and considered in relation to the presence or absence of cyanosis, the following workable, bedside classification is extremely useful.

Cyanosis Absent

Increased Pulmonary Arterial Vasculature (Pulmonary Plethora)

A. Extracardiac left-to-right shunts:
    1. Patent ductus arteriosus
    2. Aortopulmonary window
    3. Ruptured aortic sinus aneurysm
B. Intracardiac left-to-right shunts:
    1. Ventricular septal defect (VSD)
    2. Atrial septal defect
    3. Atrioventricular canal

Normal Pulmonary Arterial Vasculature

A. Right ventricular outflow obstruction—pulmonary stenosis
B. Left ventricular outflow obstruction:
    1. Coarctation of aorta
    2. Aortic valve stenosis

Pulmonary Venous Engorgement

1. Congenital mitral stenosis
2. Cor triatriatum
3. Supravalvular stenosing ring of the left atrium
4. Congenital stenosis of the pulmolnary veins
5. Congenital mitral insufficiency

Cyanosis Present

Increased Pulmonary Arterial Vasculature

A. Right-to-left shunts (Eisenmenger syndrome)
   1. Atrial septal defect
   2. Ventricular septal defect
   3. Patent ductus arteriosus

B. "Common mixing" lesions
   1. Single ventricle without pulmonary stenosis
   2. Tricuspid atresia without pulmonary stenosis
   3. Complete transposition of the great vessel without pulmonary stenosis
   4. Double outlet right ventricle without pulmonary stenosis
   5. Persistent truncus arteriosus
   6. Total anomalous pulmonary venous drainage

Decreased Pulmonary Arterial Vasculature ("Pulmonary Oligemia")

1. Tetralogy of Fallot
2. Pulmonary atresia
3. Tricuspid atresia, with pulmonary stenosis
4. Single ventricle, with pulmonary stenosis
5. Double outlet right ventricle, with pulmonary stenosis
6. Ebstein disease

Pulmonary Venous Engorgement

1. Aortic atresia
2. Aortic and mitral atresia
3. Total anomalous pulmonary venous drainage with obstruction

This approach, based on elementary clinical and radiologic findings, allows for a rapid initial step to accurate diagnosis. The more subtle clinical findings will then fit into place: The *pulmonary component of the second heart sound* will contribute to the evaluation of pulmonary hypertension, pulmonary stenosis, and pulmonary atresia. The characteristics of a *systolic murmur* will point to pulmonary or aortic valve stenosis, ventricular septal defect, or mitral insufficiency. *Ejection clicks* will assist in the diagnosis of aortic or pulmonary valve stenosis and pulmonary hypertension.

Additional *radiologic findings* will provide clues to the diagnosis of cardiac malposition, and the likelihood of complex malformations such as single ventricle, complete A-V canal, and total anomalous pulmonary venous drainage.

In dextrocardia (heart in the right side of the chest in absence of lung disease to account for the shift), associated with inversion of the other viscera (situs inversus), the incidence of heart disease is only 3%. One-fifth of these patients, however, will have Kartagener syndrome (sinusitis and bronchiectasis). When the heart is left-sided (isolated levocardia) and the abdominal viscera inverted (situs inversus) at least 90% of patients will have severe cardiac malformations.

The *situs* of an individual can be determined from the position of the liver and the main stem bronchi on an overpenetrated chest radiograph. *Situs solitus* consists of the liver and short stem bronchus on the right—the right atrium will then be on the right. *Situs inversus* will have the liver, short stem bronchus, and therefore the left atrium on the left. Exceptions to this relationship are rare and occur in the polysplenia and asplenia syndromes when the situs may be indeterminate with a transverse liver.

The presence of *splenic anomalies* is highly likely whenever levocardia and situs inversus coexist. The presence of *asplenia* may be confirmed by finding Howell-Jolly bodies in the blood film, and also by radioisotope scanning. Left axis deviation of the P wave vector suggests polysplenia and concomitant interruption of the inferior vena cava.

The *electrocardiogram* will indicate ventricular hypertrophy or hypoplasia, or conduction defects highly suggestive of individual malformations (e.g., left axis deviation in tricuspid atresia and endocardial cushion defect). It may

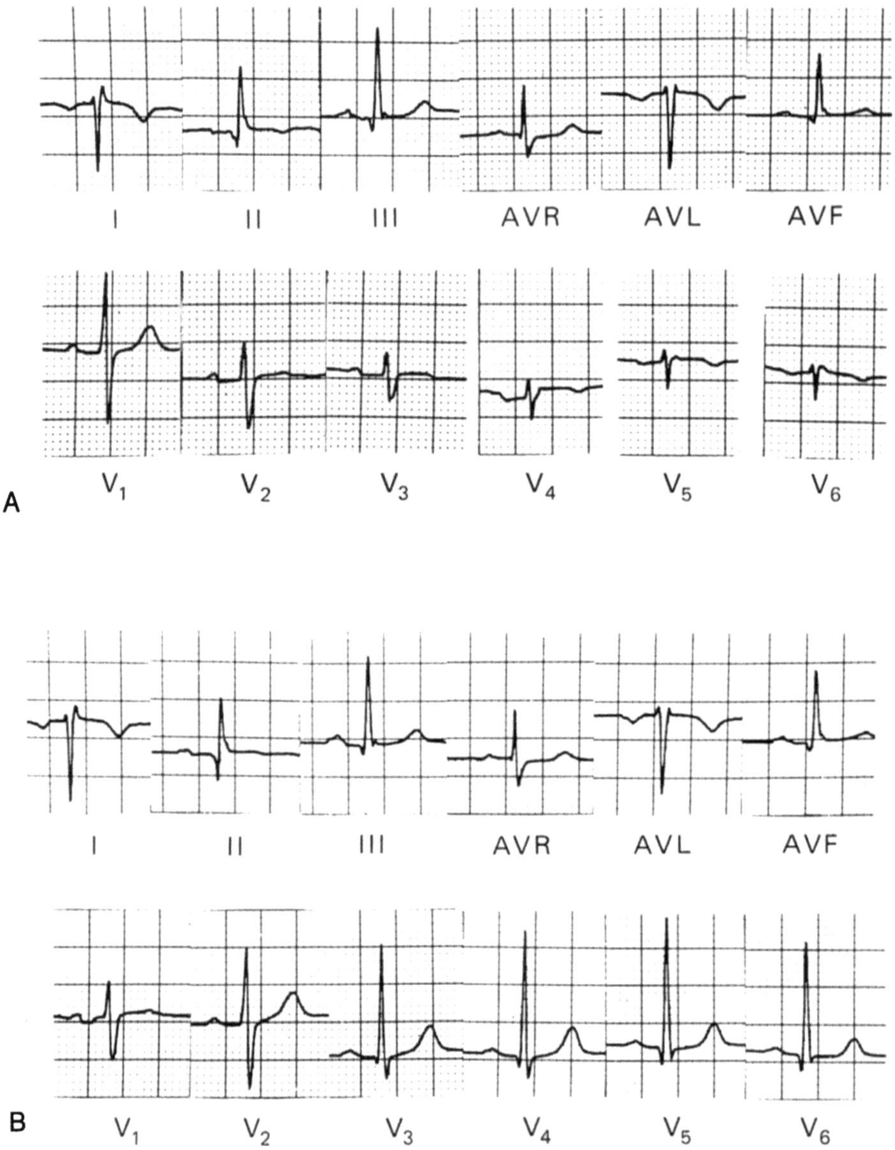

FIGURE 10.1. The electrocardiogram in mirror-image dextrocardia. (A) Precordial leads recorded over left side. (B) Precordial leads recorded over right side. In true dextrocardia lead I looks like AVR and vice versa because of the inverted atria; also P waves are *inverted* in leads V5 and V6; when the precordial leads are recorded on the right side the P waves are *upright*. When limb leads are incorrectly placed, so that AVR looks like S_1, the P wave vector is the clue—an upright P wave in V5 and V6 indicates lead reversal.

also be helpful in the diagnosis of dextrocardia (Fig. 10.1). In skilled hands noninvasive echocardiography will provide almost as much information as angiography.

As obscure, diverse, and confusing as congenital cardiac malformations may appear to be, the majority are within diagnostic reach of the clinician. Common individual malformations will now be described in view of the aforementioned approach.

Cyanosis Absent: Increased Pulmonary Arterial Vasculature: Patent Ductus Arteriosus

During fetal life the ductus arteriosus (Fig. 10.2) has the important function of diverting blood from the pulmonary circulation to the aorta so that gas exchange may take place in the placenta. About 75% of the total flow to the descending aorta is via the ductus. Normally, functional vascular closure of the ductus occurs within 15 hours after birth; permanent anatomical closure is complete within 7 days. The precise mechanism whereby ductal closure occurs is unknown, but exposure to a high oxygen concentration is important. Patency of the ductus is much more frequent at high altitude because of hypoxia.

The malformation is a common one accounting for approximately one-sixth of all cases of congenital heart disease. Females are affected twice as commonly as males. Broadly speaking, a ductus that fails to close during early infancy remains patent unless surgically corrected. Patent ductus arteriosus may occur as an isolated defect or-in combination with other anomalies.

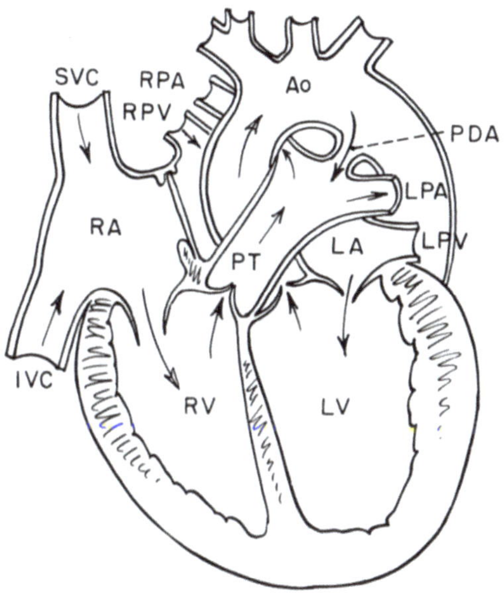

FIGURE 10.2. Central circulation in patent ductus arteriosus with left-to-right shunt and pulmonary vascular resistance less than systemic. Reprinted, with permissions, from Edwards JE: Classification of congenital heart disease in the adult. Cardiovascular Clinics 10:I, 1979, F.A. Davis Company.

As with ventricular defect, the clinical picture can be divided into those patients with normal or slightly elevated pulmonary artery pressures, those with significant pulmonary hypertension, and those with severe pulmonary hypertension.

Patent Ductus with Normal Pulmonary Arterial Pressure

Small Left-to-Right Shunt

This is by far the most frequent situation. When the communication is small, it produces a loud murmur but little disturbance of function. Patients are asymptonlatic in the absence of complications. The main danger is infective endocarditis and, for this reason, prophylactic surgery is always advised. The condition is usually discovered on routine clinical examination, often by a school doctor.

Physical Findings

The *pulse* is normal and the heart is not enlarged. A systolic, or systolic and diastolic, thrill is palpable in the second left intercostal space and just below the left clavicle. This is associated with a typical continuous or machinery-like murmur (the Gibson murmur). The systolic component is usually louder (grade 3–5) and has a late crescendo, so that it spills over and obscures the second sound, at the site of maximal intensity of the murmur. The diastolic component is more blowing and continues through diastole. Away from the site of greatest intensity, splitting of the second heart sound can usually be detected, with the normal respiratory movement. Marked fluctuation in intensity of the pulmonary component is highly characteristic. The systolic murmur, in particular, radiates fairly widely to the fourth left interspace and the apex.

The *electrocardiogram and chest X-ray* are within normal limits. Catheterization reveals normal hemodynamics and a small left-to-right shunt.

Large Left-to-Right Shunt

When the communication is large, the left-to-right shunt and the strain on the left ventricle is increased. Effort dyspnea and fatigue are present and heart failure may develop.

Physical Findings

The size of the shunt is reflected in the pulse, which is abrupt and collapsing with a high pulse pressure and low diastolic pressure, because of the aortic runoff. The left ventricle is enlarged and overactive. An apical middiastolic rumble is audible, indicating a large pulmonary venous return with increased flow across the mitral valve. The Gibson murmur is loud, radiates widely, and may obscure any associated murmur of semilunar valve incompetence, or pulmonary stenosis. Reversed splitting of the second sound may occur because of left ventricular volume overload.

The *electrocardiogram* shows diastolic overload of the left ventricle with high voltage; sometimes T wave changes and ST segment depression are found.

Radiological examination shows left ventricular and left atrial enlargement, pulmonary plethora, and increased pulmonary arterial pulsation. A prominent aortic knuckle, especially in an infant, suggests a ductus.

Diagnosis is from other conditions associated with continuous murmurs (p. 44).

Patent Ductus with Significant Pulmonary Hypertension

This is usually encountered in young infants and is a serious threat to life.

Physical Findings

An important clue is the full pulse, which indicates that a large left-to-right shunt is usually present. There is clinical evidence of right, and left, ventricular enlargement.

Because of the pulmonary diastolic hypertension and the reduced systemic diastolic pressure, a diastolic gradient between aorta and pulmonary artery may be absent, so that the diastolic component of the "continuous" murmur is much softer or absent. Therefore, only a systolic murmur is heard and since this is often loud at the fourth left intercostal space, ventricular septal defect may be suspected. A middiastolic rumble is usually present at the apex and is produced by the large left-to-right shunt. Not infrequently, functional mitral incompetence coexists. In some patients only a to-and-fro murmur of pulmonary incompetence is heard.

The *electrocardiogram* generally shows the changes of left ventricular hypertrophy and, sometimes, of left atrial overload. A particularly suggestive tracing in young infants is one showing large Q and tall R waves in the left chest leads. A tall R in V1 relative to the S with right axis deviation indicates additional right ventricular enlargement.

The Chest X-Ray

This shows biventricular and left atrial enlargement; the aortic knuckle is prominent and the main pulmonary arteries enlarged. Filling in of the angle between the aorta and the pulmonary artery in the PA view is characteristic (Fig. 10.3). Calcification of the ductus and adjoining great vessel occurs in older patients.

Cardiac catheterization confirms pulmonary hypertension and the left-to-right shunt. The catheter can frequently be passed from the pulmonary artery, through the ductus into the descending aorta. Retrograde aortography fills the pulmonary arteries.

The treatment is surgical and there is little point in procrastination once the infant has been made fit for surgery.

Patent Ductus with Severe Pulmonary Hypertension

As in ventricular septal defect, the pulmonary arterial resistance determines the hemodynamics and the clinical picture. The increased pulmonary resistance dates from early life, though occasionally in an adult progressive increase in resistance develops. Symptoms are usually present consisting of effort dyspnea, fatigue, and congestive failure; cyanosis may ultimately develop.

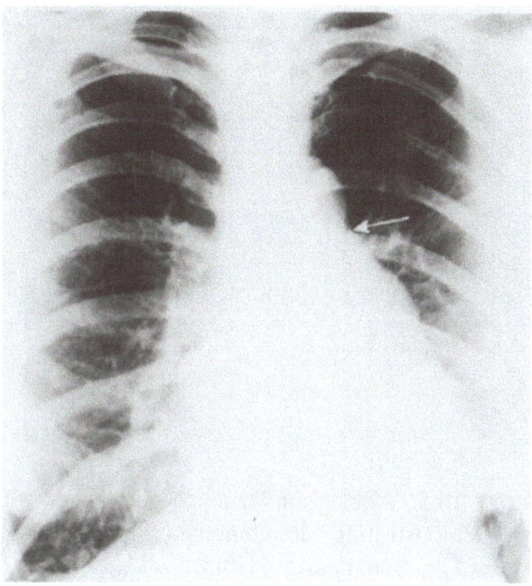

FIGURE 10.3. The X-ray in patent ductus arteriosus with large left-to-right shunt and pulmonary hypertension showing an enlarged aorta and pulmonary artery with filling in of the notch between the two (arrow).

Physical Findings

As long as the shunt is dominantly left-to-right, an ejection systolic murmur is still present, and is associated with signs of pulmonary hypertension, an atrial gallop, a pulmonary ejection click, and sometimes pulmonary incompetence. The second sound moves normally with respiration.

The *electrocardiogram* shows severe right ventricular hypertrophy and even right bundle branch block. The *X-ray* confirms the right-sided chamber enlargement and the large pulmonary arteries with peripheral "pruning."

As long as the shunt is still dominantly left-to-right, surgery is possible.

When pulmonary resistance exceeds the systemic, the shunt is reversed (*Eisenmenger syndrome*). The diagnosis can be made at the bedside, if cyanosis of the toes exceeds that of the hands (Fig. 1.10).

Indications for Surgery

Surgery is advised in all patients with patent ductus arteriosus in whom there is a dominant left-to-right shunt. When a small defect is present, surgery is a purely prophylactic elective procedure to prevent the development of bacterial endocarditis.

The problem as to whether surgery is advisable arises only in the presence of high-grade pulmonary hypertension with bidirectional shunts. Careful assessment of shunt flows using oximetry and dye-dilution curves and precise measurement of the pulmonary vascular resistance is mandatory.

Premature infants with respiratory distress syndrome and a patent ductus pose special problems. In premature infants the ductus is relatively unresponsive to increasing oxygen tensions and there is a failure of constriction. With the advent of continuous positive airway pressure to treat the respiratory distress syndrome arterial p_{O_2}s have been deliberately kept at 70–80 mm Hg to avoid retrolental fibroplasia. This p_{O_2} is not adequate to cause ductal constriction in the premature infant.

Assisted ventilation has improved survival for the respiratory distress syndrome and prevented retrolental fibroplasia, but there is an increased incidence of patent ductus. Frequently, this becomes manifest 3–5 days after birth when the respiratory distress is improving. The usual signs of heart failure are lacking. A systolic murmur, widening of the pulse pressure, and periods of apnea become manifest. Intensive medical therapy is required and if improvement is not evident in 24 hours, catheterization followed by ductal ligation is indicated.

Associated Defects

Pulmonary stenosis. This is occasionally associated with patent ductus arteriosus and must be suspected when there is a history of maternal rubella during pregnancy. It can usually be diagnosed only at catheterization or after surgery, since the signs are obscured by the ductus. The stenosis may affect the pulmonary valve and/or the pulmonary arterial branches.

In the *rubella syndrome* the heart is involved as are many other organs. Central nervous system infection leads to congenital cataract, deafness, mental deficiency, and so on. The commonest cardiac lesion is patent ductus arteriosus; pulmonary valve or distal pulmonary artery stenosis is next in frequency, with or without a patent ductus. Ventricular septal defect and supravalvular stenosis of the aorta have also been recorded.

Ventricular septal defect and patent ductus arteriosus: see ventricular septal defect (p. 44).

Coarctation and patent ductus: see coarctation of aorta (p. 220).

Complex Anomalies: In conditions such as pulmonary atresia and aortic atresia, a patent ductus is essential for the maintenance of pulmonary or systemic blood flow and is an integral part of the malformation.

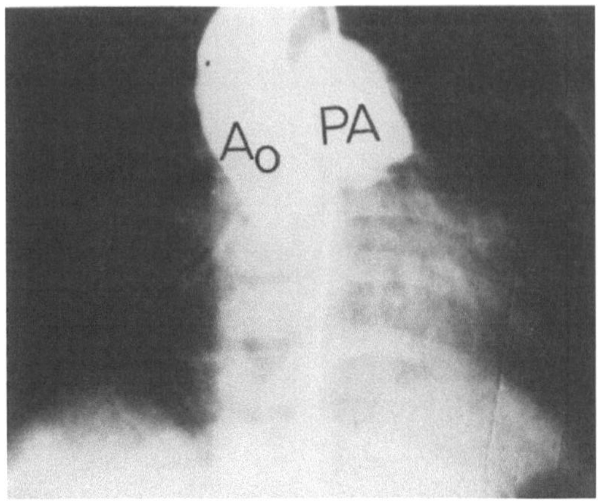

FIGURE 10.5. Aortogram in aorto-pulmonary window demonstrating simultaneous filling of aorta (A_o) and pulmonary artery (PA).

Aortopulmonary Window

Aortopulmonary window (Fig. 10.4) is a rare condition in which there is a defect in the septum that divides the truncus arteriosus into aorta and pulmonary artery, so that the aorta and pulmonary artery communicate just above the semilunar valves. The aorta and pulmonary artery are normally related but remain unpartitioned for a small length, usually 1 to 10 mm, above the aortic valve. The defect varies from 0.5 to 3 cm in diameter but is usually large.

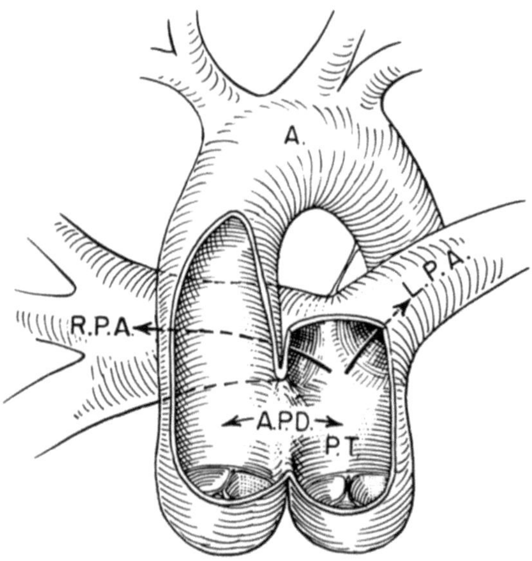

FIGURE 10.4. The anatomy of aortopulmonary widow (APD). The aortic and pulmonary valves are present and separated; the defect is usually just anterior to the ostium of the right pulmonary artery. Courtesy of Dr. Jesse E. Edwards and Dr. Edward P. Todd.

The hemodynamic changes are generally severe, both because the opening is large and because there is no length to the communication, unlike a patent ductus arteriosus. As a rule the left-to-right shunt is large and severe pulmonary hypertension is common, but irreversible arteriolar changes are infrequent.

The condition is seldom encountered after the age of 20 and there is an equal sex incidence. Heart failure is the usual cause of death.

Clinical Features

The symptoms are those associated with any large left-to-right shunt and consist mainly of dyspnea, fatigue, frequent respiratory infections, and failure to thrive. The signs of a large aortic runoff are usually present and the heart is enlarged with biventricular hypertrophy. The systemic and pulmonary diastolic pressures are equal, most of the left-to-right shunt

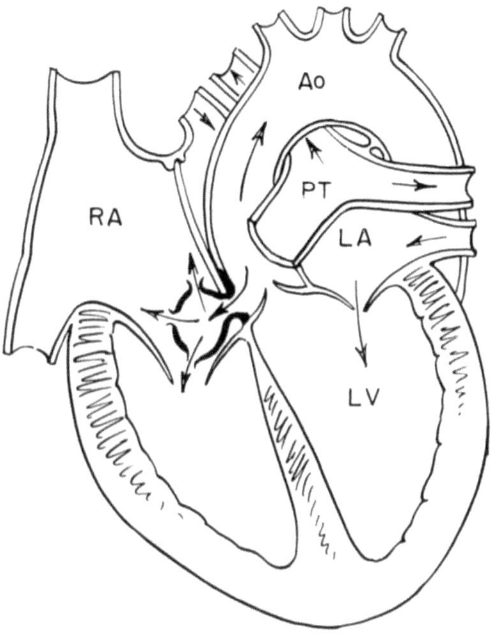

FIGURE 10.6. Diagram of rupture of an aneurysm of the posterior aortic sinus into the right atrium. Reprinted, with permission, from Edwards JE: Classification of congenital heart disease in the adult. Cardiovascular Clinics 10:I, 1979, F.A. Davis Company.

Ruptured Aneurysm of the Sinuses of Valsalva

The right and noncoronary sinuses are sometimes congenitally weakened, resulting in aneurysmal dilatation. Usually asymptomatic and silent, they may occasionally deform the aortic valves and produce aortic incompetence (Figs. 10.6 and 10.7).

Generally speaking, symptoms and signs first appear with rupture of the sinus into one or other camber of the heart (right atrium, right ventricle, left atrium, or left ventricle). The aneurysms burrow into the myocardium and, when they rupture into a cardiac chamber, sudden symptoms and often rapid heart failure develop. Rupture of the sinus may be spontaneous or the result of infective endocarditis. Occasionally, a fistula may be found during taking place during systole. Consequently, a basal systolic murmur is generally present and a continuous murmur rare, and when present, the site may be a little lower than usual for a patent ductus.

The *electrocardiographic* and *radiological* appearances are often indistinguishable from patent ductus, but the aortic knuckle is usually not prominent. A right-sided aorta and a patent ductus arteriosus are occasional associations.

The *diagnosis* is usually made by cardiac catheterization performed for study of an atypical ductus, large left-to-right shunts, severe pulmonary hypertension, or Eisenmenger syndrome (Fig. 10.5). Occasionally it is made at operation for suspected patent ductus. The treatment is closure of the defect, provided the pulmonary vascakis resistance is less than 10 units.

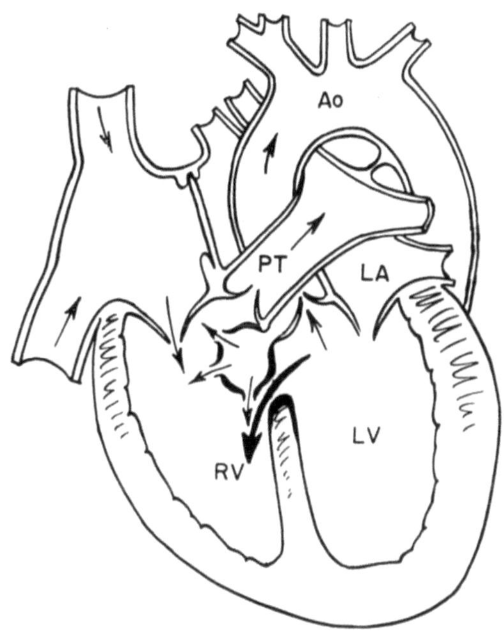

FIGURE 10.7. Diagram of rupture of an aneurysm of the right aortic sinus into the right ventricle. A ventricular septal defect is also present. Reprinted, with permissions, from Edwards JE: Classification of congenital heart disease in the adult. Cardiovascular Clinics 10:I, 1979, F.A. Davis Company.

routine examination without any symptoms and with no antecedent history of infection. The right sinus is most commonly affected and rupture into the right ventricle occurs most frequently. Involvement of the left sinus is extremely rare.

Clinical Features

The characteristic finding are the signs of an aortic runoff and a continuous murmur usually maximal lower down than a patent ductus. If the shunt is of any size and the right heart is affected, congestive cardiac failure with marked jugular venous pulsation and pulmonary plethora is found. The diagnosis must be made from other conditions producing continuous murmurs and particularly from ventricular septal defect with aortic incompetence, and aortic incompetence with tricuspid incompetence.

The electrocardiogram and X-ray do not help in differentiation but the diagnosis can be established by catheterization and angiocardiography. The treatment is surgical once the precise pathology has been established.

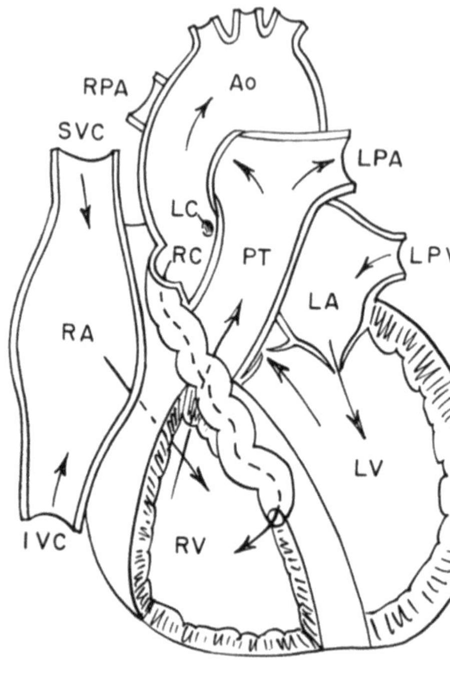

FIGURE 10.8. Diagram of congenital fistula between the right coronary artery and the right ventricular cavity. Reprinted, with permission, from Edwards JE: Classification of congenital heart disease in the adult. Cardiovascular Clinics 10:I, 1979, F.A. Davis Company.

Coronary Arteriovenous Fistulae

A fistulous communication may be present between a coronary artery and any chamber of the heart, or between a coronary artery and a vein (Fig. 10.8).

A continuous, murmur is usually situated at a level lower than a patent ductus, or at some unusual site (e.g., to the right of the sternum). It may appear superficial and often the accentuation of the murmur is in diastole and not in systole. The treatment is surgical once the pathological anatomy has been established by angiocardiography.

Ventricular Septal Defect

Ventricular septal defect is the commonest congenital cardiac anomaly. It may be isolated or combined with other malformations, such as pulmonary stenosis.

Anatomy

The ventricular septum consists of a thick muscular portion and a thin oval-shaped membranous portion (Figs. 10.9 and 10.10). Viewed from the right side the membranous septum lies just anterior to the orifice of the coronary sinus. It is crossed obliquely by the septal leaflet of the tricuspid valve; the portion of the septum above this line of attachment separates the left ventricle from the right atrium, whereas the portion below separates the two ventricles. The bundle of His traverses the posteroinferior margin of the membranous septum along the superior edge of the muscular septum, a factor of great importance in surgical repair.

Viewed from the left side, the membranous septum is related to the posterior and right cusps of the aortic valve. The membranous septum therefore separates the two ventricles and also partitions the left ventricle from the

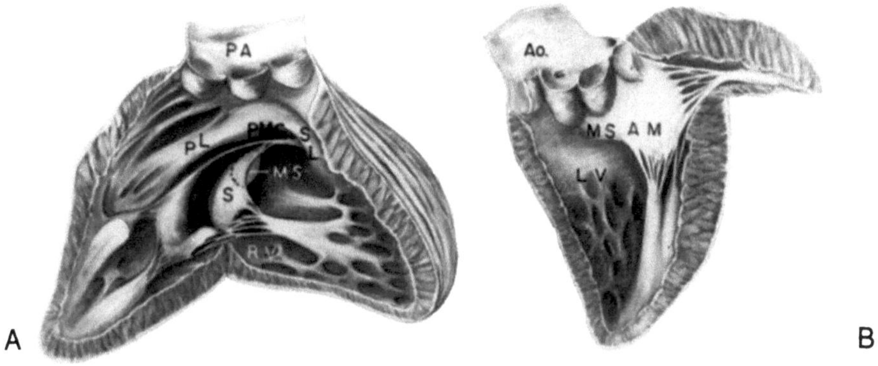

FIGURE 10.9. (A) The internal architecture of the right ventricle showing the membranous septum (MS) underneath the septal leaflet of the tricuspid valve. (B) Internal architecture of the left ventricle showing relationship of membranous septum to the right and non-coronary cusps of the aortic valve. PL and SL, parietal and septal limbs of the crista supraventricularis; PMC, papillary muscle of the conus; AM anterior mitral leaflet. Reprinted, with permission from Korns M, et al: The pathology of ventricular septal defect. Seminars in Roentgenology 1:2–33, 1966.

right atrium. Therefore, defects of the septum have the potential to produce communication between the ventricles, or the left ventricle and the right atrium (left ventricular–right atrial communication).

The body of the right ventricle is divided into an inflow portion and outflow portion by a structure known as the crista supraventricularis. The crista is a muscular structure made up of the parietal and the septal limbs. The latter blends with the ventricular septum. The inflow portion of the ventricle extends from the tricuspid valve orifice to the crista and the outflow portion from the crista to the pulmonary valve.

Almost three-fourths of all ventricular septal defects are *infracristal* and have a high tendency to involve the membranous portion of the

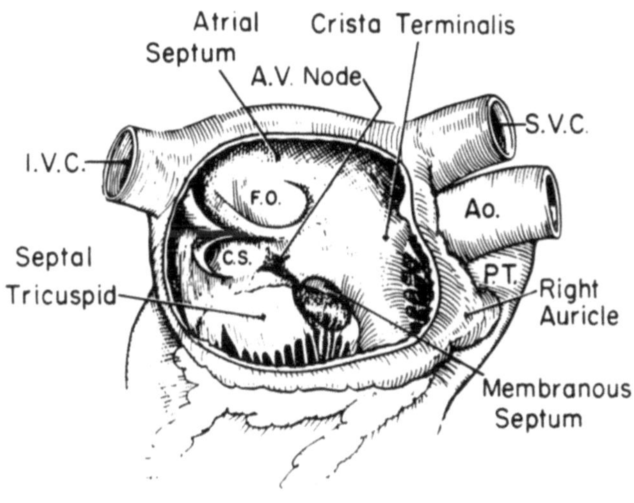

FIGURE 10.10. The membranous ventricular septum seen through the right atrium (see text). Reprinted, with permission, from Chesler E: Aneurysms of the left ventricle. Cardiovascular Clinics 9:188, 1972, F.A. Davis Company.

ventricular septum. Approximately 10% of defects lie above the crista, frequently just below the pulmonary valve on the right side and on the left side immediately below the aortic valve ring. The poor support of aortic cusps in this type of defect accounts for the development and progression of aortic incompetence among cases of supraventricular septal defect.

Muscular defects can occur at any site, particularly near the apex, and vary in size and number. A particularly difficult variety from the surgical point of view is the "Swiss-cheese" type, consisting of multiple muscular defects between the septal trabeculae. Combinations of all the defects described above may occur.

Defects should not be classified as membranous or muscular but rather as *supracristal* or *infracristal*.

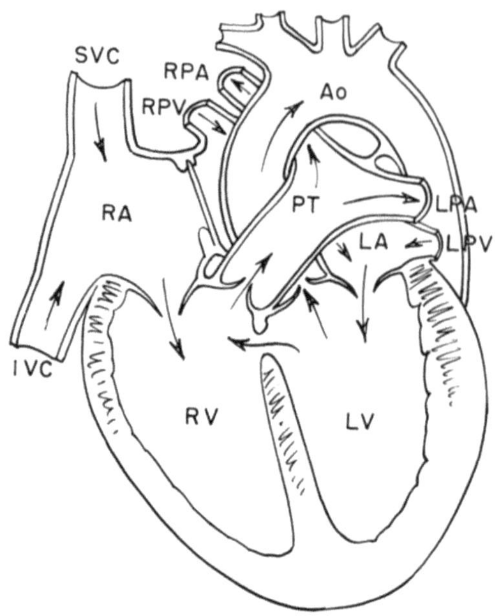

FIGURE 10.11. Diagram of central circulation in a restrictive ventricular septal defect with a left-to-right shunt. Reprinted, with permission, from Edwards JE: Classification of congenital heart disease in the adult. Cardiovascular Clinics 10:I, 1979. F.A. Davis Company.

Hemodynamics of Ventricular Septal Defect

The hemodynamics depend on two factors: (1) the size of the defect and (2) the resistance to flow within the right side of the heart. The latter includes the infundibulum of the right ventricle, the pulmonary valve, the main pulmonary arteries, and the pulmonary arterioles.

The size of the ventricular septal defect is critical in relation to the amount of blood shunted through it. When the defect is small, the resistance offered by the defect is far greater than the systemic arterial resistance, and therefore restricts flow through it (*a restrictive defect*). When the defect is restrictive, the pulmonary artery pressure cannot reach systemic levels and left-to-right shunting is therefore moderate. The defect may vary in size from a pinpoint to a centimeter or more, the shunt being proportional to the size of the defect (Fig. 10.11).

When the defect is approximately the size of the aortic valve it offers less resistance to flow than the systemic resistance (*a nonrestrictive defect*). This immediately results in equalization of ventricular pressures and a large left-to-right shunt, depending on resistance to outflow in the right ventricle and the pulmonary vascular resistance.

Right Ventricular Outflow Obstruction

In some patients, hypertrophy of the crista supraventricularis may be sufficiently prominent to produce a pressure gradient between the right ventricle and the pulmonary artery, thus restricting the left-to-right shunt. When the obstruction to flow is marked and equals the systemic resistance, there may be minimal or no left-to-right shunt with progressive cyanosis leading to the clinical picture of Tetralogy of Fallot. The development of infundibular hypertrophy is unpredictable but it is one of the factors that may account for spontaneous improvement of cardiac failure in an infant with a large ventricular septal defect.

Pulmonary Vascular Resistance

With a nonrestrictive ventricular septal defect there is equalization of pressures in both ventricles, the aorta, and the pulmonary artery.

Postnatally, there is a rapid reduction in the high fetal pulmonary vascular resistance and as this falls there is a preferential flow across the defect into the right ventricle and the pulmonary artery. Continuing reduction in pulmonary vascular resistance during the first few months of life increases the left-to-right shunt leading to a progressive elevation of pulmonary blood flow, pulmonary venous return, and left ventricular filling. This may be sufficient to eventually lead to left ventricular failure with elevation of the left ventricular end-diastolic, left atrial, and pulmonary capillary pressures resulting in pulmonary edema. When this stage is reached, the left ventricle may also be incapable of maintaining adequate systemic blood flow and there is poor peripheral circulation.

Failure of the right ventricle may supervene after the onset of left ventricular failure. The magnitude of shunting is directly related to the rapidity with which the pulmonary vascular resistance falls. Several factors influence this phenomenon. Severe cardiac failure is unusual in infants born at higher altitudes because of hypoxic pulmonary vasoconstriction. On the other hand, premature infants may develop cardiac failure within 4 weeks of birth because of a very rapid fall in pulmonary vascular resistance. The smooth muscle in the pulmonary artery normally becomes increasingly thick in the last 3 months of gestation. Therefore, in premature infants, the pulmonary arteries have less smooth muscle than the mature child and the pulmonary vascular resistance thus drops more rapidly.

The response of the *pulmonary vasculature* to increased pulmonary blood flow and pulmonary hypertension (*hyperkinetic pulmonary hypertension*) is variable. In some patients there is a progressive rise in pulmonary vascular resistance due to retention of a thick medial coat and this is subsequently replaced with hyaline material and later fibrous tissue. There is also a proliferation of the intimal layer, which in severe cases may eventually compromise the size of the lumen.

The time sequence for the development of pulmonary vascular disease is variable and there is also much variation from patient to patient. The changes probably develop because of shearing forces resultant from a high velocity of increased blood flow. When these changes are severe the pulmonary vascular resistance rises, decreasing the left-to-right shunt, the pulmonary blood flow, and the venous return to the left atrium. When the pulmonary resistance exceeds the systemic resistance, a right-to-left shunt develops across the ventricular septal defect with resultant cyanosis.

Spontaneous Closure of Ventricular Septal Defects

The exact incidence of this phenomenon has not been established with certainty. There is probably a 50% closure rate within 10 years. The fact that ventricular septal defects are frequently encountered in infancy and so rarely either clinically or at autopsy in adults strongly suggests that most defects close spontaneously because so few patients die of ventricular septal defect beyond infancy.

Hypertrophy of the muscular portions of the ventricular septum surrounding a defect with subsequent fibrous closure is a documented way in which spontaneous closure may occur. Apposition of the septal leaflet of the tricuspid valve against a defect may also produce closure. Where this mechanism is operative, the high pressure in the left ventricle may produce an *aneurysm of the membranous septum* that may bulge into and even obstruct the outflow tract of the left ventricle (Fig. 10.12).

Clinical Assessment of Ventricular Septal Defect

Group I: Ventricular Septal Defect with Normal Pulmonary Artery Pressure

The patient is usually an asymptomatic young child who is normally developed. Attention is drawn to the heart during routine physical examination because of a murmur, often accompanied by a thrill.

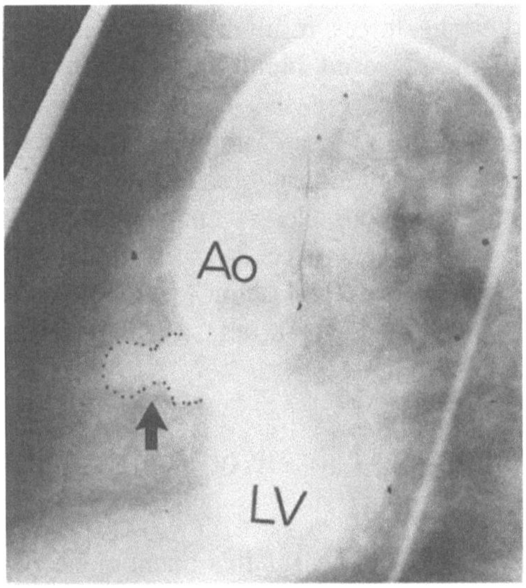

FIGURE 10.12. Left ventricular cine angiogram showing opacification of the right ventricle through a defect in an aneurysm of the membranous ventricular septum (Arrow).

Minute Ventricular Septal Defects

The *murmur* usually is localized to the left third or fourth intercostal space parasternally, and is grade 3/6 in intensity; it radiates poorly and varies little with respiration. The most unusual feature of the murmur is its shortness; it commences immediately with the first heart sound, reaches a crescendo by the first third of systole, and then softens rapidly, so that a completely normal second heart sound is unobscured. The murmur should be distinguished from mild pulmonary or infundibular stenosis, mild aortic or subaortic stenosis, pulmonary ejection murmurs due to increased flow, and the vibratory systolic murmur. It behaves like a regurgitant murmur, softening with amyl nitrite and intensifying with phenylephrine.

The *electrocardiogram* is normal as is the chest X-ray. Routine right heart catheterization usually reveals no abnormality, but with special dye-curve techniques and selective left ventricular cineangiography, a small defect at the ventricular level can be demonstrated.

The defect is of no hemodynamic significance and requires no treatment, apart from prophylaxis to prevent the development of subacute bacterial endocarditis. It is rarely encountered in adults, since spontaneous closure and natural cure occurs.

Small Ventricular Septal Defect (Maladie de Roger)

This defect is somewhat larger than the minute ventricular septal defect and the physical signs are more obtrusive so that attention is drawn to the heart more readily.

The *murmur* is characteristically regurgitant (pansystolic), commencing with the first sound, and continuing through systole to the aortic component of the second heart sound, which may be obscured, particularly if there is a late systolic crescendo. It is very loud, usually grade 4–5/6, associated with a thrill, maximal in the fourth and third left interspaces parasternally, radiating widely anteriorly, and into the back. Although usually maximal at the fourth left space, in a one-fifth of patients the murmur is maximal at the pulmonary area and closely simulates mild pulmonary valve stenosis.

Supracristal Ventricular Septal Defect

The anatomical configuration of such a defect is such that aortic and pulmonary valves are almost in contiguity and left ventricular blood is ejected directly into the pulmonary artery. The resultant murmur may mimic that of pulmonary stenosis. The clues to the presence of a ventricular septal defect are a narrowly split second sound, with a readily audible pulmonary component, findings that are incompatible with the diagnosis of pulmonary stenosis with such a long murmur. Additionally, a third heart sound is often heard at the apex.

The *electrocardiogram* also provides a valuable clue in that it does not reveal evidence of right ventricular hypertrophy, which would be anticipated with such a long murmur were it a result of pulmonary stenosis. Radiological examination confirms a normal-sized heart but the pulmonary vessels may be a little prominent.

Apart from a supracristal ventricular septal defect the differential diagnosis includes infundibular stenosis, aortic stenosis, mitral incompetence, and tricuspid incompetence.

Cardiac catheterization demonstrates a slight increase in pulmonary blood flow because of a left-to-right shunt ventricular level and a calculated pulmonary/systemic blood flow ratio of less than 50%.

Apart from the danger of infective endocarditis, which is uncommon, there is no disability and spontaneous closure is probably the rule. Surgery is not advised.

Moderate Ventricular Septal Defect

Here the defect is larger (circumference 1 cm) resulting in a significant shunt. Despite this, symptoms are absent or mild in childhood and development is normal.

Clinical evidence of increased flow is provided by a slightly enlarged left ventricle and a slight lift over the right ventricle because of volume overload. The characteristic regurgitant murmur and thrill are present but there is also a short middiastolic rumble at the apex. The pulmonary component of the second heart sound is normal in intensity.

The *electrocardiogram* is normal in more than half the patients. In some there is evidence of left ventricular enlargement with prominent Q waves in leads V5 and V6. In others, mild right ventricular hypertrophy (increased ratio of R/S in V1), or incomplete right bundle branch block is present. The mean frontal axis is usually normal; occasionally left axis deviation in the vicinity of -30 to $-40°$ is present. Left atrial enlargement may be present.

The *chest X-ray* demonstrates slight cardiomegaly with pulmonary plethora and an enlarged left atrium. *Cardiac catheterization* shows a pulmonary to systemic blood flow ratio of less than 50%.

In most centers surgery is not advised because of the tendency to spontaneous closure.

Group II: Ventricular Septal Defect with Moderate Pulmonary Arterial Hypertension

The defects are usually large and therefore lead to considerable shunting of blood into the pulmonary circulation, but there is no cyanosis.

Symptoms are present but are usually mild. Physical development tends to be retarded. Central bulging of the sternum is associated with an increase in heart size. Clinical evidence of right ventricular enlargement and pulmonary hypertension is present and there is a lift over the right ventricle, best felt in the third and fourth left intercostal spaces parasternally. Pulsation may be visible in the second left interspace because an enlarged pulmonary artery and the pulmonary component of the second heart sound may be palpable.

The characteristic regurgitant systolic murmur and thrill are present parasternally and there is a short apical rumbling middiastolic flow murmur follwing the third sound. The pulmonary component of the second heart sound is accentuated but splitting of the second sound persists.

The *electrocardiogram* is rarely normal. Usually, there is evidence of hypertrophy of the left, right, or both ventricles. Large Q waves similar to those found in a patent ductus arteriosus may be found. Abnormal P waves indicative of left, right, or combined atrial hypertrophy may be present. The mean frontal plane QRS axis may be normal, frequently deviated to the right and occasionally to the left.

The chest X-ray shows moderate to considerable cardiomegaly pulmonary plethora, and an enlarged pulmonary artery and left atrium. *Cardiac catheterization* demonstrates pulmonary hypertension and the pulmonary artery pressure may approach 80% of the systemic pressure. Because the shunt is large (pulmonary blood flow more than twice systemic blood flow) the pulmonary resistance is therefore normal or only slightly elevated.

Surgical repair is usually indicated.

Group III: Ventricular Septal Defect with Similar Systemic and Pulmonary Arterial Pressures

The defects are sufficiently large to equalize pressures in the ventricles. The direction of shunt flow, and thus the clinical picture, is dependent on the relative resistances in the two circulations.

Pulmonary Arteriolar Resistance Lower Than Systemic

In infancy this may lead to severe cardiac failure requiring therapy with morphine, Digoxin, and diuretics.

In older infants and children the symptoms and signs are those associated with chronic ill health, a predisposition to pulmonary infections and stunting of growth. Cyanosis is absent. A central chest bulge with active precordial pulsations is visible. On palpation, the signs of pulmonary hypertension and right ventricular enlargement overshadow left ventricular hypertrophy.

Auscultation

A loud pansystolic regurgitant murmur no longer dominates the findings. The regurgitant murmur is now shorter in over half the patients and may in fact be absent. Because it is so short, it is often mistaken for a pulmonary systolic murmur, which is frequently also present. The murmur can be recognized by its quality and because it intensifies with amyl nitrite inhalation and softens with phenylephrine injection. This so-called paradoxical response is due to the marked increase in smooth muscle in the pulmonary arterioles: amyl nitrite leads to relaxation of the pulmonary arteriolar tone and thus promotes left-to-right shunting (the VSD murmur lengthens and becomes louder); phenylephrine increases muscle tone, reduces the left-to-right shunt, and therefore shortens and softens the murmur.

A pulmonary ejection click and accentuated pulmonary second sound are frequently accompanied by the murmur of pulmonary insufficiency. The persistence of a loud *apical middiastolic rumble* is often a crucial finding indicating a dominant left-to-right shunt.

A normal *electorcardiogram* or one showing isolated left ventricular hypertrophy is rare. Most commonly, right ventricular hypertrophy or incomplete right bundle branch block is present. The R/S ratio in V1 is generally increased but a QR complex is rare. Evidence of left atrial and left ventricular hypertrophy (deep S waves in the right chest leads and tall R waves and deep Q waves in the left chest leads) is often present. Right axis deviation is most commonly found, but occasionally the axis is normal; rarely is it deviated to the left.

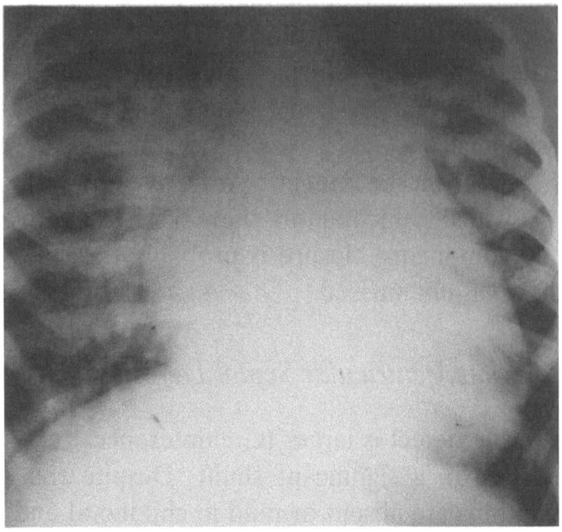

FIGURE 10.13. X-ray in ventricular septal defect with large left-to-right shunt and pulmonary hypertension.

The chest X-ray confirms a dominant left-to-right shunt with increased pulmonary arterial vasculature, a prominent pulmonary artery, biventricular, and left atrial enlargement (Fig. 10.13).

Cardiac catheterization shows equal or near-equal pulmonary and systemic pressures, with normal peripheral arterial saturation and a large left-to-right shunt (PBF twice more than twice SBF). The diagnosis is from other left-to-right shunts associated with pulmonary hypertension.

Treatment

When the pulmonary vascular resistance is less than 10 units and the pulmonary blood flow twice that of the systemic blood flow, surgery is advised to avoid the risk of irreversible pulmonary vascular disease. When this hemodynamic situation is encountered in infancy, close supervision of the patient is required because severe pulmonary vascular disease may develop as early as 3 years of age. However, even with careful clinical, radiologic, and electrocardiographic monitoring it may be difficult to detect increases in the pulmonary vascular resistance. Therefore catheterization should be repeated 6 to 9 months after the original study. Should there be evidence that pulmonary vascular resistance is increasing, surgery should be recommended.

Pulmonary Resistance Equal to or Higher than Systemic

This condition is recognized more often because of symptoms and the presence of cyanosis, rather than because of a murmur. The signs of pulmonary hypertension dominate the examination. On palpation right ventricular heave and pulmonary diastolic shock are usually marked, without recognizable cardiomegaly: there is no middiastolic murmur or murmur of ventricular septal defect. The second sound is single or narrowly split and the pulmonary component markedly accentuated. There is a soft pulmonary systolic murmur, a pulmonary ejection click, and often an early diastolic murmur of pulmonary insufficiency.

The *electrocardiogram* almost invariably demonstrates right ventricular hypertrophy, often severe, or incomplete right bundle branch block with marked right axis deviation. Right atrial overload is sometimes found.

The *chest X-ray* shows enlargement of the main pulmonary arteries with attenuation and peripheral pruning of the distal branches. Generalized cardiomegaly is no longer a feature.

Cardiac catheterization shows equal systemic and pulmonary artery pressures with an equal or dominant right-to-left shunt. When the pulmonary resistance exceeds the systemic the shunt is completely right-to-left and persistent cyanosis is present—the so-called *Eisenmenger syndrome*.

Surgery is hazardous in these patients and not advised.

Associated Defects

Patent Ductus Arteriosus. This may coexist, in up to 10% of cases. When the pulmonary artery pressure is normal, the typical continuous murmur is obvious below the left clavicle, in addition to the murmur of the VSD in the fourth left intercostal space. However, when there is severe pulmonary hypertension, the ductus murmur is completely obscured and the auscultatory signs are those of a hypertensive ventricular septal defect. Occasionally, a brisk pulse may be suggestive of an associated ductus, but this sign is unreliable. The association is of considerable importance, since the ductus must be ligated before the patient is placed on cardiopulmonary bypass. The presence of a ductus must be confirmed by cardiac catheterization.

Atrial Septal Defect. A coexistent atrial septal defect of the secundum type cannot be diagnosed clinically and is usually found at surgery or cardiac catheterization. A secundum atrial septal defect, left ventricular–right atrial communication, ventricular septal defect with tricuspid incompetence, and complete endocardial cushion defect all produce highly saturated right atrial samples at cardiac catheterization and have to be differentiated angiographically. An unusually large right atrium radiologically, and sometimes electrocardiographically, is suggestive of a left ventricular–right atrial communication, but this also occurs in the above-mentioned conditions. Left axis deviation with a counterclockwise loop with a mean axis in the vicinity of -90 to $-150°$ strongly favors the presence of an endocardial cushion defect.

Aortic Incompetence. When progressive, this is a serious complication. As the cusps of the aortic valve prolapse through the septal defect, severe aortic insufficiency results with progressive cardiac enlargement and heart failure. Occasionally, a prolapsing cusp may protrude into the defect, decreasing the left-to-right shunt and also producing right ventricular outflow obstruction. The sinus of Valsalva often becomes dilated so that it may be difficult to decide whether the primary defect is a sinus of Valsalva aneurysm with prolapse of a cusp or primary prolapse of a cusp with secondary involvement of the sinus.

Aortic insufficiency is more commonly a complication of supracristal as compared to infracristal ventricular septal defect. However, since infracristal defects are much commoner than supracristal, in any given case an infracristal lesion is more likely.

The physical signs of aortic insufficiency are superimposed on the signs of a large ventricular septal defect. Occasionally, functionally small defects are encountered with moderate to severe aortic incompetence. Also, small septal defects with slight aortic incompetence are not rare, and do not necessarily progress.

The physical signs of an aortic runoff, such as a large pulse pressure, large dilated collapsing arteries, and left ventricular enlargement, are readily recognized clinically. The diagnosis must be made from other types of aortic runoff, particularly patent ductus arteriosus, and ruptured sinus of Valsalva, pulmonary incompetence with ventricular septal defect, and rheumatic aortic valve disease.

Mitral Incompetence. Rheumatic or congenital mitral incompetence may be associated with a ventricular septal defect. Usually it is due to an endocardial cushion defect with a cleft mitral valve and occasionally to an incompentent Ebstein's valve in corrected transposition. Mitral stenosis is generally a result of a supravalvular stenosing ring, parachute mitral valve, or maldevelopment of the papillary muscle.

Pulmonary Stenosis. The coexistence of valvar, infundibular, or pulmonary artery stenosis makes the diagnosis and treatment of ventricular septal defect more difficult. Ventricular septal defect with pulmonary outflow obstruction produces a wide spectrum of clinical syndromes, depending on the size of the ventricular septal defect and the severity of the pulmonary stenosis. Furthermore, the auscultatory signs of pulmonary stenosis are accentuated by the increased flow produced by the left-to-right shunt. Cardiac catheterization is the only way of making a precise diagnosis.

All gradations and combinations may occur:

1. *Mild Pulmonary Stenosis.* As long as the valve stenosis offers less resistance than the systemic resistance, a large left-to-right shunt is present unless the ventricular septal defect is very small.
2. *Severe Pulmonary Stenosis.* If the ventricular septal defect is small, the condition behaves like severe pulmonary stenosis with intact ventricular septum.
3. *Severe Pulmonary Stenosis and Large Ventricular Septal Defect (VSD).* If the systemic resistance is greater than the resistance to pulmonary flow, a large left-to-right shunt is present (i.e., *VSD with pulmonary stenosis*). If the pulmonary resistance is greater, a right-to-left shunt is present (i.e., *Tetralogy of Fallot*). If the resistances are balanced, *acyanotic tetralogy* is present.

The clinical differentiation of VSD with severe pulmonary stenosis and Tetralogy of Fallot is thus purely one of semantics. Moreover, even in an individual patient, the hemodynamic state is not steady. An infant may have the hemodynamics of a VSD with left-to-right shunt but when hypertrophy of crista supraventricularis leads to severe infundibular stenosis, the left-to-right shunt diminishes, the heart becomes smaller, the right ventricle hypertrophies, and ultimately a right-to-left shunt and the picture of Tetralogy of Fallot develops.

Atrial Septal Defect

Embryology

About the fifth week of intrauterine life, the heart is a simple tube. The atrioventricular cushions then develop in the middle of the tube, dividing it into two chambers, one of which is destined to become the atria and the other the ventricles. The cushions themselves form the atrioventricular valves (mitral and tricuspid). The common atrium is divided into two by a ridge—the septum primum—which grows downward from the dorsal and cephalic wall of the atrium toward the atrioventricular cushions. The opening between the ridge and the cushions is known as the ostium primum. Eventually, the two limbs of the septum primum fuse with the cushions, obliterating the ostium primum and forming thereby the two atrial chambers. While this fusion is taking place a new opening appears in the septum primum some distance from the fused septum and cushions—the ostium secundum—maintaining communication between the two atria. At the same time, from a second ridge on the dorsal and cephalic wall of the right atrium to the right of the septum primum, another crescentic septum develops—the septum secundum—which grows downward, fusing with the atrioventricular cushions. The part overlying the ostium secundum ceases to grow, leaving an opening—the foramen ovale. This is an oblique passage, allowing blood to flow during fetal life, from right-to-left atrium.

A *patent foramen ovale* is found in 30% of otherwise normal adult hearts, more frequently in children. Normally, the opening is kept closed by the valve of the foramen ovale, left atrial pressure being higher than right. Occasionally, when right atrial pressure exceeds the left, blood is shunted from the right to left atrium, for example, in severe pulmonary stenosis. During routine catheterization, the catheter may be passed from the right to left atrium, through a patent foramen ovale.

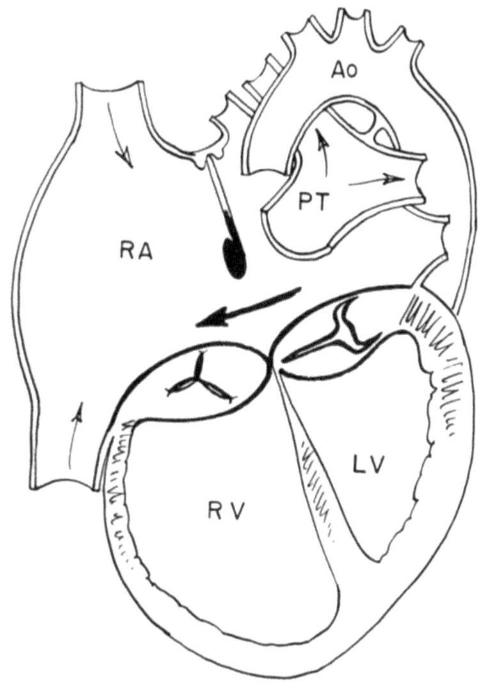

FIGURE 10.14. Diagrammatic representation of the anatomy of the ostium primum type of atrial septal defect with a cleft mitral valve.

1. *Secundum type of atrial septal defect* (defects in the region of the foramen ovale). Deficiency of the atrial septum, in the region of the foramen ovale, constitutes the common form of atrial septal defect. This may be due to an inadequate flap of septum primum, defective development of the septum secundum, or abnormal fenestration in the septum primum.
2. *Sinus Venosus defect*. These defects occur high in the septum, near the entrance of the superior vena cava in the right atrium, and are usually associated with anomalous pulmonary venous drainage.
3. *Primum type of atrial septal defect* (Fig. 10.14). Defects involving the caudal portion of the atrial septum are less frequent, and are due to failure of the septum primum to fuse with the endocardial cushions, which are maldeveloped. This leads to a communication between the two atria just above the mitral and tricuspid valves. There is almost always an associated malformation (clefts) of the atrioventricular valves (usually the mitral), resulting in incompetence of the mitral and tricuspid valves. There are two types of endocardial cushion defects: (1) with ventricular septal defect and (2) without ventricular septal defect.

Hemodynamic Effects of Atrial Septal Defect

Blood flow through an atrial septal defect is determined, to some extent, by the size of the defect. In the rare case in which the defect is small the shunt will be insignificant. However, the defect is usually large, and the magnitude of the shunt and its direction will be determined by the relative filling resistances of the right and left ventricles and the pulmonary vascular resistance. Usually, the right ventricle is more compliant than the left, so that the shunt is from left to right, resulting in increased pulmonary blood flow. The left-to-right shunt occurs mainly during late ventricular systole and early ventricular diastole. The systemic output is usually normal, whereas pulmonary flow may exceed systemic by as much as sixfold.

Despite the increased pulmonary flow, the pulmonary arterial pressure is usually normal, or only slightly elevated, because of a normal or subnormal pulmonary vascular resistance. Occasionally, changes occur in the small muscular arteries and arterioles in the lungs, resulting in an increased resistance to flow and pulmonary hypertension. Pressure overload results in right ventricular hypertrophy, which increases diastolic filling resistance and reduces the left-to-right shunt. When the right-sided compliance is less than the left, the shunt becomes predominantly right-to-left, leading to arterial desaturation. Similarly, tricuspid stenosis, right ventricular hypoplasia, infundibular or pulmonary valvular stenosis, and Ebstein's anomaly will reduce the left-to-right shunt and may even produce a right-to-left shunt.

Right heart failure may result from prolonged volume overload without the development of pulmonary hypertension and is usually associated with atrial fibrillation. Before this can be diagnosed left ventricular failure, due to hypertension or other causes, must be excluded. Since both atria are in free communication, left ventricular failure can be detected at the bedside by elevation of the jugular venous pressure.

Also, in mitral stenosis left atrial hypertension is dissipated through both atria and pulmonary venous hypertension is not prominent.

Ostium Secundum and Sinus Venous Defects

Characteristically, these defects have a higher incidence in women (3:2). They are rarely discovered in infancy and symptoms in the first three decades of life are mild or absent. Disability occurs in the third and fourth decades, because of heart failure and severe pulmonary hypertension. Occasionally, the disease is discovered for the first time in the sixth or seventh decade. Failure to appreciate this leads to frequent errors in diagnosis in persons beyond middle age, and in the elderly.

Most patients are young and referred because of incidental murmurs noted during routine physical examination or during an intercurrent illness. Occasionally, there is a familial incidence. Often, routine radiological examination of the chest leads to the discovery of heart disease. Early symptoms are usually mild effort dyspnea, repeated respiratory tract infections in childhood, fatigue, palpitation (particularly attacks of paroxysmal tachycardia), and some retardation of growth. Often, supposedly symptom-free patients appreciate their preoperative limitations only after the defect has been surgically corrected.

Physical Findings

Body development and stature are usually normal, although a high arched palate, arachnodactyly, and a gracile habitus have been described. The jugular venous pressure is normal. Atrial septal defect is the one congenital heart condition in which atrial fibrillation occurs with some degree of frequency. This is probably related to the age of the patient and seldom occurs before the fourth decade. When present at an early age, associated mitral valve disease (Lutembacher's syndrome) should be suspected.

Palpation of the chest shows evidence of diastolic overload of the right ventricle. The forceful, often heaving type of apex can be mistaken for an overactive left ventricle. The apex, however, is formed by the enlarged right ventricle, which can be recognized by the parasternal lift, which is continuous with the apical thrust. In the absence of severe pulmonary hypertension the parasternal lift is diastolic in timing (similar to that of tricuspid insufficiency). Pulsation of the right ventricular outflow tract and the main pulmonary artery may be visible and palpable, and an accompanying pulmonary systolic thrill may be felt when the chest wall is thin. The chest wall may be deformed by a left parasternal bulge.

On auscultation, a pulmonary ejection murmur is almost always present, usually grade 2–3/6. Occasionally, it is louder and associated with a thrill, which often (but not necessarily) is due to a gradient across the pulmonary valve. This is frequently functional and produced by the large stroke volume. The murmur is well heard in the back, below tne scapulae, presumably because of downward conduction in the pulmonary arteries and because of slight pulmonary arterial narrowing, which frequently coexists. Loud murmurs audible in the back should suggest the presence of peripheral pulmonary artery stenosis.

A most important auscultatory finding is a *tricuspid middiastolic murmur*, attributed to increased flow across the valve, heard maximally in the tricuspid area and increasing remarkably on inspiration, often only audible during inspiration. The murmur is not necessarily produced at the tricuspid valve. In some patients the murmur may actually arise at the site of the defect. At times the murmur is widespread, radiating to the apex, where it can be mistaken for a mitral murmur. However, it has a higher pitch than the usual mitral murmur, and occurs slightly earlier in diastole. In fact, it may be confused with pulmonary incompetence, but this is uncommon in the absence of pulmonary hypertension. A tricuspid opening snap is sometimes audible.

Fixed splitting of the second sound is one of the cardinal physical signs of atrial septal defect. The width of splitting is not the feature, since splitting is usually no more than 0.4 seconds on held expiration. The fixity of splitting to the ear is characteristic. Normally, the second sound closes completely on expiration and widens to a variable degree on inspiration and it is this change from a split to a single sound that can be readily appreciated in health. Although a slight change in the degree of splitting is often present phonocardiographically in atrial septal defect, it is extremely difficult to appreciate this with the ear. Accentuation of the tricuspid component of the first heart sound and a pulmonary ejection click are often present.

If tricuspid incompetence develops a pansystolic murmur appears and since this may radiate widely over the front of the chest; it may mimic mitral incompetence or ventricular septal defect.

The *electrocardiogram* is of crucial importance, both in confirming the diagnosis and in differentiating this condition from endocardial cushion defect. The mean QRS vector in the frontal plane lies between +90 and +150 (right axis deviation) and the loop is clockwise. A normal axis is uncommon. This is in striking contrast to the left axis deviation and the counterclockwise loop of endocardial cushion defects. A typical RSR, rSR, or rR pattern (incomplete right bundle branch block), is found in V1, and an Rs in V6. With the development of pulmonary hypertension, however, the pattern of right ventricular hypertrophy with a tall R in V1, or complete right bundle branch block develops. Atrial fibrillation is not uncommon in older patients.

The chest X-ray almost always shows cardiomegaly, because of enlargement of the right heart and main pulmonary artery. The cardiothoracic ratio is generally over 50%; the greater the shunt, the greater the ratio. The lung fields show the classical features of pulmonary plethora, with wide dilated pulmonary arteries, especially in the upper lung zones. The size of the shunt can be fairly accurately gauged from the radiological appearances. Small shunts are characterized by presence of plethora in the upper or midzones, whereas large shunts are characterized by plethora throughout the lung fields. Peripheral pruning indicates pulmonary hypertension, and massive enlargement of the pulmonary arteries with thrombosis may be a late complication.

Cardiac catheterization generally shows a large left-to-right shunt at atrial level of more than 50%. In fact, small atrial septal defects are rare, and it is exceptional to find shunts as small as 20%. Despite torrential pulmonary flow, the pulmonary resistance is nearly always low. Sinus venous defects and partial anomalous pulmonary venous drainage are usually diagnosed only at catheterization or surgery, though certain radiological features have been described.

Indications for Surgery

In a condition that is generally as benign as uncomplicated sinus venosus or ostium secundum defect, a remarkably low mortality and morbidity rate is obligatory before operation can be recommended. In most centers the risk is negligible. Operation is advised in patients with a left-to-right shunt of 50% or over, and age is no barrier. When severe pulmonary hypertension is present, the operative risks are greater, but provided the shunt is still predominantly left-to-right, operation is advised. Surgery is contraindicated when the shunt is reversed. Sinus venosus defect or anomalous pulmonary venous drainage is easily dealt with at operation.

The optimal time for surgery is between the ages of 7 and 30 years. Surgery is generally not recommended in children under the age of 3 years. Symptoms are rare in infancy and when present conditions such as cor triatriatum should be suspected.

Associated Abnormalities

Mitral Valve Disease

Acquired

Atrial septal defect may be associated with rheumatic mitral disease, usually mitral stenosis (Lutembacher syndrome). This combination promotes left-to-right shunting, decompresses the left atrium, and reduces mitral valve flow. The diagnosis is often difficult, but should be suspected when there is atrial fibrillation, left atrial enlargement, and cardiac failure without severe pulmonary hypertension. The diagnosis is often first made at surgery.

Mitral incompetence is recognized by the pansystolic apical murmur, which must be distinguished from the pulmonary ejection murmur and from tricuspid incompetence. It is often associated with a middiastolic rumble. An endocardial cushion defect is the main differential diagnosis and the telltale diagnostic clue is the presence of left axis deviation electrocardiographically.

Congenital

Congenital mitral valve disease and an atrial septal defect usually indicate an endocardial cushion defect. However, a secundum defect may on occasion be associated with congenital mitral valve deformity (cleft mitral valve) producing mitral incompetence.

Pulmonary Stenosis

The presence of a long, loud systolic murmur and thrill in the pulmonary area suggests pulmonary valve stenosis. Catheterization confirms the gradient but does not indicate whether the stenosis is organic or functional because of high flow. Even with a gradient of over 50 mm Hg, surgery and postoperative catheterization may fail to show organic stenosis. As with ventricular septal defect complicated by pulmonary stenosis a wide variety of combinations occur. These vary from large left-to-right shunts with mild pulmonary stenosis on the one hand, to severe pulmonary stenosis with riyht-to-left shunt on the other.

Anomalous Pulmonary Venous Drainage

Partial anomalous pulmonary venous drainage is usually associated with an atrial septal defect and occurs in 85% of cases with a sinus venosus defect. Single or multiple veins may drain anomalously, the right lung usually being involved.

Ventricular Septal Defect

Usually, the clinical picture is dominated by the VSD. The atrial septal defect is detected by a rise in oxygen saturation at right atrial level.

Pulmonary Hypertension

When pulmonary vascular resistance increases, the physical signs alter. As pulmonary hypertension increases, the signs of left-to-right shunt diminish. The pulmonary and tricuspid murmurs are reduced or abolished. The second sound becomes loud, and the splitting narrows but is still detectable. A pulmonary systolic ejection sound is almost always present and pulmonary incompetence is frequent. When a right-to-left shunt is established (Eisenmenger Syndrome) there is cyanosis and clubbing. Usually the process takes a number of years to develop but occasionally it is accelerated, particularly following pregnancy.

Episodes suggesting acute pulmonary arterial thrombosis frequently occur in the late stages of the disease and occasionally massive thrombosis of the main branches occur and can be recognized in the plain chest X-ray film.

Complex Anomalies

Atrial septal defect (or patent foramen ovale) may be an integral component of certain cardiac malformations. It is essential to maintain the circulation in conditions such as total anomalous pulmonary venous drainage, tricuspid atresia, pulmonary atresia with intact ventricular septum, and certain varieties of transposition of the great vessels. Closure of the defect in these conditions is contraindicated. It decompresses the right heart in Ebstein anomaly, tricuspid stenosis, and hypoplastic right ventricle.

Infective Endocarditis

This is never a complication of ostium secundum atrial septal defect.

Endocardial Cushion Defects (Syn. Atrioventricular Canal)

Defects involving the formation of the endocardial cushions exist in varying degrees of severity. With rare exceptions this malformation has as its common denominator an ostium primum atrial septal defect and a cleft mitral valve. In the complete form (total A-V canal) there is also a common, cleft atrioventricular valve, and large ventricular septal defect. The hemodynamics, and therefore the clinical picture, depend on the competency of the A-V valves, the size of the ventricular septal defect, and the magnitude of the left-to-right shunt.

In about a quarter of patients, the complete variety is present. There is a strong association with Down's syndrome and, characteristically, an early presentation in infancy with physical retardation, congestive cardiac failure, and signs of pulmonary hypertension. The early development of pulmonary vascular disease is not uncommon (Eisenmenger syndrome).

In another quarter of patients, the ventricular septum is intact, the tricuspid valve normal, and the mitral valve cleft but not incompetent. A left-to-right shunt through the primum defect is the principal abnormality.

In approximately 50% of patients, the ventricular septum is intact, the tricuspid valve is normal, and the mitral valve is cleft and incompetent. The degree of mitral insufficiency is variable and determined by the extent of valve deformity and mild scalloping of the uppermost portion of the ventricular septum. The nature of the valve deformity determines the direction of the regurgitant jet, which in some instances may produce a left ventricular–right atrial shunt, in addition to the mitral insufficiency. Thus systolic murmurs are frequently audible medially rather than laterally, and may readily be mistaken for ventricular septal defect.

The clinical findings in endocardial cushion defect may be categorized into four fairly well-defined groups. In all groups the electrocardiogram shows left axis deviation and a counterclockwise loop.

1. Those of *classical atrial septal defect*, as in ostium secundum, with signs of increased flow across the pulmonary and tricuspid valves, fixed splitting of the second sound, and no evidence of atrioventricular valve disease or ventricular septal defect.
2. Those of *atrial septal defect, with mitral incompetence*. The mitral murmur tends to be medial and may mimic ventricular defect. In some cases a continuous murmur may be heard at the pulmonary area due to the mitral incompetent murmur in systole and a murmur produced across the atrial septal defect in diastole.
3. Those of *ventricular septal defect, with or without tricuspid and mitral incompetence*. There is a murmur and thrill at the fourth left intercostal space, a pulmonary systolic murmur, and a mitral middiastolic murmur. The degree of splitting of the second sound and the intensity will depend on the pulmonary artery pressure. The size of the defect will determine the clinical findings.
4. Those of *Eisenmenger syndrome*. When there is central cyanosis and evidence of pulmonary hypertension at systemic level the electrocardiogram is of major help in

the diagnosis. Left axis deviation is present, with a mean QRS axis in the frontal plane between −30° and −120° and a counterclockwise loop, often figure of eight in shape. The PR interval is frequently prolonged and abnormal widening of the P wave (left atrial abnormality) may be present. In less than 5% of patients right axis deviation is found and occasionally other electrocardiographic abnormalities such as left or right bundle branch block, or complete heart block, may complicate the picture.

The *radiological findings* are usually indistinguishable from those of secundum defects, but left atrial enlargement has been more frequently noted by some authors.

Cardiac catheterization confirms a left-to-right shunt at atrial level. In the primum defect without mitral insufficiency, the pulmonary artery pressure may be minimally elevated. When there is a ventricular septal defect, the magnitude of rise in pulmonary artery pressure is related to the size of the defect. The most helpful finding is the "gooseneck" deformity of the left ventricular outflow tract visualized by cineangiography (Fig. 10.15).

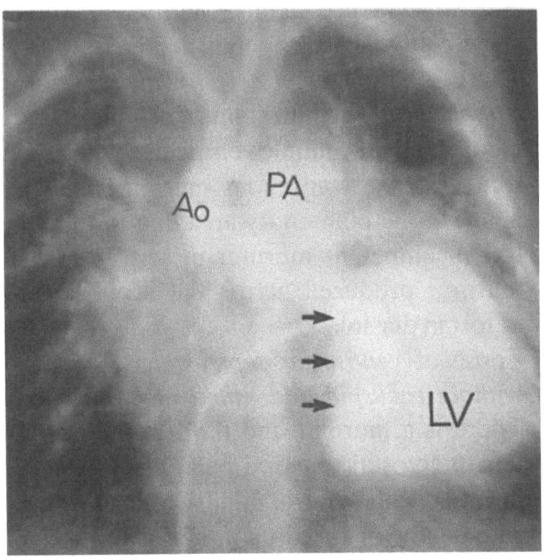

FIGURE 10.15. Left ventricular cine angiogram in AP projection demonstrating the "gooseneck" deformity of the left ventricular outflow tract in an ostium primum atrial septal defect. The arrows indicate the vertical orientation of the cleft mitral valve: a left-to-right shunt is present at atrial level.

Associated Conditions

These are similar to those encountered in ostium secundum defects. The most frequent are pulmonary hypertension and pulmonary stenosis. Endocardial cushion defect may be part of a complex malformation such as double outlet right ventricle. Unlike secundum defects there is a liability to bacterial endocarditis that involves the mitral or tricuspid valve.

It is particularly important to differentiate these defects from *rheumatic heart disease*. Patients with this condition frequently masquerade as mitral valve disease, attention being shown to the heart because of murmur heard during an illness that is often misinterpreted as rheumatic fever. The electrocardiogram is diagnostic.

Surgical Treatment

Ostium primum defects may be closed with as little risk for a secundum defect provided there is not significant mitral insufficiency. Minor degrees of mitral insufficiency are best left alone because attempting to repair the cleft usually aggravates regurgitation. When symptoms are not severe the operation is best performed at 6 years of age.

Endocardial cushion defect associated with a large ventricular septal defect, cleft atrioventricular valves, and elevated pulmonary vascular resistance pose a formidable surgical problem. The operative mortality is high and correction is not advisable under 3 years of age if conservative treatment is at all possible.

Cyanosis Absent: Normal Pulmonary Arterial Vasculature

Pulmonary Stenosis with Intact Ventricular Septum

Pulmonary stenosis with ventricular septal defect (Fig. 10.16) has always been recognized as

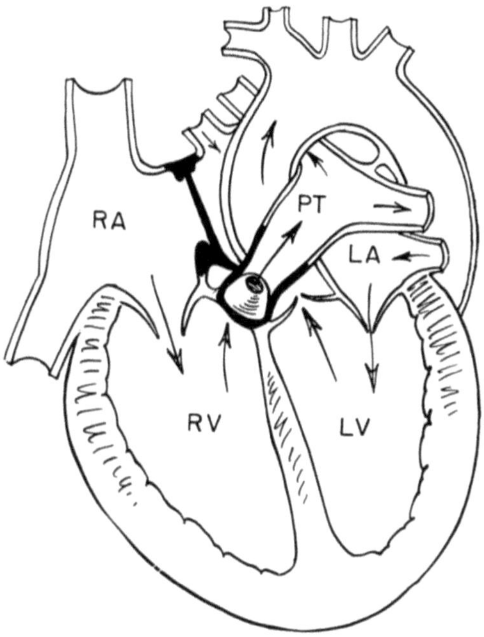

FIGURE 10.16. Diagram of the central circulation in pulmonary stenosis with a dome-shaped valve and intact ventricular septum. Reprinted, with permission, from Edwards JE: Classification of congenital heart disease in the adult. Cardiovascular Clinics 10:I, 1979, F.A. Davis Company.

a common condition. Isolated pulmonary stenosis, however, was once considered rare. It is now known that this is true for isolated infundibular stenosis, but not for isolated pulmonary valve stenosis. Pulmonary stenosis is about as common as atrial septal defect and patent ductus arteriosus.

In pulmonary valve stenosis, the cusps are fused, forming a dome or diaphragm, with a central perforation. Poststenotic dilatation of the main pulmonary arteries is often associated. The symptoms and signs depend on the hemodynamics.

Hemodynamic Effects of Pulmonary Stenosis

The hemodynamic findings depend upon severity of the stenosis, the competency of the tricuspid valve, and the patency of the atrial septum.

When stenosis is *mild*, pulmonary blood flow and pulmonary arterial pressure are normal. When the stenosis is *severe*, right ventricular pressure may equal left ventricular pressure but the hemodynamic adjustments are usually adequate, so that pulmonary blood flow and normal pulmonary arterial pressures are maintained.

When the stenosis is *extreme*, the pressure in the right ventricle may far exceed that of the left, pulmonary blood flow is usually reduced at rest, though pulmonary arterial pressures are maintained. If tricuspid incompetence is associated, the right ventricle is decompressed. When the foramen ovale is closed, heart failure without cyanosis results. If the foramen ovale is patent a right-to-left shunt at atrial level with cyanosis results. Associated tricuspid stenosis or right ventricular hypoplasia will have the same effect without right ventricular hypertension.

Clinical Features

Mild Pulmonary Stenosis

There are no symptoms or interference with development. Attention is drawn to the heart by the detection of a murmur. The intensity of the murmur varies from grade 2–4/6 and a thrill may be present. The murmur is maximal at the pulmonary area, has a crescendo in midsystole, and ends before, or at A_2. Wide splitting of the second sound on expiration (0.05 sec), with P_2 of normal intensity is found. A pulmonary ejection sound is heard in about half the cases.

The *electrocardiogram* may be normal, or may show slight right ventricular hypertrophy, or incomplete right bundle branch block. *Chest X-ray* shows a normal heart, with normal vascularity. Poststenotic dilatation of the main pulmonary artery is often present. However, the degree of pulmonary artery dilatation bears no relationship to the severity of the stenosis. *Cardiac catheterization* confirms stenosis at pulmonary valve level, with normal pulmonary artery pressure and a right ventricular pressure of under 60 mm Hg.

No restrictions are necessary apart from prophylactic precautions against infective endocarditis. Periodic reevaluation is essential, since the stenosis may increase, but this is rare.

Moderate and Severe Pulmonary Valve Stenosis

The symptoms are associated with reduced cardiac output and consist of fatigue, reduced effort tolerance, and dyspnea. Growth and development may be retarded and hyperteleorism is often present. Finally, in the late stages of the disease, congestive cardiac failure develops. The presence or absence of central cyanosis depends on the patency of the atrial septum (usually patent foramen ovale, uncommonly a secundum defect). If there is a defect in the atrial septum right-to-left shunt develops, producing cyanosis and clubbing (sometimes called Trilogy of Fallot see Table 10.1).

Physical Findings

A dominant, or giant "a" wave in the jugular pulse is an important clue to the diagnosis; it is often associated with a right atrial gallop.

The cardiac apex is formed by the right ventricle, but gross cardiomegaly is not a feature in the absence of heart failure. A systolic thrill can nearly always be felt in the pulmonary area and third left intercostal space. The systolic murmur is loud (grade 4–6/6) and long, with a late systolic crescendo; phonocardiographically it is "kite-shaped." At the site of maximal intensity (usually pulmonary area or first left space) A_2 may be partially or completely buried, so that the degree of splitting is difficult to determine at the bedside. However, splitting is always wide, sometimes extreme (up to 0.14 sec). P_2 is diminished in intensity and may be inaudible and in extreme cases the loud long murmur obscures all sounds. A pulmonary ejection sound is present in milder cases but as stenosis becomes more severe, the click occurs earlier in systole and is superimposed on the first heart sound.

The *electrocardiogram* shows varying degrees of right atrial and right ventricular hypertrophy, and partial or complete right bundle branch block.

Chest X-ray (Fig. 10.17) shows right atrial and right ventricular enlargement. Decreased pulmonary vasculature occurs only in high-grade stenosis. Poststenotic dilatation of the main and left pulmonary arteries is present.

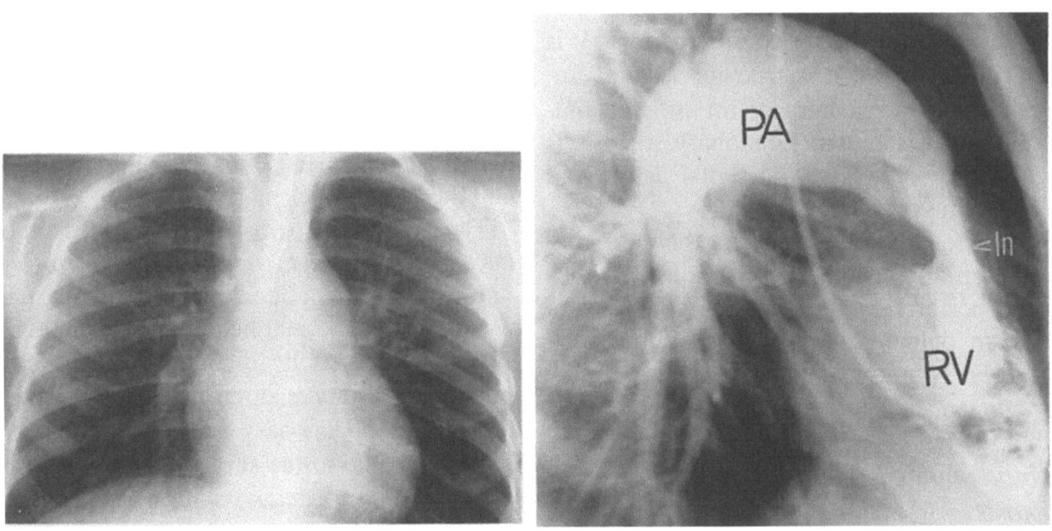

FIGURE 10.17. Chest X-ray in pulmonary valve stenosis demonstrating an enlarged main pulmonary artery that is a result of poststenotic dilatation seen in the lateral right ventricular cineangiogram, which demonstrates a thickened pulmonary valve (PV) and hypertrophied infundibulum (IN).

The size of these vessels again bears no relation to severity of the stenosis. This size of these vessels again bears no of the right atrium and right ventricle, which enlarge with heart failure.

Cardiac catheterization demonstrates a right ventricular pressure exceeding 60 mm Hg and in severe cases may be well above systemic level. The pulmonary arterial pressure is usually normal and the obstruction is demonstrated at valve level. Subvalvar muscular hypertrophy can be detected only after valvotomy. A right-to-left shunt at atrial level can be proved by dye-dilution methods, or by angiocardiography when systemic desaturation is present. A dominant or giant "a" wave is present in the right atrium.

Infundibular Stenosis

Isolated infundibular stenosis is rare. Usually infundibular stenosis is associated with ventricular septal defect and a right to left (Tetralogy of Fallot), or left to right (ventricular septal defect with pulmonary stenosis). Occasionally, a ventricular septal defect is present that has no functional effect. This may be due to (1) occlusion of the defect by the tricuspid valve during ventricular systole, (2) occlusion of a defect in the muscular septum during systole, or (3) a defect so small that it has no hemodynamic significance.

In *isolated* infundibular stenosis, or infundibular stenosis with a functionally intact ventricular septum, the symptoms and signs vary according to the severity of the obstruction, as in valve stenosis. However, an ejection click is absent and splitting of the second sound may be unusually wide. The site of maximal intensity of the murmur is sometimes of help, since the murmur tends to be maximal at the tricuspid area and not the pulmonary area of first left space, as in pulmonary valve stenosis. Pulmonary artery dilatation is absent on the chest X-ray.

Pulmonary Valve and Infundibular Stenosis

Organic stenosis of both may coexist. More commonly, however, hypertrophy of the crista supraventricularis and the subvalvar musculature occurs secondary to valve stenosis, and is functional.

Following pulmonary valvotomy hypertrophic infundibular stenosis may become hemodynamically significant producing severe obstruction ("suicidal right ventricle"), which in rare instances requires urgent surgical resection. Usually, however, maintenance of a high venous pressure will maintain an adequate right ventricular output. As time passes, the obstruction regresses spontaneously.

Assessment of the Severity of Pulmonary Stenosis

In organic stenosis from any cause the stenotic orifice remains fixed, but pressures will vary with cardiac output. The severity of pulmonary stenosis can best be determined at cardiac catheterization by calculating the valve size, once the gradient and cardiac output have been measured. Assessment of severity from the electrocardiogram and X-ray is unreliable.

However, the severity of the stenosis can often be very accurately determined clinically by determining the length of the systolic murmur, before and after amyl nitrite inhalation, and the degree of splitting of the second heart sound. In general, the longer the murmur and the wider the splitting, the greater the degree of stenosis. This is due to the fact that right ventricular systole become prolonged whereas left ventricular systole remains normal. Unless there is an escape route through the ventricle (Tetralogy of Fallot) or the atrium (Trilogy of Fallot), the right ventricle must eject all the blood it receives through the stenosed valve. As the stenosis increases, right ventricular systole becomes prolonged, the murmur lengthens, obscures A_2, and the A_2–P_2 interval increases.

Amyl nitrite increases venous return and if the right ventricle has sufficient reserve, right ventricular output is increased. The increased flow is associated with an increased velocity of ejection across the stenosed valve. In mild dnd moderate pulmonary stenosis this leads to prompt intensification of the murmur, which persists until the effects of amyl nitrite wear off. In severe stenosis, the hypertrophied muscle ("muscle bound right ventricle") cannot accommodate more venous return. The effect of amyl nitrite is thus less striking, murmur intensification is not as remarkable, and, in fact, it may actually soften.

The *electrocardiogram* has some value in assessing severity. When the stenosis is mild the record may be normal; a normal tracing is rare in severe stenosis. When the tracing is abnormal in mild pulmonary stenosis, the abnormality usually consists of slight right axis deviation, R/S ratio in V1 is 1 or less, and in V6 is greater than 1. In severe stenosis the axis becomes much more rightward (more than +120°), the R/S ratio in V1 is greater than 1 and less than 1 in V6. A qR in V1 suggests severe pulmonary stenosis with right ventricular pressure above that of systemic. Deeply inverted T waves in the right precordial leads indicate severe RVH and if these extend to V5 or V6 the stenosis is usually severe and the ventricular septum usually intact.

Differential Diagnosis

Diagnosis of isolated pulmonary stenosis must be made from ejection murmurs due to other causes, particularly tetralogy, aortic stenosis, functional pulmonary systolic murmurs, ventricular and atrial septal defects, and rare conditions such as Ebstein anomaly and hypoplastic right ventricle. Occasional causes of acquired pulmonary stenosis such as obstructive cardiomyopathy, carcinoid tumor, intracardiac tumor, aortic aneurysm, and pulmonary arteritis (part of the aortic, arteritis syndrome) may have to be considered.

Peripheral Pulmonary Artery Stenosis

Stenosis of one or both pulmonary arteries distal to the bifurcation of the main pulmonary artery may occur. Occasionally, the smaller pulmonary vessels in the lungs are affected. Pulmonary hypertension proximal to the stenosis is found on catheterization.

Peripheral pulmonary artery stenosis can be suspected when a systolic ejection murmur is heard equally loudly in both parasternal regions at the base, in the axillae and interscapular areas. Occasionally a "continuous" murmur may be heard over the lung fields. Peripheral pulmonary artery stenosis is particularly common in association with left-to-right shunts such as patent ductus arteriosus. The latter combination is especially likely to result from maternal rubella. Peripheral pulmonary artery stenosis may also be associated with supravalvar aortic stenosis combined with mental retardation and a characteristic facial appearance.

Double Chambered Right Ventricle

Occasionally anomalous muscle bundles in the right ventricle divide the cavity into two chambers. These bundles lie proximal to the infundibulum and have their septal attachments near the tricuspid valve (Fig. 10.18). The right ventricle is-thereby subdivided into proximal and distal portions. This anomaly is usually associated with a ventricular septal defect but occasionally occurs with isolated pulmonary stenosis.

Clues to the diagnosis of double chambered right ventricle are (1) murmur maximal at left second to fourth intercostal spaces, (2) pul-

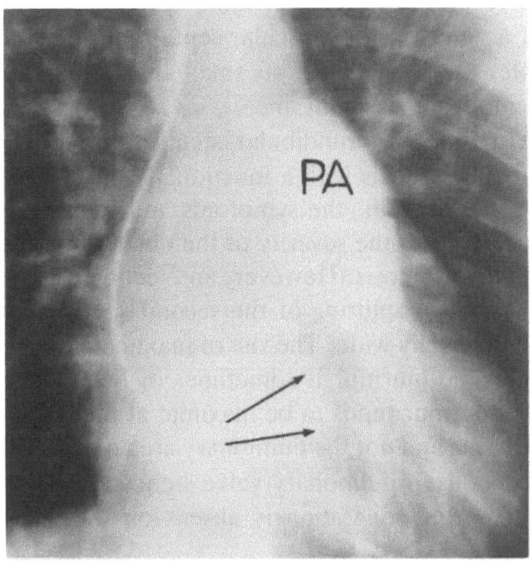

FIGURE 10.18. Right ventricular cineangiogram in a case of double-chambered right ventricle produced by anomalous muscle bundles in the right ventricular cavity (arrows).

monary component of the second sound may be normal in intensity, and (3) precordial ECG leads show less right ventricular hypertrophy than anticipated and lead AVR which "faces" the proximal chamber shows a dominant R wave.

Aortic Stenosis

When aortic stenosis is combined with pulmonary stenosis the former may well be overlooked. It should be suspected when evidence of left ventricular enlargement is found in a patient with severe pulmonary stenosis. Radiation of the murmur to the right of the sternum and into the neck may be suggestive. Aortic incompetence occasionally coexists.

Complications

Infective endocarditis is an occasional occurrence that may lead to pulmonary incompetence. *Congestive cardiac failure* ultimately ensues in the severe cases and is rapidly fatal.

Indications for Valvotomy

In most patients the indications for valvotomy are severe stenosis and a right ventricular pressure approaching or exceeding that of the left. A gradient of at least 50 mm Hg under basel conditions of cardiac catheterization should be present before valvotomy is advised. With gradients below 50 mm Hg there is no special need but prophylactic therapy against infective endocarditis.

Valvotomy is best performed after the age of three and before adulthood and should not be delayed too long once clearcut indications are present. In untreated, severe pulmonary stenosis, permanent right ventricular fibrosis with reduction in compliance and ventricular performance may develop.

When heart failure is absent the operative results are good and the immediate risks low. Prophylaxis against infection must always be continued, especially before dental treatment. The long-term effects of residual stenosis or incompetence still have to be assessed.

Operation with cardiopulmonary bypass was the method of choice with pulmonary valvotomy performed through the pulmonary artery. This has been replaced in most centers by percutaneous balloon valvotomy and the results are excellent.

In young infants valvotomy is often lifesaving and an emergency procedure. Valvotomy with inflow stasis and hypothermia is the method of choice in these desperately ill cyanotic infants.

Aortic Stenosis

Congenital aortic stenosis is common and may be valvular, subvalvular or supravalvular. Many adult cases of aortic stenosis are really congenital in origin on the basis of a bicuspid valve. The lesion is progressive, and it may take many years before critical stenosis develops. Males are more frequently affected than females.

Valvular

A congenital bicuspid valve may occur as an isolated congenital anomaly or be associated with other congenital defects. It is the commonest form of congenital heart disease. The most common association is with coarctation of the aorta. Bicuspid valves are poorly constructed to withstand the constant trauma of a high-pressure system over a prolonged period. As time passes the valve cusps become thickened, incompetent, or stenotic. Calcification is common and bacterial infection is an ever-present hazard. Adult aortic stenosis may thus develop on a congenital basis, taking many years to produce hemodynamic changes. Serious aortic stenosis in infancy is usually a result of a unicuspid unicommissural aortic valve.

Subaortic Stenosis

The site of stenosis is below the aortic valve. The obstruction may be caused by a fibrous diaphragm, by abnormal muscular hypertrophy, or by anomalous insertion of the mitral valve.

Discrete Membranous Subaortic Stenosis

In this condition there is a fibrous membrane forming a crescent-shaped ridge across the left ventricular outflow tract just below the aortic valve. The membrane is continuous with the aortic annulus and the anterior leaflet of the mitral valve. The aortic valve is usually normal and the ascending aorta is normal in size. The degree of left ventricular enlargement depends on severity of the stenosis. Occasionally, subvalvar stenosis is associated with valve ring stenosis and thickening and fusion of the valve cusps. In long-standing subvalvar stenosis the effects of the jet leads to secondary involvement of the aortic valve leaflets leading to aortic insufficiency. Occasionally, the subaortic membrane has a fibrous extension into the outflow tract of the left ventricle producing a funnel-shaped zone of constriction.

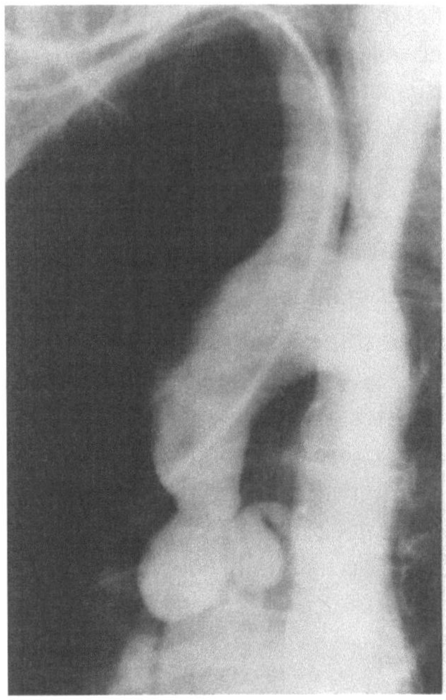

FIGURE 10.19. Aortogram (left anterior oblique projection) in a case of supravalvular aortic stenosis demonstrating a localized narrowing immediately above sinuses of Valsalva.

Mitral Valve Anomalies

Obstruction of the left ventricular outflow tract by abnormally attached mitral valve leaflets has been described. The left ventricular outflow is characteristically deformed in endocardial cushion defects.

Supravalvular Aortic Stenosis

This usually occurs in children who have mental retardation, abnormal teeth, peripheral pulmonary arterial stenoses, and abnormal facies. The syndrome may be associated with idiopathic infantile hypercalcemia or may follow excessive maternal ingestion of vitamin D during pregnancy. The involvement of the aorta is just above the valve and may take the form of a localized narrowing or a diffuse area of hypoplasia (Fig. 10.19).

Idiopathic Hypertrophic Subaortic Stenosis

This is a form of cardiomyopathy (discussed on p. 317).

Clinical Features

In aortic stenosis, the symptoms and signs depend on the severity of the obstruction. A common presentation is one of an asymptomatic patient with a systolic murmur and thrill at the base, to the right and left of the sternum, conducted into the suprasternal notch and great vessels of the neck. Attention is drawn to the heart because of the murmur, the stenosis being mild or moderate, with normal cardiac output and little or no left ventricular enlargement.

When the stenosis is severe the symptoms are effort dyspnea, angina, and syncope. Sudden death may occur with little or no previous disability. Dyspnea on effort is associated with significant stenosis and is progressive, with orthopnea and paroxysmal dyspnea occurring late. When congestive cardiac failure develops patients seldom survive more than 2 years. It is striking how rapidly patients with aortic stenosis deteriorate, often over a period of days or weeks, once the limit of physiological adjustment has passed and often without a clear precipitating factor.

Angina pectoris usually indicates severe stenosis, especially in childhood and adolescence. Nocturnal angina may be distressing and is often relieved by sitting up in bed and leaning forward. *Syncope* on effort is characteristic of left ventricular obstruction. Occasionally, it takes the form of dizziness or visual disturbance with effort. Syncope may occur at rest, after coughing, after completion of effort or may be orthostatic.

Physical Findings

The *pulse* is characteristically of small volume and has a slow rate of rise with a palpable notch—"the anacrotic pulse." This is a helpful sign in young people. In elderly patients it is often masked by a rapid rate of rise of sclerotic vessels. The *jugular venous pulse* is normal in mild stenosis. In severe stenosis the right ventricular cavity is encroached on by the hypertrophied septum, interfering with inflow, resulting in a prominent "ha" wave. A systolic thrill can be felt in the majority of patients. It is basal in situation, to the right of the sternum, often also to the left, and conducted into the vessels of the neck. The apex is left ventricular in type with a sustained heave and may be considerably displaced. A palpable presystolic impulse may be present.

The *first heart sound* is characteristically soft or inaudible in aortic stenosis. An *aortic ejection click* occurs almost exclusively in valvular stenosis but is rare when the valves are calcified; it is almost always present in congenital aortic valve stenosis in children. An aortic ejection click is rare in supra- and subvalvular stenosis.

An *ejection systolic murmur* accompanies all forms of left ventricular outflow obstruction. It is typically loud (grade 3–5), maximal at the base, and radiates into vessels of the neck. The site of the stenosis cannot be diagnosed with any degree of certainty from the position of the murmur. In advanced cases with heart failure and patients with thick chest walls, or chronic airways obstruction, the murmur may be soft or even absent. In infants, on the other hand, the murmur is often best heard low to the left of the sternum and may be mistaken for a ventricular septal defect.

The *second heart sound* is usually single or narrowly split and cannot be relied on as an index of severity. However, reversed splitting occurs only in severe stenosis. This is a difficult sign to detect at the bedside and requires phonocardiographic confirmation.

An *early diastolic murmur*, high-pitched blowing in character, is heard in the minority of patients with valve stenosis, but in a significant number with supravalvar or discrete subvalvar stenosis.

The *electrocardiogram* is helpful, showing varying degrees of left ventricular hypertrophy roughly related to the severity of the obstruction. However, it must be emphasized that high grade, even fatal, congenital stenosis can occur, with a normal electrocardiogram, particularly under the age of 10 years. Occasionally even in adults, severe acquired valve stenosis may be associated with a normal tracing. The site of the stenosis cannot be predicted from the electrocardiogram.

The *chest X-ray* in childhood shows that the heart is usually normal size. Occasionally, it shows left ventricular enlargement of varying degree and left atrial enlargement. The normal heart size contrasts sharply with the ascending aorta, which is particularly dilated in valve stenosis (poststenotic dilatation) but only mildly dilated in subaortic stenosis. Calcification of the aortic valve occurs particularly in older patients.

Systemic embolism may occur in the absence of infection and is a result of fragmentation of a calcific valve. Infective endocarditis is an occasional complication of all forms of aortic stenosis but is very rare in the hypertrophic variety.

Clinical Differentiation of Valvular from Subvalvular and Supravalvular Aortic Stenosis

Four distinctive features are the pulse, the ejection sound, the valve calcification, and the effect of prompt squatting on the murmur.

In *congenital valvular stenosis* the physical appearance is normal, the pulse anacrotic, the systolic murmur ejection in type, often associated with a thrill, maximal to right of sternum, and an ejection sound is highly characteristic unless the valve is calcified. Dilatation of the ascending aorta is present radiologically and valve calcification is diagnostic. The murmur becomes louder or remains unchanged on squatting.

In *congenital subvalvar stenosis* of the discrete variety, the above features are present except that an ejection click is exceptional and an early diastolic murmur more common. Valve calcification is absent.

In hypertrophic obstructive cardiomyopathy there is a familial incidence in some patients, the pulse has a quick jerky upstroke, often bisferiens, the systolic murmur is often maximum at the apex, longer, sometimes pansystolic; a click and early diastolic murmur are exceptional and valve calcification is absent. In at least 75% of the patients the murmur softens appreciably with squatting.

In *supravalvar stenosis* the physical appearance is often characteristic. Inequality of the brachiocephalic pulses is an important diagnostic clue. This usually results from selective acceleration of flow into and amplification of pulsations in the right subclavian and right common carotid vessels (the Keanda effect). Less commonly, there is organic occlusion because of intimal fibrosis producing so called "reversed coarctation."

An ejection click and early diastolic murmur are uncommon and aortic dilatation and valve calcification are absent. Peripheral pulmonary artery stenosis with appropriate murmurs is frequently present.

Indications of Surgery

The natural history of aortic stenosis is very variable depending on the degree of the stenosis and the state of the myocardium. Mild stenosis is compatible with a full normal life span. Physical activities, however, should always be curtailed and the patient should be advised against taking part in competitive sport or strenuous exercise. In severe stenosis, sudden death is always a danger, even though symptoms during ordinary daily activities are minimal.

There is no problem about advising surgery when severe symptoms such as progressive effort dyspnea, paroxysmal dyspnea, angina pectoris, and syncope are present and the aortic valve area is 0.7 cm^2 or less. Surgery is lifesaving under these circumstances and produces rewarding results, even in these patients with poor left ventricular function (left ventricular ejection fraction less than 20%). The results of operation are best in the discrete subvalvar type where excision produces cure.

Doppler echocardiography is the ideal method for diagnosis of the type and severity of aortic stenosis in children. It is also ideal for follow-up of such patients. In children with valve areas of more than 0.7 cm^2 physical activity should be restricted and the child followed every 6 months.

Coarctation of the Aorta

Coarctation of the aorta is a localized or diffuse constriction of varying from almost complete obstruction to trivial narrowing of the lumen. The usual site is above or below the insertion of the ductus arteriosus; rarely, it is in the thoracic or abdominal aorta. Associated congenital defects are frequently present. The condition occurs fairly frequently and is more common in men than women.

The hemodynamics depend on

1. The size of the narrowed lumen.
2. The site and length of the narrowed segment.
3. The effect of associated defects.

Size of the Narrowed lumen

When the aorta is narrowed to one-third its original size hypertension proximal to the obstruction and hypotension distal to it will result. The usual finding is a lumen reduced to 0.5 to 2 mm diameter; rarely is it completely obstructed.

The circulation to the body below the coarctation depends largely on the adequacy of the collateral circulation. The mechanical effect of the coarctation is the main cause of hypertension. There is no evidence that the kidneys are responsible.

Site and Length of the Coarctation

This determines the location and extent of collateral circulation. Since the common site is above, at, or below the insertion of the ductus, the collaterals develop from branches of the carotid and subclavian arteries. If the left subclavian artery is involved collaterals develop from the carotids and right subclavian only. If the coarctation is in the thoracic aorta, collaterals are derived from lower intercostals only and, likewise, in coarctation of the abdominal aorta, collaterals arise even lower.

The Presence or Absence of Associated Defects

Patent Ductus Arteriosus

This is the most common and most important associated defect. Usually the coarctation occurs distal to the origin of the ductus (postductal coarctation—adult type of coarctation). Particularly in infants the coarctation may occur proximal to the origin of the ductus (preductal coarctation, or infantile type).

In *postductal coarctation*, the hemodynamic consequences depend on the pulmonary arterial resistance. When the ductus is widely patent heart failure may develop, after 2 months of age as pulmonary resistance falls and pulmonary blood flow increases. Rarely, pulmonary hypertension at systemic level produces a right-to-left shunt.

In *preductal coarctation*, especially after infancy, blood flow is still normal from aorta to pulmonary artery. When pulmonary resistance in infants is high and coarctation severe, the distal aorta may be entirely perfused by the right ventricle. This leads to cyanosis of the lower extremities, increased right ventricular output, and rapid development of heart failure. Coarctation with heart failure in the first few weeks of life is usually due to this association.

Ventricular Septal Defect

The effects of a coexisting ventricular septal defect depend on the size of the defect and the pulmonary vascular resistance. When the defect is restrictive, the left-to-right shunt is small. When the septal defect is nonrestrictive the effects are determined by the pulmonary vascular resistance.

Ventricular Septal Defect and Patent Ductus Arteriosus

This combination is not uncommon, especially in infancy. The hemodynamics depend on the severity of the coarctation, the size of the ventricular septal defect, the size of the patent ductus, and the pulmonary vascular resistance. The diagnosis can frequently be made only by cardiac catheterization and angiocardiography.

When the ventricular septal defect is large, the coarctation severe, and the pulmonary resistance not unduly elevated, the picture is much the same whether a ductus is present or not. When the patent ductus is *proximal* to the coarctation the systolic and diastolic pressures in the systemic and pulmonary arteries are the same and a large, often torrential left-to-right shunt is present. The ductus is silent and can be detected only by investigation or surgery.

When the patent ductus is distal to the coarctation there is a large left-to-right shunt at ventricular level, with equalization of ventricular pressures and a right-to-left shunt at ductus level, with equalization of pulmonary artery and descending aortic pressures. There is no delay in femoral artery pulsation but the pressures in the legs is usually lower than in the arms. Both the ductus and the coarctation can be missed because it is so difficult to take the blood pressure in infants. The picture is that of an unrestricted ventricular septal defect. Because of the highly saturated blood in the pulmonary arteries the lower limbs are not noticeably bluer than the upper.

When the ventricular septal defect is small the murmur of this defect is superimposed on the signs of coarctation and patent ductus. A small VSD has little additional hemodynamic effect.

Other Defects

Bicuspid aortic valve frequently coexists, the reported incidence varying from 27 to 85%. The bicuspid valve is usually competent but occasionally aortic regurgitation develops, aggravating the strain on the left ventricle, already stressed by hypertension. Bicuspid valves also have a tendency to calcify and narrow, so that aortic stenosis in later life is not infrequent; aortic incompetence is less common.

Associated, anomalies of the aorta frequently coexist (e.g., aortic hypoplasia, dilatation and aneurysm formation, aneurysm of the aortic sinuses with dilatation of the aortic valve ring, and aortic incompetence).

Preductal coarctation is frequently complicated by other defects, such as transposition, single ventricle, endocardial cushion defect, and fibroelastosis, which may predispose to rapid development of heart failure.

Clinical Presentation

Under 1 Year of Age

Because of the aforementioned associated defects more than half the cases of coarctation of the aorta present with the signs and symptoms of heart failure in the first year of life. The association with a large ventricular septal defect and patent ductus arteriosus is particularly lethal.

Cyanosis usually denotes associated defects and a particularly striking variety occurs with transposition of the great vessels and preductal coarctation where the upper extremities are cyanosed and the lower pink so-called "reversed differential cyanosis." Interruption of the aortic arch, and the hypoplastic left heart syndrome may be associated. Murmurs are generally not very helpful since they are produced by the associated defects. The femoral pulses are usually impalpable, but even this may be misleading when there is preductal coarctation with a right-to-left shunt into the descending aorta. The diagnosis must be made by cardiac catheterization.

Over 1 Year of Age

The majority of patients are asymptomatic, the condition being discovered during routine examination. With advancing age, however, symptoms due to hypertension and inadequate collateral circulation are encountered: A highly suggestive complaint is intermittent claudication, or tiredness in the legs when running. A characteristic bodily physique is one with well-developed, muscular, powerful upper extremities and thin, spindly legs.

Symptoms usually develop as a result of complications. Thus, congestive failure is usually associated with coexisting aortic valve disease; less commonly, it is secondary to hypertension. In young children, a large patent ductus arteriosus is particularly important. Rupture of the aorta or dissection is found in approximately one-fifth of necropsy cases. Postcoarctation aortic aneurysm, often calcified, may develop. Cerebrovascular accidents due to rupture of an associated berry aneurysm is another hazard. Infective endocarditis may involve a bicuspid valve or the coarctation itself.

Physical Examination

Systolic and diastolic hypertension of the upper limbs is present. The pressure should always be recorded in both upper limbs, since the left subclavian may be involved in the coarctation, or may arise distal to it. The right subclavian may arise anomalously below the coarctation.

In children and adolescents the blood pressure is often normal. Hypertension increases gradually with age and there is no sudden acceleration, presumably because the renal arteries are protected. The systolic blood pressure in the lower limbs is always lower than that of the upper limbs. The femoral pulses are diminished and delayed. It is important to measure the blood pressure after exercise since this may reach very high levels in some patients.

Collaterals become visible as the child grows older. The dilated, tortuous vessels cannot be seen in the neck and scapular regions. The carotids are prominent and pulsate vigorously. The dilated interscapular and intercostal arteries on the back are best seen when the patient bends forward with arms hanging at the sides. The fundi may show mild retinopathy, but not papilledema.

Cardiomegaly is commensurate with the degree of hypertension, unless valve defects are present. The following murmurs may be heard.

Aortic Ejection Murmur. This is produced by flow across a normal aortic valve and is often found in hypertension of any cause; typically it is early, stopping before the second sound. When aortic valve stenosis is present, the murmur is loud, radiates more widely, but maintains the same characteristics. An aortic ejection click is commonly heard in coarctation, usually widely conducted and well separated from the first heart sound. The click may arise from a bicuspid valve or the aortic wall.

Systolic Murmur from Collaterals. This murmur varies in intensity from grade 2/6 to grade 4/6, begins in early systole, clearly separated from the first sound, and has a late crescendo ending in the second sound. It is widely distributed over collaterals and can be heard in the neck, under the left clavicle, on both sides of the chest anteriorly, and in the epigastrium and the lower sternal edge. It can also be heard posteriorly over dilated interscapular arteries. These murmurs are particularly loud in complete coarctation.

Systolic Murmurs from the Coarctation. When the coarctation is less than 2.5 mm in diameter, a continuous murmur is heard over the spine between the scapulae. It may occasionally be heard anteriorly under the left clavicle and cannot be differentiated from a patent ductus. When the coarctation is more than 2.5 mm in diameter, the murmur is systolic only. In mild coarctation there is no murmur. The localization of the murmur is extremely important, since it indicates the site of the stricture. In abdominal coarctation, the murmur is heard in the epigastrium and there may be no visible collaterals.

Aortic Incompetent Murmur. This is due to associated valve disease.

Patent Ductus Arteriosus Murmur, depending upon pulmonary vascular resistance.

Mitral Diastolic Murmur. A low-pitched, soft, middiastolic murmur is occasionally heard at the apex in the absence of organic mitral stenosis.

Electrocardiogram

This is usually normal, though occasionally left ventricular hypertrophy may be present, especially in the presence of aortic valve disease. Right bundle branch block, as an independent congenital anomaly, is encountered occasionally.

Chest X-ray

In the absence of aortic valve disease or other defects, the heart size is usually normal. Diagnostic signs are found in the appearance of the aorta. The ascending aorta and the aortic knuckle are elongated with loss of the aortic

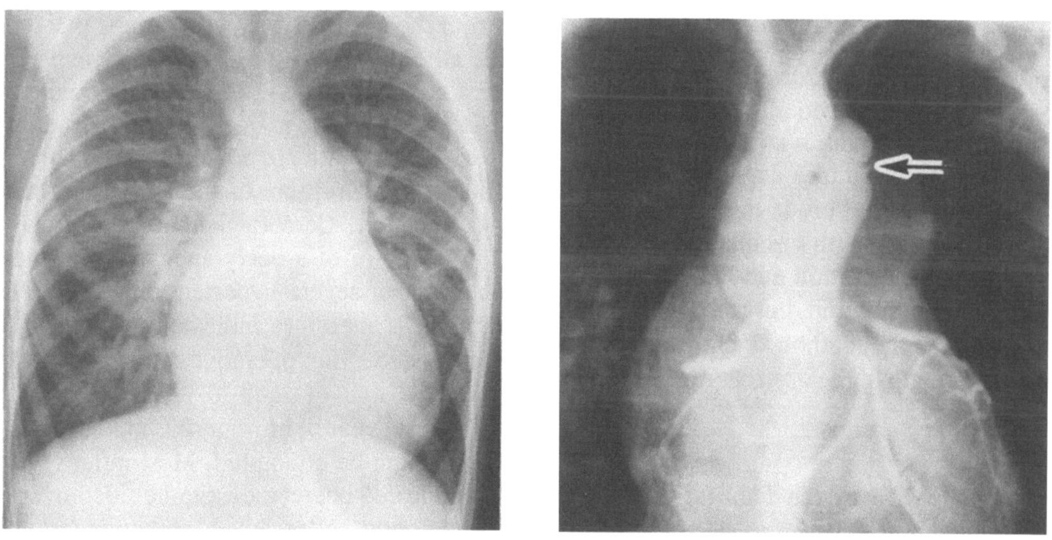

FIGURE 10.20. Chest X-ray (left) in a case of large ventricular septal defect and large left-to-right shunt associated with coarctation of the aorta demonstrated by angiography. (right)

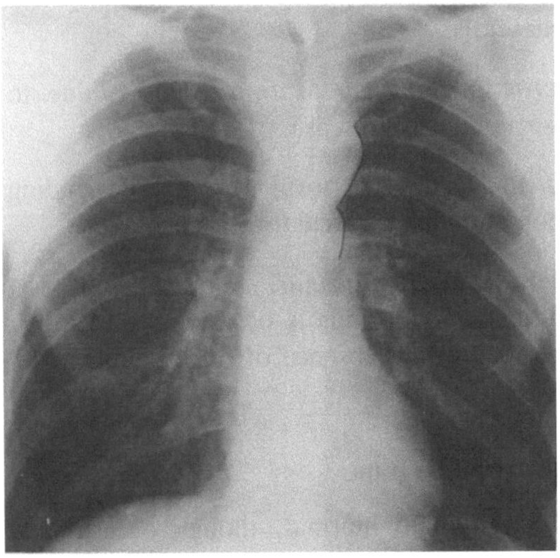

FIGURE 10.21. Chest X-ray in coarctation of the aorta demonstrating the "arabic 3" appearance produced by dilatation of the aorta proximal and distal to the coarcted segment. The left subclavian artery is also dilated. Rib notching is indicated by the arrows.

knob, the left upper border being formed by a prominently pulsating left subclavian artery, which broadens the upper mediastinum. Poststenotic dilatation of the aorta is frequently of considerable magnitude so that the dilated left subclavian artery overlapping the poststenotic dilatation produces a characteristic picture, described as a double aortic knuckle in the shape of an Arabic 3 (Figs. 10.20 and 10.21).

Notching of the ribs does not usually appear before the age of 5 and, is a frequent finding in adults. It is produced by enlarged, tortuous intercostal arteries that erode the lower margins of the third to the eighth ribs bilaterally.

Cardiac catheterization and angiocardiography are seldom required, but retrograde aortic angiography is the method of choice in determining the length of the obstruction.

Diagnosis

Routine palpation of the femoral arteries in every patient will detect most cases of coarctation. Occasionally, femoral pulsation may be quite good but the clue is the delay.

Arteritis of the aorta most closely mimics congenital coarctation. It can usually be differentiated because of the patchy involvement of several branches of the aorta, particularly the carotid and subclavian arteries. Thus, the two carotid arteries are often strikingly discrepant, and one or other subclavian absent. The degree of hypertension is often considerable and appears at an early age; congestive cardiac failure may be marked and not necessarily related to the degree of hypertension. Since arteritis usually affects the lower thoracic or abdominal aorta, collaterals are palpable low down, involving the lower thoracic intercostal vessels. The X-ray shows a normal aortic knuckle, and calcification of the thoracic aorta may be present. Aortography is quite distinctive.

In older patients, hypertension associated with aortic atherosclerosis and abdominal aortic occlusion simulates coarctation but collateral channels in the thorax are absent.

Prognosis and Treatment

The natural history of coarctation of the aorta is poor. Half the patients are dead before the age of 1 year, with the heaviest mortality in the first 2 months of life. The complexity of the deformities and the lack of adaptation to the abnormal hemodynamic state account for this heavy loss.

From the age of 1 to 20 years, most patients are well adjusted to the abnormality and relatively asymptomatic. Thereafter, the mortality rises steeply, the majority dying before 50. The causes of death are equally divided among cardiac failure, rupture of the aorta, and bacterial infection. Cerebral hemorrhage usually follows rupture of a berry aneurysm but may be a result of severe hypertension. Operative treatment is therefore indicated in almost all patients since the operative risk, especially between the ages of 6 and 20, is less than 5%.

In the first year of life vigorous medical therapy must first be attempted. Most infants with uncomplicated coarctation can be tided over a critical period, after which spontaneous improvement occurs so that elective surgery can be performed. If the infant cannot be managed with adequate medical therapy, operation is justified. In complicated defects usually associated with severe heart failure in infancy successful surgery is uncommon, except in centers specializing in neonatal and infant surgery.

The optimal age for surgery is between 7 and 10 years of age when the risks are minimal. The vessels have good elasticity and the aortic lumen is sufficiently large to maintain normal hemodynamics throughout adult life.

Some patients respond well to balloon dilatation of the coarctation, but there is a high incidence of aneurysm.

After the age of 20 the risks rise progressively, and by 35 vascular changes may be so marked that operation is difficult. The presence of aortic aneurysms, tortuous enlarged collateral vessels, severe hypertension, valve defects, and heart failure creates special problems. In such patients, conservative therapy for hypertension and cardiac failure may be preferable.

Coarctation of the Aorta and Pregnancy. The risk of rupture of the aorta and dissection is increased during pregnancy. Elective caesarean section at term without sterilization is advisable. Asymptomatic pregnant patients without valve disease can usually be successfully managed by medical means and surgical resection during pregnancy is not indicated, unless severe complications develop. After pregnancy the coarctation should be electively repaired.

Complications of Surgery. Reactive hypertension following resection of the coarctation is not uncommon. The rise in pressure may occur within 12 hours of operation or be delayed, commencing about 48 hours later. Hypertension must be controlled immediately with reserpine, hydralazine, or intravenous nitroprusside.

Postoperative abdominal pain due to mesenteric vasculitis is an occasional complication 2 to 4 days after operation. This is associated with reactive hypertension and rarely occurs independently. Severe abdominal pain, increased peristaltic sounds, abdominal distension, tenderness, vomiting, fever, and leukocytosis are followed by varying degrees of ileus. Bowel infarction and melena may ensue and resection of bowel may occasionally be necessary. Adequate control of the hypertension is the most important treatment.

Recoarctation. In some patients the gradient between the proximal and distal aorta recurs after operation. Apart from technical factors associated with the operation, recoarctation is usually attributable to failure of continued growth at the anastomotic line, or to narrowing from fibrosis occurring in the ductal tissue incorporated into the aorta at the coarctation. Most commonly, recoarctation occurs in patients first operated on under 3 years of age. Progressive signs and symptoms of obstruction develop so that the clinical picture of coarctation reappears. It has been suggested that reoperation is indicated when a gradient of 40 mm or more is demonstrated. Balloon dilatation is a suitable alternative to surgery.

Results of Surgery. Restoration of femoral pulses immediately after surgery indicates satisfactory anastomosis. The blood pressure usually returns to normal but occasionally mild residual hypertension persists, particularly in the older age group. The prognosis after surgery depends on associated lesions particularly of the aortic valve.

Vascular Rings and Other Aortic Anomalies

Significant malformations of the aorta and great vessels are encountered chiefly in the early years of life. The most important involve the aortic arch, the great vessels (innominate, carotid, and subclavian) and the ligamentum arteriosum.

Embryology

The origin of the aorta and pulmonary arteries from the brachial arch arteries is shown in Figure 10.22. The two ventral aortae arise separately from the truncus and are connected to the dorsal aortae by the six branchial arch arteries. Caudally, the paired dorsal aortae fuse into a single vessel. Division of the truncus separates the aorta from the pulmonary artery, but connection of these two vessels is main-

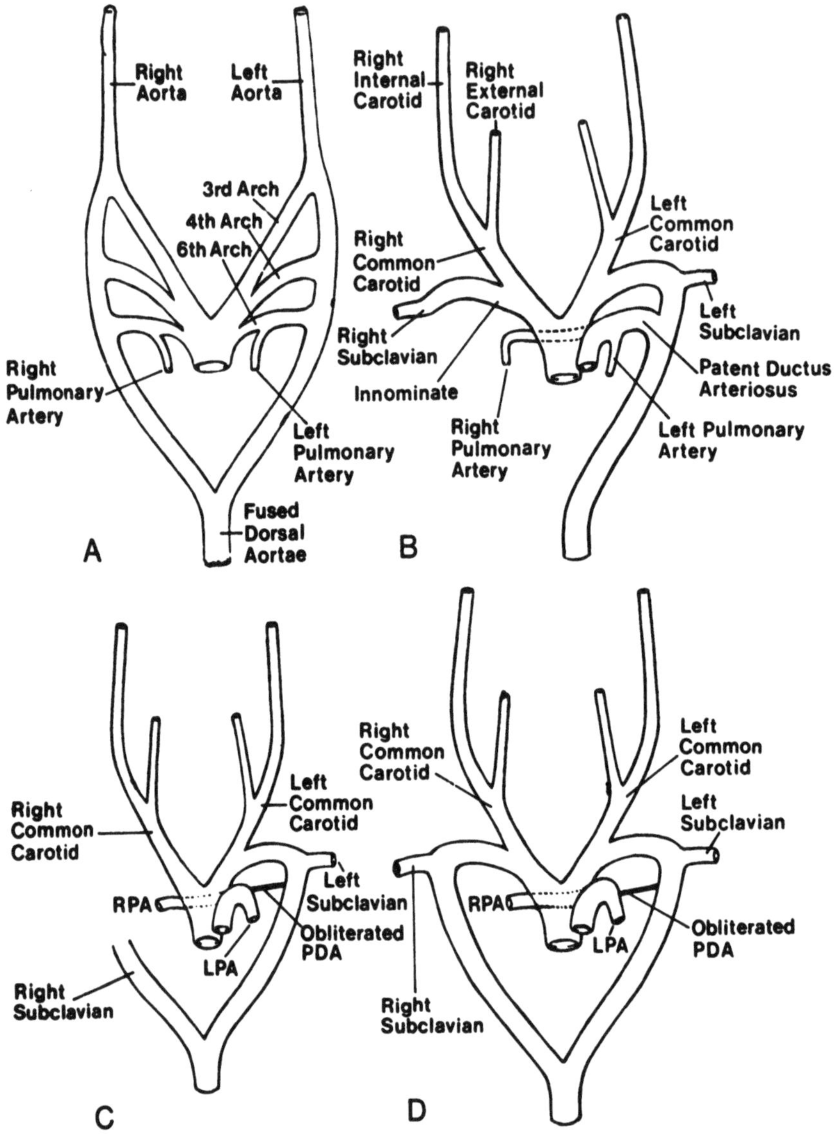

FIGURE 10.22. Embryological development of the great arteries and their branches from the dorsal aorta and the branchial arches. In (A) the primitive arrangement of the truncus, branchial arches, and aorta is shown. In (B) development has been normal with atrophy of many of the right-sided vessels. The ductus is still patent and is a very large structure in fetal life. In (C) the right dorsal aorta has persisted as the right subclavian artery, which arises anomalously from the thoracic aorta below the subclavian. In (D) a double aortic arch is present because of failure of obliteration of the right dorsal aorta.

tained by the ductus arteriosus. Normally, the right dorsal aorta atrophies and disappears; the ductus joins the aorta near the origin of the right subclavian artery. There are numerous variations and a ductus may persist on each side. When a right-sided arch develops, the great vessels are mirror image of normal with left-sided innominate, right common carotid, and right subclavian. Normally, the right subclavian arises from the innominate, which is formed by the proximal part of the right dorsal aorta. Occasionally, the right subclavian artery arises from the distal part of the right aorta and is aberrant. Similarly, an aberrant left subcla-

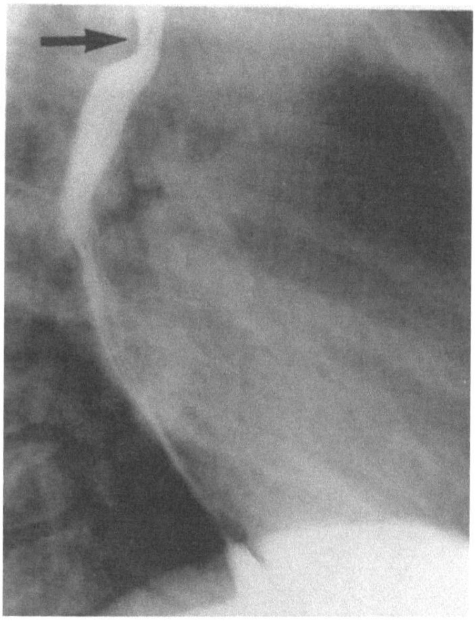

FIGURE 10.23. Barium swallow showing posterior indentation of the esophagus produced by a vascular ring in a case of double aortic arch (arrow).

vian arises from the lower left aorta when a rightsided aorta is present.

Right Aortic Arch with Right-Sided Descent of Descending Aorta

The aortic crosses behind the esophagus, which is pushed forward. The abrupt change in direction may be due to persistence of the left-sided ductus (or ligamentum), a double aortic arch, or an aberrant left subclavian artery. It is the retroesophageal crossing that causes trouble in infancy (Fig. 10.23). The trachea and esophagus are surrounded by a vascular ring. In later life arteriosclerotic changes in the aorta distort the esophagus and may interfere with swallowing.

Double Aortic Arch

Both right and left aortic arches persist, so that the ascending aorta fiburcates into two branches: one of which is anterior and to the left of the trachea, and the other is to the right and behind the trachea and esophagus. The two branches then fuse, completely surrounding these two structures, before continuing on the left as the descending aorta. In most patients the anterior limb is the smaller. Usually the space between the two limbs is too small, with the result that the trachea and esophagus are compressed.

Right Aortic Arch with Persistent or Obliterated Ductus

The ascending aorta ascends on the right of the trachea and esophagus, the arch crosses behind the esophagus; the descending aorta continues on the left of these structures. The patent or obliterated ductus runs from the left pulmonary artery in front of the esophagus and trachea to join the descending aorta encircling the trachea and esophagus.

Clinical Picture

Symptoms are encountered early in infancy and concern tracheal obstruction mainly; the slight dysphagia produced is unimportant. Airways obstruction with stridor, "crowing" respiration, tachypnea, and overactivity of accessory muscles of respiration with recession of the chest occurs. The diagnosis can usually be made by barium swallow; angiography is generally unnecessary and the treatment is surgical.

Aberrant Right Subclavian Artery

This is usually an incidental finding during barium swallow. In the middle-aged or elderly, dysphagia appearing for the first time has been attributed to arteriosclerotic changes in the great vessels (dysphagia lusoria). Conservative management is indicated.

Anomalous Innominate and Carotid Arteries

Occasionally the trachea may be compressed by an artery crossing anomalously. The arch of the aorta may rarely present as a pulsating swelling in the neck. Redundant unfolding of the aorta occurs in coarctation and may mimic coarctation (pseudocoarctation).

Idiopathic Dilatation of the Pulmonary Artery Idiopathic Pulmonary Incompetence

Idiopathic pulmonary artery dilatation produces no symptoms and it is frequently recognized on a routine chest X-ray. Only the main pulmonary artery is affected. A pulmonary ejection click and murmur and sometimes wide splitting of the second sound may lead to the suspicion of mild pulmonary stenosis, or atrial septal defect. The clinical distinction may be impossible. The electrocardiogram shows incomplete right bundle branch block. Catheterization may in fact show a very slight gradient across the pulmonary valve with a normal right ventricular pressure.

Idiopathic pulmonary incompetence can be recognized by a diastolic murmur localized to the pulmonary area, without evidence of pulmonary hypertension, or a left-to-right shunt. Radiologically, pulmonary arterial dilatation and slight right ventricular enlargement may be present. The electrocardiogram is normal, or may show incomplete right bundle branch block. The presence of pulmonary incompetence does not appear to adversely affect the right ventricle.

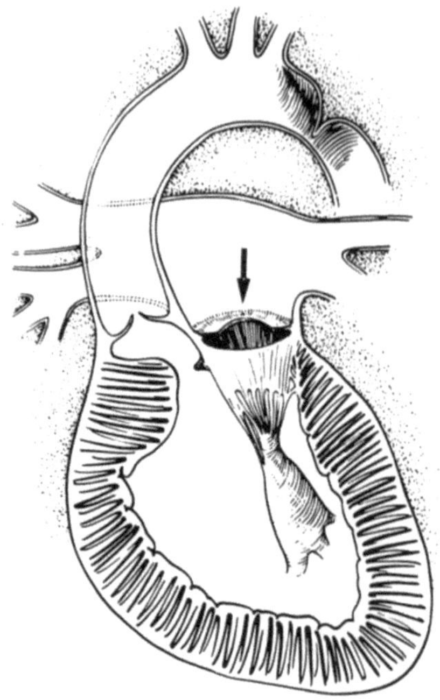

FIGURE 10.24. Supravalvular stenosing ring of the left atrium (arrow) immediately above the mitral valve, which in this case is abnormal and of the "parachute" type. Coarctation of the aorta and subaortic stenosis is also demonstrated as a component of the syndrome described by Shone et al.: "The developmental complex of 'parachute mitral valve', supravalvular ring of left atrium, subaortic stenosis, and coarctation of the aorta." Am J Cardiol 11:714, 1963. Reprinted, with permssions.

Cyanosis Absent: Pulmonary Venous Engorgement

Pulmonary venous engorgement without cyanosis is the result of left atrial hypertension produced by either an obstructive lesion in the left atrium or high end-diastolic pressure in the left ventricle associated with left ventricular failure.

Congenital Mitral Stenosis

Congenital mitral stenosis as the sole lesion is uncommon. The clinical radiological and electrocardiographic features are much the same as those occurring in the adult. Pathologically, obstruction of the mitral valve may be a result of fibrotic leaflets, commisural fusion, and shortened chordae, producing a picture indistinguishable from that of acquired rheumatic heart disease.

Alternatively, the valve may be deformed and obstructive when the chordae from both leaflets insert into a single papillary muscle leading to so-called *parachute* mitral valve. A parachute mitral valve is frequently associated with the other anomalies, the most common of which are supravalvular stenosing ring of the left atrium, subaortic stenosis, and coarctation of the aorta. Any of these anomalies, depending on their individual severity, may be responsible for producing the presenting clinical features and the other malformations may therefore be occult (Fig. 10.24).

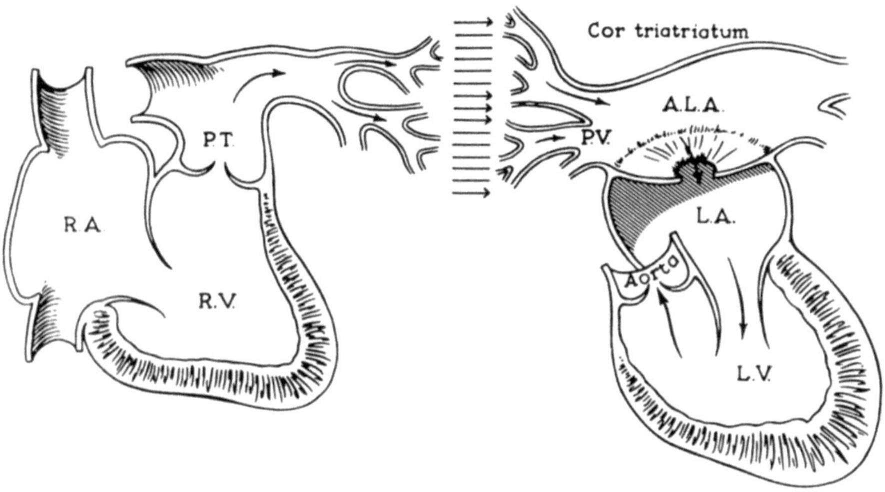

FIGURE 10.25. Diagrammatic representation of a cor triatriatum where the left atrium is divided into two chambers by a fibrous membrane; the pulmonary veins drain into the proximal chamber with resultant pulmonary venous hypertension. Reprinted, with permissions, from Lucas R et al.: Ped Clin N Am 10:781, 1967.

Supravalvular Stenosing Ring of the Left Atrium

This lesion may occur as an isolated anomaly and consists of a circumferential ring of fibrous tissue immediately above the mitral valve. Its effects are much the same as mitral stenosis (i.e., pulmonary venous hypertension and pulmonary edema).

Cor Triatriatum

This condition exists when the pulmonary veins drain into an accessory left atrial chamber superior to the left atrium (Fig. 10.25). The chamber communicates with a true left atrium through an orifice of varying size. The hemodynamic abnormality depends on the position of the accessory atrial chamber in relation to the foramen ovale and size of opening in the anomalous septum.

There are two varieties of cor triatriatum. In the first, the partitioning membrane lies above the foramen ovale and separates pulmonary veins from the foramen ovale and left atrial appendage. Thus, all pulmonary venous flow must pass through the opening in the anomalous septum. When this is inadequate, pulmonary venous hypertension and pulmonary edema develop, mimicking mitral stenosis very closely. In the less common variety, the membrane lies between the foramen ovale and the left atrial appendage. When the foramen ovale is closed, the picture resembles mitral stenosis, but when patent, the functional abnormality is that of left atrial hypertension with a left-to-right shunt at atrial level, producing in effect, the Lutembacher syndrome.

The *symptoms and signs* are determined by the degree of pulmonary venous hypertension, severity of pulmonary arterial hypertension, severity of heart failure, and size of the left-to-right shunt at atrial level. Most patients die within the first year of life and the condition is rarely compatible with a normal life span. Males are affected a little more frequently than females. Dyspnea, orthopnea, and pulmonary edema are results of pulmonary venous hypertension.

Sweating, pallor, and syncope are prominent in infants. The *physical signs* are those of pulmonary hypertension with right ventricular enlargement and a loud pulmonary component of the second heart sound. In older subjects the signs are more like those of atrial septal defect with disproportionate pulmonary hypertension. Radiologically, evidence of right-sided enlargement is present with the features of pulmonary arterial and venous hypertension.

Stenosis of Individual Pulmonary Veins

This is a rare condition that may exist as the sole anomaly. The hemodynamic effects are the same as for cor triatriatum, mitral stenosis, and other forms of pulmonary venous obstruction with the important exception being that left atrial pressure is normal.

In the investigation of patients manifesting evidence of pulmonary venous obstruction, echocardiography plays an important part prior to cardiac catheterization. The demonstration of a normal mitral valve echo clearly excludes the diagnosis of mitral valve stenosis and points to some other causes as listed above.

Endocardial Fibroelastosis

The primary from of endocardial fibroelastosis occurs in approximately 1% of births and is responsible for left ventricular failure, pulmonary venous hypertension, and edema. The condition affects the left ventricle primarily and in the common, or *dilated* type, the chamber is markedly enlarged with a thickened smooth shiny endocardium. The *contracted* type is relatively uncommon, the endocardial abnormalities less pronounced, and the left ventricular chamber size is contracted. The cause is unknown.

Symptoms occur in the first year of life and the presentation is one of heart failure with dyspnea, cough, and respiratory difficulty. A gallop rhythm is frequent, as is a soft systolic murmur of functional mitral insufficiency. The electrocardiogram provides evidence of severe left ventricular hypertrophy and left atrial enlargement.

The differential diagnosis is from other forms of left ventricular disease such as anomalous origin of the left coronary artery from the pulmonary artery, viral myocarditis, and the various forms of pulmonary venous obstruction. The prognosis is poor and the majority of victims do not survive the second year of life.

Congenital Mitral Insufficiency

Mitral insufficiency may result from intrinsic abnormalities of the leaflet such as clefts, accessory commissures with abnormal insertion of papillary muscles, and double orifice. Mitral insufficiency may also be functional as a component of left ventricular failure in endocardial fibroelastosis, myocarditis, or anomalous origin of the left coronary artery from the pulmonary artery. Volume overload of the left ventricle from ventricular septal defect may also result in mitral insufficiency. Mitral insufficiency may be the presenting features of corrected transposition of the great vessels. With ventricular inversion the right-sided tricuspid valve is subject to Ebstein malformation and resultant mitral insufficiency.

Anomalous Origin of the Left Coronary Artery with Mitral Insufficiency

When the left coronary artery originates from the pulmonary trunk there is a series of anastamotic communications with the normally originating right coronary artery. Blood flow is from the right coronary artery through these channels into the left coronary artery and the lower pressure pulmonary artery (Fig. 10.26). The result is left ventricular ischemia, produced in effect by an arteriovenous fistula. The ventricular damage takes the form of frank myocardial infarction, subendocardial scarring, or even aneurysm. Ischemia of the papillary muscles results in mitral insufficiency and with concomitant left ventricular damage, left ventricular failure.

In infancy, the presentation is one of congestive cardiac failure without murmurs but with cardiomegaly. Feeding difficulties are classically associated with attacks of myocardial ischemia, which are undoubtebly angina pectoris. In older children signs of mitral insuffi-

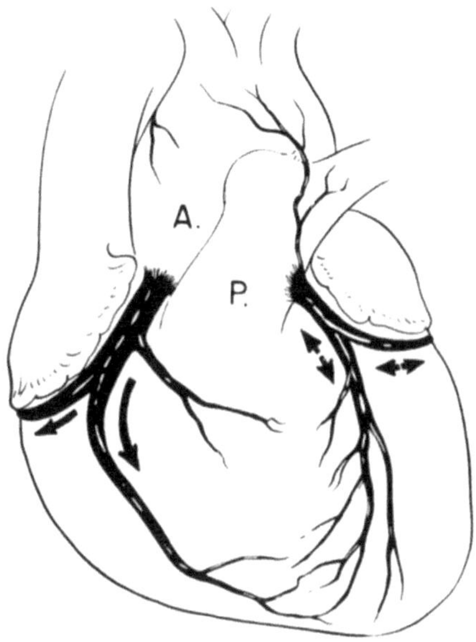

FIGURE 10.26. Anomalous origin of the left coronary artery from the pulmonary trunk. The right Coronary artery arises normally from the aorta. The fate of the left ventricle depends on the flow in the left coronary artery: when inadequate, myocardial infarction will result. Shunting of blood from the higher pressure right coronary artery to the lower pressure left coronary artery also results in ischemia. From Edwards JE: The direction of blood flow in coronary arteries arising from the pulmonary trunk. Reprinted, with permission, from Circulation 29:163–166, 1984. Copyright by the American Heart Association, Inc.

ciency and left ventricular failure are more prominent. Usually, the electrocardiogram will provide diagnostic information showing changes of anterior myocardial infarction.

Cyanosis Present: Increased Pulmonary Arterial Vasculature

Eisenmenger Syndrome

Definition

The original description of Eisenmenger complex was that of a large ventricular septal defect with cyanosis, which was erroneously attributed to streaming of right ventricular blood into an overriding aorta. It is now recognized that the cyanosis is a consequence of a right-to-left shunt at atrial, ventricular, or aortopulmonary level secondary to pulmonary hypertension.

A wide variety of malformations may therefore be associated with the syndrome. The definition given by Wood is that of pulmonary hypertension at systemic level, due to a high pulmonary vascular resistance (over 10 units or 800 dynes sec cm^{-5}) with a reversed or bidirectional shunt.

The condition is a result of failure of the high fetal pulmonary vascular resistance to drop adequately because of a large aortopulmonary or interventricular communication that maintains high pulmonary blood flow and pressure from birth. Although the shunt may originally be completely left-to-right, a right-to-left shunt occurs when the pulmonary vascular resistance rises pari pasu with organic changes in the pulmonary vascular bed. In atrial septal defect, pulmonary vascular disease develops more gradually, precipitated by thromboembolic disease later in life and affecting women in particular.

Clinical Diagnosis

Eisenmenger syndrome is fairly easy to diagnose at the bedside. Cyanosis and evidence of pulmonary hypertension are invariably present. The right ventricle is palpable parasternally, and the pulmonary component of the second heart sound is frequently palpable in the second left interspace. A left ventricular impulse is characteristically absent.

A right atrial gallop, pulmonary ejection click, short pulmonary ejection systolic murmur, early diastolic pulmonary murmur of pulmonary insufficiency, and an accentuated pulmonary component of the second heart sound with narrow splitting are the usual auscultatory findings.

The *electrocardiogram* shows right ventricular hypertrophy, right axis deviation, and occasionally evidence of right atrial enlargement. In atrioventricular canal the mean frontal plane QRS axis is leftward.

The *chest X-ray* shows prominence of the

main pulmonary artery and its proximal branches and diminution of the vascular markings distal to the hilum. Peripheral pruning of the pulmonary arteries is, however, not invariable; these may be normal or even slightly plethoric.

Although the bedside diagnosis of Eisenmenger syndrome is usually fairly easy, the identification of the particular cause is more difficult. Differential cyanosis points with certainty to *patent ductus arteriosus* and narrow splitting of the second heart sound is an additional useful clue. Calcification of the ductus is rare. *Atrial septal defect* is far more frequent in women and cyanosis and symptoms do not appear before adult life—a distinctly split second sound that does not vary with respiration is diagnostic. The definitive diagnosis of individual causes of Eisenmenger syndrome requires cardiac catheterization, dye-dilution techniques, and angiography.

The course of the disease is one of progressive cyanosis. Massive hemoptysis and ill-advised surgical intervention are the leading causes of death. Without operation death usually occurs in the fourth decade. The treatment is medical and small venesections may be helpful for polycythemia. Direct repair of the defect in cases where the pulmonary vascular resistance is over 10 units and the pulmonary blood flow less than twice the systemic leads to rapid right ventricular failure.

Common Mixing Lesions

The term "common mixing lesion" refers to those anomalies in which, by virtue of the abnormal anatomy, there is obligatory mixing of pulmonary venous and systemic blood:

1. *At atrial level*: Total anomalous pulmonary venous drainage, common atrium, tricuspid atresia, and aortic atresia.
2. *At ventricular level*: Single ventricle, double outlet right ventricle, and transposition of the great vessels.
3. *Aortopulmonary level*: Persistent truncus arteriosus.

In the absence of pulmonary stenosis, pulmonary blood flow is increased and cyanosis is present. When pulmonary vascular disease and pulmonary arterial hypertension complicate the picture, pulmonary blood flow is reduced and cyanosis becomes more intense.

Total Anomalous Pulmonary Venous Drainage

Instead of joining the left atrium, all the pulmonary veins join a venous recess above the left atrium. From here one major venous channel leaves to join a systemic vein or the right atrium (Fig. 10.27). The ultimate venous connection is either supradiaphragmatic or infradiaphragmatic. In the infradiaphragmatic type a long vein traverses the esophageal hiatus of the diaphragm to join the portal vein or the ductus venosus. These sites are intrinsically stenotic and an additional obstruction is offered by the liver.

The supradiaphragmatic type is characterized by an ascending vertical vein leaving the common venous recess to join, most commonly, the left innominate vein, the coronary sinus (Fig. 10.28), or the superior vena cava. Occasionally, the pulmonary veins enter the right atrium independently. A patent foramen ovale or an atrial septal defect is universally present

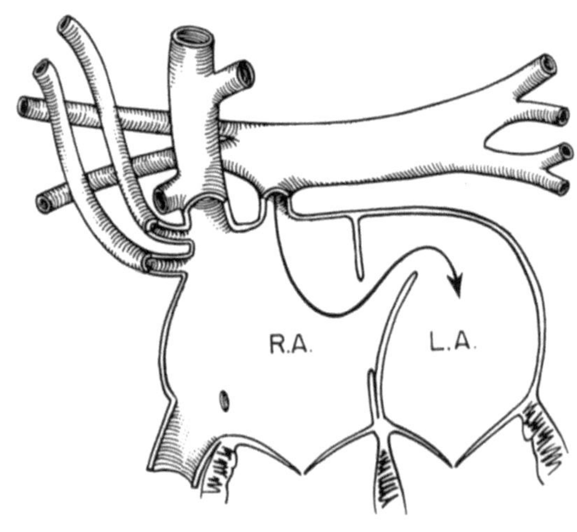

FIGURE 10.27. Total anomalous pulmonary venous drainage to the right atrium. The common pulmonary vein drains directly into the right atrium and there is right-to-left shunt at atrial level. Reprtinted, with permission, from Nakib A, et al.: Anomalies of the pulmonary veins. Am J Cardiol 20:77–90, 1967.

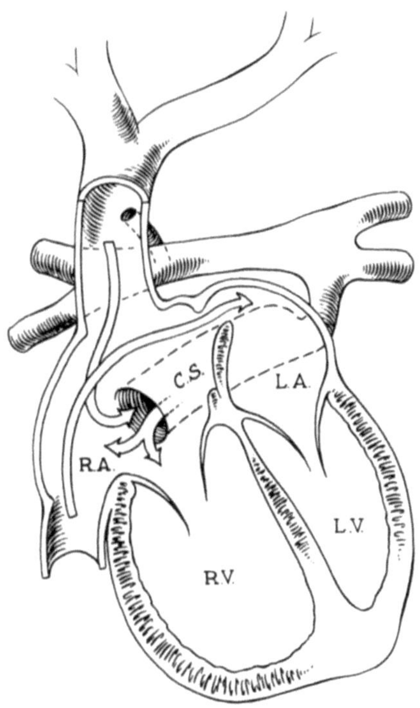

FIGURE 10.28. Total anomalous pulmonary venous drainage into coronary sinus.

and is the route by which systemic and pulmonary venous blood enters the left atrium. Obstruction to pulmonary venous drainage is universal in the subdiaphragmatic type, but may also complicate the supradiaphraglnatic type and the site of obstruction in the latter is between the left pulmonary artery in the front and the left main bronchus at the back.

Hemodynamics

When pulmonary venous obstruction is absent, the hemodynamics are very similar to that of a large atrial septal defect except for complete admixture of the pulmonary and systemic venous returns. The right atrial pressure is higher than the left to provide adequate filling of the left ventricle. Should there be any degree of obstruction at the foramen ovale the right atrial pressure will be even further elevated. The elevated right atrial pressure of necessity must increase the pulmonary venous pressure and passively the pulmonary arterial pressure.

In patients without obstruction to pulmonary venous return there is a progressive increase in pulmonary blood flow resulting in very large pulmonary-to-systemic flow ratio and therefore relatively high arterial oxygen saturation. In the absence of obstruction the changes in the pulmonary circulation are similar to those in patients with large atrial septal defect. Intimal proliferation occurs gradually and in late adolescence there is an increasing incidence of pulmonary vascular obstruction.

Clinical Features

Cyanosis is frequently present at birth and is usually followed by evidence of congestive cardiac failure within the first few weeks of life. Cardiomegaly and a prominent lift is present at the left lower sternal border as a result of the overloaded right ventricle. A systolic ejection murmur is detected at the upper left sternal border and represents increased pulmonary blood flow, as in atrial septal defect. The second sound is widely split and shows little variation with respiration. Frequently, there is a third sound and a tricuspid middiastolic rumble at the lower left sternal border. In those patients where an ascending vertical vein enters the left innominate vein, a high frequency continuous murmur may be present just below the left clavicle; it originates from turbulence in the venous connection.

The *electrocardiogram* demonstrates peaked P waves, right ventricular hypertrophy, and right axis deviation. The *chest X-ray* shows an enlarged heart because of right ventricular and right atrial prominence. The main pulmonary artery is enlarged and there is marked increase in pulmonary arterial vascular markings. In the case of drainage of the left ascending vertical vein into the innominate vein the mediastinal shadow is enlarged on both sides of the spine giving rise to the classical "figure eight" or "snowman" appearance; this sign is observed only after 4 months of age. Echocardiography may contribute to diagnosis by demonstrating paradoxical motion of the septum and an enlarged right ventricle.

The diagnosis is confirmed by cardiac catheterization which shows (1) evidence of admixture at the right atrial level leading to similar oxygen saturations in all cardiac chambers, aorta and pulmonary artery; (2) catheter may enter the anomalous trunk and angiography from this site will demonstrate its course and any site of obstruction; and (3) pulmonary angiography may show the anomalous venous connection.

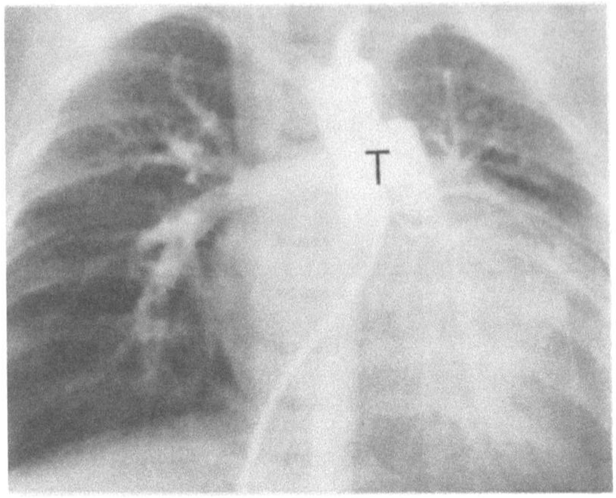

FIGURE 10.30. Aortogram in truncus arteriosus (T) demonstrating a common truncal valve, simultaneous opacification of the pulmonary arteries, which arise independently from the aorta.

Differential Diagnosis

Single atrium has virtually the identical clinical presentation but the important clue at the bedside is the presence of left axis deviation, which is almost always present. Similarly, *endocardial cushion defect* complicated by pulmonary stenosis and resultant cyanosis will be distinguished by the same electrocardiographic feature. However, with *common mixing lesions* such as single ventricle, the diagnosis must be made by echocardiography, catheterization, and angiography. The severe form of *Ebstein's disease*, particularly when associated with pulmonary stenosis, may produce a similar clinical picture. The distinguishing features are the electrocardiogram, which shows right bundle branch block with low voltage, and chest X-ray, which shows normal or decreased pulmonary vascularity.

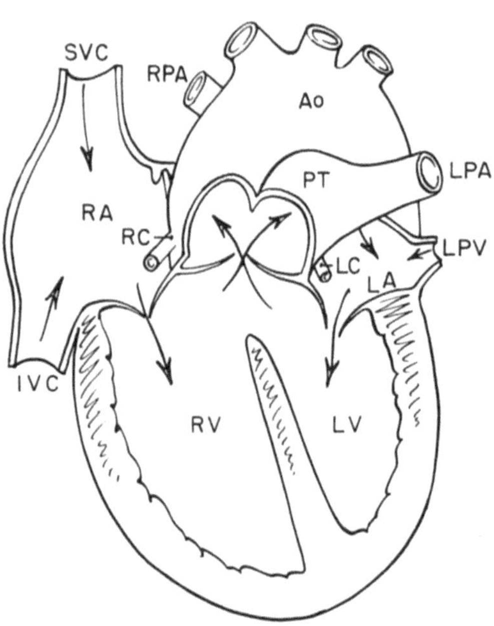

FIGURE 10.29. Diagram of anatomy of truncus arteriosus showing a common truncal valve from which the aorta and the pulmonary trunk arise. A ventricular septal defect is present. Bidirectional shunting occurs in the truncus. Reprinted, with permission, from Edwards JE: Classification of congenital heart disease in the adult. Cardiovascular Clinics 10:I, 1979, F.A. Davis Company.

Treatment of this condition is now amenable to total correction using cardiopulmonary bypass. The pulmonary venous recess is anastomosed to the left atrium, the atrial is communication closed, and the ascending vertical vein is ligated.

Truncus Arteriosus

This anomaly consists of a single great vessel with a single semilunar valve arising from both ventricles with subjacent ventricular septal defect. The pulmonary arteries arise from the truncus via a common trunk or independently (Figs. 10.29 and 10.30). Insufficiency of the truncul valve is not uncommon.

Hemodynamics

The effect of the truncus is to produce mixing of left- and right-sided blood immediately above the truncal valve. The pulmonary blood flow is determined by the pulmonary vascular resistance, which in turn determines systemic arterial oxygen saturation. In cases with high pulmonary blood flow, systemic saturation may be only mildly reduced.

Clinical Features

In the first few weeks of life severe heart failure and cyanosis are frequent because of torrential pulmonary blood flow. The pulses may be bounding in character and the pulse pressure wide. The heart is considerably enlarged and involves both ventricles.

The second heart sound is loud and single and frequently there is a murmur of truncal insufficiency. A prominent aortic ejection click is an important diagnostic clue and should lead to consideration of the diagnosis of truncus in any infant who has this finding. Most patients have a systolic murmur and thrill in the third and fourth left intercostal space, like that of a ventricular septal defect. Continuous murmurs are uncommon. A middiastolic rumble related to torrential mitral flow is frequently heard at the apex. When pulmonary blood flow is decreased, cyanosis may be a prominent finding.

The *electrocardiogram* shows a normal QRS axis and biventricular hypertrophy. The *chest X-ray* confirms cardiomegaly and demonstrates increase in the pulmonary arterial vasculature (Fig. 10.31). A right-sided aorta is present in a third of patients and is a helpful diagnostic feature.

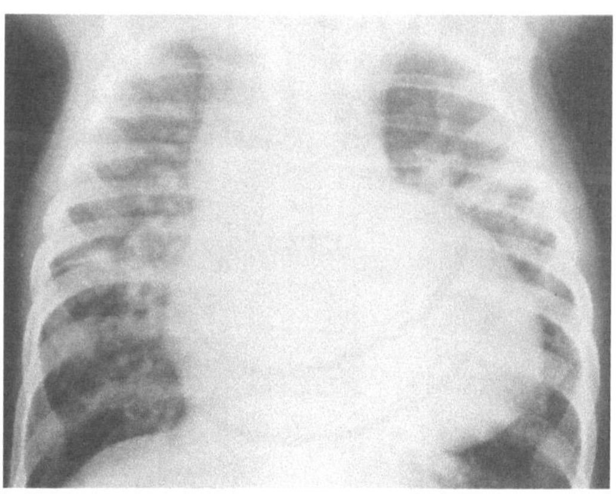

FIGURE 10.31. X-ray of the chest in truncus arteriosus demonstrating marked cardiomegaly, severe pulmonary plethora, and absence of the main pulmonary artery segment.

The differential diagnosis included other conditions associated with cyanosis, cardiac failure, and increased pulmonary blood flow. These include transposition of the great vessels, tricuspid atresia without pulmonary stenosis, single ventricle, double outlet right ventricle, and total anomalous pulmonary venous drainage.

Management

In infants with severe uncontrollable cardiac failure, banding of the pulmonary artery is the only procedure available. In older children complete repair is possible and this is done by closing the ventricular septal defect, inserting an aortic homograft and aortic valve, and connecting the right ventricle to the pulmonary artery.

Tricuspid Atresia with Increased Pulmonary Blood Flow

Hemodynamics

When tricuspid atresia is associated with a large ventricular septal defect in the absence of pulmonary stenosis, there is considerable increase in pulmonary blood flow. Provided the pulmonary vascular resistance is not high, the large pulmonary blood flow may result in a near normal arterial oxygen saturation. When these hemodynamics exist the great vessels may be normally related or transposed.

Clinical Features

This is one of mild cyanosis, considerable increase in pulmonary blood flow, and heart failure. A loud pansystolic murmur is usually present at the lower left sternal border and a middiastolic rumble is present at the apex. The second heart sound is narrowly split and the pulmonary component is increased. The *chest X-ray* demonstrates marked cardiomegaly, left atrial enlargement, and marked pulmonary plethora, but the findings are not distinctive.

The *electrocardiogram* helps distinguish the condition from other causes of cyanosis and increased pulmonary blood flow. Characteristically, there is left axis deviation with evidence of left ventricular hypertrophy and right atrial enlargment. Right ventricular forces are usually absent and are present only occasionally in instances where the great vessels are normally related. Although these features are very helpful in excluding transposition of the great vessels and total anomalous pulmonary venous drainage, they do not exclude the diagnosis of single ventricle where the electrocardiogram may be identical.

Therapy consists of a medical regime for heart failure; and banding should be avoided wherever possible because clinical improvement is not uncommon as a result of spontaneous decrease in size of the ventricular septal defect or development of infundibular stenosis.

Double Outlet Right Ventricle without Pulmonary Stenosis

In its typical form this malformation is characterized by the origin of both great vessels from the right ventricle. Both aortic and pulmonary valves are at the same level and the aorta usually lies to the right of the pulmonary artery. Characteristically, there is discontinuity between the semilunar and atrioventricular valves. A ventricular septal defect is almost invariably present and its position and the state of the pulmonary valve determine the pulmonary blood flow.

Hemodynamics

When the ventricular septal defect is below the pulmonary valve (and pulmonary stenosis is absent) streaming of left ventricular blood into the pulmonary artery, and right ventricular blood into the aorta, results in cyanosis with high pulmonary blood flow. This is known as the Taussig–Bing malformation.

When the ventricular septal defect is subaortic, the hemodynamics resemble that of a large left-to-right shunt, because there is relatively little mixing within the right ventricle and cyanosis may be absent.

The *Taussig–Bing malformation* (subpulmonary VSD without pulmonary stenosis) must be included in the differential diagnosis of cyanosis and pulmonary plethora. Patients with the condition are cyanotic from birth and have clinical evidence of severe pulmonary hypertension. The condition is particularly difficult to distinguish from transposition of the great vessels with large ventricular septal defect. Helpful features are radiological evidence of a narrow mediastinum in transposition and an electrocardiogram that sometimes shows left axis deviation in double outlet right ventricle. Usually, however, the diagnosis is made by catheterization and angiography, which in itself is difficult and rests on recognition of the single most important feature, the presence of mitral–semilunar discontinuity. Echocardiography is helpful in demonstrating this phenomenon.

Single Ventricle without Pulmonary Stenosis

In single ventricle (Figs. 10.32 A 10.33) there is one ventricular chamber receiving both

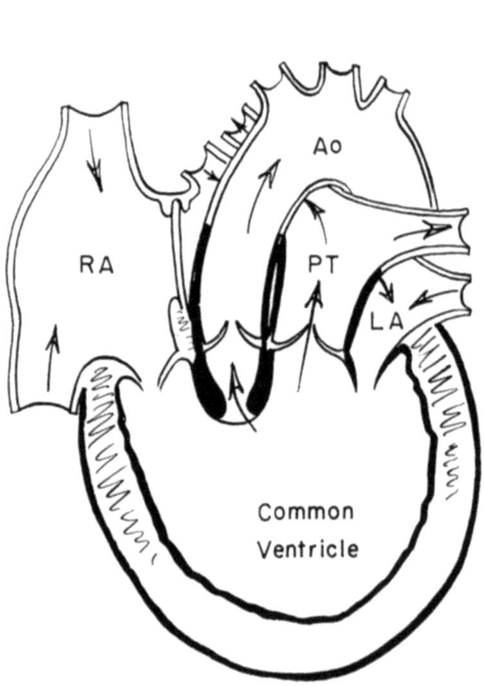

FIGURE 10.32. Anatomy of single ventricle without pulmonary stenosis, the aorta arising from a rudimentary chamber. Reprinted, with permission, from Edwards JE: Classification of congenital heart disease in the adult. Cardiovascular clinics 10:I, 1979. F.A. Davis Company.

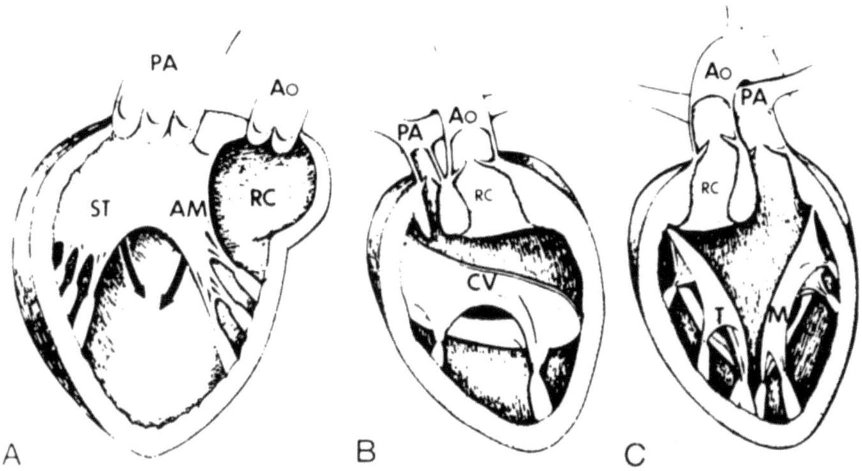

FIGURE 10.33. Anatomy of the atrioventricular valve in single ventricle (A) conjoined septal tricuspid (ST) and anterior mitral leaflets (AM), (B) a common atrioventricular valve (CV), and (C) two separate valves. RC, rudimentary chamber. Reprinted, with permission, from Chesler E, et al.: Echocardiography in the diagnosis of congenital heart disease. Ped Clin N Am 18:1163, 1971.

atrioventricular valves or a common atrioventricular valve. A small outlet chamber is present and this represents the infundibular portion of the right ventricle—the sinus portion is absent. Either the aorta or the pulmonary artery arises from the outlet chamber, thereby communicating with the body of the single ventricle. In one-fifth of patients an outlet chamber cannot be identified and the single ventricle is therefore called "primitive." Transposition of the great vessels occurs in approximately 80% of the patients.

Clinical Features

This is related to associated defects. Severe pulmonary stenosis will produce a picture similar to that of Tetralogy of Fallot. When pulmonary stenosis is absent the clinical picture is one of high pulmonary blood flow, cyanosis, and congestive cardiac failure.

Clinical examination is usually not helpful in arousing the suspicion of single ventricle. A systolic murmur may be produced by high pulmonary blood flow and is unhelpful. The *electrocardiogram* may provide a clue by demonstrating electrocardiographic features found in corrected transposition (i.e., a QR pattern in the right precordial leads and absence of Q waves in the left precordial leads). When the great vessels are in the D-transposition profile, the electrocardiogram may resemble that of tricuspid atresia with right ventricular forces and left ventricular hypertrophy.

Radiology

The identification of L-transposition (aorta anterior and to the left) is suggested by a straight or convex contour of the left upper heart border. L-transposition of the great vessels points to the diagnosis of either *corrected transposition* or *single ventricle*. *Echocardiography* demonstrates absence of a ventricular septum and a large single anteriorly moving atrioventricular valve, features that are extremely helpful in the diagnosis. The definitive diagnosis must be made by cardiac catheterization.

Transposition of the Great Vessels

This important anomaly is characterized anatomically by the aorta rising from the right ventricle and lying anteriorly to the pulmonary artery, which arises from the left ventricle. The aortic valve is situated anteriorly, superiorly, and to the right because it is supported by the normal infundibulum of the right ventricle, which is the most anterior portion of the heart.

The pulmonary valve lies posterior to the aortic valve and because there is no infundibulum (or conus) in the left ventricle, there is therefore *mitral–pulmonary continuity*. The atria and the connections of the superior and inferior vena cavae and the pulmonary veins are usually normal.

Because the transposed aorta lies anteriorly and to the right of the pulmonary artery it is frequently referred to as *dextro- or D-transposition*. Associated malformations such as ventricular and atrial septal defects, patent ductus arteriosus, and pulmonary stenosis are quite frequent and determine the hemodynamics, resultant clinical picture, and prognosis.

Hemodynamics

In the absence of a communication between the left and right sides of the heart, systemic venous blood from the vena cava will be delivered by the right heart into the aorta; pulmonary venous blood entering the left atrium will be returned to the lungs via the pulmonary artery. The potential for this situation exists when there is the normal postnatal closure of the ductus arteriosus and foramen ovale.

For survival, systemic venous blood must enter the pulmonary circulation to be oxygenated, and pulmonary venous blood must enter the systemic circulation to oxygenate the tissues (a bidirectional shunt). Bidirectional shunting permits survival, and may occur through normal channels such as the foramen ovale, and/or a patent ductus arteriosus or abnormal channels such as ventricular and/or atrial septal defects (Figs. 10.34–10.37). Usually, at birth there is patency of the foramen ovale, but the increase in pulmonary blood flow raises the left atrial pressure, which partially or completely seals the flap of the fora-

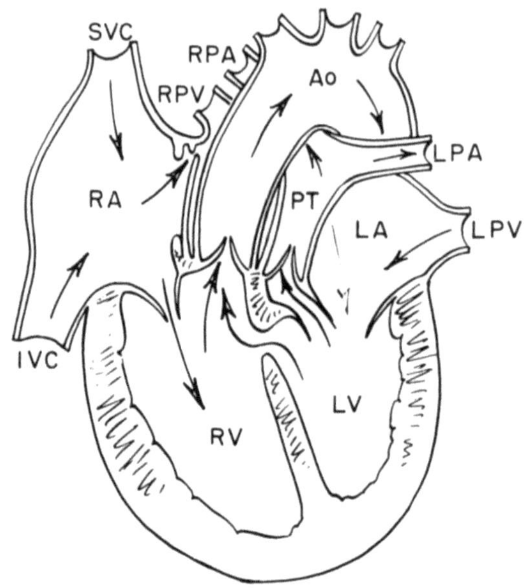

FIGURE 10.35. Diagram of complete transposition of the great vessels with subpulmonary stenosis and ventricular septal defect. There is favorable streaming of left ventricular blood into the aorta because the VSD is proximal,to the subpulmonary stenosis. Reprinted, with permission, from Edwards JE, et al.: A review of congenital anomalies of the heart and great vessels according to functional categories . Ped Clin N Am 2(1), 1964.

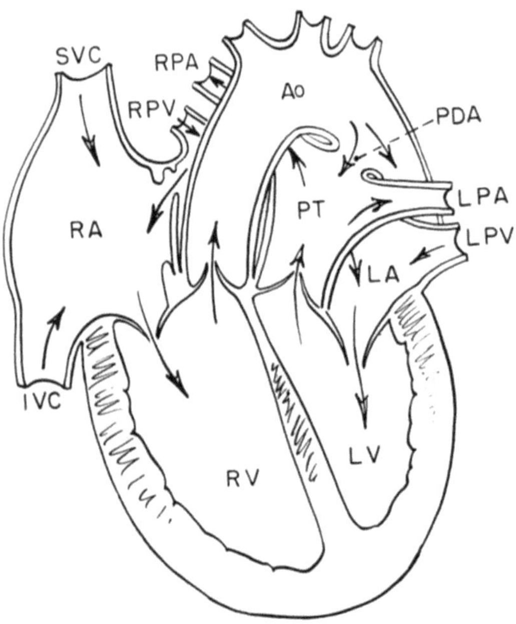

FIGURE 10.34. Diagram of complete transposition of the great vessels with patent ductus arteriosus and interatrial communication. Reprinted, with permission, from Edwards JE, et al.: A review of congenital anomalies of the heart and great vessels according to functional categories. Ped Clinic N Am 2(1), 1964.

men ovale and diminishes the shunt; severe hypoxia, acidosis, and hypoglycemia result.

When a large ventricular septal defect is present, adequate mixing occurs, cyanosis may be minimal, but severe cardiac failure is frequent when the pulmonary vascular resistance drops. Eventually, however, pulmonary vascular damage and intimal proliferation increase the pulmonary vascular resistance with amelioration of the heart failure but with progressive disability resulting from cyanosis and hypoxia.

When a large ventricular septal defect is accompanied by severe pulmonary stenosis, shunting is from the left ventricle to the right ventricle, thus delivering pulmonary venous blood to the systemic circulation; systemic venous blood is shunted from right atrium to left atrium through the foramen ovale. This favorable situation may be adversely altered by early closure of the ductus before the bronchial circulation has developed. Under these circumstances, pulmonary blood flow would be critically reduced and severe hypoxia results. When the ductus closes in the presence of a well-developed bronchial circulation, the situation is similar to that of Tetralogy of Fallot, but not as favorable, because blood entering the pulmonary artery from the left ventricle is well oxygenated and returns to the lungs, and therefore hypoxia is more severe.

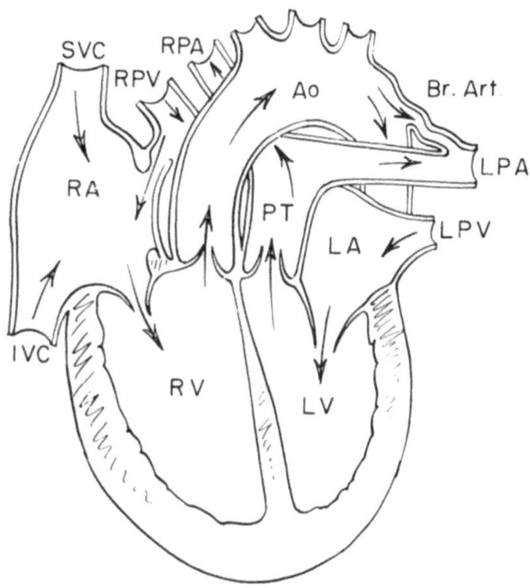

FIGURE 10.37. Diagram of complete transposition of the great vessels with an interatrial communication, intact ventricular septum, closed ductus arteriosius, and enlarged bronchial arteries. From Edwards JE, et al.: A review of congenital anomalies of the heart and great vessels according to functional categories. Reprinted, with Permission, from Ped Clin N Am 2(1), 1964.

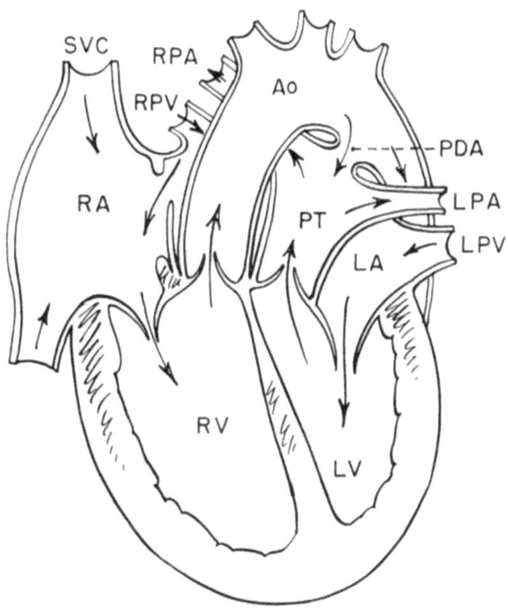

FIGURE 10.36. Diagram of complete transposition of the great vessels, intact ventricular septum, interatrial communication and patent ductus arteriosus. Reprinted, with permission, from Educarts JE, et al.: A review of congenital anomalies of the heat and great vessels according to functional categories. Ped Clin N Am 2(1), 1964.

Clinical Features

Transposition of the great vessels is the commonest cause of death in the neonatal period and is second only to Tetralogy of Fallot as a cause of cyanotic congenital heart disease. The condition is at least twice as common in the male as it is in the female.

Cyanosis in an otherwise apparently healthy infant is usually the presenting finding. At first, the physical examination and the electrocardiogram are unremarkable. By the end of the first week cyanosis becomes severe and is accompanied by hypoxia and acidosis. The pulses are readily palpable and evidence of concestive cardiac failure is uncommon. Auscultation may reveal a systolic murmur of ejection type at the left sternal border, but is otherwise unimpressive. With progressive hypoxia, the *chest X-ray* will demonstrate increasing cardiac enlargement and an increase in pulmonary vascularity. The most helpful radiological diagnostic feature is the combination of a narrow mediastinum (resulting from the posteriorly situated pulmonary artery) combined with an increase in the pulmonary arterial markings. The characteristic "egg-on-side" appearance is often difficult to detect (Fig. 10.38).

When transposition is associated with *large ventricular septal defect* marked increase in pulmonary blood flow usually leads to cardiac failure within 2 to 3 weeks. Cyanosis is less intense and there is clinical evidence of cardiomegaly and marked hepatomegaly. A gallop rhythm and a middiastolic flow murmur is present at the apex. The second sound is split and a pansystolic murmur may be heard at the left sternal border. The chest X-ray demonstrates considerably cardiomegaly, a narrow mediastinum, and marked increase in pulmonary arterial vasculature. The electrocardiogram shows right axis deviation and right ventricular hypertrophy. Progressive heart failure and pulmonary edema are characteristic and frequently lead to early death. Should infants survive the period of left ventricular failure, chronic cardiac failure, frequent respiratory infections, and the risk of a rising pulmonary vascular resistance complicate the course of the disease.

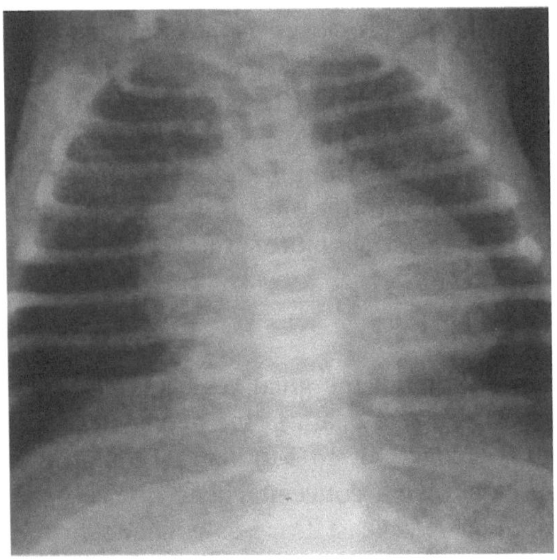

FIGURE 10.38. Chest X-ray in complete transposition of the great vessels showing the typical "egg-on-side" appearance.

Not infrequently, transposition and ventricular septal defect are complicated by the presence of severe pulmonary stenosis and the picture may then be indistinguishable from Tetralogy of Fallot. A holosystolic murmur is present at the left sternal border and the second heart sound is single. The distinction from Tetralogy of Fallot can be made only by cardiac catheterization.

The *differential diagnosis* of transposition of the great vessels includes pulmonary atresia, severe pulmonary stenosis, and Tetralogy of Fallot, which can usually be excluded by the detection of splitting of the second heart sound and the presence of decreased pulmonary vascular markings. The electrocardiogram will readily exclude tricuspid atresia and pulmonary stenosis by demonstrating left axis deviation and absence of R waves over the right chest leads. Echocardiography is helpful in excluding single ventricle and aortic atresia.

The *idiopathic respiratory stress syndrome* occurs more commonly in premature infants in contrast to babies with transposition who are frequently large and overweight. The respiratory difficulty in transposition consists of increased depth and rate of breathing and differs from the grunting respiration associated and the sternal retraction of the respiratory distress syndrome. Chest radiography in the respiratory distress syndrome shows diffuse infiltrates in the lung, areas of atelectasis, or a granular appearance. The administration of 100% oxygen to an infant with respiratory distress leads to significant increase in the arterial p_{O_2}, whereas in transposition the rise in p_{O_2} is minimal or absent.

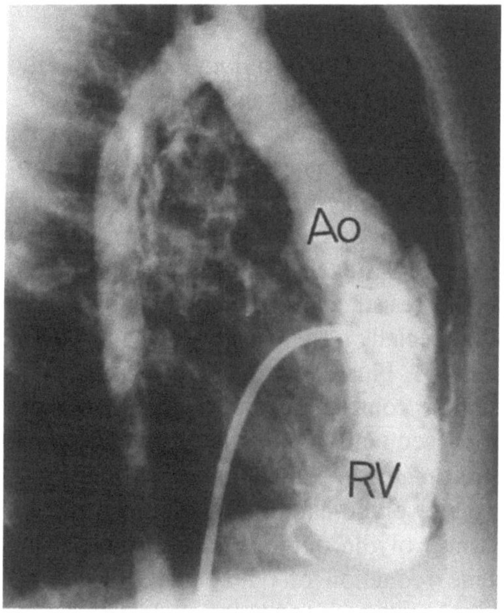

FIGURE 10.39. Lateral right ventricular and left ventricular angiograms showing aorta arising from the right ventricle and the pulmonary artery from the left ventricle in transposition of the great vessels.

Treatment

Emergency cardiac catheterization is mandatory once the suspicion of transposition of the great vessels is aroused. The procedure is both diagnostic and therapeutic (Fig. 10.39). Balloon atrial septostomy, if properly performed, will create an adequate atrial septal defect, improving mixing at atrial level, with a rapid amelioration of symptoms. Without this procedure at least one-half of the children will die within 1 month of birth and 90% within the first year. Elective repair using the *Mustard operation* is generally recommended at 18 months of age or earlier if there are signs of increasing pulmonary vascular resistance or worsening hypoxia. The operation consists of excision of the atrial septum, inserting a new atrial septum made from pericardium in a position such that pulmonary venous blood is routed to the right ventricle and aorta via the tricuspid valve. For those patients with transposition, large ventricular septal defect, and pulmonary arterial hypertension, repair should be performed within 6 months of age to avoid pulmonary vascular disease. When there is pulmonary stenosis and ventricular septal defect a shunt procedure is indicated as a palliative procedure so that elective repair may be performed at a later date.

In several centers the "arterial switch" procedure is gaining favor. This consists of transecting the aorta and pulmonary arteries and switching them to the correct position and reimplanting the coronary arteries.

Cyanosis Present: Decreased Pulmonary Vasculature

Tetralogy of Fallot

The term Tetralogy of Fallot has for almost a century been applied to the combination of ventricular septal defect, pulmonary stenosis, overriding aorta, and right ventricular hypertrophy. The important abnormalities are pulmonary stenosis and ventricular septal defect. The stenosis is infundibular in approximately two-thirds of the cases and mainly valvar in the rest. Infundibular and valvar stenosis of varying degree frequently coexist. The ventricular septal defect involves the membranous septum just below the aortic valve, which is nearly always competent. The aorta is large, carrying most of the output of both ventricles; it is more anterior than usual and apparently overrides the septal defect. A right-sided aorta is frequent (10–20%). The pulmonary arteries are small and may be hypoplastic; the bronchial collateral circulation from the aorta may be extensive.

Tetralogy of Fallot is the commonest cause of cyanotic congenital heart disease, accounting for approximately two-thirds of these cases. Males are affected about twice as frequently as females. The severity of the stenosis (hence the pulmonary blood flow), and not the overriding aorta, determines the symptoms and degree of cyanosis.

Hemodynamics

Hemodynamically (Fig. 10.40), tetralogy can be considered as a single pumping chamber

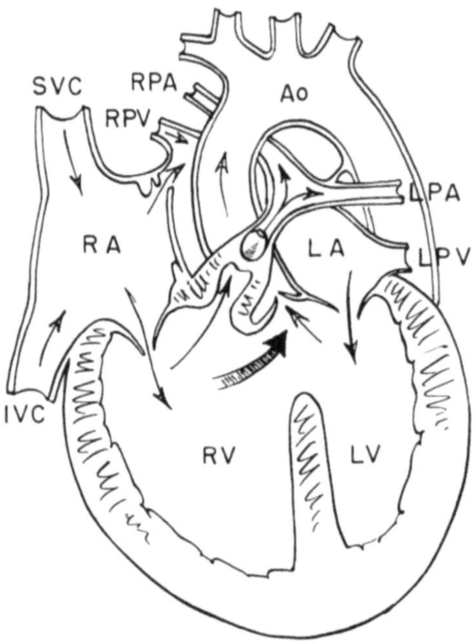

FIGURE 10.40. Diagram of the central circulation in Tetralogy of Fallot. Pulmonary blood flow is determined by the relative resistances in the pulmonary and systemic circuits since there is a large ventricular septal defect. Reprinted, with permission, from Edwards JE: Classification of congenital heart disease in the adult. Cardiovascular Clinics 10:I, 1979, F.A. Davis Company.

with two resistances: (1) systemic resistance and (2) resistance offered by the stenotic outflow tract of the right ventricle. The more severe the stenosis, the more preferential is blood flow into the aorta rather than the lungs.

Adaptation is achieved by bronchial collaterals, so that in the extreme case (pulmonary atresia) the pulmonary circulation is entirely maintained by collaterals. Unlike severe pulmonary stenosis with intact ventricular septum, pulmonary blood flow in tetralogy is limited by the systemic resistance, since the ventricular septal defect is almost always nonrestrictive. In the presence of severe pulmonary outflow tract stenosis, blood is preferentially ejected from the right ventricle into the systemic circuit—the lesser of the two resistances. In milder cases, particularly *acyanotic tetralogy*, the pulmonary outflow obstruction is less severe and offers less resistance to flow than the systemic resistance. A slight left-to-right shunt may even be present at rest.

Between extreme tetralogy and acyanotic tetralogy there is a wide spectrum. Rarely, the systemic resistance is elevated (coexisting coarctation of the aorta or systemic hypertension) and this may promote pulmonary blood flow. Squatting is beneficial by increasing the peripheral resistance. Like the systemic resistance the resistance to pulmonary flow is not fixed, expecially if there is muscular infundibular stenosis. Fluctuation in the intensity of infundibular contraction affects the resistance, and consequently pulmonary blood flow. *Cyanotic attacks*, characteristic of severe tetralogy, may well be due to increased contraction ("spasm") of the outflow tract, producing an extreme reduction of pulmonary blood flow. The earlier the infundibulum "clamps down" the more severe the obstruction. Furthermore, as the heart grows, the stenosis may remain relatively fixed, or infundibular hypertrophy may increase, aggravating the stenosis. This may account for the conversion of ventricular septal defect with pulmonary stenosis to Tetralogy of Fallot.

In Tetralogy of Fallot the murmur is produced by blood flow across the stenotic outflow tract; the septal defect is silent. The length and loudness of this murmur reflect the volume and rate of blood ejected through the stenosis.

Clinical Features

Cyanosis is usually absent at birth, except in very severe cases. It usually appears in early infancy and is progressive. Polycythemia and equal clubbing of the fingers and toes develop with increasing cyanosis. Syncopal attacks associated with intense cyanosis, convulsions, and unconsciousness are usually associated with periods of stress and effort, such as crying and feeding. The degree of cyanosis is not necessarily related to the severity of syncopal attacks. In fact, apparently well-nourished, relatively acyanotic, infants are often subject to repeated, alarming spells.

Growth and development are generally impaired and normal milestones delayed. Once the child begins to walk, squatting on effort is highly suggestive of the condition. Bacterial endocarditis, paradoxical embolism, cerebral arterial, and venous thrombosis are constant hazards. The latter is particularly liable to occur when polycythemic patients become dehydrated. Cardiac failure is extremely uncommon and is usually due to myocardial disease or associated malformations. Iron deficiency anemia is not rare and may easily be missed in the presence of a normal red cell count. Metabolic acidosis is commonly associated with severe tissue hypoxia. In extreme cases of polycythemia, gout may develop.

The *jugular venous pressure* is usually normal and a dominant "a" wave is uncommon. The pulse is normal and the extremities are warm. Cardiomegaly is usually absent, except when there is severe anemia. The apex beat is formed by the right ventricle with little or no lift over the parasternum.

Pulsation in the second and third left space is occasionally present, unlike pulmonary stenosis with intact septum, and a further important differential point is the palpable second sound of aortic valve closure. A systolic thrill accompanies loud murmurs. The aorta being large and anteroposed is responsible for these findings.

Except in cyanotic attacks, when the murmur is soft or absent, an ejection murmur is nearly always present, maximal in the second to fourth left intercostal spaces. The severity of the stenosis can be determined from the length of the murmur. In acyanotic tetralogy there is a loud long murmur and thrill, and a soft localized P_2 widely separated from A_2. Increasingly severe stenosis is associated with a shorter, earlier, and softer systolic murmur. In extreme tetralogy, the murmur is invariably short, soft and associated with an aortic click.

The use of vasoactive drugs is helpful in clinical diagnosis. *Amyl nitrite* inhalation produces a fall in both systemic and right ventricular systolic pressures, an increased venous return, an increase in right-to-left shunt, and cyanosis. The reduced right ventricular pressure results in diminution in pulmonary flow, which is reflected by a decrease in the intensity and duration of the systolic murmur. *Phenylephrine* (or other pressor drugs) elevates systemic and right ventricular pressures, increases the pressure gradient across the stenosis, augments pulmonary blood flow, and reduces the right-to-left shunt. This is reflected by marked intensification and prolongation of the murmur, intensification' of the pulmonary second sound, and diminution of cyanosis. The behavior of the murmur with these drugs clearly differentiates pulmonary stenosis with intact ventricular septum from tetralogy.

The *electrocardiogram* shows right ventricular hypertrophy with a tall R wave in V1. Commonly, there is a rapid transition to an R/S pattern in V2. It is rare to find severe right ventricular hypertrophy with inverted T waves anteriorly. Right axis deviation is generally present. Right atrial hypertrophy is a frequent finding.

The *chest X-ray* shows that the heart is normal in size and in half the patients the shape is normal. Pulmonary oligemia is present, and occasionally bronchial arterial collaterals can be recognized. A characteristic appearance is the "coeur en sabot" with an up-tilted apex, concavity in the region of the pulmonary artery, and small peripheral pulmonary arteries (Fig. 10.41). Occasionally an infundibular

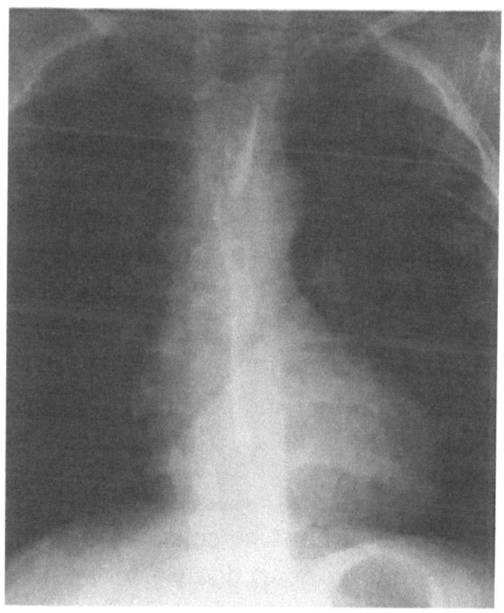

FIGURE 10.41. Chest X-ray in Tetralogy of Fallot showing the typical boot-shaped appearance of the heart and pulmonary oligemia.

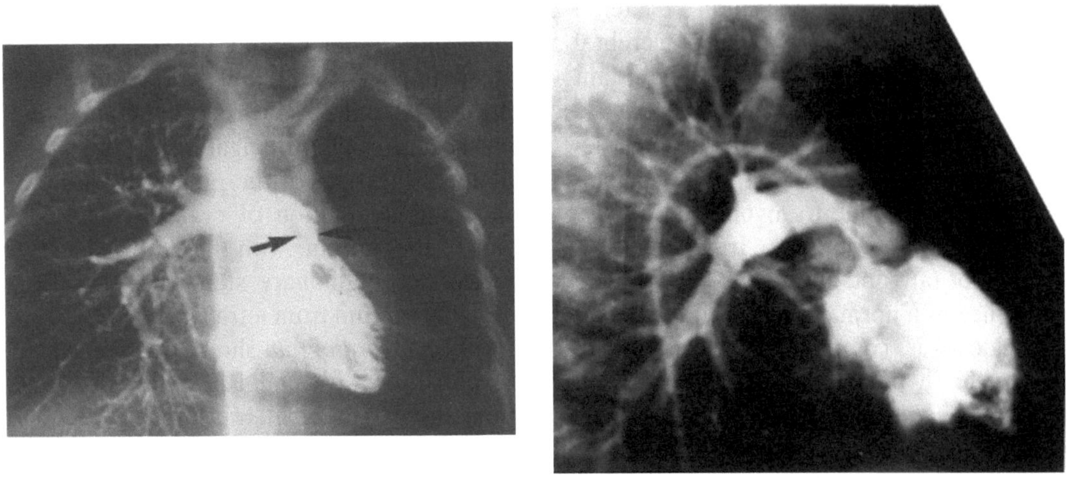

FIGURE 10.42. Biplane right ventricular angiogram in Tetralogy of Fallot demonstrating severe infundibular stenosis (arrows) and thickened pulmonary valve (above), and right-sided aorta opacified by the right-to-left shunt. The left pulmonary artery is absent.

chamber produces a slight bulge on the left cardiac border but poststenotic dilatation of the pulmonary artery is absent. A right-sided aorta is highly suggestive of this anomaly.

Cardiac catheterization shows equal systemic and right ventricular pressures and normal or low pulmonary artery pressure. The site of stenosis, whether valvar or infundibular, is sometimes difficult to determine from pressure tracings. The presence of a ventricular septal defect is proved by passing the catheter into the aorta from the right ventricle. It is difficult to assess the severity of the condition by pressures or saturation data. However, the magnitude and direction of shunts can be more easily determined by dye-dilution techniques. Angiocardiography is the method of choice for establishing the diagnosis and for depicting the abnormal anatomy (Fig. 10.42).

Diagnosis

Tetralogy of Fallot must be considered in any patient with cyanotic heart disease with normal or diminished pulmonary blood flow. It must be differentiated from pulmonary stenosis associated with other congenital anomalies and from pulmonary and tricuspid atresia.

Pulmonary stenosis with intact ventricular

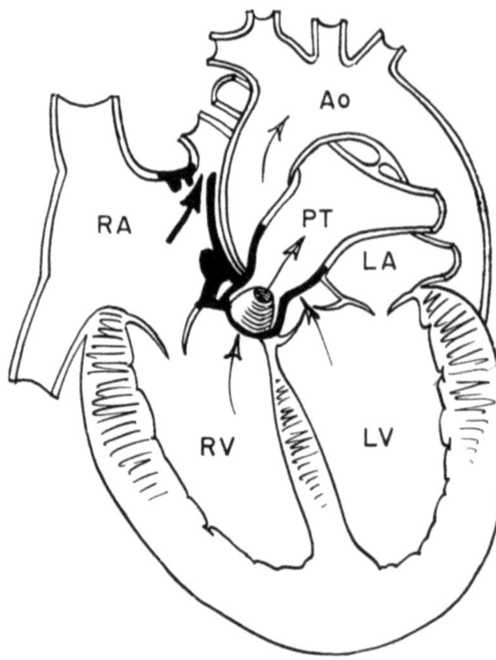

FIGURE 10.43. Diagram of the central circulation in Trilogy of Fallot. The ventricular septum in intact and cyanosis results from a right-to-left shunt at atrial level. Reprinted, with permission, from Edwards JE: Classification of congenital heart disease in the adult. Cardiovascular Clinics 10:I, 1979, F.A. Davis Company.

TABLE 10.1. Clinical distinction between tetralogy and trilogy of fallot.

	Tetralogy	Trilogy
Cyanosis and clubbing	Early	Late
Hyperteleorism	No	Yes
Cyanotic spells	Common	Uncommon
Squatting	Common	Uncommon
Heart failure	Very rare	Common
Cardiomegaly	Very rare	Common
S_4 Gallop	Very rare	Common
Giant "a" wave	Absent	Common
X-ray: pulmonary artery	Pulmonary bay	Post stenotic dilatation
Aorta	Right-sided 25%	Normal
Murmur	Short	Long
P_2	Absent	Soft and late
Ejection click	Aortic	Pulmonary
ECG	Moderate RVH	Severe RVH

septum and reversed atrial shunt (Trilogy of Fallot) generally gives rise to the most difficulty (Fig. 10.43). Helpful clues are given in Table 10.1.

In infants transposition of the great vessels with pulmonary stenosis, double outlet right ventricle, and common ventricle with pulmonary stenosis cannot be differentiated except by two-dimensional echocardiography and angiocardioyraphy.

Acyanotic tetralogy must be distinguished from isolated ventricular septal defect, pulmonary stenosis with intact ventricular septum, and tricuspid disease.

Medical Management

This is mainly directed at the treatment of cyanotic attacks, correction of anemia, dehydration, and metabolic acidosis.

Cyanotic Attack

The infant must be placed in the knee-chest position and given oxygen. For severe attacks 1 mg morphine/10 lb body weight is specific and at least half of this dose can be given intravenously if necessary. Prolonged attacks of cyanosis are associated with acidosis, which results from hypoxia. Intravenous infusion of sodium bicarbonate (1/6 molar sodium bicarbonate in 5% dextrose water) may be lifesaving. Propranolol in doses of 5–15 mg daily has been useful in prophylaxis.

Iron preparations by mouth or intramuscular injection are indicated when iron deficiency is present. It is important to remember that an increased amount of hemoglobin is required in severe tetralogy. A normal red cell count often indicates anemia and therapy is directed at producing polycythemia. On the other hand, excessive polycythemia (hematocrit over 70%) is associated with increased blood viscosity and liability to thrombosis so that venesection with plasma replacement may occasionally be required.

Adequate hydration must always be ensured, particularly in hot weather, fever, gastrointestinal infection, and before surgical procedures. This is especially important before and during cardiac catheterization.

Indications for Surgery

The prognosis in Tetralogy of Fallot is poor. Although exceptional patients have survived to the sixth decade, 90% die before age 25. During their short lives disability is considerable and limitation of effort marked. Apart from the discomfort of cyanotic attacks there is stunting of growth, paroxysmal dyspnea, thrombolic episodes, and a tendency to bleeding Cerebral thrombosis is a particular problem in children under the age of 2. Paradoxical embolism is a risk with any right-to-left shunt. Brain abscess, especially after the age of 2, is not uncommon. Bacterial endocarditis is an occasional complication and there is susceptibility to pulmonary infection.

Surgery is therefore strongly indicated in Tetralogy of Fallot. The initial palliative treatment was anastomosis of the subclavian to pulmonary artery (Blalock–Taussig operation) or aorta to pulmonary artery (Pott's operation). This was soon followed by complete repair using cardiopulmonary bypass. With increasing experience in the handling of young infants, complete correction can often be achieved below the age of 4, provided the anatomical abnormalities are not extreme.

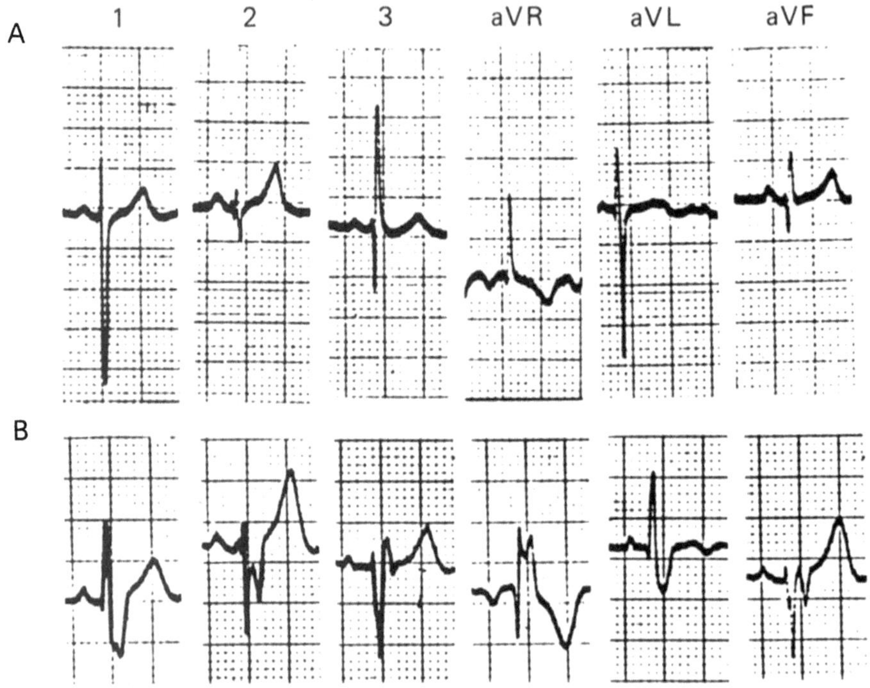

FIGURE 10.44. Conduction defect developing after complete repair of Tetralogy of Fallot. Tracing (A) shows typical preoperative right axis deviation whereas tracing (B) after operation shows complete right bundle branch block with left anterior hemiblock.

After age 4 complete correction is the method of choice. An operative risk of 2% or less can be achieved between the ages of 5 and 9. In most patients, infundibular resection with closure of the ventricular septal defect can be achieved, leaving mild residual stenosis. In some patients an outflow patch is required and this may leave significant pulmonary incompetence. A third of the patients can be restored to virtual normality. Complete right bundle branch block is common postoperatively, occasionally with left anterior hemiblock, but complete heart block is rare (Fig. 10.44). Prophylaxis against infective endocarditis must be maintained throughout life.

Pulmonary Atresia with Ventricular Septal Defect (syn. Pseudotruncus Arterosus)

This may be regarded as an extreme variety of Tetralogy of Fallot when there is no communication between the right ventricle and the

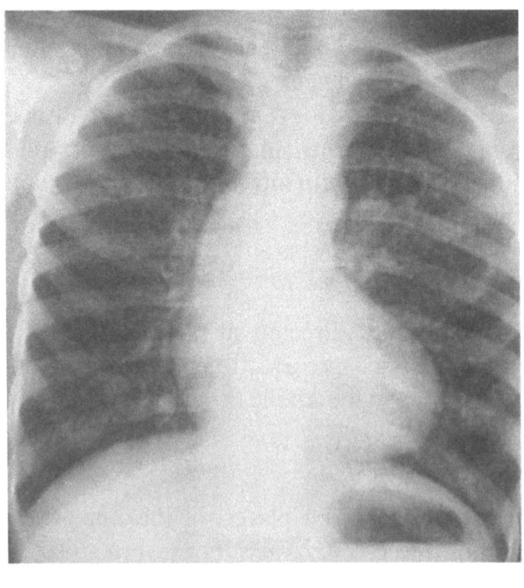

FIGURE 10.45. X-ray of the chest in pulmonary atresia. Configuration of the heart is much the same as in Tetralogy of Fallot but there is a lacey pattern in the lung fields produced by bronchial collaterals.

pulmonary artery. The pulmonary valve is atretic and there are varying degrees of hypoplasia of its branches. In some instances the branches of the pulmonary arteries are normally developed and a thin fibrous membrane (the atretic valve) separates the right ventricle from main pulmonary artery. The pulmonary circulation is maintained by bronchial collaterals which arise from the arch and descending aorta.

Clinical Features

Cyanosis is usually present, but with good bronchial collateral flow may be almost absent. An aortic ejection click is almost always present and continuous murmurs, particularly in the subclavicular region and over the back of the chest, suggest the diagnosis. The *chest X-ray* may also be helpful in that the branches of the pulmonary artery are poorly defined and a "lacey" pattern representing bronchial collaterals may be visible (Fig. 10.45).

Since effective surgical treatment is now available it is important to establish the precise anatomical details of the pulmonary arteries. This is accomplished by selective angiographic injection of bronchial collaterals (Figs. 10.46). In most patients the main pulmonary artery is present so that it is possible to restore contin-

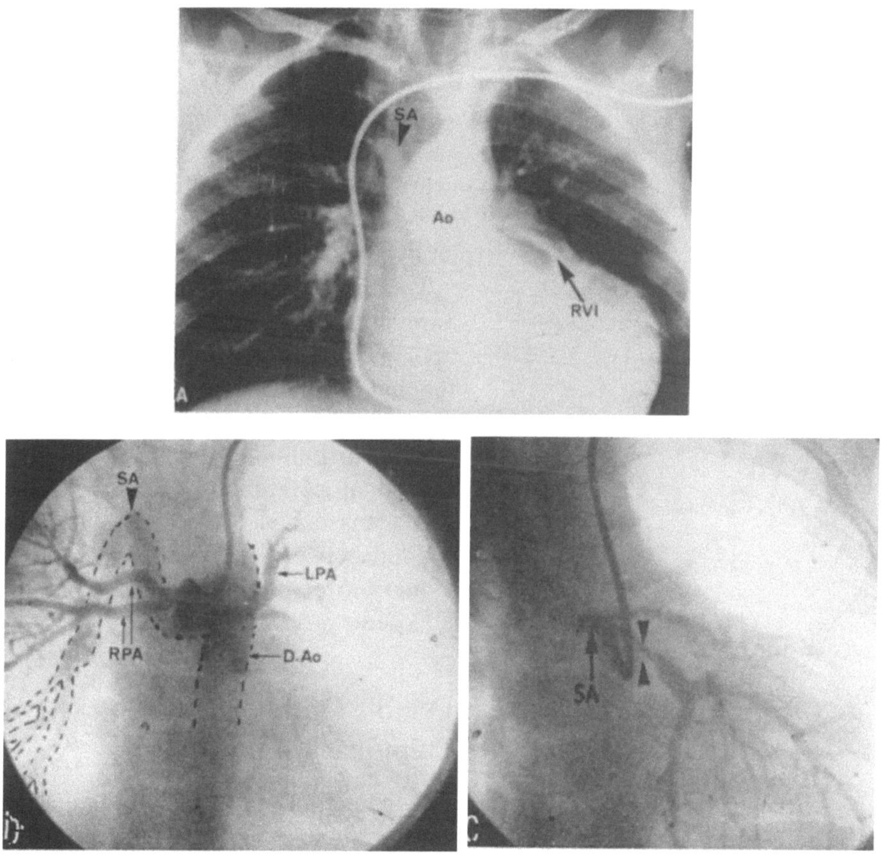

FIGURE 10.46. Angiograms in pulmonary atresia with ventricular septal defect showing (A) a blind right ventricular infundibulum and systemic artery (SA) filling from the aorta. In (B) and (C) selective angiography identifies the collateral circulation arising from the descending aorta. Reprinted, with permission, from Chesler E, et al.: The assessment of arterial supply to the lungs in pseudotruncus arteriosus and truncus arteriosus Type IV in relation to surgical repair. Am Heart J 88:542, 1974.

uity with the right ventricle using an aortic homograft and valve.

When no elements of pulmonary arteries are identifiable and the entire pulmonary circulation is via bronchial arteries, the situation is untreatable. This entity has been classified as *truncus arteriosus type IV* or *absence of the 6th arch*. Death usually results from pulmonary apoplexy when bronchial collateral vessels rupture.

Tricuspid Atresia with Pulmonary Stenosis

Obstruction to pulmonary blood flow in tricuspid atresia is particularly common when the great vessels are normally related (Fig. 10.47). The obstruction may be by a restrictive ventricular septal defect, infundibular stenosis, pulmonary valve stenosis, or atresia, individually or in combination. The right ventricle is hypoplastic. Mixing of systemic and pulmonary venous blood occurs in the left atrium and from there the circulation is to an enlarged left ventricle and the great vessels.

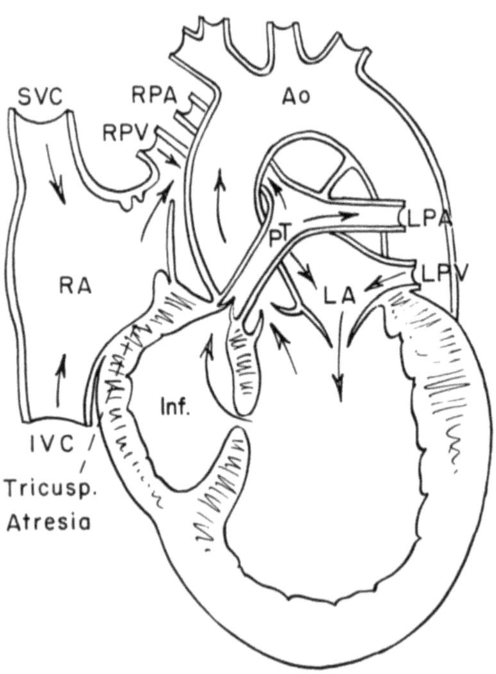

FIGURE 10.47. Diagram of central circulation in tricuspid atresia with normally related great vessels and obstruction to pulmonary blood flow. The left ventricle behaves as a single or common ventricle. Reprinted, with permission, from Edwards JE: Classification of congenital heart disease in the adult. Cardiovascular Clinics 10:I, 1979, F.A. Davis Company.

Clinical Features

There is usually severe cyanosis from infancy. Tricuspid atresia has to be distinguished from pulmonary atresia with intact ventricular septum, single ventricle with pulmonary stenosis or atresia, and Tetralogy of Fallot. There are no helpful clinical signs. Radiologically, there may be left ventricular and left atrial enlargement, but these are inconsistent findings (Fig. 10.48).

The most helpful clue is the *electrocardiogram*, which shows left axis deviation, left ventricular hypertrophy, and sometimes left atrial enlargement. Right ventricular forces are characteristically diminished (Fig. 10.49). There are few other forms of cyanotic congenital heart disease with obstruction to pulmonary blood flow that do not manifest right ventricular hypertrophy.

Treatment is palliative with an aortopulmonary shunt. Enlargement of the atrial septum opening may be required in addition, because the left atrial pressure may rise sufficiently after operation to narrow the foramen ovale leading to pulmonary edema. An alternative functional correction (Fontan procedure) is direct anastamosis of a nonvalved prosthetic conduit between the right atrium and the pulmonary artery; the interatrial communication is closed.

Double Outlet Right Ventricle with Pulmonary Stenosis

This condition may be indistinguishable clinically, radiologically, and electrocardiographically from Tetralogy of Fallot (Fig. 10.50). The ventricular septal defect is subaortic so that left ventricular blood tends to stream into the aorta. When pulmonary stenosis coexists right ventricular blood is also directed to the aorta, resulting in cyanosis.

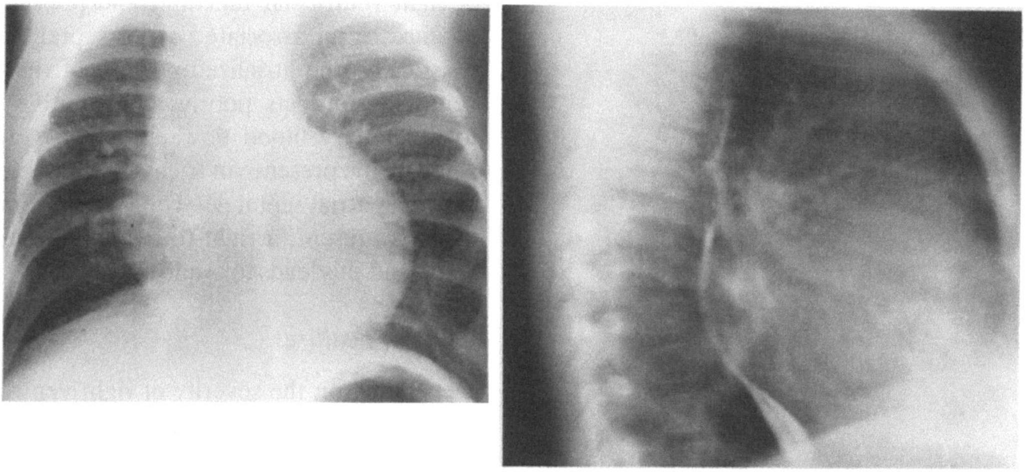

FIGURE 10.48. X-rays of the chest in tricuspid atresia with obstruction to pulmonary blood flow demonstrating left ventricular and left atrial enlargement and pulmonary oligemia.

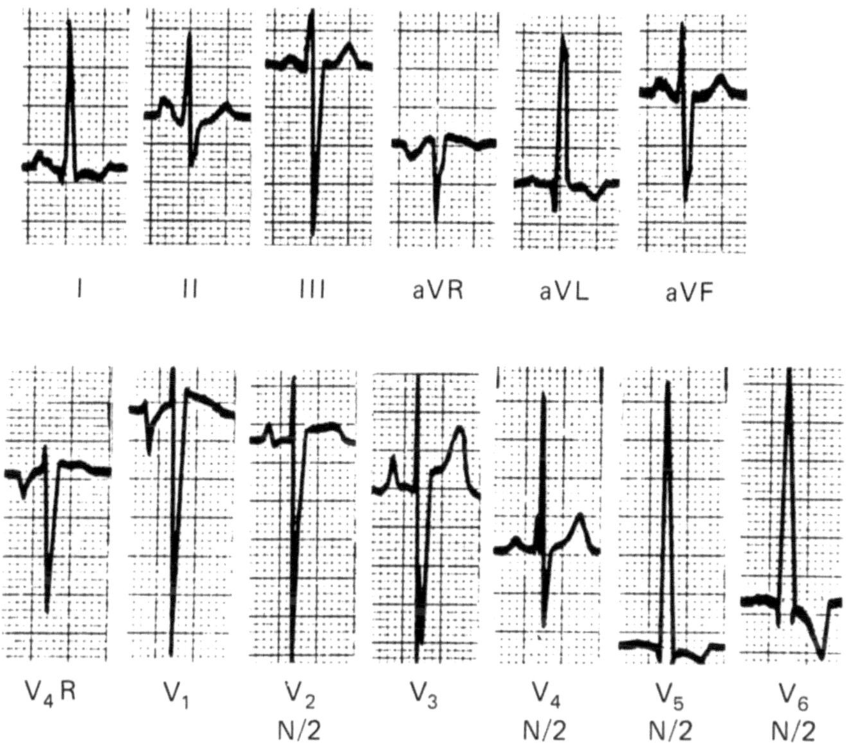

FIGURE 10.49. The electrocardiogram in tricuspid atresia in a neonate, showing a frontal plane axis of −20°, which is leftward for this age. There is marked left ventricular hypertrophy, left atrial enlargement, and an absence of right ventricular forces.

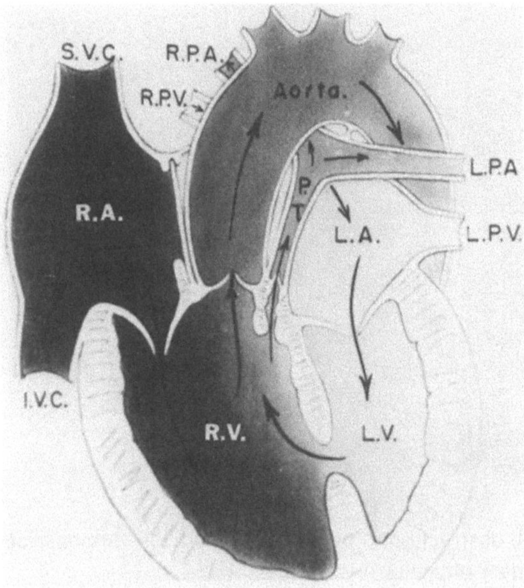

FIGURE 10.50. Diagram of the central circulation in double outlet right ventricle with pulmonary stenosis and a subpulmonary ventricular septal defect resulting in severe cyanosis.

The distinction from tetralogy is made by echocardiography and angiography, which demonstrate aortic and pulmonary values at the same level, bilateral conus, and mitral–semilunar discontinuity.

In severely cyanotic babies a palliative aortopulmonary shunt is indicated. In larger children total correction consists of resection of infundibular stenosis and closure of ventricular septal defect with a patch, which diverts left ventricular blood into the aorta.

Ebstein's Anomaly

In this malformation (Fig. 10.51) the tricuspid valve leaflets are not normally attached to the annulus. The septal and posterior leaflets are displaced into the body of the right ventricle and the valve orifice is located at the junction of the inlet and trabecular portions of the chamber.

Hemodynamics

The findings correlate with the severity of tricuspid incompetence, degree of impairment of right ventricular function, and presence or absence of an associated atrial septal defect. Classically, the atrialized portion of the right ventricle contracts poorly, contributing little to pulmonary blood flow, and this is aggravated by the presence of tricuspid icompetence. When an atrial septal defect or patent foramen ovale is present, a right-to-left shunt may develop and this leads to cyanosis.

Clinical Features

Depending on the severity of right ventricular dysfunction, patients may live into the seventh decade. In the severe form, large "CV" waves are present in the jugular venous pulse, but frequently it is the auscultatory findings that draw attention to the disease. The first heart sound is widely split due to a delayed closure of the large redundant anterior leaflet (the "sail sound"). The second heart sound is widely split because of right bundle branch block and the intensity of the pulmonary component is usually normal. Third and fourth heart sounds are

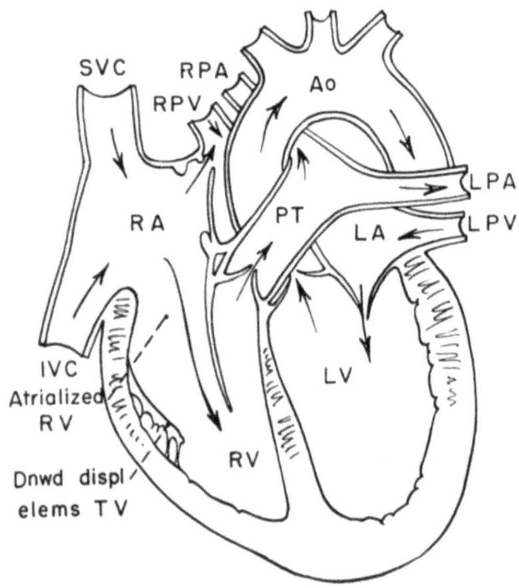

FIGURE 10.51. Diagram of the anatomy and central circulation in Ebstein disease of the tricuspid valve complicated by tricuspid insufficiency and a right-to-left shunt at atrial level. Reprinted, with permission, from Edwards JE: Classification of congenital heart disease in the adult. Cardiovascular Clinics 10:I, 1979, F.A. Davis Company.

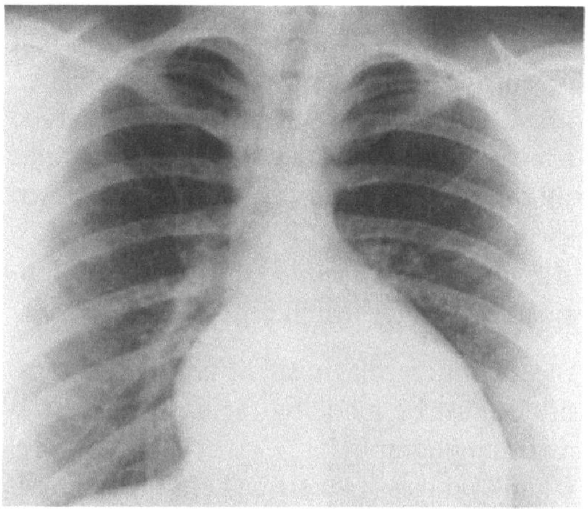

FIGURE 10.52. The chest X-ray in Ebstein disease. The cardiac silhouette resembles that of a pericardial effusion.

frequently audible and become louder with inspiration. Similarly, the murmur of tricuspid regurgitation accentuates with inspiration as does a tricuspid middiastolic murmur when mild tricuspid stenosis is occasionally present.

The *chest X-ray* is occasionally normal, but the classical picture is one of a cardiac silhouette almost indistinguishable from pericardial effusion. Most of the cardiomegaly is accounted for by right atrial enlargement (Fig. 10.52). In cyanotic patients the pulmonary vasculature is diminished because of the right-to-left shunt. The presence of increased vascularity is almost sufficient to exclude a diagnosis of Ebstein anomaly.

The *electrocardiogram* is rarely normal and the characteristic features are extremely helpful in clinical diagnosis. Type B Wolff–Parkinson–White syndrome pattern is seen in some cases and this in combination with cyanosis and a history of palpitation is highly suggestive of the diagnosis. The P waves are frequently large and peaked, reflecting right atrial enlargement. The QRS voltage is frequently low with right bundle branch block pattern. The QRS axis is usually normal, but may be deviated to the right.

The diagnosis of Ebstein malformation may be established by intracardiac electrocardiography or angiocardiography. The finding of atrial pressures in the presence of ventricular QRS complexes from the atrialized portion of the ventricle is diagnostic. Echocardiography, whether M-mode or two dimensional, is extremely helpful in making the diagnosis noninvasively.

In those individuals seriously disabled by the disease, plication of the tricuspid valve appears to be the procedure of choice.

Corrected Transposition of the Great Vessels with Pulmonary Stenosis

When accompanied by the presence of a ventricular septal defect and pulmonary stenosis, cyanosis and diminution of pulmonary arterial vasculature are characteristic, and therefore described in this section. When pulmonary stenosis is absent and there is a large ventricular septal defect the clinical picture may closely resemble that of the usual type of ventricular septal defect.

In this malformation the atria and the abdominal viscera are normally situated but the ventricles are inverted. The anatomical right ventricle is switched to the left receiving pulmonary venous blood from the left atrium through a tricuspid valve. Similarly, the morphologic left ventricle is switched to the right, receiving systemic venous blood through a mitral valve. As in the case of the normal right ventricle, its infundibulum (or conus) lies anteriorly, and therefore connects with the great vessel situated anteriorly, which, as implied by the name, is the aorta. Essentially the ventricles are in mirror-image relationship (or inversion) and the great vessels are transposed. The disposition of the great vessels is usually in the levo (L-) position (i.e., the aorta lies to the left and anterior to the pulmonary artery and forms a highly distinctive convex leftward bulge on the upper cardiac silhouette).

Were it not for the presence of associated malformations, there would be no physiological disturbance and the course of circulation would be entirely normal; pulmonary venous blood would be directed through the tricuspid valve into the anatomical right ventricle and anteriorly situated aorta.

The common malformations associated with

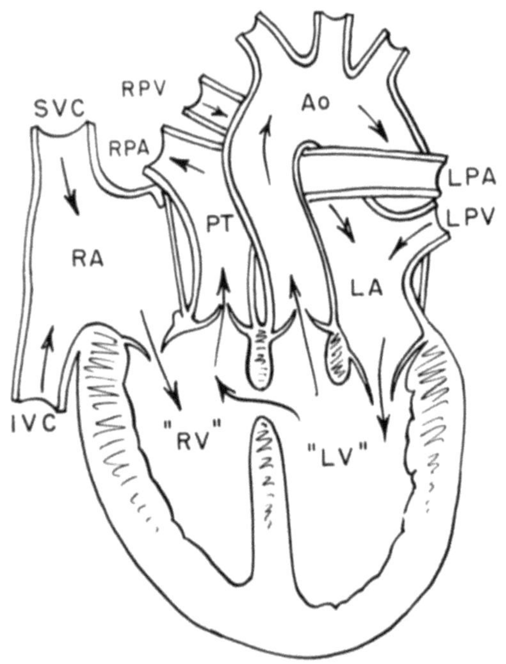

FIGURE 10.53. Diagrammatic representation of the anatomy and central circulation corrected transposition of the great vessels with ventricular septal defect. The diagram is included for reference to explain ventricular inversion in the presence of transposition. The addition of pulmonary stenosis would decrease pulmonary blood flow. Reprinted, with permission, from Edwards JE, et al.: A review of congenital anomalies of the heart and great vessels according to functional categories. Ped Clin N Am 18(4), 1971.

corrected transposition are ventricular septal defect (Fig. 10.53) with and without subvalvular or valvular pulmonary stenosis, or both. Atrioventricular regurgitation is a fairly frequent finding and results from Ebstein malformation of the left A-V valve, since this is an inverted tricuspid valve. Arrhythmias and conduction disturbances are common.

When there is a large ventricular septal defect and significant pulmonary stenosis, clinical differentiation must be made from other conditions associated with cyanosis obstruction to pulmonary blood flow and diminished pulmonary arterial vasculature.

Clues to the diagnosis are

1. *Electrocardiogram* showing varying degrees of A-V block, Q waves present in the right precordial leads but absent in the left leads.
2. *Chest X-ray* that demonstrates a curved convex border of the upper left cardiac silhouette produced by the L-transposed ascending aorta.
3. *A pansystolic murmur* suggestive of left-sided A-V valve insufficiency.

The definitive diagnosis of corrected transposition must be made by cardiac catheterization and angiography.

When cyanosis is severe a shunt procedure is usually indicated because of the difficulties of surgical repair.

Pulmonary Atresia with Intact Ventricular Septum

The pulmonary valve is represented by an imperforate diaphragm and the pulmonary circulation is maintained through a patent ductus arteriosus (Fig. 10.54 and 10.55). The size of the right ventricle appears to be determined by the functional status of the tricuspid valve. When this is competent the right ventricular cavity tends to be small, but when it is incompetent the right ventricular cavity may be normal or even enlarged. Survival is dependent on patency of the ductus arteriosus and an interatrial communication.

Clinical Features

Cyanosis is evident soon after birth. In infants with incompetence of the tricuspid valve, a pansystolic murmur of tricuspid regurgitation may be heard along the lower left sternal border. Should the infant survive, there is progressively severe hypoxia and heart failure.

The *chest X-ray* demonstrates diminution of pulmonary oligemia. The heart size will vary depending on the competency of the tricuspid valve. The *electrocardiographic changes* also depend on the size of the right ventricular cavity. When this is diminutive there is an absence of normal neonatal right ventricular dominance and there are tall peaked P waves.

However, when the right ventricular cavity is more normal in size, right ventricular forces may be present.

When this condition is suspected, immediate catheterization is indicated since closure of the ductus is fatal. The systolic pressure in the right ventricle exceeds that of the left and angiography demonstrates a blind infundibulum and emptying of the right ventricle through enlarged coronary vessels.

Once the diagnosis is established surgical treatment will depend on the size of the right ventricular cavity. When this is adequate, a pulmonary valvulotomy may be curative. When the right ventricle is diminutive, a shunt procedure is indicated.

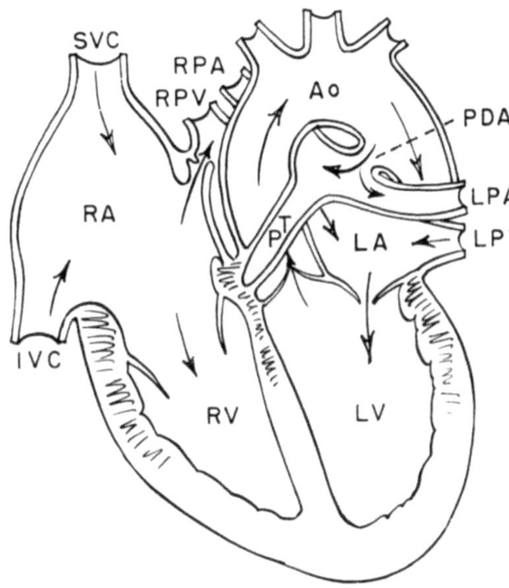

FIGURE 10.55. Pulmonary atresia with intact ventricular septum and a well-developed right ventricular cavity and tricuspid insufficiency. Reprinted, with permission from Edwards JE, et al.: A review of congenital anomalies of the heart and great vessels according to functional categories. Ped Clin N Am 2(1), 1964.

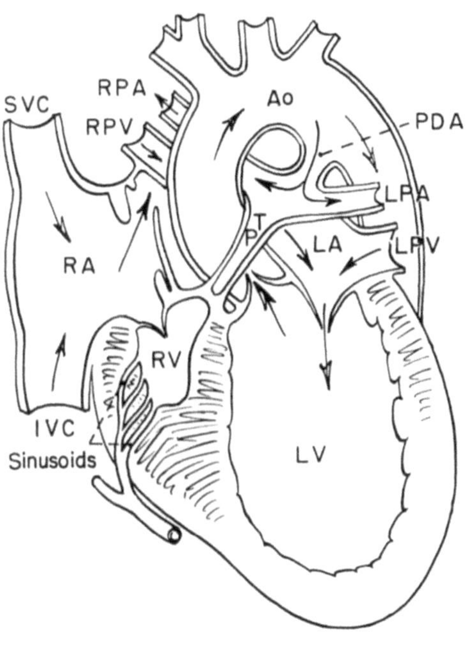

FIGURE 10.54. Diagram of anatomy and central circulation in pulmonary atresia with intact ventricular septum, competent tricuspid valve, and hypoplastic right ventricle. Enlarged intramyocardial sinusoids communicate the right ventricle cavity with the coronary artery. Pulmonary circulation is maintained by a patent ductus. From Edwards JE, et al.: A review of congenital anomalies of the heart and great vessels according to functional categories. Reprinted, with permission, from Ped Clin N Am 18(4), 1971.

Cyanosis Present: Pulmonary Venous Hypertension

Malformations characterized by obstruction to blood flow into the left side of the heart associated with a bidirectional shunt (or admixture phenomenon) produces the combination of clinical cyanosis and pulmonary venous engorgement. The admixture of pulmonary venous and systemic venous blood occurs in the right atrium.

Aortic Atresia, Mitral Atresia, and Aortic and Mitral Atresia

The Hypoplastic Left Heart Syndrome

When the left heart is hypoplastic (Fig. 10.56–10.58), effective egress for blood from the left atrium is via the foramen ovale to the right atrium. Because the foramen ovale is restric-

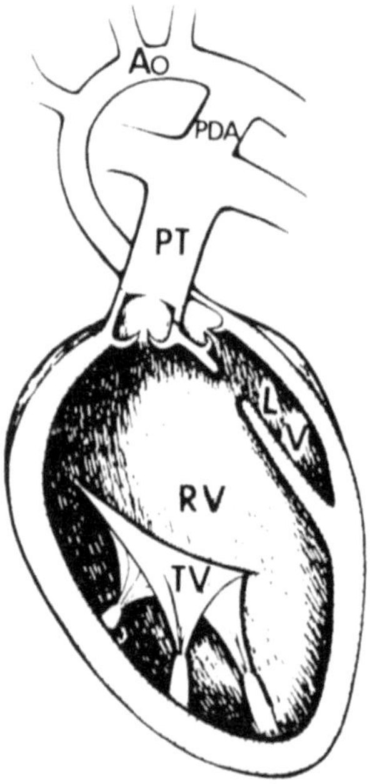

FIGURE 10.56. Mitral atresia with ventricular septal defect resulting in the hypoplastic left heart syndrome. Reprinted, with permission, from Chesler E, et al.: Echocardiography in the diagnosis of congenital heart disease. Ped Clin N Am 18(4), 1971.

with tachypnea and respiratory distress. Poor peripheral perfusion with generally weak pulses and pallor soon develop. Quite characteristically there is fluctuation in the clinical condition produced by spontaneous fluctuation in the size of the ductus arteriosus. When there is a preductal coarctation the pulses may be better felt in the lower extremities than in the upper—so-called "reversed coarctation."

The cardiac impulse is that of a hyperactive right ventricle and the second sound is loudest in the pulmonary area because aortic valve closure is absent. Murmurs are variable and an ejection systolic murmur, presumably related to flow through the pulmonary artery and ductus arteriosus, may be present. Cyanosis is not intense but as respiratory difficulty increases and peripheral perfusion fails, mottling and skin pallor are quite common.

Chest X-ray shows moderate cardiomegaly and the eventually pulmonary edema. The *electrocardiogram* shows right axis deviation, right ventricular hypertrophy, and poor left

tive, there is pulmonary venous hypertension. Following admixture in the right atrium flow is to the right ventricle, which supplies the lung via the pulmonary artery and sytemic circulation through a patent ductus arteriosus.

The right ventricle therefore behaves functionally as a "single ventricle." In aortic atresia, mitral atresia, or combined aortic and mitral atresia, the course of the circulation is quite similar. The coronary arteries are perfused retrograde from the aorta, and therefore flow is critically dependent on patency of the ductus arteriosus. When mitral atresia is accompanied by a large ventricular septal defect, the left ventricle may not be hypoplastic and there may be forward flow into the aorta.

Aortic atresia is the leading cause of death in the neonatal period. It is more common in males than females. Infants with the condition are usually normal in appearance at birth but symptoms develop within an hour or two, and are certainly present by 48 hours. Features of pulmonary congestion are typically present

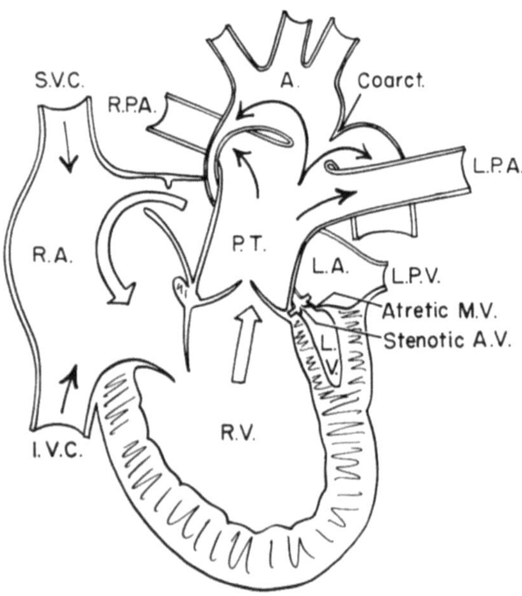

FIGURE 10.57. Hypoplastic left heart syndrome due to mitral atresia and severe aortic stenosis. The circulation is maintained by the right ventricle through the pulmonary trunk and perfusion of the aorta through the ductus arteriosus. Courtesy of Dr. Jesse E. Edwards.

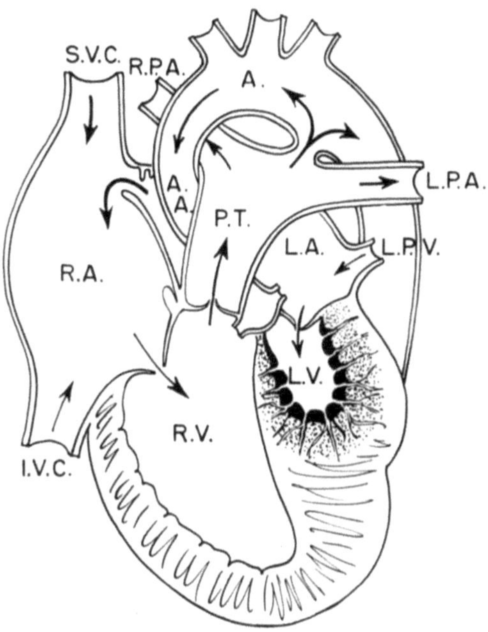

FIGURE 10.58. Hypoplastic left heart syndrome due to aortic atresia and the course of the circulation is as seen in Figure 174. Courtesy of Dr. Jesse E. Edwards.

ventricular forces. *Echocardiography* is extremely helpful in diagnosis of aortic and/or mitral atresia. Aortic and mitral valve echoes are absent and only the right ventricular chamber can be demonstrated. With skilled examination a small aortic root and small left atrial dimension may also be demonstrated.

Cardiac catheterization is usually performed to confirm the diagnosis. The principal diagnostic difficulties are with the obstructed variety of total anomalous pulmonary venous drainage where the clinicla features may be very similar. This is an important distinction that must be made by cardiac catheterization because obstructed total anomalous venous drainage is curable.

Congenital unicuspid aortic stenosis may produce a similar picture but a harsh ejection systolic murmur is usually present if the cardiac output is maintained. Catheterization will demonstrate a gradient across the dortic valve and confirm the diagnosis.

The treatment of these syndromes can only be palliative. This consists of correction of hypoglycemia and acidosis, and treatment of heart failure with digitalis and diuretics. High concentrations of oxygen may be disadvantagous because this may result in closure of the ductus with aggravation of heart failure and failure of peripheral perfusion. Surgical palliation in two stages (the Norwood procedure) is very extensive. Other centers prefer cardiac transplantation.

Obstructive Total Anomalous Pulmonary Venous Drainage

When there is total anomalous drainage of the pulmonary veins, the site of obstruction is usually infradiaphragmatic at the ductus venosus, the portal vein, or one of its tributaries (Fig. 10.59). Another variety is connection to the left innominate vein where obstruction is either due to intrinsic stenosis at the junction or to compression of the venous trunk between the left pulmonary artery and left bronchus. Blood flow is similar to cases of total anomalous pulmonary venous drainage without obstruction and all blood reaches the right atrium where there is admixture. Some of the mixed blood crosses the foramen ovale to the left side of the heart and the remainder flows across the tricusped value into the right ventricle for delivery to the pulmonary circulation.

Clinical Features

Babies with obstructed infradiaphragmatic total anomalous pulmonary venous drainage are usually normal at birth but soon develop cyanosis, increasing respiratory difficulty, and pulmonary edema. Usually the heart is not clinically enlarged but there is a hyperactive right ventricular left parasternal impulse. The pulmonary component of the second heart sound is increased in intensity because of pulmonary hypertension. Usually, the precordium is silent, but occasionally there may be a murmur of tricuspid regurgitation.

The *electrocardiogram* reflects severe right ventricular hypertrophy with right axis deviation with dominant R waves in the right precordial leads and a deep S wave in the left precor-

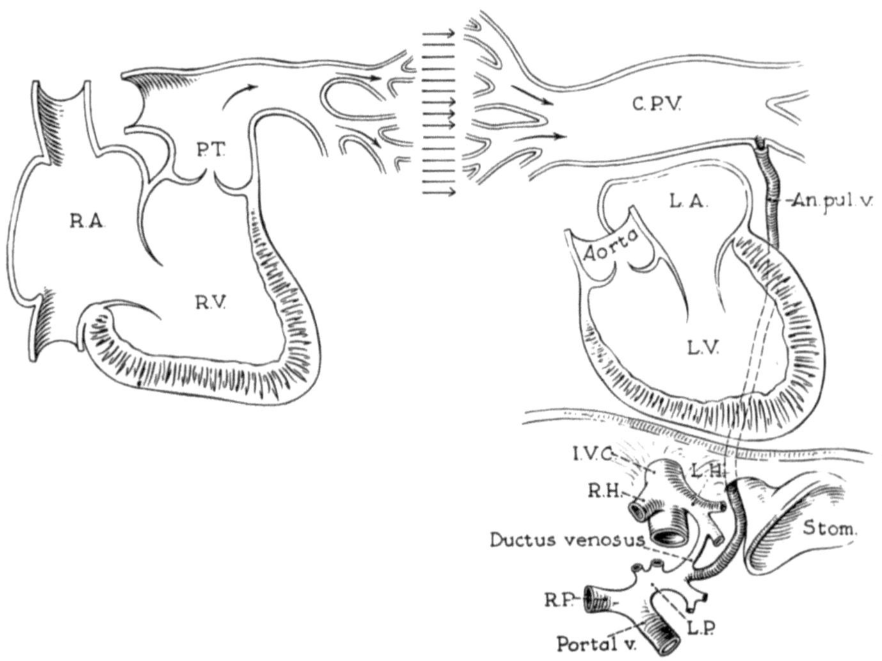

FIGURE 10.59. Course of the circulation in total anomalous pulmonary venous drainage of the obstructed infradiaphragmatic type. The anomalous pulmonary vein communicates with a ductus venosus. Courtesy of Dr. Jesse E. Edwards.

dial leads. The *chest X-Ray* shows a normal sized heart and a reticular-nodular pattern representing distended veins and lymphatic, or diffuse hazziness produced by pulmonary edema.

The differential diagnosis includes idiopathic respiratory distress syndrome, aortic and mitral atresia, and cor triatriatum. The distinction should be made by cardiac catheterization as soon as possible because surgical treatment is available for obstructed pulmonary venous drainage. This consists of anastamosing the common pulmonary vein to the left atrium.

Additional Reading

Campbell M: Natural history of patent ductus arteriosus. Br Heart J 30:4, 1968.

Campbell M: Natural history of atrial septal defect. Br Heart J 32:820, 1970.

Campbell M: Natural history of coarctation of the aorta. Br Heart J 32:633, 1970.

Edwards JE, Carey LS, Neufeld HN, Lister RG: "Congenital Heart Disease: Correlation of Pathologic Anatomy and Angiocardiography." Vols I and II W.B. Saunders, Philadelphia, 1965.

Gottsman MS, Beck W, Barnard CN, O'Donovan TG, Schrire V: Results of repair of tetralogy of Fallot. Circulation 40:803, 1968.

Hoffman JI: Natural history of congenital heart disease: Problems in its assessment with special reference to ventricular septal defects. Circulation 37:97, 1968.

Kanjuh VI, Edwards JE: A review of congenital anomalies of the heart and great vessels according to functional categories. Pediatr Clin North Am 2:55, 1964.

Keith JD, Rowe RD, Vlad P: "Heart Disease in Infancy and Adulthood." The Macmillan, New York, 1967.

Roberts, WC: "Congenital Heart Disease in Adults." F.A. Davis, Philadelphia 1980.

Rudolph AM: "Congenital Diseases of the Heart." Year Book Publishers, Chicago, 1974.

Schrire V, Vogelpoel L: Atrial septal defect. Am Heart J 68:305, 1964.

Schrire V, Vogelpoel L, Beck W, Nellen M, Swanepoel A: Ventricular septal defect. The clinical spectrum. Br Heart J 27:813, 1965.

Stanger P, et al.: Diagramatic portrayal of variations in cardiac structure. Circulation 37(Suppl 4):1, 1968.

Wood PH: The Eisenmenger's syndrome. Br Med J 2:701, 1958.

Wood PH: Congenital heart disease. Br Med J 2:I,506, 1960.

11
Rheumatic Fever

Acute rheumatic fever is an inflammatory process involving the heart, joints, central nervous system, skin, and subcutaneous tissue. Only the cardiac manifestations are important in that valvular damage leads to considerable morbidity and mortality. In its virulent form, the effects on the heart may be devastating at an early age.

Etiology

Following an episode of pharyngitis the exact pathogenesis of an attack of rheumatic fever is uncertain but an autoimmune state initiated by an immune response to Group A, β-hemolytic streptococcal infection appears to be the most likely mechanism. The site of infection is almost invariably the pharynx and the probability of an attack of rheumatic fever is proportional to the virulence of the organism and ensuing antibody response. Rheumatic fever rarely follows streptococcal pyoderma and is infrequently associated with glomerulonephritis. It appears likely that certain serotypes of Group A β-hemolytic streptococci are more liable to produce an attack of rheumatic fever than others.

Epidemiology

There is ample evidence to support the contention that rheumatic fever is primarily a socioeconomic disease. Overcrowding and squalor facilitate the spread of virulent streptococcal infection and increases the frequency and severity of rheumatic fever. Previously thought to be more prevalent in white-skinned races and in temperate climates, it is abundantly clear that rheumatic fever is a major cause of organic heart disease in tropical and subtropical areas. Data from South Africa, India, Israel, and the Phillipines clearly demonstrate the presence of a more serious variant of the disease. In these communities children are affected at a much younger age, the incidence of carditis is greater, the mortality for acute attack is much higher, and established valve disease is a frequent occurrence in children and adolescents.

In westernized countries improved living conditions led to a decline in the incidence of the disease even before the introduction of penicillin. Regardless of race, the death rate for rheumatic fever and rheumatic heart disease is higher for urban children and adolescents than for residents in rural areas. The effects of overcrowding are clearly demonstrated by epidemiological studies in military camps. With sporadic streptococcal infections, the attack rate of rheumatic fever is 0.3%, whereas in epidemics involving closed populations such as military recruits the attack rate may be as high as 3%.

Clinical Manifestations

According to the revised criteria of T. Duckett Jones, the *major* manifestations of acute rheumatic fever are (1) carditis, (2) polyarthritis,

(3) chorea, (4) erythema marginatum, and (5) subcutaneous nodules.

The *minor* manifestations are (1) previous attack of rheumatic fever or evidence of rheumatic heart disease, (2) arthralgia, (3) fever, (4) prolongation of the PR interval, and (5) elevation of the ESR or C-reactive protein.

A combination of two major, or one major and two or more minor manifestations is sufficient to establish the diagnosis, particularly when there is evidence of a preceding streptococcal infection.

Carditis

This is the most important manifestation of acute rhematic fever and affects two-thirds of patients. The mortality for the acute attack is approximately 1% and is a direct result of heart failure secondary to valvular damage.

Pericarditis

Although pericarditis has no long-term sequelae it usually signifies a severe attack of rheumatic fever with concomitant valvular damage. Acute pericarditis produces intense precordial pain and dyspnea. Rheumatic pericardial effusions are serous and although they may accumulate rapidly with dramatic enlargement of the cardiac silhouette, tamponade is uncommon. Fever, leukocytosis, and a raised sedimentation rate are usually present. Serial electrocardiograms demonstrate the evolution of the characteristic abnormalities of acute pericarditis. Echocardiography is helpful in detecting smaller effusions.

Endocarditis

The mitral valve is most commonly affected. In order of frequency, mitral regurgitation is the commonest lesion, followed by combined aortic and mitral regurgitation, and less commonly by aortic regurgitation alone. The tricuspid valve is very rarely affected alone.

A blowing pansystolic murmur is usually the first evidence of endocarditis. The murmur is maximal at the apex and conducted well to the axilla. It is usually caused by active disease of the mitral valve, rather than by dilatation of the valve ring produced by acute left ventricular failure. The first sound is frequently soft because of a long PR interval. A third heart sound is so frequently heard in normal children and accentuated by fever and tachycardia of any cause that its presence does not necessarily indicate valvulitis. However, when a third sound is followed by a short low pitched, rumbling middiastolic murmur (*Carey Coombs murmur*), valvulitis is definitely present. This middiastolic murmur may be transient and detected during only the course of the acute attack. However, it may be the forerunner of permanent mitral valve disease, persisting and ultimately merging with the presystolic murmur of established mitral stenosis.

It is important to appreciate that systolic murmurs and occasionally middiastolic murmurs detected during the course of an acute attack of rheumatic fever do not necessarily indicate permanent heart disease. Aortic ejection murmurs are usually a result of tachycardia and therefore have little significance. Long-term studies have demonstrated that approximately three-quarters of patients with loud apical systolic murmurs have no evidence of rheumatic disease 5 years later. Similarly one-third of patients with apical middiastolic murmurs have no residual murmurs after 5 years. A new aortic diastolic murmur, however, is definite evidence of valvulitis and rarely if ever disappears.

Hemodynamically severe mitral or aortic insufficiency may develop during the course of the acute illness and be responsible for heart failure.

Myocarditis

Histological evidence of myocarditis (characterized by the Aschoff node) is regularly encountered in fatal cases of acute rheumatic fever, but the clinical significance of this finding is unclear. *Myocarditis* may be assumed to be present when there is pericarditis and active endocarditis; tachycardia disproportionate to fever and anxiety may be a clue to its presence. It should be emphasized, however, that the onset of heart failure with cardiac enlargement is almost invariably a result of severe valve damage and only rarely is it possible to clearly incriminate a significant myocardial factor.

Generally, the *electrocardiogram* is not helpful in diagnosis. Prolongation of the corrected Q-T interval is a variable and nonspecific finding, as are changes in the amplitude and configuration of the T waves. First-degree heart block is common during the course of acute rheumatic fever but is not evidence of active carditis and is frequently found in other infections; it is probably a result of increased vagal tone. A-V dissociation is common, but again is a nonspecific finding. Complete heart block is of the utmost rarity.

Arthritis

Objective evidence of joint involvement occurs in approximately half the cases of rheumatic fever. It is typically polyarticular, involving the large joints and flitting from one to the other. Classically, several of the large joints are involved and usually none is affected for longer than a week. The joints are extremely painful, swollen, and hot, but respond rapidly to the administration of salicylates. Pyrexia, malaise, and raised sedimentation rate are associated.

Occasionally, prolonged involvement of a single joint may occur and after repeated attacks of rheumatic fever may be deformed much like rheumatoid artnritis. This atypical manifestation of rheumatic arthritis is referred to as *Jacoud's arthritis*. Generally, however, involvement of a single joint is a result of rheumatoid arthritis.

Chorea

Sydenham's chorea is a late self-limited neurologic complication of rheumatic fever. The condition is more common in females and may occur during pregnancy (*chorea gravidarum*). Unless arthritis or carditis is associated, there are no constitutional symptoms. The sedimentation rate is characteristically normal. About 20% of patients with chorea develop chronic rheumatic heart disease.

Usually there is an insidious onset of spontaneous, involuntary movements involving both sides of the body. Occasionally the disease is unilateral (hemichorea). Movements are uncoordinated, purposeless, and nonrepetitive and disappear during sleep. Muscular contraction is poorly sustained and the weakness and uncoordination may be elicited by asking the patient to shake hands or put out the tongue. Clumsiness, facial grimacing, and difficulty with gait are common (*St. Vitus's dance*).

Hysterical movements are more jerky and repetitive. Tics are also repetitive and not as complex as the writhing movements of chorea.

Subcutaneous Nodules

These are situated over bony prominences such as the back of the head, the knuckles, and the back of the elbow, and are also attached to fascia, tendon sheets, and joint capsules. They vary in size from less than 1 mm to over 1 cm in diameter. They differ from the nodules of rheumatoid arthritis in that they are transient and do not persist for longer than 3 months. In rheumatoid arthritis the nodules persist for many months or years.

Subcutaneous nodules were once extremely common but are now rare even in the presence of severe rheumatic fever.

Erythema Marginatum

This lesion is regarded as specific for rheumatic fever but like nodules has become uncommon. The typical rash is erythematous and is up to 5 cm in diameter, clearing in the center, so that the pale pink margins form rings, crescents, or serpentine patterns. The lesion may be very transient and detection is difficult.

Peritoneal Involvement

This occurs occasionally in children and may produce acute abdominal pain often antedating other features of rheumatic fever. It may readily simulate an acute abdomen. A markedly elevated sedimentation rate and a prompt response to a large dose of aspirin are helpful clues.

Pulmonary Involvement

Pleurisy is commonly encountered and may be dry, or associated with a serous effusion. Rheumatic pneumonia has been described in severely ill patients. There is still considerable dispute as to whether this condition represents true pneumonia or is an unusual manifestation of pulmonary edema associated with left ventricular failure. Characteristically, the physical signs are scanty in contrast to the marked radiological opacities.

Non-specific Changes

The temperature is usually elevated and the pulse rate is proportionately raised. However, sinus bradycardia may occur even in the presence of active carditis. Anemia is common and leukocytosis, splenomegaly, proteinuria, and even microscopic hematuria may be found.

Laboratory Findings

The ESR and C-reative protein tests are indicators of any inflammatory process and are almost always increased in the course of active rheumatic fever. Congestive cardiac failure may retard the sedimentation rate, but rarely to normal range. A raised antistreptolysin titer is supporting evidence of preceding streptococcal infection. Titers of 250 Todd units in adults and 500 in children are significant levels. The titers rise a week after streptococcal infection, reach a peak approximately 3 weeks later, and return to normal in 2 to 4 months. Throat cultures are positive in only one-third of patients with rheumatic fever and the test is therefore not as helpful as the antistreptolysin titer.

Treatment

Bed Rest

This is a difficult question and recommendations have always been made on an empirical basis. There is no solid evidence to indicate that prolonged bed rest abbreviates the course of acute rheumatic fever, prevents initial mortality, or ameliorates valvular damage. No definite guidelines can therefore be given and the period of bed rest should be determined by clinical judgment. Patients with severe attacks of rheumatic fever complicated by cardiomegaly, congestive heart failure, and evidence of arly valve damage dictate their own period of bed rest and this may last several months. In those instances where arthritis and the other extracardiac manifestations of rheumatic fever are the prominent findings without carditis, prolonged bed rest should be avoided since this predisposes to cardiac neurosis.

Penicillin Therapy

Although there is convincing evidence that the prophylactic use of penicillin prevents streptococcal infection and subsequent attacks of rheumatic fever, the evidence is less definite that early penicillin therapy in acute rheumatic fever will modify the course of the disease. Nevertheless, penicillin treatment is generally recommended for the acute attack in the hope that eradication of streptococci will dampen the hyperimmune state and severity of the attack. A single intramuscular injection of benzathine penicillin in a dosage of 600,000 units for children and 1.2 million units for adults is recommended.

Antiinflammatory Agents

There is no specific therapy for rheumatic fever. Salicylates and steroids are palliative; neither shortens the course of the disease and there is no evidence that they terminate rheumatic activity or prevent cardiac damage. Salicylates (100 mg/kg/day) effectively control fever and the pain of arthritis within 24 hours. Prednisone in a dose of 2 mg/kg/day should be reserved for those patients with severe carditis, cardiac failure, and pericarditis. Because of the danger of a rebound phenomenon the dose should be discontinued gradually over a period of several weeks.

Heart Failure

This is the usual cause of mortality in severe rheumatic fever and is the result of severe valve damage. When cardiac failure is resistant to the usual medical measures, valve replacement should not be delayed. Fears of a myocardial factor appear to be ill-founded, and the operative results support this contention.

Chorea

Bed rest is required during the active phase and sedatives such as phenobarbital are prescribed for symptomatic relief. Occasionally, therapy may have to be continued for several months.

Prophylaxis After the First Attack of Rheumatic Fever

The occurrence of one attack indicates a susceptibility to further streptococal infections and the danger of recurrent rheumatic fever. Whether or not carditis was present, long-term antibiotic prophylaxis should be started in all individuals and continued until the age of 40, at least. Intramuscular benzathine penicillin in a dosage of 1.2 million units may be given every 4 weeks. Alternatively, penicillin G may be given orally in a dose of 250,000 units twice a day. In patients who are allergic to penicillin, erythromycin may be given in a dosage of 250 mg twice a day.

Additional Reading

American Heart Association: Jones Criteria (revised) for guidance in the diagnosis of rheumatic fever. Circulation 32:644, 1965.

Chesler E, Levin SE, Freiman E: The pattern of rheumatic heart disease in the urbanised Bantu of Johannesburg. S Afr Med J 40:899, 1966.

Feinstein AR, Spanuolo M: The clinical pattern of acute rheumatic fever: A reappraisal. Medicine 41:279, 1962.

Wood P: Rheumatic fever and acute rhematic carditis. In, "Diseases of the Heart and Circulation," 3rd ed., Eyre and Spottiswoade, London, 1968.

12
Rheumatic Valvular Disease

Mitral Stenosis

Anatomy

The mitral valve apparatus is composed of the anterior and posterior leaflets attached by chordae tendinae to their respective papillary muscles. The anterior leaflet is triangular and has a fibrous attachment to the aortic root; the posterior leaflet is quadrangular and is attached to two-thirds of the annulus fibrosis. The two leaflets are joined by commissural tissue. Whereas the anterior leaflet is mobile, the posterior is restricted in its movement and acts as a buttress so that in systole both leaflets are firmly apposed along their margins.

Rheumatic fever produces inflammation of the leaflets with subsequent fibrosis, thickening, and fusion at the commissures. The chordae tendinae are also involved and become thick, and contracted down onto scarred papillary muscles. The end result is a funnel-shaped valve apparatus with an eccentric opening, producing marked obstruction to blood flow from left atrium to left ventricle. After the initial attack of rheumatic fever there is progressive narrowing and scarring over the years until the valve area is markedly reduced.

Hemodynamics of Mitral Stenosis

The normal mitral valve orifice in the adult is 4 to 6 cm^2. Interference to blood flow is hemodynamically not significant until the valve area is reduced to less than 2.5 cm^2. Between 2 and 2.5 cm^2, symptoms occur with moderate exertion, unless the cardiac output is increased by thyrotoxicosis, pregnancy, or anemia. When the valve area is 1 cm^2 or less, symptoms are present with mild exertion (Fig. 12.1).

With progressive narrowing of the valve orifice, a diastolic gradient develops between the left atrium and left ventricle (Fig. 12.2). The left atrium enlarges and hypertrophies in response to the increased pressure. Left atrial hypertension results in "passive" elevation of the pressures in the pulmonary veins, capillaries, and arteries. The resultant pulmonary arterial hypertension leads to right ventricular hypertrophy and right atrial enlargement.

In approximately 10% of patients with mitral stenosis there is a disproportionate rise in pulmonary arterial pressure, so-called "*reactive*" pulmonary arterial hypertension. This in fact, has a protective effect on the lungs since progressive elevation of the left atrial pressure may lead to the pulmonary capillary pressure exceeding that of the blood osmotic pressure, thus producing pulmonary edema. Reactive pulmonary arterial vasoconstriction may be accentuated by intimal hyperplasia and medial hypertrophy in the pulmonary arterioles. Although these changes in the pulmonary arteries may decrease the possibility of pulmonary congestion, pulmonary hypertension has the adverse effect of producing right ventricular enlargement and eventually congestive cardiac failure.

Pulmonary venous hypertension results in pulmonary congestion and exudation of fluid

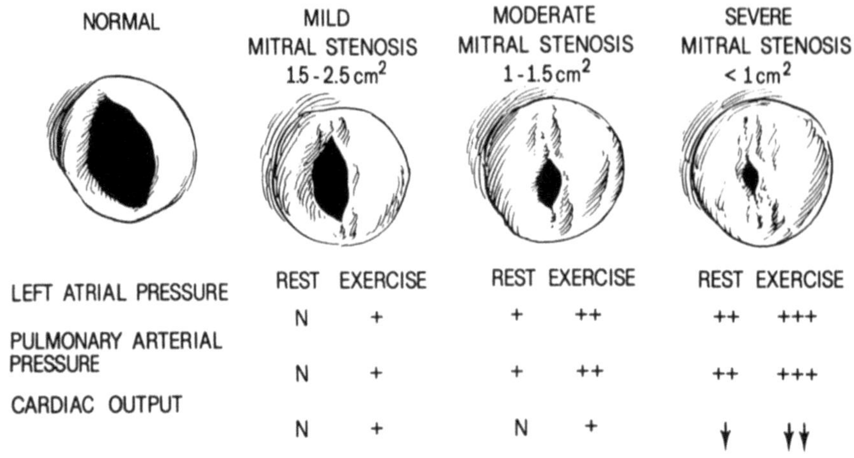

FIGURE 12.1. The hemodynamic changes at rest and exercise with varying degrees of severity of mitral stenosis.

into the alveoli with formation of interstitial pulmonary edema. This results in diminished lung compliance and an increase in the work of breathing which is directly related to the height of the pulmonary venous pressure. In mitral stenosis there is also an alteration of distribution of blood flow to the lungs. In the normal situation pulmonary blood flow is greater in the lower than in the upper lobes in the upright posture. In mitral stenosis constriction of the lower lobe pulmonary arterioles redistributes blood to the upper lobes producing pulmonary venous distention and subsequent edema in this location.

The ultimate result of pulmonary venous obstruction is a disturbance in the ventilation/

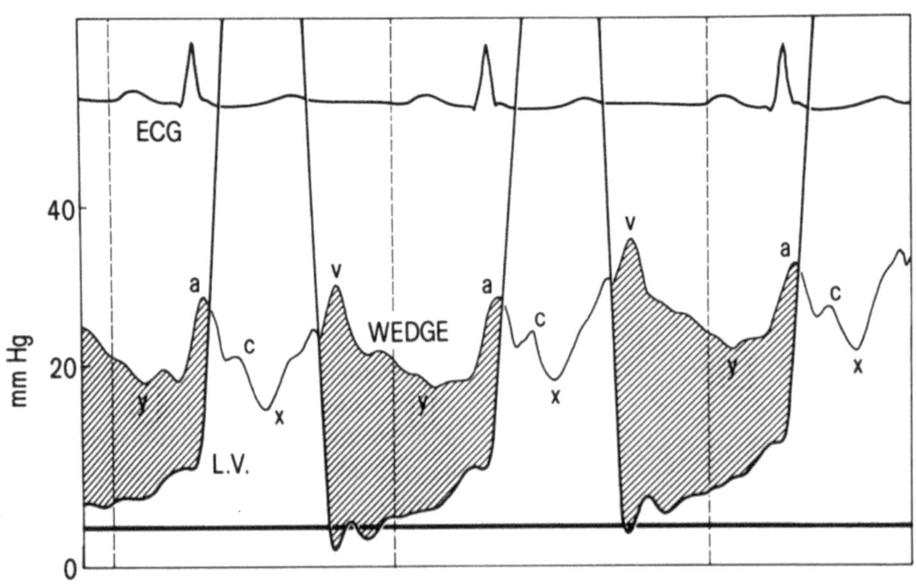

FIGURE 12.2. Simultaneous wedge and left ventricular pressures in a case of mitral stenosis showing the diastolic gradient (shaded) between the left atrium and left ventricle.

perfusion ratio, which leads to venous admixture—"physiological shunting" and desaturation of pulmonary venous blood. This results in central cyanosis, typically found in advanced cases complicated by pulmonary edema. More usually, cyanosis is peripheral and is a result of reduced cardiac output, peripheral vasoconstriction, and increased extraction of oxygen from the arterial blood.

Clinical Manifestations

Women are affected approximately twice as frequently as men. Since it usually takes about 20 years for significant stenosis to develop following an acute attack of rheumatic fever, symptoms appear in the twenties and it may take another 10 years for these to become incapacitating.

In countries where rheumatic fever exists in severe form, critical mitral stenosis develops at a much earlier age. In South Africa among the Black population 21% of valvotomies are performed on patients less than 20 years of age whereas in the United Kingdom and the United States the comparable figure is less than 1% for this age group.

Dyspnea

Dyspnea is an important symptom and is directly related to the height of the pulmonary venous pressure. With mild mitral stenosis dyspnea may be a feature only during severe exertion. With critical mitral stenosis, when the valve area is less than 1 cm^2, dyspnea may be present with minimal effort or at rest. Precipitating factors such as pregnancy, intercurrent infection, and atrial fibrillation may produce attacks of pulmonary congestion in an otherwise asymptomatic patient.

Paroxysmal Nocturnal Dyspnea and Orthopnea

These are produced by aggravation of the pulmonary venous congestion when postural changes increase venous return and the left atrial pressure rises in the recumbent position. These symptoms may occur, however, in any form of left ventricular failure.

Fatigue

When there is severe pulmonary hypertension the resting cardiac output is reduced and the cardiac output fails to rise adequately during exercise. Inadequate systemic perfusion produces fatigue, which may be a more prominent symptom than dyspnea.

Hemoptysis

Mild blood staining of the sputum is a frequent occurrence during episodes of acute bronchitis and attacks of acute pulmonary edema. More severe hemorrhage may occur, however, in those patients with pulmonary venous, but not pulmonary arterial hypertension. Here, rupture of an anastamosis between the pulmonary and bronchial venous systems may result in *pulmonary apoplexy*, which is occasionally life-threatening. Among those patients with pulmonary arterial hypertension and right ventricular failure, hemoptysis is not uncommonly a result of pulmonary infarction secondary to deep venous thrombosis in the lower extremities.

Systemic Embolism

This complication occurs in approximately 20% of patients with mitral valve disease. The cerebral circulation is affected in two-thirds of the cases. Atrial fibrillation appears to be the most important contributory factor and is present in 70% of cases. Emboli are also more common in elderly patients. Some degree of left atrial enlargement is always present but the frequency of embolism cannot be closely correlated with the severity of mitral stenosis or left atrial size.

Stroke may be the presenting symptom in an otherwise asymptomatic patient and mitral valve disease should always be considered in the differential diagnosis of stroke.

Congestive Cardiac Failure

This follows right ventricular hypertrophy and dilatation secondary to severe pulmonary hypertension. Tricuspid insufficiency is frequently present and there is systemic venous congestion and hepatomegaly.

The physical signs of pulmonary hypertension and right ventricular enlargement may mask the auscultatory features of mitral stenosis because of the reduction in cardiac output. A diagnosis of primary pulmonary hypertension should not be entertained until mitral stenosis has been excluded by echocardiography.

Recurrent Pulmonary Infection

Chronic bronchitis and recurrent pulmonary infections frequently complicate the pulmonary congestion associated with mitral stenosis. In the middle-aged and elderly it may be difficult to determine the relative importance played by mitral stenosis and/or chronic chest disease in relation to the patient's disability.

Chest Pain

Typical angina pectoris resulting from occlusive atherosclerosis is not uncommon in older patients. Pain indistinguishable from typical angina occurs in those patients who have developed severe pulmonary hypertension with reduced cardiac output; right ventricular ischemia has been postulated to be the responsible factor.

Pleuritic Pain

This is usually a result of complicating pulmory infarction.

Hoarseness

Allegedly a result of recurrent laryngeal nerve paralysis produced by left atrial enlargement, hoarseness is an oft-quoted symptom of mitral stenosis. It is so rare clinically that it is of no significance.

Syncope

Syncope on effort is an occasional symptom.

Infective Endocarditis

This is a rare complication of *pure* mitral stenosis. *Left atrial myxoma* is a more likely diagnosis when a patient presents with a middiastolic murmur and systemic manifestations suggestive of infective endocarditis.

Epilepsy

The incidence of seizures in patients with mitral stenosis is increased and this has been attributed to small cerebral emboli.

Physical Signs

Mitral Facies

This refers to persistent cyanotic patches involving the cheeks, frequently associated with a tinge of icterus. Usually it occurs when there has been persistent right ventricular failure with tricuspid insufficiency.

Jugular Venous Pressure

In the absence of pulmonary hypertension, this is usually normal. When right heart failure or severe pulmonary hypertension is present a large "A" wave is found. Atrial fibrillation and tricuspid insufficiency (functional or organic) are associated with large "CV" waves and frequently systolic pulsation of the liver. A "tricuspid rock" may be detected by careful palpation.

The Heart

The apex is usually in normal position and a mild systolic left parasternal lift may be present. Pulmonary valve closure may be palpated in the second left intercostal space and mitral valve closure at the apex. Not infrequently, a diastolic thrill is present at the apex.

Important auscultatory abnormalities include (1) accentuation of the mitral component of the first heart sound, (2) the opening snap, and (3) an apical rumbling middiastolic murmur.

The First Heart Sound

The normal first heart sound is produced by coaption of the mitral leaflets shortly after the onset of ventricular systole. In mitral stenosis, the leaflets of the mitral valve at the onset of ventricular systole are well within the left ventricular cavity because of the pressure gradient between the left atrium and left ventricle. When this gradient is reversed the leaflets move rapidly with a wide excursion to the closed position. This accentuates the first heart sound provided the leaflets are mobile. With atrial fibrillation the intensity of the accentuated first sound varies with the preceding cycle length: a short RR interval results in a loud first heart sound, whereas a long RR interval is followed by a softer first heart sound. The intensity of the first heart sound provides a good index of leaflet mobility but not of severity of mitral stenosis.

The Opening Snap

This sound occurs at the time of the maximum opening movement of the anterior mitral leaflet. Its timing after the aortic component of the second heart sound is directly related to the left atrial pressure and therefore to the severity of mitral stenosis. When mitral stenosis is critical the interval between the aortic component of the second heart sound and the opening snap is 80 msec or less. In atrial fibrillation this interval varies with the length of the preceding diastolic interval: following a long pause, the snap occurs later because there is more time for left atrial emptying.

The presence of an opening snap is a fairly good sign of mobility of the anterior mitral leaflet. Its presence does not preclude significant mitral insufficiency. The sound is quite common in cases of mitral insufficiency where there is shrinkage of the posterior leaflet and some degree of commissural fusion and rigidity of the anterior leaflet.

The snap is best heard just medial to the apex and at the lower left sternal border. When loud it may radiate to the second right intercostal space.

The Middiastolic Rumble

This murmur has a characteristic rumbling quality with a decrescendo–crescendo cadence that can be recognized by these features alone. In pure tight mitral stenosis the murmur starts shortly after the opening snap, and runs throughout diastole culminating in a presystolic crescendo and ending with the accentuated first heart sound. In mild mitral stenosis only the pre-systolic murmur may be present. As the stenosis becomes more severe, a middiastolic murmur becomes audible and its length is a good predictor of the severity of mitral stenosis since this reflects the duration of the gradient between the left atrium and the left ventricle. When the cardiac output is increased by effort or amyl nitrite, diastole is shortened and the murmur becomes full length.

In atrial fibrillation the typical presystolic accentuation is lost. However, when the cycles are short the middiastolic rumble may continue right up to the first heart sound and simulate a presystolic murmur. This is the classical teaching. In fact a "presystolic murmur" may occur even in the presence of atrial fibrillation. The explanation for this finding is controversial. The "murmur" actually occurs at the very onset of ventricular systole and is probably an accentuation of the initial low-frequency component of the first heart sound called "M."

The murmur of mitral stenosis is reduced and in fact may be inaudible when there is severe pulmonary hypertension, rapid atrial fibrillation, congestive cardiac failure, particularly when tricuspid insufficiency coexists, and a thick chest wall. However, it is very rarely absent and careful auscultation with the bell of the stethoscope applied very lightly to the skin directly at the apex will facilitate its detection. With careful clinical examination there are, in fact, few examples of so-called "silent mitral stenosis."

With pure mitral stenosis a systolic murmur is usually absent. An apical systolic murmur does not necessarily mean that mitral insufficiency is present. In the presence of severe pulmonary hypertension, the right ventricle underlies most of the precordium and a tricuspid systolic murmur may be audible at the apex; it is recognized by its accentuation with inspiration.

In the pulmonary area, an ejection click is frequently heard when there is severe pulmonary hypertension. Unlike an aortic ejection click this is localized to the second left interspace and becomes markedly softer or disappears with inspiration. Not uncommonly, a short superficial crackling ejection systolic murmur is heard in this area and this is most likely produced by a dilated pulmonary artery rubbing against the pericardium.

An early diastolic murmur in the second left interspace (Graham–Steel murmur) indicates the presence of functional pulmonary insufficiency consequent on pulmonary hypertension. This murmur is differentiated from the murmur of aortic insufficiency by the fact that it does not radiate well toward the apex, accentuates slightly with inspiration, is not associated with the peripheral signs of aortic insufficiency, and is heard only when there is other clear-cut evidence of pulmonary hypertension.

Electrocardiogram

Left atrial overload is the commonest abnormality and is usually found when there is significant stenosis. When there is associated pulmonary hypertension, right atrial enlargement is also present.

The combination of left atrial overload and severe right ventricular hypertrophy is highly suggestive of mitral stenosis. Right ventricular hypertrophy indicates pulmonary hypertension and the severity of the changes roughly parallels the increase in pulmonary vascular resistance. Right bundle branch block with right axis deviation is occasionally found. Changes in the left ventricular leads are usually due to digitalis and are rarely encountered in isolated mitral stenosis. Atrial fibrillation is the commonest arrhythmias and occurs in approximately one-third of patients.

Radiologic Findings

In the anteroposterior view, the characteristic features are small aorta, prominent pulmonary artery and left atrial appendage, hilar congestion, prominence of upper lobe pulmonary veins, and Kerley B-lines. When there is pulmonary arterial hypertension the pulmonary arteries are prominent and the right atrium is enlarged.

The enlarged left atrium produces a characteristic double density, and in the left lateral projection there is posterior displacement of the barium column. The size of the left atrium is not related to severity of the stenosis. However, aneurysmal dilatation of the left atrium is uncommon in pure mitral insufficiency. Marked cardiomegaly with right atrial, right ventricular, and left atrial enlargement is found when there is long-standing heart failure associated with atrial fibrillation, severe pulmonary hypertension, and tricuspid insufficiency.

Calcification of the mitral valve is fairly common, especially in the older patient, but left atrial calcification is rare. Mitral valve calcification, is best detected by fluoroscopy but may also be seen on an overpenetrated lateral view of the chest.

Pulmonary hemosiderosis is not uncommon in long-standing cases with prolonged elevation of the pulmonary venous pressure.

Echocardiography

This is a helpful technique in the diagnosis of mitral stenosis where there is difficulty in elucidation of the physical signs. With 2D and Doppler measurement of the mitral flow half-time, it is a good predictor of severity. It is particularly useful when there is difficulty in evaluation of a loud middiastolic murmur at the apex in cases of severe aortic insufficiency. Additionally, in those congenital malformations associated with large left-to-right shunts and torrential mitral blood flow, a loud diastolic murmur mimicking mitral stenosis is frequently audible at the apex; a normal mitral valve echogram is helpful in excluding associated cor triatriatum and supravalvular stenosing ring of the left atrium. Similarly, a normal mitral valve echogram is helpful in excluding mitral valve disease among the casues of pulmonary venous hypertension such as congenital stenosis of the pulmonary veins.

The characteristic M-Mode echocardiographic features found in mitral stenosis are (1) an E-F slope of less than 35 mm/sec with loss of the atrial reopening movement, (2) abnormal movement of the posterior leaflet of the mitral valve parallel to that of anterior leaflet, (3) thickening of the echoes recorded from both leaflets, and (4) decreased amplitude of movement.

Two-Dimensional Echocardiogram

This shows thickening and doming of the leaflets, depending their pliability. Doming indicates adhesion of the leaflets and this distinguishes a stenotic valve from one that opens poorly because of low cardiac output.

Doppler Echocardiography

Using continuous wave, the rate of decline of early diastolic flow is decreased and increased with atrial systole. The pressure half-time correlates with severity of stenosis.

Cardiac Catheterization

This is not usually required in the young symptomatic patient with isolated, noncalcific mitral stenosis who has clinical evidence of a mobile mitral valve. Catheterization is useful, however, when there is (1) clinical difficulty in assessing the severity of mitral regurgitation, (2) associated tricuspid and aortic valve disease, the severity of which is difficult to determine clinically, electrocardiographically, and radiologically, (3) disproportion between symptoms and physical signs, and (4) unexpected left ventricular enlargement, suggesting the possibility of associated cardiomyopathy or ischemic heart disease.

Left ventricular cineangiography provides an accurate assessment of the degree of mitral regurgitation and the mobility and thickening, if any, of the mitral valve apparatus. It also gives an accurate assessment of left ventricular function and measurement of the ejection fraction.

Treatment

The prognosis for patients with mitral stenosis depends on the severity of symptoms. For patients who are in the New York Heart Association functional class III, the survival rate 5 years after diagnosis is 62% and approximately 38% at 10 years. Patients who are in class IV have only a 15% survival rate after 5 years and no survival after 8 years. In a random series of patients with mitral stenosis diagnosed initially at different stages of the disease approximately 80% will be alive after 5 years and approximately 60% alive after 10 years.

Patients who are asymptomatic may remain so for periods of 10 to 20 years. In contrast, once a patient becomes seriously symptomatic with mitral stenosis, progressive disability and death follow relatively rapidly. Asymptomatic patients are therefore not usually considered as surgical candidates, whereas those in classes III and IV need early surgical intervention. Difficulties in decision arise most commonly in patients with class II disability; the decision to operate must be made on an individual basis. It is important to make a careful assessment of so-called "asymptomatic" patients when there is evidence of critically tight mitral stenosis with severe pulmonary hypertension. It is common clinical experience that after successful operation "asymptomatic" patients acknowledge that they were in fact previously disabled but had learned to live with their symptoms.

Cardiologists do not agree as to whether to recommend surgery for the asymptomatic patient who suffers a single systemic embolus. However, patients who suffer recurrent emboli in spite of careful long-term anticoagulation are certainly candidates for surgery.

Patients must be carefully selected for closed mitral valvulotomy in that pure stenosis must be present and the valve must be mobile. This information is available from a thorough physical examination, the electrocardiogram, chest X-ray, and echocardiogram. In these patients there is no advantage to performing so-called "open" valvulotomy provided the surgeon has had sufficient experience with the "closed" technique. Patients with heavy calcification of the mitral valve, usually middle-aged males, are not candidates for valvulotomy and should have mitral valve replacement.

The presence of other valve disease also has a bearing on the nature of the surgical procedure. When there is significant aortic insufficiency requiring therapy in its own right, valvulotomy is best done as an open procedure at the time of aortic valve replacement. When tricuspid insufficiency is present a careful decision must be made as to whether this is functional or organic. In the majority of patients, tricuspid insufficiency is secondary to severe pulmonary hypertension and this disappears after successful mitral valvulotomy. However, when tricuspid insufficiency is due to organic disease of the valve, the increase in cardiac output following successful valvulotomy may seriously aggravate tricuspid insufficiency and lead to severe right-sided congestion. Tricuspid valve replacement may be required subsequently. Severe pulmonary hypertension is not a contraindication to surgery and there is usually satisfactory reduction in the pulmonary artery pressure following successful surgery.

Mitral valvotomy provides dramatic relief of symptoms but restenosis occurs in approximately 15% of patients within 5 years of operation. The operation also provides a significant improvement in the life span of individuals in classes III and IV. Actuarial survival curves show that whereas 85% of patients who undergo this procedure survive 5 years, only 48% survive a similar period with medical treatment.

Following successful mitral valvulotomy the opening snap usually persists but is well separated from the aortic component of the second heart sound. The diastolic rumble rarely disappears completely but becomes very much shorter. The E-F slope of the mitral echogram and the Doppler pressure half-time become more rapid following successful valvulotomy but uncommonly return to normal values. Cardioversion for atrial fibrillation can be attempted 2 weeks postoperatively whether the patients are receiving anticoagulants or not. Cardioversion is most successful if this arrhythmia develops in the early postoperative period or if it was present for less than a year prior to surgery.

Mitral Regurgitation

Mitral regurgitation is a result of scarring and contracture of the valve leaflets, shortening of the chordae, and scarring of the papillary muscles. The posterior leaflet is frequently more severely affected than the anterior.

Hemodynamics

Pure mitral regurgitation is an uncommon manifestation of rheumatic fever; almost invariably some degree of stenosis is present. When regurgitation is the most important hemodynamic feature this is a result of inadequate leaflet coaption. The severity of the regurgitation determines the degree to which the left ventricle must compensate to maintain forward flow into the aorta. The important adaptive feature that occurs in chronic mitral insufficiency is progressive increase in diastolic compliance of the left ventricle in response to increasing degrees of insufficiency. The Frank–Starling mechanism comes into effect and the left ventricle is therefore able to expel a large forward stroke output (the sum of the regurgitant and-the forward stroke volume). Importantly, the increase in volume end-diastole does not result in an increased end-diastolic pressure because of the change in diastolic compliance. The result is that severe left atrial and pulmonary capillary hypertension is not present and the patient may remain free of congestive pulmonary symptoms for a long time.

Systolic unloading of the ventricle may permit the patient with chronic mitral insufficiency to survive many years with relatively little disability. Because regurgitation into the left atrium begins immediately with the onset of systole, isovolumetric contraction is absent and the ventricle is protected from excessive tension on its walls, sparing myocardial oxygen consumption and allowing the energy of contraction to be used for fiber shortening.

Eventually, left ventricular function becomes impaired and there is a reduction of forward flow and an increase in left ventricular enddiastolic pressure. Pulmonary venous hypertension then passively raises the pulmonary artery pressure and reactive pulmonary hypertension may also supervene. Severe pulmonary hypertension, however, is generally less frequent and less severe than in mitral stenosis. Atrial fibrillation may exacerbate the symptoms, but this is not as severe as in mitral stenosis. Similarly, acute pulmonary edema is less frequent in mitral regurgitation.

Clinical Features

Symptoms

If the degree of regurgitation is mild, there are no symptoms. A major hazard, however is the development of infective endocarditis, which may seriously aggravate the insufficiency. Systemic embolism is less common than in mitral stenosis and, when it occurs, atrial fibrillation is usually present.

Among patients with more severe degrees of mitral insufficiency there is gradual progression of symptoms leading eventually to severe incapacity. Symptoms are a result of pulmonary congestion and effort dyspnea progresses to orthopnea, paroxysmal cardiac dyspnea, and attacks of acute pulmonary edema. Hemoptysis, angina pectoris, and embolism are less frequent than in mitral stenosis. Patients are frequently aware of the overactive, hyperdynamic left ventricle and may complain of palpitation. Fatigue and loss of energy are common.

Physical Signs

The pulse is usually normal, but occasionally has a slight collapsing quality, producing the so-called "jerky" pulse. Atrial fibrillation is frequent. The jugular venous pressure and wave form are normal in the absence of right heart failure. A prominent "A" wave may be found when there is pulmonary hypertension. In the late stages when there is tricuspid insufficiency, jugular venous distention and hepatomegaly are present.

Palpation of the precordium is of great value. Considerable left ventricular enlargement is present producing a displaced hyperactive apical impulse sustained through systole.

Careful evaluation of the pulsations in the left parasternal region is of diagnostic value in mitral insufficiency. A common clinical error is to attribute pulsations in this area to right ventricular hypertrophy when in fact it is usually a result of expansion of the left atrium by the regurgitant jet. *The left parasternal lift* of left atrial expansion starts early in systole, and rises slowly to have a peak amplitude in late systole near the timing of the second heart sound, followed by a precipitous collapse. In contrast, the pulsation of right ventricular hypertrophy starts at the onset of systole, is of small amplitude, and is sustained throughout systole. In severe cases of mitral insufficiency the left atrial lift may be present to the right of the sternum.

The left atrial lift should be carefully distinguished from the left parasternal lift of tricuspid insufficiency. The latter lift is *diastolic* in timing and is produced by volume overloading of the right ventricle by an overdistended right atrium.

Auscultation

A loud apical pansystolic regurgitant murmur is the auscultatory hallmark of significant mitral insufficiency. The murmur commences with the soft first heart sound, which it may obscure especially when insufficiency is severe. When mitral insufficiency is mild the first heart sound may be normal or even accentuated. The murmur runs through systole to the aortic component of the second heart sound, or even beyond it. It is maximal at the apex, high-pitched, blowing in quality and usually radiates to the axilla and posteriorly, since this is the usual direction of the regurgitant jet.

Less commonly the regurgitant jet is directed medially, so that the murmur radiates up to the fourth left space and even to the second right intercostal space, thus masquerading as aortic stenosis. This is more common, however, in the acute forms of mitral regurgitation when the posterior mitral leaflet is flail. The severity of mitral insufficiency cannot be assessed from the intensity of the murmur, though it is generally true that the loudest murmurs are present when insufficiency is severe and the patient is symptomatic.

Careful clinical evaluation of the murmur helps to distinguish it from other systolic murmurs. The murmur of mitral regurgitation varies little with the cycle length in atrial fibrillation and does not increase in intensity following a postectopic pause. This is a helpful feature in the distinction from the systolic murmur of left ventricular outflow obstruction where the murmur becomes much louder following a postectopic pause. *Amyl nitrite* softens the murmur of mitral insufficiency but intensifies the murmur of aortic or subaortic stenosis. Unlike the murmur of tricuspid insufficiency the murmur of mitral insufficiency is not accentuated by inspiration and is markedly softened by amyl nitrite and intensified by phenylephrine.

The *second heart sound* is usually closely or normally split but wide splitting may occur because of early aortic valve closure when left ventricular systole is markedly shortened due to severe regurgitation. A third heart sound is usually present at the apex and usually precedes a short middiastolic murmur. The middiastolic murmur is a result of a middiastolic gradient across the mitral valve because of some degree of commissural fusion and also high flow produced by the regurgitant volume. A presystolic murmur is not present. An opening snap may occur with predominant mitral regurgitation and signifies a thickened but mobile anterior leaflet; regurgitation is a result of a shrunken posterior leaflet. When significant pulmonary hypertension coexists, a pulmonary ejection sound, accentuation of the pulmonary component of the second heart sound, a tricuspid insufficiency murmur, and a right ventricular gallop may be present.

Electrocardiogram

The *electrocardiogram* may be normal or may show left atrial overload. Diastolic overloading of the left ventricle results in the pattern of left ventricular hypertrophy. Atrial fibrillation and supraventricular ectopic beats are frequent. The mean frontal plane QRS axis is usually normal or deviated to the right. Left axis deviation is uncommon and should alert one to the possibility of congestive cardiomyopathy with functional mitral insufficiency or endocardial cushion defect.

Radiology

This shows left atrial enlargement, which may reach aneurysmal proportions even protruding beyond the right cardiac border (Fig. 12.3). The aorta is not prominent. Fluoroscopy demonstrates systolic pulsation of the left atrium and an enlarged hyperactive left ventricle. Color Doppler echocardiography helps in the assessment of severity by detecting how much and how far the regurgitant jet fills the left

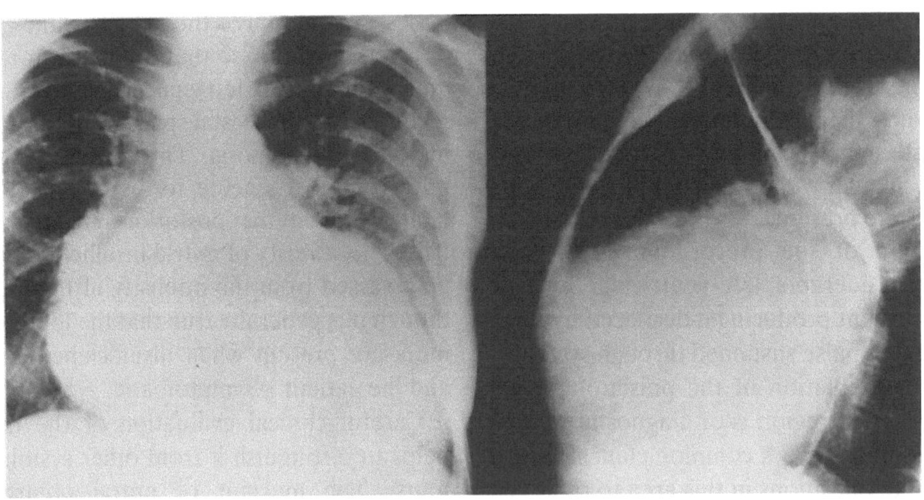

FIGURE 12.3. Chest X-ray in a case of gross mitral insufficiency demonstrating an aneurysmal left atrium protruding beyond the right cardiac border.

atrium and also in evaluating left ventricular function.

Cardiac catheterization is useful for estimation of the degree of mitral insufficiency and evaluating left ventricular function. The left ventricular enddiastolic pressure is frequently elevated but this does not necessarily imply left ventricular dysfunction and may occur with a reasonable ejection fraction. Simultaneous left ventricular and left atrial pressures demonstrate a middiastolic gradient, which disappears in late diastole.

Treatment

Survival statistics for patients with mitral insufficiency show that approximately 80% are alive 5 years after the diagnosis is established and approximately 60% are alive after 10 years. Mitral valve replacement is the procedure of choice for rheumatic mitral regurgitation and this results in symptomatic improvement in most patients. The risks of operation and the long-term complications of prosthetic cardiac values, such as thromboembolism, disintegration of ball valves, hemolytic anemia, and infective endocarditis, must be weighed against the degree of disability (Fig. 12.4). The indication for surgical intervention is a deterioration in effort tolerance and left ventricular function measured noninvasively. Operation should not be delayed for patients who are in functional class IV. When operation is performed in function classes II and III the operative mortality is less than 10%.

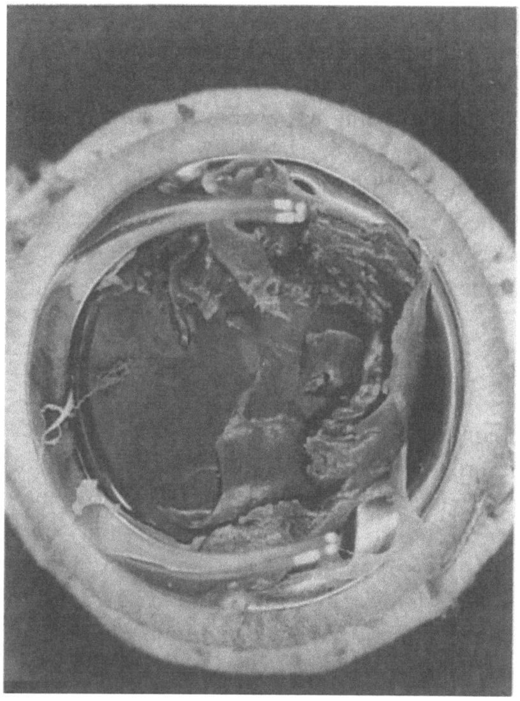

FIGURE 12.4. Thrombosis of Lillehei–Kaster prosthesis.

Mixed Mitral Stenosis and Insufficiency

This is far commoner than pure mitral insufficiency, but less common than pure mitral stenosis. Pathologically the valves are always more seriously damaged. Distortion and heavy calcification of the leaflets, shortening of the chordae tendinae, and scarring of the papillary muscles produce a so-called "washer" valve. There is a wide spectrum, of severity of the disease, which relates to the hemodynamics. When there is significant stenosis, the left atrial pressure is often as high as in mitral stenosis: The hemodynamics are also affected by volume overloading of the left ventricle.

Clinical Features

Dominant mitral insufficiency is associated with left ventricular enlargement, a left atrial lift, a loud pansystolic regurgitant murmur and a significantly long middiastolic murmur; a presystolic murmur is generally absent. *Dominant mitral stenosis* has a normal apex, right ventricular enlargement with long rumbling middiastolic and presystolic murmur, and a soft apical pansystolic murmur.

Some help may be obtained from the electrocardiogram and chest X-rays. Right ventricular hypertrophy, electrocardiographically is unusual in severe chronic mitral regurgitation and the sign would favor predominant mitral stenosis. Similarly, left ventricular hypertrophy would favor mitral regurgitation and militate against the diagnosis of pure mitral stenosis. Radiologically, little can be deduced from the size of the left atrium. Changes in pulmonary vascularity are helpful, the most marked redistribution to the upper lobes occurring with mitral stenosis.

Cardiac catheterization is useful in assessing the hemodynamics and for angiographic assessment of the degree of mitral insufficiency and mobility of the mitral valve apparatus.

Treatment

In contrast to pure chronic mitral insufficiency the prognosis for mixed mitral valve disease is worse. Only two-thirds of these patients may be expected to be alive 5 years, and only one-third 10 years after making the initial diagnosis. Prosthetic valve replacement is required and recommended when symptoms are present and there is evidence of significant hemodynamic impairment.

Aortic Stenosis

Aortic stenosis follows an attack of acute valvulitis. Fusion of the commissures occurs in the healing phase, and frequently the valve becomes bicuspid. It is generally possible to distinguish this acquired type of bicuspid valve from the congenital variety by the presence of a characteristic raphe in the latter condition. The raphe extends from the edge of one of the leaflets of the congenital bicuspid valve to the aortic wall. Slow, but progressive narrowing and calcification of the orifice ultimately lead to significant aortic stenosis. This generally tends to occur later than in patients with mitral stenosis.

Hemodynamics

The normal cross-sectional area of the adult aortic valve is 2.6 to 3.5 cm^2. Significant aortic stenosis is present when the valve area is reduced to less than 0.7 cm^2 and the gradient between the left ventricle and the aorta is 50 mm Hg or more (Fig. 12.5). Obstruction to left ventricular emptying results in an increase in left ventricular muscle mass by concentric left ventricular hypertrophy. Left ventricular dilatation even with pressures of 250 mm Hg is not part of the compensatory mechanism. The thick ventricle is less distensible than normal and this elevates the enddiastolic pressure even at rest; in the presence of severe aortic stenosis therefore this does not imply that heart failure is present.

Atrial contraction (the so-called "atrial kick") is important in contributing to ventricular filling by increasing ventricular pressure and myocardial fiber length at the end of diastole and this assists ventricular emptying by the Frank–Starling mechanism. The left atrial "A" wave may reach 35 mm Hg to accomplish adequate filling of the ventricle. Elevation of the left atrial pressure to this magnitude is usually sufficient to cause pulmonary edema, but since this occurs only during the brief period of atrial contraction, pulmonary edema will not occur. When, however, the mean left atrial pressure is elevated above 25 mm Hg pulmonary edema is imminent. The left atrial kick thus provides a means whereby increased enddiastolic stretch may occur without chronic elevation of pulmonary capillary pressure and consequent pulmonary edema. Thus, loss of atrial contraction in atrial fibrillation is an important factor contributing to the reduction of cardiac output and heart failure in severe aortic stenosis.

When obstruction of the aortic valve is significant the arterial pulse is small with a slow rate of rise and a distinct anacrotic shoulder on the ascending limb. The rate of rise of arterial pressure is reduced and the systolic ejection period is increased. This type of pulse has been referred to a "pulsus parvus et tardus."

Clinical Features

Isolated clinically severe aortic valve stenosis, particularly in a male without a history of rheumatic fever, is usually a result of nonrheumatic disease such as d congenital bicuspid valve. A history of rheumatic fever and evidence of mitral valve disease indicate rheumatic etiology.

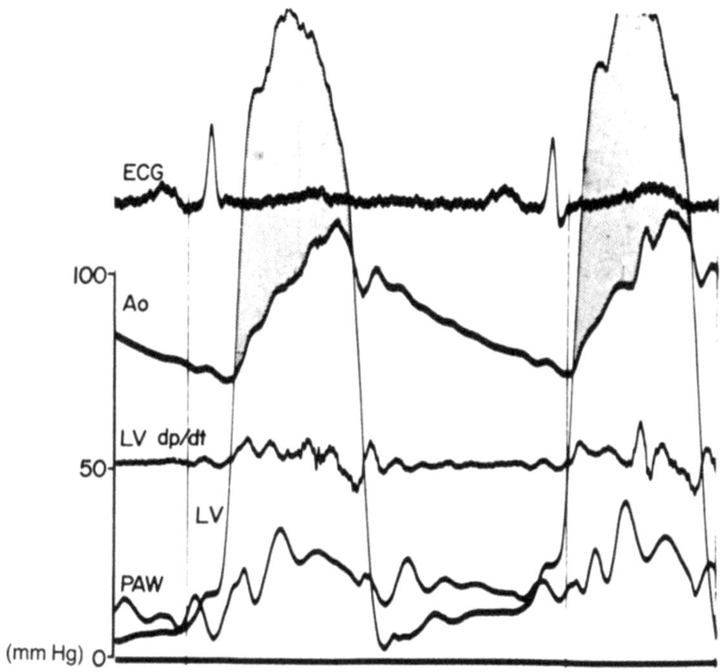

FIGURE 12.5. Simultaneous electrocardiogram, aortic, left ventricular, and wedge pressures in a case of severe rheumatic aortic stenosis. Systolic gradient between the left ventricle and aorta is shaded.

Symptoms cannot be used to identify those patients with hemodynamically significant aortic stenosis. When the stenosis is mild, there are no symptoms and attention is drawn to the heart because of the murmur. When symptoms do occur, they do so late when the disease is well advanced. Patients with significant aortic stenosis are frequently asymptomatic and undetected for many years. On the other hand mild aortic stenosis may be associated with prominent symptoms when coronary artery disease is associated.

Dyspnea is usually the first symptom and occurs with exertion. It does not have the same grave prognostic significance as nocturnal dyspnea or frank attacks of pulmonary congestion. Usually attacks of left heart failure occur spontaneously and once this has occurred the course is generally rapidly downhill with an average survival of less than 2 years.

Angina pectoris occurs in up to three quarters of patients with severe aortic stenosis. In the majority of patients there is no evidence of occlusive atherosclerosis, and angina is a result of imbalance between myocardial oxygen demand and availability. Nitroglycerin is effective in alleviating angina even in the presence of normal coronary arteries because it decreases left ventricular systolic pressure and also shortens the duration of systole. It also decreases the dimensions of the left ventricle, which, by the law of Laplace, reduces transmural tension and therefore myocardial oxygen requirements. However, in at least one-half of patients with aortic stenosis there is significant coronary artery disease, which contributes to the inadequacy of oxygen supply to the myocardium.

For the majority of patients the onset of angina pectoris implies an average life expectancy of only 5 years.

Syncope characteristically occurs with effort and is an omnious sign; survival beyond 4 years is unusual. It follows a fall in cardiac output produced by a marked decrease in arterial pressure when the systemic vascular resistance fails to increase appropriately.

Physical Signs

Pulse

The pulse is normal when the stenosis is mild. With severe stenosis, an anacrotic or slow rising pulse is classical. This is best felt in the carotid, left brachial, and femoral arteries. The pulse pressure is usually narrow (30–40 mm Hg) because of a low systolic blood pressure.

In the elderly patient, sclerotic vessels may normalize the carotid upstroke time; a fairly rapid upstroke time thus does not exclude severe aortic stenosis. For the same reason the systolic blood pressure may reach 180 mm Hg in the elderly in the presence of severe aortic stenosis, levels that would exclude the condition in the younger age groups. However, significant aortic stenosis is unlikely when the diastolic pressure exceeds 100 mm Hg.

Jugular Venous Pressure

This is usually normal except in heart failure, or when there is associated mitral or tricuspid valve disease. Prominent "A" or "H-A" waves are known to occur in aortic stenosis and were previously ascribed to the so-called "Bernheim" phenomenon. Deviation of the ventricular septum into the right ventricular cavity was thought to produce right ventricular outflow obstruction. A more likely mechanism is that the prominent "A" wave is the result of reduced right ventricular compliance because the ventricles share a common septal wall.

Precordial Palpation

In thin-chested individuals there is a sustained holosystolic apical impulse. Additionally, there is frequently a palpable presystolic pulsation produced by atrial systole. A basal systolic thrill is a helpful clue indicating the presence of significant aortic stenosis.

Auscultation

The *aortic ejection murmur* is characteristic and is louder in the second right intercostal space than the left. It radiates to the vessels of the neck and to the apex. Sometimes it is loudest at the apex and may even be confined to this area, in which case it has to be distinguished from the murmur of hypertrophic cardiomyopathy, which softens with squatting, whereas that of valvular aortic stenosis is little changed. The most helpful feature in assessing the severity of the stenosis is the timing of the crescendo of the murmur. The later the crescendo, the more severe the stenosis. Characteristically, the murmur intensifies following a postectopic pause and the administration of amyl nitrite.

An *aortic ejection click* is frequently heard when the aortic valve is not heavily calcified. It is almost invariably present in children with severe aortic stenosis but is unusual in the elderly with heavily calcified valves. When present it is a helpful clue that the left ventricular outflow obstruction is located at the valve.

The aortic component of the second sound is delayed because of the prolongation of left ventricular systole and this may result in a single or reversed split second sound. When the valve is heavily calcified the aortic component of the second sound becomes soft. A soft early diastolic murmur at the third or fourth left interspace reflecting mild aortic insufficiency is quite common. A presystolic gallop, particularly in the left decubitus position, is frequent and indicates significant aortic stenosis.

The Electrocardiogram

This is extremely valuable in assessing the severity and progression of aortic valvular stenosis. In mild cases, the electrocardiogram is normal but when stenosis is significant, left ventricular hypertrophy is almost a constant finding. A fairly characteristic pattern is that of "systolic overload," manifested by deep S waves in the right precordial leads and tall R waves in the left precordial leads: ST segment depression and T wave inversion are commonly found in the leads showing tall R waves. Pathological left axis deviation, left bundle branch block, or nonspecific intraventricular conduction defects are common in advanced cases and result from patchy subendocardial fibrosis.

As in congenital aortic stenosis, the electrocardiogram is rarely normal in severe rheumatic aortic stenosis. Sinus rhythm is the usual finding; atrial fibrillation in young patients usually suggests the presence of associated mitral valve disease. Left atrial enlargment characterized by a negative terminal deflection of the P wave in V1 is supportive evidence of severe stenosis.

Radiological Findings

Characteristically, the cardiothoracic ratio is within normal limits but left ventricular hypertrophy may be suggested by some bulging of the lower third of the left cardiac border. Poststenotic dilatation of the ascending aorta is common but its extent cannot be correlated with the severity of the stenosis. Calcification of the aortic valve should always be searched for with fluoroscopy; its absence in a patient over 45 years of age should raise the suspicion that outflow tract obstruction is not at valve level.

Phonocardiography and External Carotid Pulse Recording

These may be helpful in diagnosis. The most sensitive indices are prolongation of the ejection time, diminution of the maximum rate of arterial pressure rise, and prolongation of the interval from the Q wave to the peak of the systolic ejection murmur. When all these findings are present severe aortic stenosis is almost invariable.

Echocardiography

In valvular aortic stenosis this technique demonstrates multiple, thick poorly mobile linear leaflet echoes within the aortic root, which are frequently thicker than echoes from the aortic wall itself. Doppler echocardiography utilizing the Bernoulli equation provides an accurate measurement of aortic valve area. It has proved so reliable that it is no longer absolutely necessary to measure the gradient at cardiac catheterization.

Cardiac Catheterization

This is indicated when any of the symptoms described are present. The goal of the procedure is to calculate the valve area using the Gorlin formula by measuring the gradient across the aortic valve and the cardiac output. When the left ventricle cannot be entered the Doppler measurement is used. A valve area of less than 0.75 cm^2 is generally accepted as an indication for valve replacement. Left ventricular angiography is performed during the same procedure to assess left ventricular function. Coronary angiography will determine whether coronary atherosclerosis is present.

There is no problem about advising surgery when severe symptoms such as progressive effort dyspnea, paroxysmal dyspnea, angina pectoris, and syncope are present. Catheterization under these circumstances will generally confirm that the valve area is critically narrowed. Valve replacement is life-saving and the long-term results rewarding. The management of the *asymptomatic* patient with significant aortic stenosis is a difficult question since the condition tends to progress, becoming more severe, and there is also a tendency to sudden death. The immediate and late risks of valve replacement have not been demonstrated to favor valve replacement in such patients. Medical management of the asymptomatic patient with mild aortic stenosis includes prophylaxis against infective endocarditis and avoidance of competitive sports and strenuous exercise.

Aortic Insufficiency

Rheumatic aortic insufficiency is the result of fibrosis and contracture of the valve cusps without significant adhesion between the cusps at the commissures. The murmur of aortic insufficiency is frequently first detected during the acute attack of rheumatic fever and, following this, never disappears.

Hemodynamics

Depending on its severity, aortic insufficiency is characterized by a latent period of up to 10 years before symptoms are manifest. The hemodynamic effect of the incompetent valve is diastolic reflux from the aorta to the left ventricle. Since the left ventricle is then filled through both mitral and aortic valves, the chamber is overloaded and the enddiastolic volume is increased. The increased volume is accommodated by left ventricular dilatation and hypertrophy. The magnitude of the aortic reflux is determined by the size of the aortic valve orifice in diastole and by the systemic resistance. The importance of the latter is demonstrated by the fact that severe reflux may occur even when the regurgitant orifice is small but the total peripheral resistance is high. Similarly, a reduction in the peripheral resistance produced by the inhalation of amyl nitrite enhances left ventricular ejection and reduces the regurgitant volume. Exercise also reduces the peripheral vascular resistance and this accounts for the excellent effort tolerance maintained by some patients with severe aortic insufficiency.

Left ventricular dilatation increases the stroke volume ejected by the left ventricle by the Frank–Starling mechanism. The regurgitant volume may reach 80% of the total output of the left ventricle. Like mitral insufficiency, this is accomplished without significant increase in the left ventricular enddiastolic pressure because of a significant increase in diastolic compliance of the ventricle as it enlarges over the years. The hypertrophy that develops with regurgitation keeps ventricular wall stress within normal range and diminishes oxygen consumption; ultimately, however, cardiac decompensation will occur.

Clinical Features

Following the initial attack of rheumatic fever the majority of patients with aortic regurgitation develop symptoms in the age group 20 to 50 years. This long incubation is related to a latent period of 7 to 10 years following the acute attack and the development of "free" aortic insufficiency. The term "free" insufficiency is used when a wide pulse pressure and bounding pulses are present. Following this latent period, symptoms occur 7 to 10 years later.

This latent period may not occur in those countries where rheumatic fever is virulent in nature and free aortic insufficiency develops during the acute attack, or when otherwise mild aortic insufficiency is complicated by infective endocarditis.

Symptoms

The early symptoms are related to forceful cardiac action and the patient becomes aware of visible pulsations in the precordium or neck. Frequently, there is a gradual decrease in effort tolerance leading to symptoms of pulmonary congestion, orthopnea, paroxysmal cardiac dyspnea, and eventually frank pulmonary edema.

Angina pectoris is less common in aortic insufficiency than in aortic stenosis. It also has a tendency to occur at night and is frequently associated with dyspnea and palpitation, forcing the patient to sit up and lean forward. It occurs in young patients with normal coronary arteries and is thought to be a result of the low aortic diastolic pressure and increased oxygen demand of a hypertrophied dilated left ventricle.

Right heart failure ultimately results from passive elevation of the pulmonary capillary pressure and pulmonary arterial hypertension. Sudden death has also been noted after vigorous exercise in apparently healthy asymptomatic subjects. Embolism is rare but infective endocarditis is always a danger, often converting mild to severe incompetence. The sudden development of torrential regurgitation into an unprepared ventricle produces acute pulmonary congestion and heart failure.

Physical Signs

Mild aortic insufficiency is diagnosed by hearing the early diastolic murmur and not from symptoms; it is not infrequently found during a routine physical examination. The murmur is blowing in character, commencing with aortic component of the second sound. Because of its high pitch and softness it is the most frequently missed organic murmur.

With increasing degrees of insufficiency the murmur becomes louder, longer, and radiates more widely. However, there are exceptions to this. Occasionally, loud murmurs have little hemodynamic significance and conversely murmurs may be absent during the low cardiac output of congestive failure, or when aortic insufficiency is suddenly aggravated because of infective endocarditis. The early diastolic murmur is heard better to the right.

An early diastolic murmur heard better to the right of the sternum than the left suggests that the cause of regurgitation is associated with dilatation of the ascending aorta produced by syphilitic aortitis or dissecting aneurysm. Occasionally, it has a high-pitched musical character resembling a "cooing-dove." This suggests that the valve has an unusual deformity produced by laceration, perforation, or eversion of the edges. A loud systolic murmur does not necessarily indicate significant aortic stenosis. The murmur is produced by a large stroke volume ejected across the aortic valve.

At the apex, a pansystolic murmur may represent functional or organic mitral insufficiency. An apical third sound followed by a middiastolic murmur (Austin–Flint murmur) is frequent with significant aortic insufficiency; it may be difficult to distinguish this from that of true mitral stenosis. Amyl nitrite characteristically softens the Austin–Flint murmur but intensifies the murmur of true mitral stenosis, whereas squatting increases the peripheral vascular resistance and intensifies the Austin–Flint murmur. The presence of an opening snap is diagnostic of rheumatic mitral valve disease. A loud first heart sound is of no value in differentiation. A very large pulse pressure favors the Austin–Flint murmur but a moderately increased pulse pressure with a reasonably high diastolic pressure does not exclude this murmur. Radiological examination may be helpful in that significant left atrial enlargement favors organic mitral valve disease.

Echocardiography is invaluable in the diagnosis of an Austin–Flint murmur: a fast fluttering movement of the anterior leaflet is observed during diastole. Additionally, the diastolic closure rate of the mitral valve leaflets is extremely rapid and mitral valve closure may occur prior to the onset of the QRS complex; thickening of the mitral valve leaflets is absent. Diastolic fluttering is the most specific of the echocardiographic signs used for the diagnosis of the Austin–Flint murmur. When mitral stenosis is present the E to F slope is characteristically slow.

The mitral component of the first heart sound is usually normal. A long PR interval, unrelated to the administration of digitalis, is frequently associated with aortic insufficiency and this tends to soften the first heart sound. The aortic component of the second heart sound is softer than normal when regurgitation is severe.

Pulse

The pulse becomes full and collapsing and arterial pulsation appears in the neck (Corrigan's sign). Pistol shots can be heard over the femoral arteries and capillary pulsation is visible. Duroziez's sign refers to a systolic and diastolic bruit detected by applying mild pressure with a stethoscope over the femoral artery. In normals, compression of the femoral artery will elicit a systolic bruit only; the presence of a diastolic bruit reflects rapid regurgitation toward the heart in diastole. This is a valuable sign of aortic "runoff" but is not exclusive to aortic insufficiency and may occur in other causes of high cardiac output. A bisferiens pulse is a manifestation of aortic incompetence. A basal systolic thrill conducted into the vessels of the neck occurs in pure aortic insufficiency and is not necessarily suggestive of aortic stenosis.

Blood Pressure

Blood pressure correlates roughly with the degree of insufficiency in that the larger the pulse pressure and the lower the diastolic pressure the more severe is the insufficiency. The diastolic pressure, however, is difficult to measure and a reading of zero is frequent. The diastolic pressure is best recorded where the sounds alter and both this point and the disappearance point should be recorded. In the late stage of the disease when the end-diastolic pressure in the left ventricle is markedly raised, the diastolic pressure in the aorta rises correspondingly and the pulse pressure therefore does not reflect the severity of the diastolic leak. The systolic pressure may often be quite markedly elevated to levels of up to 200 mm Hg. This does not necessarily imply associated systemic hypertension since readings return to normal following valve replacement.

Precordial Palpation

Left ventricular enlargement is readily detected and the apical impulse has a sustained, thrusting character displaced inferiorly and laterally. It has a hyperactive character due to the overfilled left ventricle.

Electrocardiogram

Usually there is sinus rhythm. Atrial fibrillation suggests coexisting mitral valve disease or left ventricular failure. First degree heart block is not uncommon, but pathological left axis deviation, left bundle branch block, and widening of the QRS complex are less common than in aortic stenosis. Characteristically, the QRS amplitude is increased and the ST segments are depressed with inverted T waves in the left precordial leads. Left atrial overload is often present.

Radiological Findings

The left ventricle is enlarged and fluoroscopy demonstrates marked pulsation of the left ventricle and the aorta. The ascending and descending aorta is commonly enlarged, in contrast to aortic stenosis, which involves only the ascending portion.

Cardiac Catheterization

This is employed to assess the degree of regurgitation, evaluate left ventricular function, and exclude concomitant valvular or coronary artery disease.

Treatment

Infective endocarditis is a hazard in all degrees of severity of aortic insufficiency. Antibiotic prophylaxis is essential before any possible precipitating procedure.

Most data would suggest that among patients with chronic aortic insufficiency, three-quarters of chose treated medically will be alive at 5 years, and one-half at 10 years after the diagnosis has been made. Thus, free aortic insufficiency has a relatively good prognosis and the approximate 10-year survival rate is 50%. When the insufficiency is milder, 95% of patients will be alive after 10 years. However, once aortic insufficiency is complicated by heart failure, deterioration is rapid and most patients will die within 2 years of the onset of heart failure. The excellent survival rate for patients with moderate aortic insufficiency would seem to preclude early surgical intervention in an asymptomatic patient despite the recent improvement in mortality and morbidity for valve replacement. Ideally, surgery should be performed as soon as there is a clear indication of deterioration in symptoms, or decreasing left ventricular function and increasing left ventricular size assessed noninvasively by echo and MUGA but well before the development of congestive heart failure.

Aortic Stenosis and Incompetence

Combined aortic stenosis and incompetence produces a variable clinical picture dependent on whether stenosis or incompetence is the dominant lesion, or whether both lesions are equally significant.

The Clinical Findings

These consist of bisferiens pulse, an overfilled enlarged hyperactive left ventricle with a thrusting apex beat, and systolic and early diastolic murmurs. Predominant stenosis or predominant incompetence is readily differentiated. When the lesions are equally significant it is difficult to assess their relative contribution. From the practical standpoint, however, this determination is unimportant. Therapeutic measures are dictated by close supervision of the patients symptoms and left ventricular function.

Tricuspid Valve Disease

Based on necropsy evidence there is a 25% incidence of tricuspid valve involvement in rheumatic heart disease. However, clinical recognition lags behind, and the differentiation of functional from organic tricuspid valve disease still remains a problem. Organic tricuspid disease is always associated with multivalvular, severe rheumatic heart disease.

Tricuspid Incompetence

Functional tricuspid incompetence occurs with right heart failure because dilatation of the right ventricle stretches the valve ring. *Organic* tricuspid incompetence is a result of shortening and thickening of the tricuspid leaflets so that they are imperfectly sealed during ventricular systole.

Hemodynamics

The normal drop in right atrial pressure during ventricular systole is replaced by an increase in pressure because of regurgitation of right ventricular stroke volume into the right atrium. This produces an increase in the mean right atrial pressure, the contour of which is characterized by systolic elevation ("CV" waves) frequently referred to as "ventricularization" of the atrial pressure. When the right atrial pressure rises sufficiently, systemic venous congestion and hepatomegaly result.

Clinical Features

Tricuspid incompetence is almost always associated with mitral valve disease and often with aortic valve disease. Atrial fibrillation is present in 90% of patients and may contribute to the development of tricuspid incompetence. The tricuspid valve normally closes after atrial contraction just before the onset of right ventricular systole. With fibrillating atria the valve

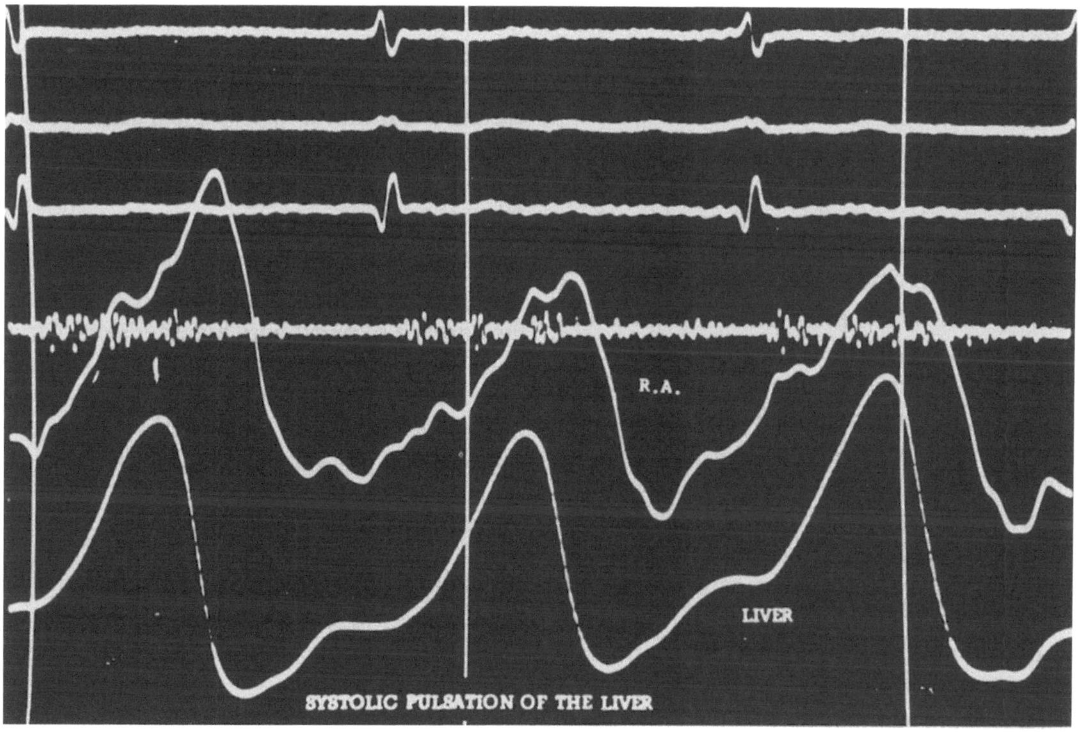

FIGURE 12.6. Electrocardiogram (top panel), phonocardiogram (second panel), kinetocardiogram of the right atrial pulsation (third panel), and of the liver (fourth panel) demonstrating systolic expansion of the right atrium and the liver in severe tricuspid insufficiency. A pansystolic murmur of tricuspid insufficiency is demonstrated.

may still be open at the onset of systole. Not infrequently, tricuspid regurgitation frequently becomes first evident with the onset of atrial fibrillation.

Tricuspid incompetence contributes to and aggravates chronic congestive cardiac failure, producing hepatomegaly, ascites, and dependent edema. When tricuspid incompetence is severe important abnormalities are present in the jugular venous pulse. The mean pressure is elevated with "CV" waves producing a sustained systolic pulsation, with a marked "Y" collapse. Systolic *pulsation of the liver* is an expression of the same phenomenon (Fig. 12.6). In the presence of atrial fibrillation, incompetence is always more marked. These features serve to differentiate the condition from chronic constrictive pericarditis where the signs and symptoms of chronic heart failure are comparable.

Arterial Pulse

Like the blood pressure this is influenced by associated valve lesions.

Heart

The right ventricle is enlarged and in severe incompetence may form the apex. A triple rhythm may be palpable and audible. Auscultation detects a systolic murmur at the tricuspid area. The characteristic feature is accentuation of this murmur with inspiration. Sometimes the murmur has a peculiar "honking" quality that is almost specific. With marked right ventricular dilatation the murmur is widespread and easily heard at the apex, so that it is readily confused with mitral incompetence, which may coexist. It is particularly important to recognize the origin of the murmur, however, since an erroneous diagnosis of mitral incompetence may mean that mitral stenosis of considerable severity may be overlooked and operation deferred.

The systolic murmur may be the only sign of tricuspid incompetence, but when the lesion is severe there is little turbulence across the valve and the characteristic murmur may be absent or very soft indeed. The murmur is often recognized as functional because it disappears with treatment as the signs of congestive failure disappear. It can be remarkably transient, being precipitated by effort and disappearing with rest, or it may appear on inspiration only. Not infrequently when patients are admitted to hospital a loud murmur is interpreted as mitral incompetence and this disappears overnight with bedrest and diuretics. At other times the murmur disappears only many weeks after operation on the mitral valve.

A delayed *tricuspid early diastolic murmur* does not necessarily imply the presence of tricuspid stenosis, and that a coexisting systolic murmur is therefore due to organic disease of the valve. It may also be functional when incompetence is severe and results in high forward flow across the valve. This tricuspid diastolic murmur is often confused with the murmur of aortic insufficiency because it sometimes has a softer blowing quality than a mitral middiastolic murmur and also because it occurs somewhat earlier in diastole. Characteristically, it also increases markedly with inspiration and may even become musical. When the right atrium is grossly dilated tricuspid murmurs may be heard best to the right of the sternum in the third and fourth intercostal spaces and not in the xiphisternal (or tricuspid) area.

Electrocardiogram

When there is sinus rhythm, right atrial overload may be helpful in diagnosis especially in the absence of pulmonary hypertension. Atrial fibrillation, however, is the rule. Complete right bundle branch block is also a frequent finding. A QR pattern in lead V1 is also highly suggestive of tricuspid incompetence.

Radiology

Right atrial enlargement may be detected from the chest X-ray but coexistent findings associated with mitral and aortic valve disease dominate the picture.

Tricuspid Stenosis

The normal tricuspid valve area is greater than 7 cm^2 and reduction of this orifice size to less than 1.5 cm^2 results in hemodynamic impairment. Rheumatic tricuspid stenosis is almost invariably associated with mitral valve disease. Tricuspid stenosis without insufficiency is a relatively uncommon condition and since the diagnosis is difficult to make, it is often undetected.

Clinical Features

The symptoms are much the same as those occurring with tricuspid incompetence.

The most important diagnostic clue is the *jugular venous pulse*. When sinus rhythm is present a "giant A wave" is the most striking finding. It is particularly helpful if evidence of severe pulmonary hypertension is absent. The A wave is far more easily recognized than the slow Y descent. At the tricuspid and xiphisternal areas there is a middiastolic murmur with presystolic accentuation that intensifies remarkably with inspiration. A tricuspid opening snap frequently precedes the middiastolic murmur but is difficult to distinguish from a mitral opening snap. The tricuspid middiastolic murmur may have to be distinguished from the early diastolic murmur of aortic incompetence as previously discussed.

Electrocardiogram

This is usually dominated by effects of associated valve lesions. Marked right atrial overload in the absence of right ventricular hypertrophy is a valuable clue, but this is lost when there is atrial fibrillation. A prolonged PR interval is frequently associated.

Radiological Findings

Marked dilatation of the right atrium without significant right ventricular or pulmonary artery enlargement is the most characteristic finding.

Cardiac Catheterization

This is helpful in establishing the diagnosis and is best accomplished by simultaneous double-lumen recording of the right ventricular and right atrial pressures. A valve area of less than 1.5 cm^2 indicates significant stenosis. *Echocardiography* will demonstrate the thick leaflets and the enlarged right atrium, and exclude a myxoma. Angiography demonstrates an enlarged right atrium and a jet through the stenotic tricuspid valve. It also is helpful in excluding a right atrial myxoma.

Treatment of Tricuspid Valve Disease

Minor involvement of the tricuspid valve is best left alone. For severe tricuspid stenosis, blind valvotomy is more difficult than in mitral stenosis. When mitral stenosis coexists, both valves are probably best dealt with by open valvulotomy using cardiopulmonary bypass. In the case of significant tricuspid regurgitation that persists after adequate bedrest and diuretic therapy inspection of the tricuspid valve is indicated at the time of operative correction for associated valve disease.

When the tricuspid valve is found to be relatively normal, most surgeons favor tricuspid annuloplasty since the postoperative course is smoother. When organic tricuspid disease is present with leaflet shortening, tricuspid valve replacement should be carried out as part of the procedure for associated mitral and/or aortic valve disease. Prosthetic tricuspid valves are relatively stenotic and mild persistent venous hypertension and hepatomegaly frequently result. An aortic homograft or porcine heterograft provides more satisfactory hemodynamics in the tricuspid position.

Additional Reading

Armstrong TG, Mitha AS, Weir EK, Chesler E: Non-invasive observation on the initial low frequency vibrations of the first heart sound—correlations with the "presystolic murmur" in mitral stenosis. Br Heart J 40:750, 1978.

Bland EF, Jones TD: Rheumatic fever and rheumatic heart disease. A twenty year report on 1000 patients followed since childhood. Circulation 4:836, 1951.

Criley JM, Hermer AJ: The crescendo presystolic murmur of mitral stenosis with atrial fibrillation. N Engl J Med 285:1284, 1971.

Dack S, Bleifer S, Grishman A, Donoso E: Mitral stenosis: Auscultatory and phonocardiographic findings. Am J Cardiol 5:815, 1960.

Lakier JB, Pocock WA, Gale GE, Barlow JB: Haemodynamic and sound events preceding first heart sound in mitral stenosis. Br Heart J 34:1152, 1972.

Levy MJ, Edwards JE: Anatomy of mitral insufficiency. Prog Cardiovasc Dis 5:119, 1962.

Olson KH: The natural history of 271 patients with mitral stenosis under medical treatment. Br Heart J 24:349, 1962.

Perloff JK, Harvey WP: Clinical recognition of tricuspid stenosis. Circulation 22:346, 1960.

Rahimtoola, SH: Perspective on valvular heart disease: An update. J.A.C.C. 14:1:1–23, 1989.

Rapaport E: Natural history of aortic and mitral valve disease. Am J Cardiol 35:221, 1975.

Spaynuolo M, Kloth N, Taranta A, Doyle E, Pasternack B: Natural history of aortic regurgitation: Criteria predictive of death, congestive heart failure and angina in young patients. Circulation 44:368, 1971.

Wood P: An appreciation of mitral stenosis: I Clinical features. II Investigations and results. Br Med J 1:1051, 113, 1954.

Wood P: Aortic stenosis. Am J Cardiol 1:553, 1958.

13
Nonrheumatic Valvular Disease

The Mitral Valve

Most acquired nonrheumatic conditions affecting the mitral valve have mitral insufficiency as their important manifestation. The components of the mitral valve consist of the papillary muscles, chordae tendinae, annulus, and leaflets, all of which play an important and complex part in maintaining valve competence. Involvement of any of these structures may lead to varying degrees of mitral insufficiency.

Myxomatous Mitral Valve [Syn. "Click-Murmur Syndrome," "The Billowing Mitral Leaflet Syndrome" (BMLS), "Barlow's Syndrome"]

This syndrome consists of voluminous mitral leaflets, a nonejection click, frequently followed by a late systolic murmur of mild mitral regurgitation, electrocardiographic abnormalities, and a familial incidence. With the decline in incidence of rheumatic fever, the BMLS has emerged as the most frequent form of valve disease.

Pathology

The primary lesion is an increase in the centrally situated spongiosa component of the normal mitral valve. This leads to interruption of the outer fibrous layer that weakens the leaflet producing first, abnormal interchordal hooding followed by progressive ballooning of the entire leaflet toward the left atrium (Fig. 13.1).

The posterior leaflet is particularly affected, especially in its central third, but the posteromedial portion of anterior mitral leaflet is also occasionally involved. Friction lesions of the mural endocardium of the posterior ventricular wall occur because of contact with the chordae in diastole. These may become fibrous and calcified and may be important in the genesis of ventricular arrhythmias (Fig. 13.2). Contact between the posterior leaflet and the left atrial wall leads to fibrin deposition, which may be a source of systemic embolism (Fig. 13.3).

Myxomatous degeneration of the mitral valve is common in patients with Marfan's and Ehlers–Danlos syndrome and pectus excavatum. The degree of regurgitation is variable, some patients having mild insufficiency manifested by a click and late systolic murmur and others having severe regurgitation associated with voluminous leaflets and elongated or even ruptured chordae tendinae.

Mitral valve prolapse detected by echocardiography does not mean that the valve is myxomatous. In atrial septal defect and hypertrophic cardiomyopathy prolapse of *normal* leaflets may occur when there is disproportion between the volume of the left ventricle and the size of the mitral annulus. Similar false associations have been described in inferior myocardial infarction. cardiomyopathy, and myocarditis where failure of chordal systolic

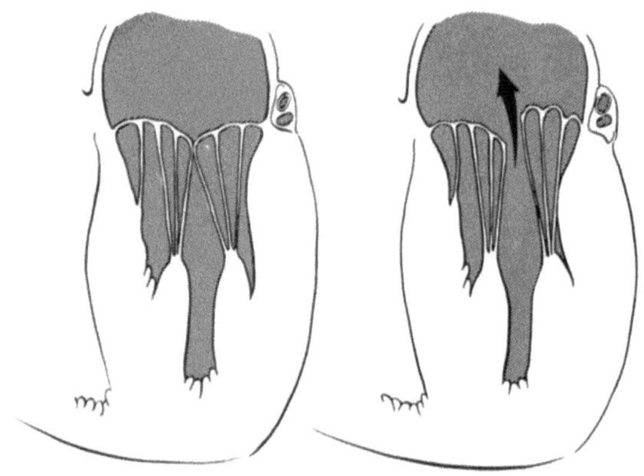

FIGURE 13.1. Diagrammatic representation of the billowing mitral leaflet syndrome. During left ventricular systole mitral regurgitation occurs as the posterior mitral leaflet billows into the left atrium and fills to appose with the anterior leaflet.

tension also leads to prolapse of normal leaflets.

Since myxomatous valves occur in approximately 5% of the population it is not surprising that there will be *coincidental* association with other common conditions (e.g., migraine thyrotoxicosis).

Clinical Features

The condition occurs in patients of all ages and is more common in females. There is an unquestioned familial incidence and an autosomal dominant mode of inheritance is evident. The exact prevalence is uncertain but it probably occurs in 4–5% of the normal population.

Atypical Chest Pain

This is a common symptom and usually is not exercise related. Typically it is sharp, knifelike, transitory, and may disappear spontaneously for months. It is almost certainly a result of iatrogenic cardiac neurosis.

Psychological Manifestations

Many patients with this syndrome are extremely anxious and have been labeled "hyperadrenergic." Their symptoms have been attributed to autonomic imbalance and "neuroendocrine imbalance." Like atypical chest pain these symptoms are a result of anxiety and fear of serious heart disease.

Physical Findings

The typical auscultatory features appear to be more common among subjects with pectus

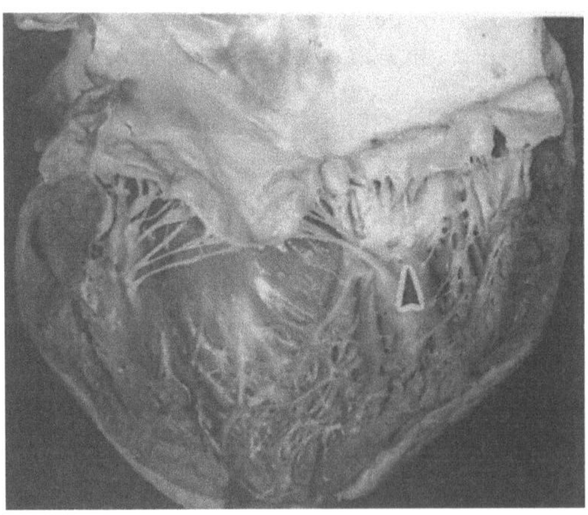

FIGURE 13.2. Mitral valve prolapse, both leaflets. The chordae are thickened and the subjacent endocardium shows confluent fibrosis (arrow).

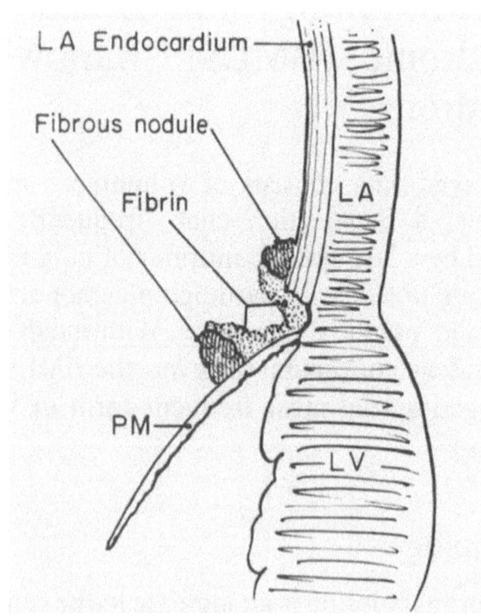

FIGURE 13.3. The "angle lesion" associated with myxomatous mitral valve. The lesion is a source of systemic emboli.

excavatum and other chest wall deformities. Generally, however, the physical appearance is normal.

Auscultation

The clinical hallmark of the condition is the combination of a nonejection click (or clicks) followed by a late systolic murmur. The click occurs toward the middle of systole and is usually loudest at the apex or along the left sternal border. The murmur is crescendo–decrescendo and extends to the aortic component of the second heart sound. The click and late systolic murmur may be manipulated by various interventions and will occur earlier in systole with maneuvers that decrease the volume of the left ventricle.

The systolic murmur becomes softer and earlier following the inhalation of amyl nitrite or during the straining phase of the *Valsalva maneuver* because both left ventricular volume and pressure are decreased. During *standing*, left ventricular enddiastolic volume is also decreased but left ventricular pressure is maintained and myocardial contraction is more vigorous because of catecholamine secretion: the systolic murmur becomes earlier, louder, longer, and occasionally pansystolic. *Squatting* results in a later onset click and softens the murmur. Frequently the nonejection click is intermittent and can be detected only by prolonged careful auscultation in the standing, supine, left lateral, and squatting positions.

The Electrocardiogram

This demonstrates abnormalities in approximately one-third of patients. The commonest pattern is inverted, or partially inverted T waves in leads II, III, AVF, and V4–V6. The T waves usually become upright following strenuous effort. The ST segment is usually normal.

The etiology of the electrocardiographic abnormalities is not understood. They are certainly not a result of coronary artery disease because coronary arteriograms are normal. They may be a result of endocardial scarring and chordal friction lesions (Fig. 13.2).

Premature ventricular contractions are the most frequent form of arrhythmia, but supraventricular tachycardia, atrial fibrillation or flutter, and atrial ectopic beats may also occur. The ventricular premature beats may also be the result of friction lesions on the posterior ventricular wall. They may be important in the mechanism of rare but unexplained cases of sudden death.

Echocardiography

This is a useful diagnostic and confirmatory test. The characteristic features are either an abrupt midsystolic posterior movement of the thickened mitral leaflet echo or a pansystolic prolapse producing so-called "hammocking."

Cardiac Catheterization and Angiography

The hemodynamics are normal unless there is significant mitral regurgitation. Left ventricular cineangiography demonstrates prolapse of the posterior, and occasionally the anterior mitral leaflet. Maximal excursion of the leaflets coincides with the timing of the nonejection click. The technique also clearly demonstrates that the late systolic murmur is a result of mitral regurgitation. Segmental abnormalities of left ventricular wall contraction are not uncommon. In the right anterior oblique projection the "hourglass" or "ballerina-foot" configuration is a result of the voluminous leaflet stretching the chordae and the papillary muscles producing traction on the inferior ventricular wall (Fig. 13.4).

Complications

In the overwhelming majority of patients the prognosis for this condition is excellent. There are, however, several important complications.

Sudden Death

This complication is presumed to be a result of ventricular arrhythmias. It is so rare that patients should not be told of this. However, when there is a history of syncope and evidence of high grade ventricular ectopy, antidysrhythmic treatment is justified.

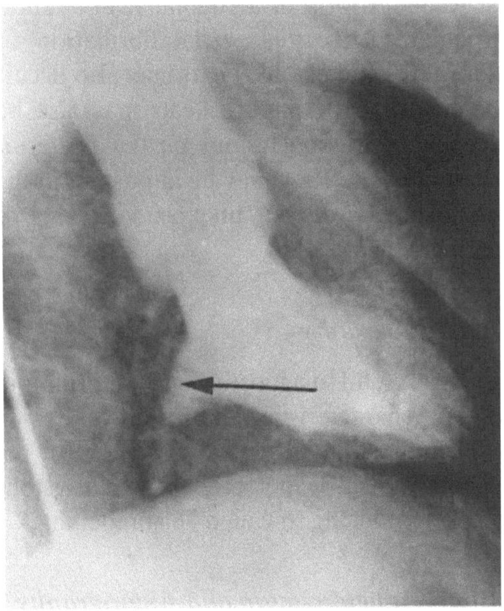

FIGURE 13.4. Left ventricular angiogram in the right oblique view demonstrating protrusion of the posterior mitral leaflet.

Rupture of Chordae Tendinae

For the majority of patients with myxomatous valves there is little tendency for mitral regurgitation to increase with the passage of time. There is, however, pathological evidence among patients with "spontaneous" rupture of the chordae, of myxomatous change involving not only those segments devoid of their chordal support, but also those segments of the valve with intact chordae. This supports the clinical suggestion that in some patients with the BMLS progressive billowing may produce sufficient traction-on the chordae to produce eventual rupture.

Infective Endocarditis

This is a definite potential complication affecting the valve at the contact area of the prolapsing segment. For patients with the click *and late systolic murmur*, antibiotic prophylaxis is therefore recommended. It is uncertain, however, whether patients with a click but without a murmur should receive prophylaxis or not.

Neurological Disorder

Apart from the psychological findings mentioned previously, there is a predisposition to cerebral embolism. Fibrin thrombi arising from the contact surface of the prolapsing leaflets is the presumed site of origin.

Pure Severe Mitral Regurgitation: Rupture of the Chordae Tendinae

Recognition of this highly characteristic clinical syndrome is important since it is surgically remediable. It accounts for a significant number of patients who have acute mitral regurgitation. This is a recognized complication of bacterial endocarditis. More usually, it occurs spontaneously in apparently normal people who have myxomatous valves. The condition affects men more commonly than women and is most common in the ages of 40 to 60 years. The syndrome should be distinguished from acute mitral regurgitation complicating myocardial infarction where it is the papillary muscle itself, rather than the chordae that rupture.

Clinical Picture

This is dependent on the number of chordae ruptured. When a single chorda ruptures the patient may be asymptomatic and the only evidence is the characteristic murmur. When several chordae rupture suddenly and simultaneously there is a dramatic onset of dyspnea, often associated with tightness in the chest and a rapid progression to severe left ventricular failure and pulmonary edema.

In contrast to chronic rheumatic mitral regurgitation, sinus rhythm is the rule. The apical impulse is formed by the left ventricle and is hyperactive; a left atrial parasternal lift may be present.

Auscultation

The murmur of acute mitral regurgitation is crescendo–decrescendo with accentuation in midsystole. An important finding is its tendency to be conducted to the base and to the vessels of the neck—a feature that has frequently led to an incorrect diagnosis of aortic stenosis. Important clinical clues in making this distinction are as follows:

1. The *first heart sound* is abnormally loud because of the snapping, flail leaflet. In aortic stenosis the first sound is normal.
2. The *second sound* in aortic stenosis is paradoxically split, whereas in severe mitral incompetence the second sound is normally or widely split.
3. A loud *apical third sound* is a characteristic finding in acute mitral regurgitation. In aortic stenosis it is a fourth sound that is audible.
4. In severe aortic stenosis, the *peripheral pulses* are slow rising whereas in severe mitral regurgitation the pulses are normal or slightly waterhammer in quality.
5. *Radiologically*, prominence of the ascending aorta and calcification of the aortic valve point to aortic stenosis. Mild left atrial enlargement, a normal aorta, and pulmonary edema favor ruptured chordae.

Careful auscultation will distinguish the murmur of acute mitral regurgitation from that of predominant mitral regurgitation resulting from rheumatic involvement of the posterior leaflet. In the latter condition there may be an opening snap but, most importantly, there is a middiastolic rumble indicating commissural fusion.

Chest X-ray

This demonstrates a heart of normal size, little or no left atrial enlargement, and evidence of pulmonary edema.

The Electrocardiogram

This is normal and characteristically shows sinus rhythm.

Echocardiography

This technique is extremely helpful in confirming the diagnosis. The findings are posterior systolic protrusion of one or both flail mitral leaflets into the left atrium.

Cardiac Catheterization

The hemodynamic findings are giant V waves in the left atrial, or wedge pressure, which may be so large that they are superimposed on the pulmonary artery pressure trace. In contrast to rheumatic mitral regurgitation there is no diastolic pressure gradient between the left atrium and left ventricle. Left ventricular cineangiography demonstrates normal or hyperactive wall motion, severe mitral regurgitation, and with careful scrutiny, the leaflet may be observed to prolapse into the left atrium.

Treatment

When patients are markedly symptomatic because of severe regurgitation, operation provides good results. In those cases where only one or two chordae to the posterior leaflet are involved, conservative plication or shortening of the leaflet with annuloplasty may be all that is required. When, however, there is extensive rupture of the chordae to the anterior leaflet in addition, most surgeons would favor mitral valve replacement.

Mitral Regurgitation Resulting from Ischemic Heart Disease

Papillary Muscle Dysfunction

This is the commonest type of mitral regurgitation resulting from myocardial ischemia. Mitral regurgitation occurs when there is ischemic fibrosis and atrophy not only of the papillary muscles but also of the adjacent posterior ventricular wall. The regurgitation is usually mild and the symptomatology is largely related to associated left ventricular dysfunction.

The murmur of papillary muscle dysfunction may be noted during the course of acute myocardial infarction, and occasionally may be evident only during an attack of angina pectoris. It varies considerably in its timing and intensity. Usually, it is soft, crescendo–decrescendo in shape, and commences following a short interval after the first heart sound. Frequently, there is associated clinical evidence of left ventricular dysfunction such as a dyskinetic precordium and an apical gallop sound. There are no specific electrocardiographic findings to confirm the diagnosis. Similarly, radiology, echocardiography, nuclear angiography, and cardiac catheterization will usually simply reflect the degree of myocardial damage.

Medical management includes propranolol and nitrates for the control of angina pectoris and digitalis and diuretics when there is evidence of heart failure. It is uncommon for papillary muscle dysfunction to be sufficiently severe to warrant mitral valve replacement, but revascularization surgery and aneurysectomy may be indicated for associated lesions.

Rupture of the Papillary Muscle

This is almost invariably a complication of myocardial infarction, but occasionally follows chest trauma. The condition complicates approximately 5% of cases of myocardial infarction and leads to fulminating pulmonary edema and death in 75% of the victims within a week following the episode of infarction.

Clinical Features

Typically, there is sudden onset of pulmonary edema quite refractory to medical treatment. A pansystolic murmur of varying degree of intensity is present at the apex. This may radiate quite widely and gives rise to considerable difficulty in the differential diagnosis from a postinfarction ventricular septal defect. In the latter condition, the systolic murmur is usually audible at the left sternal border but there is a considerable degree of overlap.

In the presence of shock and hypotension the apical murmur may be deceptively soft. Under such circumstances it is essential to pass a Swan-Ganz catheter to confirm the diagnosis and exclude postinfarction septal rupture. The characteristic findings are giant V waves, frequently detectable on the pulmonary artery tracing, and an absence of oxygen saturation step-up in the right ventricle. The distinction from ventricular septal rupture may be made at the bedside with Doppler-color flow echocardiography.

Cardiac catheterization and left ventricular cineangiography are essential and may have to be performed with the assistance of intraaortic balloon counterpulsation. This will document the severity of mitral regurgitation and occasionally even identify a highly mobile filling defect in the left ventricular cavity produced by the flail belly of the papillary muscle. The findings at catheterization will determine the type of surgery involved, which may include not only mitral valve replacement but also aneurysectomy and coronary artery bypass grafting. The prognosis will obviously depend on the severity of associated myocardial damage.

Calcification of the Mitral Annulus

This condition is frequent in those over the age of 45 years and is more common in women. Heavy calcification follows degeneration and fibrosis of the mitral annulus particularly related to the posterior leaflet. Usually, the condition is detected by routine chest radiography or echocardiography as a heavy U-shaped calcific bar between the left ventricle and the left atrium.

Significant disturbance of mitral valve function is unusual. When calcification is severe, restricted mobility of the posterior leaflet may result in a minor degree of mitral regurgitation. A crescendo–decrescendo murmur is present at the apex and may radiate to the axilla. Patients are generally asymptomatic and no specific therapy is required or indicated.

Mitral Valve Disease Associated with Lupus Erythematosus

In its classical form this is known as *Libman–Sachs endocarditis*. Verrucous lesions composed of damaged valve tissue are most commonly found underneath the basal portion of the mitral vlave. Prior to the advent of steroid therapy for the underlying disease these lesions were rarely significant enough to interfere with valve function. With improved survival, healing of these lesions may result in fibrosis and binding of the posterior mitral leaflet to the underlying myocardium. In some instances valve replacement has been necessary.

Marantic (Nonbacterial Thrombotic Endocarditis)

In its typical form this condition is thought of as affecting those individuals with terminal malignancy and profound cachexia. It is now recognized that the condition may occur in any serious systemic illness and may have early important clinical manifestations. Although the mitral valve is most commonly affected, vegetations may also be found on the aortic and tricuspid valves.

The classical pathological lesions on the mitral valve are large verrucous, fibrinous masses, several millimeters in diameter occurring at the coaptation line of the valve leaflets. It is distinguished from the vegetations of rheumatic fever by the absence of chordal thickening and shortening, and the lack of commissural fusion. Similarly, the vegetations of infective endocarditis are associated with destruction of valve tissue and bacterias are found with light microscopy.

The lesions may be sufficiently large to produce mitral systolic murmurs, which may be erroneously attributed to rheumatic heart disease or a senile aortic ejection murmur. The importance of marantic endocarditis is for its potential to cause peripheral emboli, which usually involve the cerebral circulation.

The condition should be thought of in an elderly patient suffering from malignancy who develops psychosis, stroke, or systemic embolus. The vegetations are large enough to be visualized by echocardography. There is no specific therapy for the condition.

The Aortic Valve

Congenital Aortic Valve Disease

Brief mention is made of those congenital malformations of the aortic valve that have a proclivity to produce aortic stenosis. The severity of the stenosis determines the hemodynamics and the consequent clinical, radiological, and electrocardiographic features as described in the section under rheumatic aortic stenosis.

Congenital deformities of the aortic valve that may result in aortic stenosis are of two types: (1) a *unicuspid* aortic valve and (2) a *bicuspid* aortic valve.

The *unicuspid* aortic valve is a unicommissural domed valve. It has a single leaflet starting at the aortic wall and extending across the annulus without making contact with the opposing aortic wall, returning to reconnect to the aortic wall at the site of origin, thus forming a single commissure. The attachment of this type of valve to the aortic wall is via a raphe. The valve is intrinsically stenotic and usually responsible for significant aortic stenosis at birth or shortly thereafter. Unicuspid valves may produce aortic stenosis up to the age of 30 and they may become calcified. Like congenital bicuspid aortic valve disease there is a stong tendency for male involvement.

The *bicuspid aortic valve* is a more common malformation than the unicuspid valve and, indeed, is the commonest form of congenital abnormality, occurring in 2% of the population. Eighty-five percent of patients with coarctation of the aorta have an associated congenital bicuspid valve.

Unlike the unicuspid variety the bicuspid valve is not as intrinsically stenotic. Frequently, however, the valve becomes fibrotic and calcified because the bicuspid configuration is subject to hemodynamic stresses. By the age of 55 most stenotic congenital bicuspid aortic valves have undergone calcification and it is therefore unusual to hear an aortic ejection click. Usually a bicuspid valve occurs as the sole abnormality and in the absence of significant stenosis the only physical finding in a young person is an aortic ejection click. The valve is prone to infective endocarditis and aortic insufficiency may result.

Senile Degeneration and Calcification of the Aortic Valve

Degeneration, thickening, and even calcification of the aortic valve leaflets are almost a normal part of the aging process. When calcification is severe, significant aortic stenosis results. Systolic murmurs in the elderly are a common result of senile stenosis. The ejection systolic murmur in the elderly patient sounds very much like that of aortic stenosis and has the same radiation. Because of the frequency of transient ischemic attacks and dizzy spells resulting from caroticovertebral disease in this age group the distinction from valvular aortic stenosis is important and may be difficult. Systolic hypertension and an audible atrial sound are common findings in the elderly, and therefore serve to confuse the issue.

The character of the peripheral pulse is also of little help in making the distinction because critical aortic stenosis may exist with a relatively rapid carotid upstroke time. The only helpful feature is the timing of the crescendo of the systolic murmur. The later the crescendo, the more likely is the presence of aortic stenosis. If serious doubt exists, echocardiography and cardiac catheterization to assess the gradient are essential, because valve replacement may have gratifying results even in the elderly.

Ankylosing Spondylitis

Aortic insufficiency is a well-recognized complication of longstanding ankylosing spondylitis. Occasionally, the cardiac manifestations may precede the arthritis. Aortic insufficiency occurs because of thickening and shortening of the leaflets and dilatation of the aortic root. Were it not for involvement of the basal portion of the leaflets with fibrosis and scarring extending into the outflow tract of the left ventricle, the lesion is almost indistinguishable from syphilitic aortitis. Fibrosis of the outflow tract includes the basal portion of the ventricular septum and, therefore, conduction defects (including complete heart block) are well recognized complications.

The combination of *aortic insufficiency and an electrocardiographic conduction* defect includes the following differential diagnosis:

1. Ankylosing spondylitis.
2. Mycotic aneurysms of the left ventricle during the course of infective endocarditis.
3. Congenital aneurysms of the sinus of Valsalva with extension into the interventricular septum.
4. Rheumatoid arthritis.
5. Reiter's syndrome.

Aortic insufficiency complicating ankylosing spondylitis shortens the lifespan of these patients and valve replacement may be necessary.

Rheumatoid Arthritis

Typical rheumatoid granulomas are often found in the aortic and mitral valves at autopsy. Granulomatous involvement may also lead to pericarditis and an interstitial myocarditis.

Aortic regurgitation is usually mild but heart failure disproportionate to the regurgitant leak may occur because of myocardial involvement. *Complete heart block* is also a well-recognized complication that may require electrical pacing.

Reiter's Syndrome

In the long-standing form of this disease aortic regurgitation and complete heart block are potential complications. The pathological lesion is identical to that of ankylosing spondylitis. The diagnosis is suggested by a long history of sacroiliac arthritis, iritis, and skin rashes.

The Tricuspid Valve

Nonrheumatic organic tricuspid valve disease is unusual. The most important conditions are (1) the carcinoid syndrome, (2) infective endocarditis in drug addicts, and (3) endomyocardial fibrosis.

The Carcinoid Syndrome

Involvement of the pulmonary and tricuspid valves is a well-recognized complication of this syndrome. Right-sided congestive cardiac failure is a result of pulmonary stenosis and tricuspid insufficiency and stenosis. Tricuspid is more common than pulmonary involvement.

The diagnosis is suggested by the typical history of paroxysmal flushing, diarrhea, edema, and wheezing. Elevation of the urinary excretion of 5-HIAA establishes the diagnosis. Treatment consists of chemotherapy for the malignant carcinoid in the intestine or ovary, and the associated hepatic metastases. Pulmonary valvotomy and tricuspid valve replacement may be necessary.

Infective Endocarditis

Isolated tricuspid valve disease, particularly when associated with recurrent pulmonary infiltrates, should immediately arouse a suspicion of intravenous drug addiction. The condition is discussed in the section on infective endocarditis.

Endomyocardial Fibrosis

Binding down of the tricuspid valve is common in endomyocardial fibrosis and Loeffler's parietal endocarditis and involvement of the right side may precede left-sided involvement (see chapter 15).

Additional Reading

Barlow JB: "Perspectives on the Mitral Valve." F.A. Davis, Philadelphia, 1987.

Barlow JB, Bosman CK, Pocock, WA, Marchand P: Late systolic murmurs and non-ejection ("midlate") systolic clicks: Analysis of 90 patients. Br Heart J 30:203, 1968.

Chesler E, Gornick CC: Maladies attributed to myxomatous mitral valve. Circulation 83:1;328, 1991.

Chesler E, King RA, Edwards JE: The myxomatous mitral valve and sudden death. Circulation 67:632, 1983.

Chesler E, Weir EK, Braatz GA, Francis GS: Normal catecholamine and hemodynamic responses to orthostatic tilt in subjects with mitral valve prolapse. Am J Med 78:754, 1985.

Edwards JE: Pathologic aspects of cardiac valvular insufficiencies. Arch Surg 77:634, 1958.

Edwards JE: On the etiology of calcific aortic stenosis. Circulation 26:817, 1962.

Jeresaty RM: Mitral valve prolapse-click syndrome. Progr Cardiovasc Dis 15:623, 1973.

Roberts WC, Dangiel JC, Bulkley BH: Nonrheumatic valvular cardiac disease: A clinicopathologic survery of 27 different conditions causing valvular dysfunction. In Likoff W (guest ed.), "Valvular Heart Disease," Caradiovasc Clin 5:333, 1973.

Roberts WC, Perloff JK, Constantino T: Severe valvular aortic stenosis in patients over 65 years of age. A clinico-pathologic study. Am J Cardiol 27:497, 1971.

Selzer A, Kelly JJ, Jr, Vannitamby M, Walker P, Gerbode F, Kerth WJ: The syndrome of mitral insufficiency due to isolated rupture of the chordae tendinae. Am J Med 43:822, 1967.

14
Infective Endocarditis

Definition

Infective endocarditis is a disease produced by direct infection of a natural or prosthetic heart valve, certain congenital defects of the heart and aorta, or acquired surgical shunts such as the Blalock–Taussing anastomosis. Prior to the advent of antimicrobial agents a distinction was made between *acute* and *subacute* bacterial endocarditis on the basis of the length of survival of the patient. Survival beyond 8 weeks was said to indicate subacute endocarditis whereas death within 8 weeks was a result of acute bacterial endocarditis. Additionally, acute and subacute bacterial endocarditis was sometimes distinguished by the size of the vegetations and the presence or absence of previous valvular disease. The use of powerful antibiotics has made these classifications more of historical interest than of practical value. A classification by causative microorganisms is probably a superior method since the identity of the organism determines (1) the clinical course, (2) the presence or absence of underlying heart disease, and (3) the type of antibiotic regimen to be used.

Pathogenesis

Endocarditis usually affects an abnormal valve. The most common valvular abnormalities are congenital bicuspid aortic valve, rheumatic valve disease, myxomatous mitral valve, and senile calcific sclerosis of the aortic valve. Normal valves are involved in intravenous drug abusers and in most cases it is the tricuspid valve that is infected. Following cardiac surgery, endocarditis most commonly involves a prosthetic valve.

The disease is characterized by infected thrombi ("vegetations") on the endocardial surface of the valve leaflets and cusps. The mechanism of infection during a bacteremia is either (1) seeding of microorganisms into the interstitium of the valves through their intrinsic blood supply, or (2) direct implantation on the endocardial surface by surface contact. The latter is the most widely accepted view, and it seems likely that microorganisms adhere to preexisting bland thrombi situated on the endocardial surface of the valve. These thrombi adhere to a subendocardial inflammatory reaction, which may result from conditions such as rheumatic fever or disseminated lupus erythematosus. They are also found on prosthetic valves and on intravascular surfaces traumatized by foreign bodies such as catheters.

Velocity and turbulence of blood flow also play a role. Infection occurs in those areas characterized by a high velocity of blood flow from a high- to a low-pressure chamber through a narrow orifice. Thus, endocarditis is located on the right side of a ventricular septal defect and just beyond the constriction in coarctation of the aorta. When the pressure gradient is negligible (secundum atrial septal defect, large ventricular septal defect, or widely patent ductus arteriosus) endocarditis is rare. Infection of valves is more common when they are insufficient rather than stenotic. Characteristically, the atrial surface of the mitral valve and the ventricular aspect of the aortic valve are the areas of predilection. In order of frequency, the mitral valve is affected most commonly, followed by the aortic, tricuspid, and pulmonary, respectively.

Microorganisms may enter the bloodstream from many sources. Manipulation of infected foci in the bone, tonsils, teeth, gastrointestinal tract, and genitourinary tract may produce transient bacteremia. Usually the episode of bacteremia is asymptomatic. Bacteremia occurs commonly after tooth brushing or oral irrigation. Following dental surgery bacteremia is much more likely in the presence of periodontitis, but may also occur when multiple teeth are extracted.

Bacteremia may also follow sigmoidoscopy, barium enema, transurethral prostatic resection, cytoscopy, prostatic massage, urethral dilatation, and catheterization. Operative intervention or instrumentation of the female genitourinary tract, including the placement of an intrauterine contraceptive device, may result in bacteremia. Endocarditis has followed self-administration of intravenous drugs and may also occur with prolonged use of intravenous catheters.

There is clear evidence of a preceding precipitating cause of bacteremia in only 40% of cases of infective endocarditis.

Infecting Microorganisms

The antibiotic era has brought about a change in infecting organisms; there has been a marked reduction in the occurrence of pneumococci and gonococci with a simultaneous increase in the frequency of staphylococcal and enterococcal infections.

Streptococci

These are the causative agents in 60–80% of cases of infective endocarditis and *Streptococcus viridans* is the most important variety, particularly in young patients.

Following *S. viridans*, group D enterococci are the next most frequent streptococci responsible and are incriminated in approximately 10% of cases. The enterococcus group includes the organisms *S. faecalis* (varieties *zymogenes* and *liquefaciens*), *S. faecium*, and *S. durans*. Most enterococci causing endocarditis are *S. faecalis* (*liquefaciens* variety). Enterococcal endocarditis is more frequent in men than women, and men are affected at an older age. This male predominance is related to risk factors and in approximately 50% of patients there is a history of a preceding operative manipulation that includes cystoscopy, urethral catheterization, prostatectomy, and prostatic massage. Abortions, pregnancy, and gynecologic surgery are risk factors in women.

The remaining streptococci include microaerophilic, anerobic, nonhemolytic, and group A β-hemolytic varieties. Enterococci and group A β-hemolytic streptococci may attack normal or previously damaged heart valves and cause rapid destruction. The other streptococci are more likely to cause endocarditis on previously damaged heart valves and rarely cause rapid destruction.

Staphylococci

Staphylococci are the second most common cause of endocarditis. Both coagulase-positive and coagulase-negative varieties may be responsible. The incidence has increased over the past 30 years and this may be attributed to drug addiction and the increasing use of prosthetic cardiac valves. Coagulase-positive staphylococci may infect normal or previously diseased heart valves and cause rapid destruction. Characteristically, the course is fulminant leading to death within weeks. Coagulase-negative staphylococci, however, usually affect normal heart valves and do not cause rapid destruction; the course of the disease is subacute.

Staphylococcus epidermidis (formerly *S. albus*) is responsible for more than one-third of prosthetic valve infections, but causes only 1%, of endocarditis in nonsurgical patients. This organism is the commonest cause of infection in the early postoperative period. It is possible that those infections presenting more than 60 days after operation may actually have been acquired in the immediate perioperative period.

Pneumococci

Diplococcus pneumoniae is now a rare cause of endocarditis and this is probably related to the early antibiotic treatment of pneumococcal pneumonia. The organism is capable of attacking normal or previously damaged heart valves and is characterized by rapid destruction and a fulminant course.

Nessieria gonorrhoeae

This organism was a common cause of endocarditis of the right side of the heart but since the advent of penicillin has become rare.

Other Bacteria

Almost any variety of bacteria is known to cause endocarditis. Gram-negative bacilli are responsible for infections in drug addicts and prosthetic valve endocarditis. Diphtheroid infections are far more likely to involve a prosthetic than a natural cardiac valve.

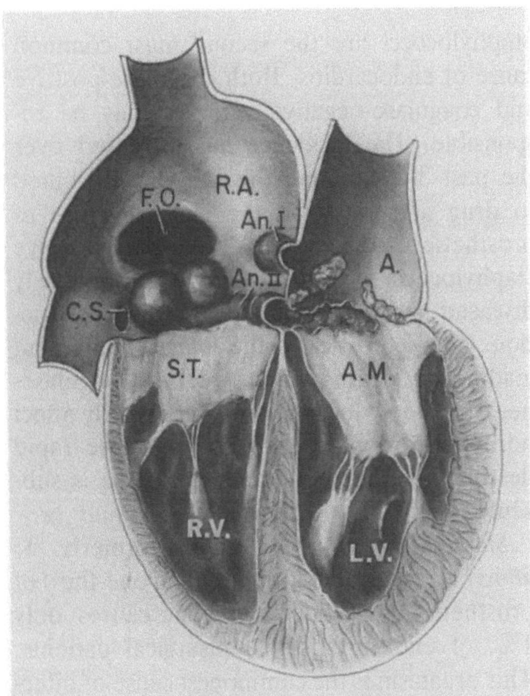

FIGURE 14.1. Aortic root (A) endocarditis with aneurysms (An. I and II) presenting into right atrium (RA).

Fungi

Candida and *Aspergillus* infections often occur in patients with intravascular catheters who have received corticosteroids, broad spectrum antibiotics, or cytotoxic agents. These infections are also common in narcotic addicts and in patients who have received prosthetic cardiac valves.

Rickettsiae

Coxiella burnetti, the causative agent of Q fever, is a fairly recently recognized cause of infective endocarditis. This infection usually occurs in patients with underlying heart disease who have been exposed to infected animals. It is characterized by great chronicity and frequently involves the aortic valve.

Pathology

The Heart

The characteristic feature is vegetations on a valve leaflet. They vary in size from a few millimeters to several centimeters and are usually located along the line of closure of the leaflet. They are composed of a mass of fibrin, platelets, leukocytes, and colonies of bacteria. The destructive effect of the vegetation leads to perforation of the valve leaflets, rupture of chordae tendinae, aneurysms of the sinuses of Valsalva, abscesses of the aortic valve annulus with fistula formation, and obstruction to valve orifices. Involvement of the pericardium is rare and an ominous sign. It usually results from perforation of an aortic root or myocardial abscess (Fig. 14.1).

Embolism

Emboli are encountered in approximately 60% of cases studied at autopsy and involve many organs. Embolic occlusion of vessels may produce myocardial, splenic, renal, or cerebral infarction.

Mycotic aneurysms result from septic emboli

to the bacterial wall and frequently occur at arterial bifurcations. The intracranial vessels, in particular the middle cerebral, are most commonly affected. Their rupture leads to intracerebral and subarachnoid hemorrhage.

Kidney

Three types of lesions are associated with endocarditis: (1) renal infarcts, (2) diffuse glomerulonephritis, and (3) focal "embolic" glomerulitis. Large emboli occlude a major division of the renal artery and produce frank infarction. Diffuse glomerulonephritis associated with endocarditis is a result of immune complex disease similar to that occurring in lupus erythematosus, syphilis, malaria, and so on. Deposits of immunoglobulin and complement along the glomerular basement membrane are characteristic findings. Frequently, the serum complement is reduced and the rheumatoid factor increased. Renal failure may complicate the lesions but is usually reversible when the underlying infection is treated.

Focal embolic nephritis ("flea-bitten kidney") is the commonest renal lesion in infective endocarditis. Originally thought to be a result of small bacterial emboli, this lesion is now also considered to be a form of immune complex disease. It is rarely responsible for renal failure.

Spleen

Enlargement is frequent and related to the duration of the illness. Usually splenomegaly is a result of lymphoid hyperplasia but embolism may result in splenic infarction, abscess formation, and even rupture of the organ.

Lung

Pulmonary embolism and infarction are almost always the result of tricuspid valve endocarditis and septic emboli may also result in recurrent pneumonia.

Clinical Features

The clinical manifestations of infective endocarditis are so variable that early diagnosis may be extremely difficult.

Endocarditis caused by *S. viridans* frequently has an insidious onset with malaise, anorexia, and low-grade fever, which is easily mistaken for a virus infection; symptoms may persist for several weeks before medical attention is sought. On the other hand, staphylococcal and other types of acute endocarditis may present with dramatic manifestations such as stroke, congestive cardiac failure, uremia, splenic infarction, or the sudden onset of peripheral gangrene.

The absence of a cardiac murmur does not exclude the presence of infective endocarditis and apparently insignificant murmurs may in fact be a manifestation of acute infection of the mitral and tricuspid valves, or a congenital bicuspid aortic valve. The differential diagnosis should include atrial myxoma and acute rheumatic fever. Infective endocarditis may be superimposed on the acute attack of rheumatic carditis.

The clinical picture depends on (1) infection, (2) embolism, and (3) cardiac involvement.

Infection

A history of dental extraction, abortion, or surgery is frequently present. This is followed by gradually progressive malaise, fever, anorexia, sweating, and occasionally rigors. Fever is almost invariably present during the course of the disease but may be absent in the elderly, or when there is uremia or heart failure. The temperature chart usually shows a remittent fever, rarely exceeding 103°F, except in acute gonococcal, pneumococcal, or staphylococcal infections. The administration of antibiotics in inadequate dosage may partially suppress the disease and prolong the phase of generalized ill health or produce intermittent symptoms. Steroid administration mistakenly administered for rheumatic arthritis may produce an acute exacerbation with florid complications.

Clubbing of the fingers and toes usually develops within a few weeks and is progressive. Slight clubbing is found in uncomplicated rheumatic heart disease and must be interpreted with caution.

A mild normochromic normocytic anemia resembling the type seen in other chronic infections is the rule; a hematocrit below 30% is, however, rare. A leukocytosis in excess of 13,000/mm^3 is found in staphylococcal and other types of acute endocarditis but is less common in infections produced by *S. viridans*. The erythrocyte sedimentation rate is almost always elevated and returns to normal with antibiotic treatment. A normal ESR would be strong evidence against a diagnosis of infective endocarditis. Rheumatoid factor is present in 50% of patients and initially high titers will return to normal when the condition is successfully treated. Serum complement levels are depressed when there is renal involvement.

Embolism

Petechiae are common in the skin, mucous membranes, conjunctivae, and fundi, particularly when the illness is prolonged. However, petechiae are not uncommon in elderly persons without evidence of infection, and may also occur in normal people with poorly fitting dentures, and in the conjunctival sac of women using eye makeup.

Splinter hemorrhages under the nails occur so frequently in health as a result of local trauma that their significance must be interpreted with caution. Fresh red hemorrhages, especially at the base of the nails, are much more significant than brown linear streaks near the tips of the fingers.

Osler's nodes occur in approximately 25% of cases and are thought to be a result of an acute vasculitis rather than embolism. They are not specific for endocarditis and have been reported in other conditions such as sytemic lupus erythematosus, typhoid fever, and gonorrhea. The lesions are firm, raised, and painful, vary from 2 to 15 mm in diameter, and are most frequently found on the finger and toe pads.

Janeway's lesions are nontender macular or hemorrhagic areas present on the palms and soles. In a few cases microorganisms have been cultured from the lesion; they are most frequently encountered in acute bacterial endocarditis.

Roth's spots in the retina are oval hemorrhagic lesions containing a pale center. They are not pathognomonic of bacterial endocarditis and may occur with any severe anemia and in the collagen diseases.

Major thromboembolic episodes have now decreased in incidence following the introduction of antibiotics. Usually they are late complications of the disease but may be the initial symptom. Septic embolism may lead to mycotic aneurysms of the intracranial vessels, abdominal aorta, and splenic and coronary arteries. Embolism to the spleen is found frequently at autopsy but clinical signs of infarction are infrequently recognized. The classic symptom is pain in the left upper quadrant radiating to the shoulder aggravated by inspiration associated with a splenic friction rub and a left pleural effusion. Coronary artery emboli are most frequently a complication of aortic valve endocarditis and occasionally may be sufficiently large to produce myocardial infarction. Usually, however, the emboli are too small to be recognized during life.

Pulmonary embolism with infarction is often the presenting symptom of tricuspid valve endocarditis and occurs most frequently in narcotic addicts. Recurrent episodes of pulmonary infection in an addict should suggest the diagnosis. In children the same finding may occur with infective endocarditis or a patent ductus arteriosus.

Retinal artery emboli may produce sudden, complete, or partial loss of vision but this complication is now uncommon in the antibiotic era. Obstruction of a major limb artery is uncommon and usually the result of fungal or rickettsial endocarditis, which characteristically produce large friable vegetations; the diagnosis may be made by microscopic examination following removal of the embolus. Major cerebral emboli occur in approximately one-third of all patients and the middle cerebral artery is the vessel usually involved. Mycotic aneurysms are less common and characteristically are located at the bifurcation of small peripheral arteries, in contrast to the congenital aneurysms, which involve the circle of Willis. These aneurysms are small and may result in catastrophic subarachnoid hemorrhage. Toxic encephalopathy and brain abscesses are also well-recognized complications and may even be the presenting symptom.

Systemic emboli to the kidney are common

and produce renal infarction with loin pain, renal colic, hematuria, and pyuria. Microscopic hematuria is present in 50% of cases and usually results from focal or diffuse glomerulonephritis.

Murmurs

Mitral or aortic murmurs are usually present. Particularly in the elderly, the significance of an aortic ejection murmur may not be appreciated since this is such a common finding. There may, however, be no murmur in as many as 15% of patients with infective endocarditis. A changing heart murmur has been taught to be a major diagnostic finding. Actually, this is an uncommon physical sign and the development of a *new* murmur, particularly an early diastolic aortic murmur, is a much more reliable sign. In the early stages, heart failure is uncommon but sudden cusp perforation or rupture of chordae may produce acute pulmonary edema.

In aortic valve endocarditis when there is sudden perforation or detachment of a leaflet, the early diastolic murmur and wide pulse pressure disappear as aortic and left ventricular end-diastolic pressures equilibrate and pulmonary edema ensues. The left ventricular end diastolic pressure may be so high that the aortic leaflets may actually open in diastole. Under these circumstances Durozier's sign is extremely useful. The diastolic murmur heard over the femoral arteries is the equivalent of retrograde aortic flow detected by Doppler studies.

Electrocardiogram

The electrocardiogram may yield important clues in aortic valve endocarditis. Invasion of the ventricular septum produces first-degree A-V block, which may progress to complete heart block.

Diagnosis

Active rheumatic fever gives rise to the greatest problem in diagnosis. Arthritis, valve lesions, mild clubbing of the fingers, anemia, and fever occur in both conditions. Hematuria, proteinuria, and splenomegaly may occur in rheumatic fever and bland embolism is not uncommon in established valve disease. A raised sedimentation rate and elevation of the antistreptolysin titer is of no help. Pericarditis strongly favors a diagnosis of rheumatic fever. A failure of response to antibiotic therapy with a prompt response to salicylates strongly suggests the diagnosis of rheumatic fever.

Other causes of a pyrexial illness must be differentiated from infective endocarditis and these include brucellosis virus infections (especially cytomegalic infection), protozoal infections, and so on. Pyrexia, splenomegaly, and anemia are found in the lymphomas and blood dyscrasias such as leukemia. Anemia may closely mimic the picture of endocarditis since cardiac murmurs Roth spots, and petechial hemorrhages are common to both. The clinical picture may be closely mimicked by collagen diseases such as systemic lupus erythematosus, since there is arthritis, fever, heart murmurs, renal involvement, anemia, and vascular occlusions. Carcinoma and occult purulent infections (perinephric or pelvic abscess) are also occasional problems. Atrial myxoma should be considered, particularly when blood cultures are negative.

The following entities deserve special mention.

Infective Endocarditis in the Elderly

Endocarditis is becoming more common among older individuals, particularly in men. Although the causative organisms are similar to those producing endocarditis in the young, the disease differs in that the presenting symptoms are often atypical chiefly because central nervous system manifestations such as cerebral vascular accidents, hemiplegia, encephalopathy, and psychosis dominate the presentation. Additionally, underlying debilitating disease such as diffuse arteriosclerosis or neoplastic disease make clinical diagnosis difficult. The latter factors also contribute to a poorer prognosis in the elderly. The prognosis is particularly ominous in infections caused by *Staphylococcus aureus* and gram-negative bacilli. The most important factor contributing to the poor prognosis in the elderly patient is delay in diagnosis and treatment. The presence of an aortic ejection murmur and fever should alert one to the possibility and early treatment should improve the prognosis.

Endocarditis After Cardiac Surgery

This is rare with closed mitral valvotomy but complicates 2 to 4% of valve replacements. Endocarditis occurring within the first two months following valve replacement, is usually a result of S. Epidermidis (25%) S. Aureus (20%), gram-negative organisms and fungi (14% each). Late postoperative infections are the result of *Streptococci viridans* infection (40%), *Staphylococcus epidermidis* (20%), and gram-negative and *Staphylococcus aureus* (about 12%). *S. fecalis* may also cause late endocarditis.

The diagnosis of infective endocarditis must be entertained in all patients who are febrile in the postoperative period. The symptoms must be differentiated from those of other complications such as the postcardiotomy and postperfusion syndrome, pneumonia, wound sepsis, and thrombophlebitis. Early postoperative endocarditis is characterized by the appearance of a regurgitant murmur, and cardiac failure is related to prosthetic valve dysfunction or dehiscence. The subsequent course is frequently complicated by intractable cardiac failure and pulmonary edema. Emboli to the cerebral, coronary, and splenic vessels are common and occlusion of major peripheral arteries is characteristic of fungal endocarditis. The mortality for early endocarditis is approximately 75% but is somewhat lower for late infections (45%).

Blood Cultures

The most definitive finding in patients with endocarditis is bacteremia or fungemia. Unfortunately, negative blood cultures may occur in 5% of patients and treatment may have to be instituted without laboratory confirmation when the diagnosis appears likely on clinical grounds. This applies particularly to patients with endocarditis caused by fungi such as *Aspergillus* or *Histoplasma*. The diagnosis may be made by staining and culturing emboli surgically removed from peripheral vessels.

It is recommended that five or six blood cultures be obtained to minimize the problem of interpretation of a questionable single contaminated culture. This will also detect a very high percentage of those patients having a significant bacteremia. The skin should be prepared with 70% alcohol and iodine and the area should be punctured without retouching. Blood should never be withdrawn from an indwelling catheter because of contamination and only one series of blood cultures should be grown from one venipuncture. The blood should be immediately innoculated into broth or pour plates at the bedside. When penicillin has been administered to the patient before the cultures are drawn, penicillinase should be added to the culture.

Routine disc sensitivity tests do not discriminate organisms resistant to low levels of antibiotics, and ideally more quantitative results may be obtained with broth-dilution sensitivity tests. Additionally, modification of the broth-dilution tests should be employed to estimate the serum antimicrobial activity during antibiotic therapy.

Echocardiography

The 2D, and in particular the transesophageal technique are important advances in diagnosis. Good quality images will identify vegetations and the complications of infective endocarditis.

Vegetations larger than 4 mm in diameter may be identified in approximately 80% of cases of infective endocarditis (Figs. 14.2 and 14.3). They are particularly easy to identify when the valve leaflets are relatively normal and the vegetation mobile. Redundancy and thickening of a myxomatous mitral valve may make identification difficult. Similarly, the echo-dense valve characteristic of senile aortic sclerosis obscures vegetations. The diagnosis of endocarditis on a prosthetic valve is difficult for the same reasons unless the vegetation is mobile and protrudes into the cavity of the left ventricle. Echocardiography cannot distinguish between an infected vegetation and that of bland marantic endocarditis. Also, it is important to remember that vegetations may persist long after bacteriologic cure.

Color flow Doppler echocardiography is

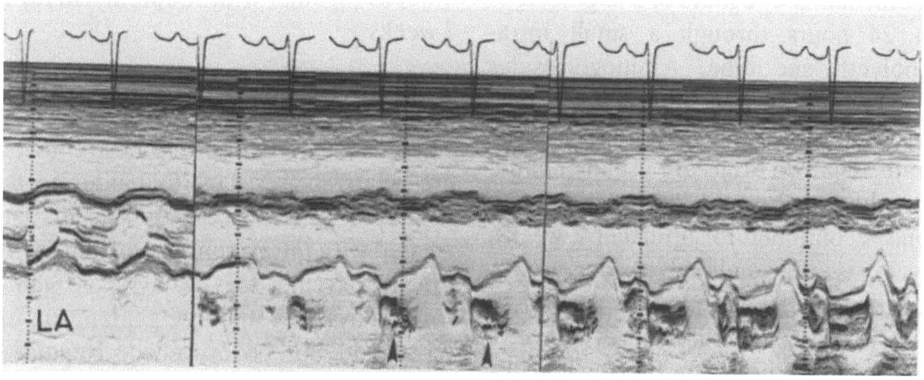

FIGURE 14.2. M-Mode echocardiogram showing vegetation on mitral valve (arrow) prolapsing into left atrium (LA).

valuable in quantifying and following the severity of valvular regurgitation. Also, the ability of this technique to identify aortic root abscess penetrating the ventricular septum, fistulae between the aortic root and cardiac chambers, has made planning of operation much easier. There is now less reliance on invasive catheterization and angiography.

Treatment

Successful therapy depends on early diagnosis, and survival is directly related to the appropriate use of effective antibiotics. Infective endocarditis is not cured with bacteriostatic antibiotics despite high dosage for prolonged periods. The parenteral route is the most effective in achieving concentration of bactericidal antibiotics in the serum. Absorption of penicillin G or V orally is variable, and this form of therapy should not be used routinely. Treatment must be prolonged, and should never be less than 2 weeks for penicillin-sensitive streptococci or less than 4 weeks for enterococcal infections. Once the appropriate therapy is instituted, daily blood cultures and frequent monitoring of serum bacteriocidal activity are advisable. A serum bactericidal activity at a one-in-eight or greater dilution is acceptable.

Streptococcal Endocarditis

This is the commonest cause of infective endocarditis and the majority of strains are highly susceptible to penicillin. The susceptibility of streptococci does not appear to have changed since the introduction of penicillin. Given alone for 4 weeks, penicillin achieves bacteriological cure in 95% of patients. The dosage should be at least 4–5 million units of penicillin daily and 0.5 g probenecid 3–4 times a day. Penicillin may be given as procaine penicillin intramuscularly at six hourly intervals but when the dosage becomes too great for repeated intramuscular injections, the intravenous route must be used, changing the site of venipuncture every 48 hours. Twenty-million

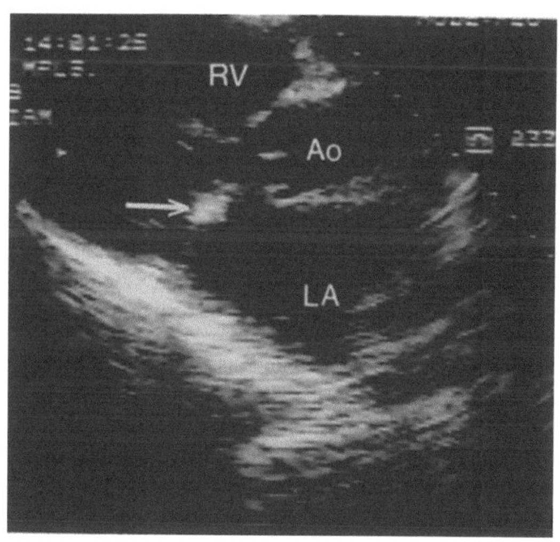

FIGURE 14.3. Two-dimensional echocardiogram showing vegetation on anterior leaflet of the mitral valve (arrow).

units of penicillin in 1–2 liters of 5% glucose is given in 24 hours through a small intravenous polyethylene tube. Aminoglycosides act in synergism with penicillin against most strains of streptococci and may decrease the relapse rate. The two drugs are usually administered for the first 2 weeks, after which penicillin alone is continued for a further 2 weeks: Gentamycin is the aminoglycoside usually used. Low dosage (80 mg b.i.d.) is synergistic and avoids toxicity. Patients with evidence of renal failure should be treated with penicillin alone. Should the patient be hypersensitive to penicillin, cephalothin or cefazolin may be given in a dosage of 2 g every 4 hours in conjunction with gentamycin for the first 2 weeks. Patients who are hypersensitive to penicillin may also react to cephalosporins and if these cannot be used, vancomycin may be given intravenously in a dose of 0.5 g every 6 hours for 4 weeks together with streptomycin for the first 2 weeks.

TABLE 14.1. Cardiac condition.[a]

Endocarditis Prophylaxis Recommended
Prosthetic cardiac valves, including bioprosthetic and homograft valves
Previous bacterial endocarditis, even in the absence of heart disease
Most congenital cardiac malformations
Rheumatic and other acquired valvular dysfunction, even after valvular surgery
Hypertrophic cardiomyopathy
Mitral valve prolapse with valvular regurgitation
Endocarditis Prophylaxis Not Recommended
Isolated secundum atrial septal defect
Surgical repair without residua beyond 6 mg of secundum atrial septal defect, ventricular septal defect, or patient ductus arteriosus
Previous coronary artery bypass graft surgery
Mitral valve prolapse without valvular regurgitation[b]
Physiologic, functional, or innocent heart murmurs
Previous Kawasaki disease without valvular dysfunction
Previous rheumatic fever without valvular dysfunction
Cardiac pacemakers and implanted defibrillators

[a]This Table lists selected conditions but is not meant to be all inclusive.
[b]Individuals who have a mitral valve prolapse associated with thickening and/or redundancy of the valve leaflets may be at increased risk for bacterial endocarditis, particularly men who are 45 years of age or older.
Reprinted, with permission, from Prevention of bacterial endocarditis. JAMA 264(22):2919–2921, 1990.

Enterococci

These is a variety of group D streptococci that are relatively resistant to moderate doses of penicillin. Enterococcal endocarditis should be treated with intravenous ampicillin for 14 days, oral amoxycillin for 14 days, and gentamycin for 28 days. A total dose gentamycin of 2 mg/kg should not be exceeded. Regular assessment of renal, hepatic, and vestibular function is necessary. Cephalosporin should not be used in the treatment of enterococcal endocarditis since these organisms are highly resistant to this antibiotic.

Staphylococcal Endocarditis

The majority of hospital, and many home-acquired staphylococcal infections are resistant to penicillin because of the production of penicillinase. Treatment should be instituted with penicillinase-resistant penicillins (methycillin, cloxicillin, or nafcillin) or the cephalosporins. A minimum of 6 weeks therapy is required.

Gram-Negative Endocarditis

These organisms are generally resistant to treatment and are fortunately uncommon. Therapy consists of bactericidal antibiotics, usually a penicillin or cephalosporin, with an aminoglycoside such as gentamicin.

Fungal Endocarditis

Amphotericin B is fungicidal for *Histoplasma* and other varieties of fungi. It must be given intravenously and is slowly excreted in the urine. The most serious complication is nephrotoxicity, and the creatinine clearance should be performed twice weekly. The drug is diluted in 5% dextrose water and given as a slow intravenous infusion over 6 hours. Treatment is started with a dose of 0.25 mg/kg and increased until 1 mg/kg is reached. Impairment of renal function develops routinely, but is reversible when therapy is discontinued. When

TABLE 14.2 Dental or surgical procedures.[a]

Endocarditis Prophylaxis Recommended
Dental procedures known to induce gingival or mucosal bleeding, including professional cleaning
Tonsillectomy and/or adenordectomy
Surgical operations that involve intestinal or respiratory mucosa
Bronchoscopy with a rigid bronchoscope
Sclerotherapy for esophageal vances
Esophageal dilatation
Gallbladder surgery
Cystoscopy
Urethral dilatation
Urethral cathetenzation if urinary tract infection is present[b]
Urinary tract surgery if urinary tract infection is present[b]
Prostatic surgery
Incision and drainage of infected tissue[b]
Vaginal hysterectomy
Vaginal delivery in the presence of infection[b]

Endocarditis Prophylaxis Not Recommended[c]
Dental procedures not likely to induce gingival bleeding, such as simple adjustment of orthodontic appliances or fillings above the gum line
Injection of local intraoral anesthetic (except intraliga mentary injections)
Shedding of primary teeth
Tympanostomy tube insertion
Endotracheal intubation
Bronchoscopy with a fllexible bronchoscope, with or without biopsy
Cardiac catheterization
Endoscopy with or without gastrointestinal biopsy
Caesarean section
In the absence of infection for urethral catheterization, dilatation and curettage, uncomplicated vaginal delivery, therapeutic abortion, sterilization procedures, or insertion or removal of intrauterine devices

[a]This table lists selected procedures but is not meant to be all-inclusive.
[b]In addition to prophylactic regimen for genitourinary procedures, antibiotic therapy should be directed against the most likely bacterial pathogen.
[c]In patients who have prosthetic heart valves, a previous history of endocaritis, or surgically constructed systemic-pulmonary shunts or conducts, physicians may choose to administer prophylactic antibiotics even for low-risk procedures that involve the lower respiratory, genitournary, or gastrointestinal tracts.
Reprinted with permission, from Prevention of bacterial endocarditis. JAMA 264(22):2919–2921, 1990.

TABLE 14.3. Recommended standard prophylactic regimen for dental, oral, or upper respiratory tract procedures in patients who are at risk.[a]

Drug	Dosing regimen[b]
	Standard Regimen
Amoxicillin	3.0 g orally 1 hr before procedure; then 1.5 g 6 hr after initial dose
	Amoxicillin/Penicillin—Allergic Patients
Erythromycin or Clindamycin	Erythromycin ethylsuccinate, 800 mg, or erythromycin stearate, 1.0 g, orally 2 hr before procedure; then half the dose 6 hr after initial dose 300 mg orally 1 hr before procedure and 150 mg 6 hr after initial dose

[a]Includes those with prosthetic heart valves and other high-risk patients.
[b]Initial pediatric doses are as follows: amoxicillin 50 mg/kg; erythromycin ethylsuccinate or erythromycin sterate, 20 mg/kg; and clindamycin, 10 mg/kg. Follow-up doses should be one-half the initial dose. Total pediatric dose should not exceed total adult dose. The following weight ranges may also be used for the initial pediatric dose of amoxicillin: <15 kg, 750 mg; 15 to 30 kg, 1500 mg; and >30kg, 3000 mg (full audit dose).
Reprinted with permission, from Prevention of bacterial endocarditis. JAMA 264(22):2919–2921, 1990.

the blood urea rises above 50 mg% the intervals between injections are increased. Most patients develop nausea, vomiting, malaise, and rigors, which may be controlled by antihistamines. Phlebothrombosis is also a troublesome complication. 5-Fluorocytosine is a promising new drug given orally with few side-effects. Surgical removal of vegetations and valve replacement may be necessary.

Rickettsial Endocarditis

Tetracycline is the drug of choice and prolonged therapy is required. The aortic valve is usually involved and in many cases surgical removal is required to achieve a cure.

Endocarditis with Negative Cultures

This is a not uncommon problem and the management of these patients is difficult. The hazards of waiting until a firm diagnosis is established outweighs the risks and discomforts of therapy. The wisest course, albeit empirical, is to treat these patients as for enterococcal endocarditis with penicillin and gentamicin for 6 weeks. A penicillinase-resistant penicillin should be added if the infection is not controlled.

Surgical Treatment

When relapse occurs after appropriate therapy is discontinued, or when positive blood cultures continue on adequate therapy, valve excision and replacement with a prosthesis should be considered. Without surgical intervention the chances of cure of a fungal or rickettsial infection are remote. The onset of sudden medically uncontrollable heart failure is an indication for prompt valve replacement to avoid an almost certainly fatal outcome. In the case of an infected prosthetic valve, an aggressive surgical approach is appropriate when there is evidence of a new periprosthetic leak or repeated systemic embolism and evidence of resistant infection after 2 weeks of adequate antibiotic therapy. Valve replacement may also be indicated when relapse occurs following a successful course of optimal medical therapy. Paravalvular abscess and cardiac fistulae are indications for replacement of an infected aortic valve. Tricuspid endocarditis may be treated by excision of the leaflets without valve replacement provided the pulmonary artery pressure is normal. The indications are recurrent sepsis, embolization, and fungal infection in intravenous drug abusers.

TABLE 14.4. Alternate prophylactic regimens for dental, oral, or upper respiratory tract procedures in patients who are at risk.

Drug	Dosing regimen[a]
Patients Unable to Take Oral Medications	
Ampicillin	Intravenous or intramuscular administration of ampicillin, 2.0 g, 30 min before procedure; then intravenous or intramuscular administration of ampicillin, 1.0 g, or oral administration of amoxicillin, 1.5 g 6 hr after initial dose
Ampicillin/Amoxicillin/Penicillin—Allergic Patients Unable to Take Oral Medications	
Clindamycin	Intravenous administration of 300 mg 30 min before procedure and an intravenous or oral administration of 150 mg 6 hr after initial dose
Patients Considered High Risk and Not Candidates for Standard Regimen	
Ampicillin, gentamicin, and amoxicillin	Intravenous or intramuscular administration of ampicillin, 2.0 g, plus gentamicin, 1.5 mg/kg (not to exceed 80 mg), 30 min before procedure; followed by amoxicillin, 1.5 g, orally 6 hr after initial dose; alternatively, the parenteral regimen may be repeated 8 hr after initial dose
Ampicillin/Amoxicillin/Penicillin—Allergic Patients Considered High Risk	
Vancomycin	Intravenous administration of 1.0 g over 1 hr, starting 1 hr before procedure; no repeated dose necessary

[a] Initial pediatnc doses are as follows: ampicillin, 50 mg/kg; clindamycin, 10 mg/kg; gentamicin, 2.0 mg/kg; and vancomycin, 20 mg/kg. Follow-up doses should be one-half the initial dose. Total pediatric dose should not exceed total adult dose. No initial dose is recommended in this table for amoxicillin (25 mg/kg is the follow-up dose).

Criteria for Cure of Infective Endocarditis

Among patients with antibiotic-sensitive organisms receiving adequate antibiotic treatment, the temperature usually drops to normal in 48 hours and this is subsequently followed by a feeling of well-being and an increase in appetite. A good response is judged by a gain in weight, return of the hemoglobin to normal, and a drop in the sedimentation rate. Fresh emboli may, however, persist for sometime after bacteriological cure and do not necessarily indicate a recrudescence of infection. After completion of treatment the patient should be kept under observation for at least

4 weeks, since most relapses occur within this period. Prompt reinstitution of treatment for further prolonged periods is required should this occur.

Prognosis

Before the introduction of antibiotics infective endocarditis was always fatal in a period from 6 months to 2 years. Since the introduction of antibiotic therapy the average cure rate is approximately 80%. Only exceptionally, is death a result of uncontrolled sepsis. The long-term prognosis depends on the underlying cardiac lesions. If valve disease has been seriously aggravated by the infection resulting in congestive cardiac failure, the prognosis is poor unless operative correction can be performed. Systemic embolism, rupture of mycotic aneurysms, and intractable heart and renal failure account for the remaining deaths. The long-term survival rate for patients cured of endocarditis is approximately 75% for 5 years, with the highest mortality occurring during the first 2 years.

Prophylaxis of Bacterial Endocarditis

The recommendations of the American Heart Association for the prevention of bacterial endocarditis are reproduced in Tables 14.1 through 14.4 with permission.

Additional Reading

Dressler FA, Roberts WC: Infective endocarditis in opiate addicts: Analysis of 80 cases studied at necropsy. Am J Cardiol 63:1240–1247.

Garvey GJ, Neu HC: Infective endocarditis—an evolving disease. Medicine 57:105, 1978.

Kaplan EL, et al.: Prevention of bacterial endocarditis. AHA Committee Report. Circulation 56:139A, 1977.

Kaye D: "Infective Endocarditis." University Park Press, Baltimore, 1976.

Weinstein L, Schlesinger JJ: Pathoanatomic, pathophysiologic and clinical correlations in endocarditis. N Engl J Med 291:832, 1974.

15 Cardiomyopathy

The term "cardiomyopathy" refers to "heart muscle disease of unknown cause or association," a definition proposed by Goodwin and Oakley. The cardiomyopathies may be classified into three types based on the physiological disturbances and pathological features.

Congestive Cardiomyopathy

Clinically, the recognition of heart failure is generally easy, but this is not an etiological diagnosis and a search for the *cause* is mandatory. Hypertensive, valvular, and ischemic heart disease are usually readily identifiable and careful clinical examination will reveal the less frequent and less obvious causes including infective endocarditis, recurrent pulmonary embolism, and states of high cardiac output produced by thyrotoxicosis, beriberi, anemia, or arteriovenous fistula.

Additionally, there are systemic diseases including virus infections, sarcoidosis, amyloidosis, and collagen disorders in which the myocardium may be damaged by inflammation or infiltration. These conditions will be described so that they may be considered in the diagnostic approach to this problem. When they are identified and excluded, there remains the largest group where mycardial disease is unexplained, and in the current state of our knowledge this idiopathic group is best classified as dilated or congestive *cardiomyopathy* (Fig. 15.1). A great deal of semantic confusion has resulted through deviation from this approach.

Previously thought to be rare, congestive cardiomyopathy is now more frequently recognized, though not as commonly as hypertensive, ischemic, or rheumatic heart disease. Among the black population of South Africa, congestive cardiomyopathy is one of the leading causes of heart failure. The disease usually occurs alone, but may also complicate pregnancy (peripartum cardiomyopathy) and even obfuscate the presentation of concurrent hypertensive, rheumatic, and congenital heart disease.

Pathology

Characteristically, the heart is hypertrophied and dilated, and this usually involves all chambers. The atrioventricular and semilunar valves are intrinsically normal and the coronary arteries free of atherosclerosis. Intracavitary thrombus occurs in approximately half of the cases, the left ventricle being involved twice as commonly as the right. Organization of this thrombus, which results from stasis, leads to a mild degree of subendocardial fibrosis with the formation of avascular plaques. The underlying myocardium shows hypertrophied muscle fibers and absence of inflammation. The subendocardial fibrosis is patchy and quite different from the severe confluent endocardial thickening seen in endomyocardial fibrosis.

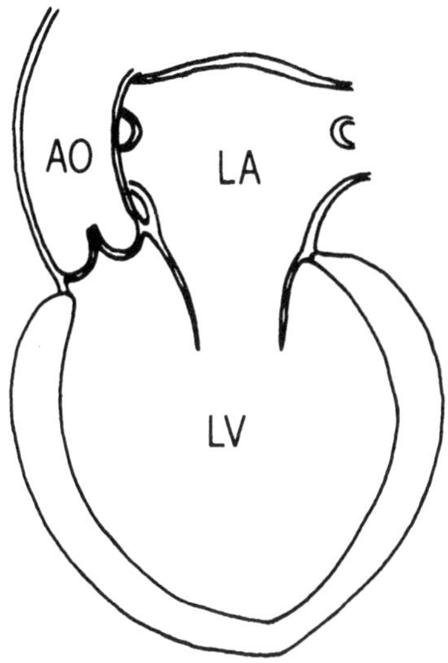

FIGURE 15.1. Congestive cardiomyopathy. Characteristically, the heart is dilated with only moderate hypertrophy.

Clinical Features

The onset of the disease is usually in the third and fourth decade and men are affected twice as commonly as women. In populations where the disease is common it may be encountered before the onset of symptoms in the form of unexplained cardiomegaly or an abnormal electrocardiogram found during a routine physical examination or intercurrent illness.

The majority of patients present with a gradual onset of biventricular failure manifested by pulmonary and systemic venous congestion. Dyspnea and fatigue usually occur early, followed by orthopnea, paroxysmal cardiac dyspnea, hepatic pain, and edema. Occasionally, acute pulmonary edema or systemic embolism is the presenting symptom.

On examination there is evidence of congestive cardiac failure: The jugular venous pressure is always elevated, occasionally showing prominent "ha" wave and brisk "y" descent, and inspiratory filling of the neck veins ("Kussmaul's sign"). These may suggest impaired ventricular filling and the possibility of effusive constrictive pericarditis when the heart size is large on chest X-ray. The pulse is small and when pulsus paradoxus occurs, it is generally less than 10 mm Hg. Pulsus alternans may be found and is indicative of advanced disease.

Systemic hypertension is a frequent finding when cardiac failure is at its worst and is the result of peripheral vasoconstriction secondary to low cardiac output. The hypertension usually settles to normal levels with bed rest and treatment, but may persist in advanced cases. An important clue to the etiology is obtained by examination of the fundi: hypertensive heart disease of sufficient severity to produce congestive cardiac failure is invariably associated with advanced stages of retinopathy whereas the fundi are normal in cases of congestive cardiomyopathy. Failure to appreciate the significance of this clinical sign has led to confusion between hypertensive heart failure and congestive cardiomyopathy.

The apex beat is generally displaced outward and is hypodynamic. The heart sounds are normal or soft and wide splitting of the second sound may be present because of left bundle branch block. Gallop rhythm is usual, the extra sound being a third or summation sound. Pansystolic mitral and/or tricuspid murmurs of functional atrioventricular valve insufficiency are often present.

Radiology

This confirms generalized cardiac enlargement, varying degrees of hilar and upper lobe venous congestion, and frequent pleural effusions. Evidence of pulmonary arterial hypertension and significant left atrial enlargement are characteristically absent and this aids in the distinction from rheumatic mitral incompetence.

The Electrocardiogram

This is invariably abnormal showing a fairly uniform pattern of left ventricular hypertrophy and left atrial enlargement. The electrocardiogram reflects the imbalance of electrical forces produced by left ventricular hypertrophy since the left ventricle bears the major hemodynamic load. Right ventricular hypertrophy is absent and right axis deviation rare in the absence of pulmonary embolism.

Conduction defects are restricted to the left

bundle branch of the conducting system and are found in 25% of cases. Left bundle branch and left anterior hemiblock occur with equal frequency. These findings are related to fibrosis of the divisions of the left bundle branch. The left bundle immediately divides into two main networks, widely interconnected, lying entirely in the subendocardium, where they are susceptible to fibrosis. The right bundle, however, follows a long intramyocardial course within the ventricular septum before supplying the Purkinje system and is thus spared by subendocardial fibrosis, which, in any event, is less common in the right ventricle. This immunity of the right bundle does not pertain in virus myocarditis.

Pathological Q waves indicative of myocardial necrosis are rare; when encountered in a case of congestive cardiac failure of obscure etiology they would strongly indicate a diagnosis of either cardiomyopathy complicated by coronary embolism, virus myocarditis, or occult ischemic heart disease.

Echocardiography

This has greatly simplified the diagnosis and quickly rules out pericardial effusion when the heart size is very large. The characteristic findings are (1) four chamber enlargement, (2) global left ventricular hypokinesis with depressed ejection fraction, (3) E point septal separation and "floating mitral valve," (4) left ventricular mural thrombus, and (5) color-Doppler confirming mitral and tricuspid regurgitation through intrinsically normal leaflets (Fig. 15.2).

Cardiac Catheterization

This establishes the diagnosis of heart failure and excludes coronary artery disease as the cause. Left ventricular cineangiography is quite characteristic and shows a large dilated poorly contractile chamber. There is generalized hypokinesis, quite distinct from the segmental abnormalities of wall motion that are seen in ischemic heart disease. Selective coronary angiography demonstrates patent widely splayed vessels and is diagnostic in excluding occlusive atherosclerosis as occurs in the so-called "ischemic myopathy." The latter term is a misnomer and should not be used since the muscle damage related to coronary artery disease clearly has a cause. Recognition of an ischemic etiology may prove difficult in the absence of a typical history of chest pain and when an electrocardiographic interventricular conduction defect masks the telltale Q waves. Mitral insufficiency is not uncommon in advanced cardiomyopathy and left ventricular angiography will usually distinguish this from primary rheumatic valve disease where left ventricular contractility is usually normal. However, in long-standing rheumatic mitral insufficiency with poor left ventricular function the distinction may be difficult.

Confirmation of the diagnosis of congestive cardiomyopathy may be made by endomyocardial biopsy of the right ventricle, which is a safe procedure. The morphological features found in specimens obtained from congestive cardiomyopathy are not specific, but myocarditis and degenerative and infiltrative diseases of the myocardium may be excluded fairly confidently.

Peripartum Cardiomyopathy

A variant of congestive cardiomyopathy with a special tendency to occur in relationship to childbirth occurs more commonly in black than white people. Pathologically, it is indistinguishable from congestive cardiomyopathy but does differ clinically in that it may be reversible. Unfortunately, there is a tendency to recurrence with subsequent pregnancies. It is probable that this is not a specific disease but simply congestive cardiac failure precipitated by the hemodynamic load of pregnancy in patients with occult cardiomyopathy. Among the black populations of South Africa it appears to be correlated with multiparity, twin pregnancy, and prolonged lactation.

The onset of the disease is usually in the last trimester of pregnancy or within the first 10 weeks of the puerperium. The mortality is much higher in patients who are left with persistent cardiomegaly and subsequent pregnancies have a poor prognosis.

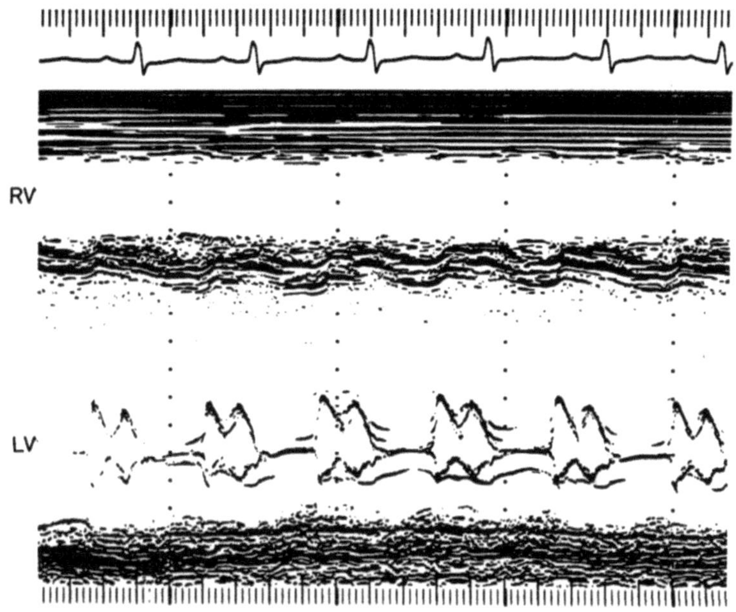

FIGURE 15.2. Echocardiogram in congestive cardiomyopathy showing detailed ventricles, "floating mitral valve" with E point septal separation.

Alcoholic Cardiomyopathy

When the clinical picture of congestive (or dilated) cardiomyopathy occurs in abusers of alcohol, the condition has been called "alcoholic cardiomyopathy." The symptoms, physical signs, and noninvasive tests and pathological findings are identical in both conditions.

Usually, this cardiomyopathy is not accompanied by other features of chronic alcoholism such as neuropathy, pancreatitis, and avitaminosis. Indeed, victims are frequently well-nourished. It is also very difficult to produce alcoholic cardiac damage in experimental animals. This author believes that "alcoholic cardiomyopathy" may not be a separate entity but, as in the case of peripartum cardiomyopathy, alcohol may be a conditioning factor in the development of heart failure.

Among "binge drinkers," the effect of acute alcoholism may be to precipitate supraventricular dysrhythmia, particularly atrial fibrillation—so called "Holiday Heart." Dysrhythmias are probably induced by catecholamines released in response to acetaldehyde, which is a metabolite of alcohol.

Certainly, when excessive alcohol consumption is recognized in a patient with congestive heart failure, abstinence should be recommended.

Cardiomyopathy Complicating Other Diseases

Among populations in whom congestive cardiomyopathy is prevalent there may be a coincidental association with other forms of heart disease. Superimposition of myopathic heart failure modifies the clinical presentation and management of conditions such as Tetralogy of Fallot, ventricular septal defect, pulmonary stenosis, rheumatic heart disease, and thyrotoxicosis.

Tetralogy of Fallot is a good example. In the differential diagnosis of cyanotic congenital heart disease the presence of congestive cardiac failure is said to preclude the diagnosis of Tetralogy. Occasionally, heart failure may occur in infants with Tetralogy when there is superadded bacterial endocarditis, aortic insufficiency, absence of the pulmonary valve, or functional obstruction of the ventricular septal

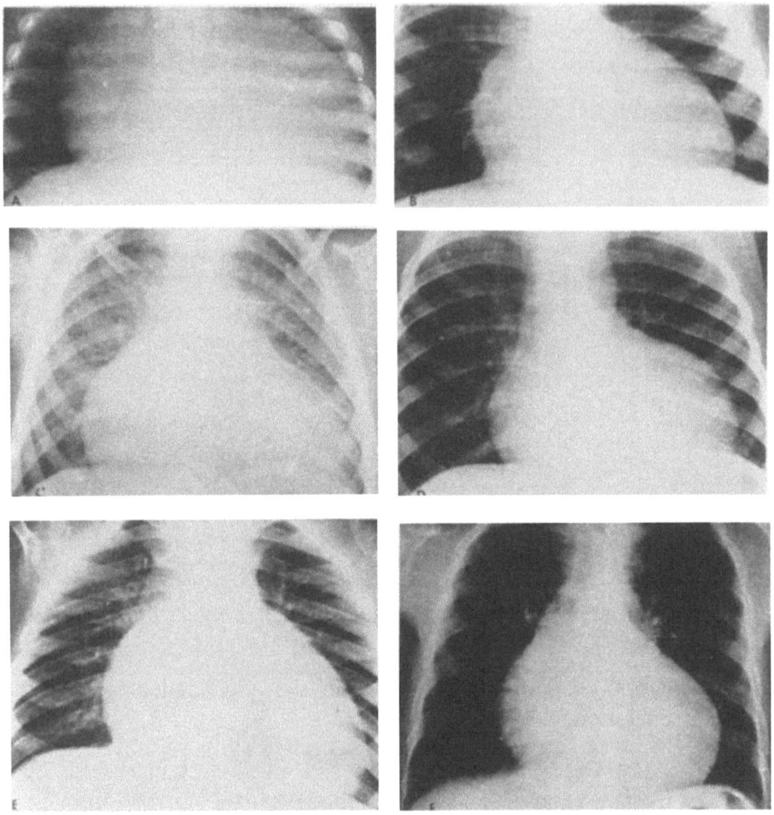

FIGURE 15.3. X-rays of the chest in Tetralogy of Fallot complicated by cardiomyopathy (see text).

defect by the tricuspid valve. Additionally, some examples have been ascribed to systemic hypertension. We encountered cases of Tetralogy of Fallot where the clinical presentation was dominated by the presence of severe protracted congestive cardiac failure (Fig. 15.3). At catheterization or autopsy none of the aforementioned predisposing factors was operative and histological examination of the myocardium showed the nonspecific changes of congestive cardiomyopathy. These patients are frequently hypertensive as a manifestation, and not a cause of their heart failure. Similarly, we have encountered severe heart failure disproportionate to the degree of hemodynamic disturbance in mild pulmonary valvular stenosis, small ventricular septal defect, and double outlet right ventricle.

Mild aortic insufficiency has been thought to be a complication of cardiomyopathy but we believe this to be mild rheumatic aortic insufficiency, complicated by superimposed cardiomyopathy. Also, heart failure encountered in thyrotoxicosis in young patients without atrial fibrillation is thought to have the same cause.

An awareness of this phenomenon is imperative in the practice of clinical cardiology in these areas where congestive cardiomyopathy is prevalent. Failure to identify impaired myocardial function in conditions such as Tetralogy of Fallot may lead to disastrous results when total anatomic correction is embarked on.

Treatment

As may be expected, the treatment of a disease of unknown cause is unsatisfactory. Control of the heart failure with digitalis and diuretics is essential and in resistant cases vasodilator therapy may be useful. Factors thought to be important in the genesis of congestive cardiomyopathy include thiamine deficiency, excessive consumption of alcohol, and chronic general malnutrition. There is, however, no firm evidence to suggest that modification of the dietary and alcoholic habits has any influence on the course of this disease.

Prognosis

Untreated, the course is usually progressively downhill with death in heart failure affecting at least three-quarters of the victims within 5 years. Afterload reduction using vasodilators may improve this prognosis.

Specific Diseases of the Myocardium

Numerous conditions may involve the heart muscle and produce a clinical picture resembling dilated cardiomyopathy. A diagnosis of congestive cardiomyopathy implies that they have been excluded.

Myocarditis

Bacterial

Although occasional examples have been reported, myocarditis is so rare as to be of little clinical significance in tuberculosis, typhoid fever, scrub typhus, poliomyelitis, infective hepatitis, infective mononucleosis, virus pneumonia, and other respiratory tract infections. Histological evidence of myocarditis may be present in these conditions but there is usually no clinical counterpart. This discrepancy between the pathological and clinical findings may not necessarily be resolved by routine electrocardiography since ST and T wave changes may be nonspecific and vagal bradycardia and prolongation of the PR interval are not uncommon in the convalescent state.

For practical purposes, clinically significant myocarditis may occur in the following groups.

Toxic

Diphtheria

Myocarditis is the most lethal complication of diphtheria and is a result of circulating exotoxin. It occurs in about 10% of cases and carries a mortality rate of approximately 60%.

Pathological examination shows diffuse hyaline degeneration and necrosis of cardiac muscle and the tissues of the conduction system. Diphtheria exotoxin interferes with cellular respiration by competing with the cytochrome enzymes and has a high degree of affinity for the conduction system.

The onset is in the second week of the disease and presents with sinus tachycardia, gallop rhythm, cardiomegaly, and hypotension. There is a combination of congestive cardiac failure and circulatory collapse resulting from vasomotor paralysis. The electrocardiographic abnormalities are useful in diagnosis and fall under two heads:

1. Tracings showing evidence of diffuse myocardial damage: low voltage, prolongation of the Q-T interval, and T wave flattening or inversion.
2. Tracings showing evidence of damage to the conduction system with all degrees of atrioventricular and fascicular block. The development of bundle branch block or complete heart block is a particularly ominous finding and the reported mortality rates vary from 54 to 100%. The presence of myocardial damage is confirmed by marked elevation of the serum transaminase levels.

Treatment consists of antibiotics such as penicillin or erythromycin to prevent secondary infection and eliminate the diphtheria organisms in the throat. Antitoxic serum should not be given at this stage because the exotoxin is already fixed and because of the risk of fatal serum reactions. Temporary transvenous electrical pacing in cases of atrioventricular block has been shown to be of value in preventing fatal asystole. Intubation and positive pressure ventilation may be required for those patients with evidence of respiratory failure.

The electrocardiogram eventually returns to

normal (in those cases that survive) but conduction abnormalities may persist for years.

Viral

Coxsackie

Numerous reports have documented the importance of Coxsackie B viruses as the commonest cause of myocarditis. The infection was first recognized in the neonate and may occur in epidemic form in the nursery. The disease is frequently sudden in onset with tachycardia, dyspnea, and cyanosis, followed by severe heart failure. Cardiomegaly is usually present and the electrocardiogram shows evidence of myocardial damage. The prognosis is poor and the mortality rate is in the region of 60%.

In adults, the disease is frequently associated with pericarditis and has a more benign prognosis. It is more common in men and usually occurs in young adults. Chest pain is usually pleuropericardial but occasionally may be indistinguishable from angina pectoris. Signs of systemic involvement such as pleural rub, encephalitis, hepatitis, orchitis, and lymphadenopathy may be present. Evidence of congestive cardiac failure and pericarditis with effusion is common.

The electrocardiogram demonstrates low voltage, ST segment, and T wave changes, atrioventricular block, intraventricular conduction defects, and occasionally pathological Q waves. Indeed, in some patients the presentation may be indistinguishable from acute myocardial infarction. Usually, pericarditis is a prominent feature and the differential diagnosis therefore includes tuberculosis, collagen diseases, sarcoidosis, and so on. Cardiac tamponade may be a complication and pericardiocentesis may yield blood-stained fluid. Constrictive pericarditis may be a long-term complication.

Ideally, the diagnosis of Coxsackie infection is established by isolation of the virus from pericardial fluid. Alternatively, virus isolation from the pharynx or feces and a fourfold rise in type-specific convalescent antibodies would also be diagnostic.

The prognosis in the adult is usually good and the mortality rate is less than 5%. A tendency for recurrence may be a troublesome feature. In a minority, there is persistent myocardial damage producing intractable cardiac failure indistinguishable from congestive cardiomyopathy; endomyocardial biopsy may be helpful in the distinction. Complete heart block has been reported and permanent electrical pacing may be necessary.

There is no specific treatment; absolute bed rest is essential until the signs regress. The value of steroids and immunosuppressive drugs is moot. Digitalis and diuretics are used for heart failure.

Rubella

Rubella is an important cause of myocarditis in the fetus and neonate. Myocardial damage is severe and there is a high mortality rate. Associated features of the rubella syndrome include retinitis, hepatitis, thrombocytopenic purpura, epiphysitis, and congenital cardiac malformations including ventricular septal defect, patent ductus arteriosus, and peripheral pulmonary artery stenoses.

Difficulties in Diagnosis of Virus Myocarditis

Proof of a viral course for myocarditis is difficult. Ideally, this is by isolation of the virus. Raised antibody titers may suggest viral myocarditis but are not diagnostic. Endomyocardial biopsy is safe but interpretation may be difficult because of small sample size, sampling error, and most importantly varying interpretation of the histological findings. The important histopathological findings are focal myocyte necrosis with surrounding inflammatory infiltrates.

Parasitic

Trypanosomiasis, "Chagas' Disease"

This is a leading form of heart disease in South America. Infection is transmitted by a bedbug vector and myocarditis occurs during the acute stage. Recovery is usual, however, and the disease is quiescent for the next 10 to 15 years. Myocardial involvement is one of the characteristic manifestations of chronic Chagas' disease. There is destruction of cardiac muscle but, more importantly, widespread damage to the conduction system. *Trypanosoma cruzi* may be found in degenerated muscle cells, especially in the right atrium.

The disease is characterized clinically by severe, protracted, congestive cardiac failure complicated by mitral and tricuspid insufficiency. Bifascicular block is present in more than 80% of cases and death from asystole and arrhythmia is common. There is no specific therapy. Heart failure and arrhythmias are treated with the usual measures.

Trichinosis

This infection is common in the United States and ingestion of infested pork may lead to *Trichinella spiralis* myocarditis. Myocarditis is responsible for most of the deaths in this type of parasitic infection. The clinical diagnosis is suggested by marked muscle tenderness, eosinophilia, and periorbital edema. Treatment is with thiabendazole and steroids to reduce allergic edema.

Toxoplasmosis

Myocarditis occurs in both congenital and acquired varieties. Cardiomegaly and complete heart block are not uncommon. The diagnosis is confirmed by complement fixation and the Sabin Feldman dye test. Treatment is with pyrimethamine and sulfonamide.

Drugs, Chemicals, and Physical Agents Affecting the Myocardium

Patients receiving drug therapy for general medical diseases may sustain myocardial damage responsible for a variety of cardiovascular complications. Some of these agents are briefly enumerated.

Emetine and Chloroquine

Both of these agents are used in the treatment of amebiasis and their cardiotoxic effects may be additive. They may result in arrhythmias, hypertension, and sudden death. Electrocardiographic abnormalities are frequent and bed rest is mandatory during therapy.

Tricyclic Antidepressant Drugs

These drugs block norepinephrine uptake and also have an important anticholinergic effect. They may cause resistance to therapy for hypertension, particularly when guanethidine and clonidine are used. Additionally, they may precipitate hypertensive crises, heart failure, myocardial infarction, cardiac arrhythmias, and sudden death.

Phenothiazines

Chlorpromazine and its various derivatives may deplete or increase myocardial catecholamines. Depletion may induce hypotension or interventriclar conduction defects. An increase in catecholamines may be associated with arrhythmias or hypertension. They are contraindicated in patients with heart disease.

Adriamycin

This antibiotic is used to treat lymphoma and solid tumors. Myocardial damage may supervene from 1 to 6 months after completion of therapy and the presentation is one of sudden, but intractable cardiac failure. A similar presentation may result from daunorubicin therapy. Patients without heart disease may safely receive 450 mg/m^2. When higher doses are required, this should be monitored by MUGA measurement of rest and exercise ejection fraction.

Heavy Metals

Arsenic, antimony, mercury, phosphorus, and so on may all produce myocardial damage.

Cobalt

This agent was used to promote frothing in beer and has been incriminated in the production of cardiomyopathy. The entity has now disappeared as a result of removal of cobalt from beer.

Radiation

This usually produces pericarditis with effusion and occasionally tamponade or constrictive pericarditis. Myocardial fibrosis may also occur.

Systemic Diseases Involving the Myocardium

Myocardial involvement in systemic disease may lead to congestive cardiac failure, arrhythmias, and systemic embolism. Occasionally, the signs of the responsible systemic disease are not always evident and the presentation in congestive cardiac failure may simulate that of idiopathic congestive cardiomyopathy.

Infiltration of the Myocardium

Amyloid

The heart may be involved in primary, familial, or senile amyloidosis but rarely in the type secondary to long-standing suppurative disease. The disease should therefore be suspected when cardiac involvement occurs in multiple myelomatosis, and when there are clinical clues such as macroglossia, purpura, peripheral neuropathy, conjunctival thickening, or the nephrotic syndromes.

Heavy deposition of amyloid in the myocardium stiffens the ventricular walls in the absence of cardiac dilatation. The clinical presentation, therefore, resembles that of restrictive cardiomyopathy. Frequently, there is a pericardial effusion. Hemodynamically, in addition to the restriction of diastolic filling there is also compromised systolic pump function with low cardiac output and reduced ejection fraction. These features are helpful in the distinction from constrictive pericarditis.

The electrocardiogram, while not specific for amyloidosis, may help in differentiation from constrictive pericarditis. Tracings show high voltage and in one-third of cases there are pathological Q waves.

Echocardiography is the most useful noninvasive test. The combination of (1) symmetric wall thickening, (2) small left ventricular cavity (3) "granular sparkling" appearance of the myocardium, (4) depression of left ventricular ejection fraction in two-third of patients, and (5) pericardial effusion in 50% of patients is indicative of diagnosis. Endomyocardial, rectal gingival, and skin biopsies may confirm the diagnosis. Treatment is palliative and the disease is fatal within a few years.

Hemochromatosis

Infiltration of the heart with iron is extremely common in hemochromatosis but clinically significant involvement occurs in only 15% of patients. Since the advent of insulin to control the associated diabetes, cardiac failure is now the leading cause of death in hemochromatosis. Deposition of iron in the myocardium produces a restrictive type of hemodynamic defect or a picture resembling congestive cardiomyopathy. Cardiomegaly, substernal pain, and congestive cardiac failure are the commonest manifestations. The electrocardiogram shows low-voltage, nonspecific T wave changes, atrial fibrillation, and occasionally A-V block.

The diagnosis is obvious when there is associated diabetes, cirrhosis, pigmentation, and loss of sexual hair. Occasionally, however, cardiac manifestations are the presenting feature. An identical syndrome may occur in the acquired hemosiderosis that follows multiple blood transfusions used for the treatment of refractory anemia. Treatment by venesections or iron-chelating agents is helpful. Untreated, the disease is usually fatal within 12 months.

Glycogen

Cardiac involvement is common in glycogenusis type II (Pompes disease). Inabilty to hydrolize glycogen to glucose because of a congenital enzyme deficiency leads to massive deposition of glycogen in the myocardium and the skeletal muscles. Heart failure usually occurs before 18 months of age. The clinical clues are hypotonia, muscle weakness, macroglassia, and positive family history. The diagnosis is confirmed by demonstration of increased glycogen and absence of α-glucosidase activity in skeletal muscle biopsy.

Myocardial Involvement in Hereditary Muscular Dystrophies and Neurological Disorders

Myocardial involvement occurs in 50% of cases of progressive muscular dystrophy and may precede skeletal muscle disease. Fibrofatty replacement of the posterobasal myocardium results in mitral insufficiency, an electrocardiographic pattern of posterior myocardial infarction, and occasionally heart failure. Heart muscle disease is less frequent in the other muscular dystrophies such as the "facioscapular-humeral" and "limb-girdle" types.

Friedreich's Ataxia

Clinically, obvious heart disease occurs in only 50% of cases although there is uniformly evidence of myocardial involvement at autopsy. Degeneration of the heart muscle leads to heart failure and electrocardiographic conduction defects.

Myotonia Atrophica

This is frequently associated with myocardial complications having a particular predilection for the conduction system. Bradycardia, A-V block, and fascicular blocks may cause sudden death.

Collagen Disorders

Heart failure is common in the collagen disorders and usually results from associated hypertension, valvular involvement, coronary artery disease, lung pathology, or pericarditis. Involvement of the myocardium itself is rarely responsible. These disorders are mentioned here so that they are thought of before the diagnosis of idiopathic congestive cardiomyopathy is made. Clues to the diagnosis are as follows:

1. *Polyarteritis nodosa*: hypertension, pericarditis, renal failure, and peripheral neuropathy.
2. *Disseminated lupus erythematosus*: hypertension, arthritis, hemolyticanemia, renal failure, butterfly rash, and pericarditis.
3. *Scleroderma*: Raynaud phenomena, dysphagia, sclerodactyly, telangiectasia, calcinosis, and renal failure.

Sarcoidosis

Sarcoid granulomas involve the myocardium and the conducting system. The disease should be thought of in the presence of unexplained heart block, ventricular aneurysm, or heart failure in a young person. Usually, however, these complications arise when the disease is well established in other organs.

Restrictive (Including "Obliterative") Cardiomyopathy

The restrictive group is the least frequent of the cardiomyopathies (Fig. 15.4 and 15.5). Variants of the syndrome occur in the tropics described as "endomyocardial fibrosis," and in the temperate zones as "Loeffler's endocarditis" or "primary restrictive cardiomyopathy."

It is likely that these conditions are part of a continuum of the same disease commencing with eosinophilia and moving to Loeffler endocarditis and eventually to the tropical type of endomyocardial fibrosis. In the burned-out phase, these diseases are histologically indis-

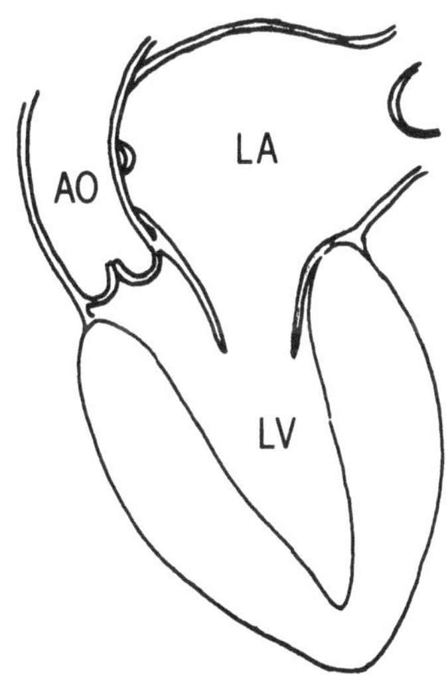

FIGURE 15.4. Diagrammatic representation of restrictive cardiomyopathy in which there is reduction of left ventricular cavity size and moderate ventricular hypertrophy.

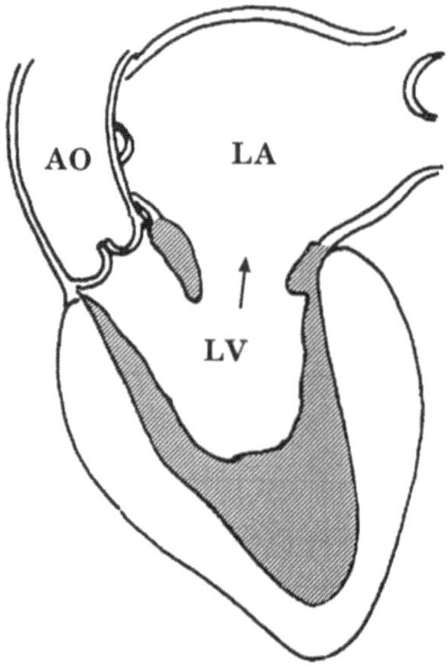

FIGURE 15.5. Diagrammatic representation of obliterative cardiomyopathy where the cavity is reduced in size by overgrowth of fibrous tissue, which extends to involve the atrioventricular valves.

tinguishable. Prolonged eosinophilia (produced by eosinophilic leukemia, tropical infestations, status asthmaticus, etc.) may produce thrombotic endocarditis and myocardial necrosis. It may be that Loeffler disease, with its serious constitutional illness and hypereosinophilia, represents the acute form of the disease, while tropical endomyocardial fibrosis and obliterative cardiomyopathy are the result of chronic involvement. Patients with milder forms (i.e. "primary restrictive cardiomyopathy") encountered in England constitute an intermediate variety with lesser degrees of subendocardial fibrosis.

Pathology

There are varying degrees of subendocardial eosinophilic infiltrates, necrosis and fibrosis, frequently associated with mural thrombus. The papillary muscles may be bound down by fibrous tissue and the chordae adherent to the ventricular wall. In the extreme stage when there is *obliterative cardiomyopathy* the cavity of the ventricle is occupied entirely by fibrous tissue and superimposed thrombus. The disease may involve either or both ventricles and be complicated by pericarditis with effusion (Fig. 15.6).

Clinical Findings

Like congestive cardiomyopathy the clinical picture may be one of pulmonary and systemic venous congestion with atrioventricular valve incompetence. The dominant physical findings,

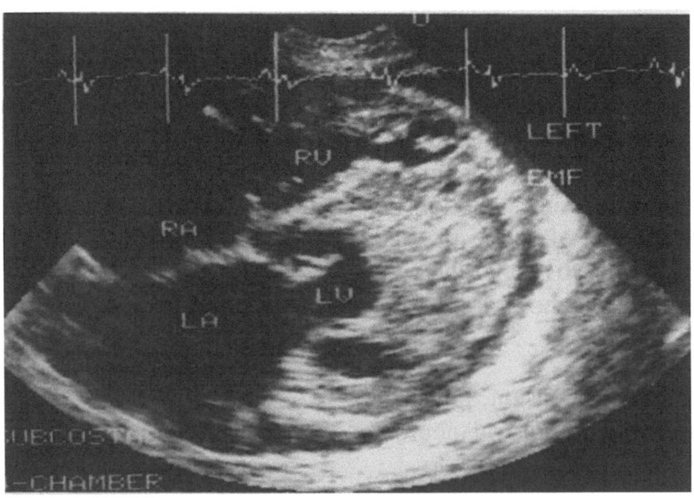

FIGURE 15.6. Echocardiogram in restrictive cardiomyopathy showing cavity obliteration enlarged left artuim (LA) and small pericardial effusion. Right ventricle (RV) and left ventricle.

however, are produced by restriction to diastolic ventricular filling and therefore resemble constrictive pericarditis.

The clinical manifestations of right-sided restrictive cardiomyopathy are similar to those of constrictive pericarditis with ascites, hepatomegaly, pulsus parodoxus, and an early third sound. In contradistinction to constrictive pericarditis, however, there is frequently a murmur of tricuspid incompetence. Radiography may demonstrate an enlarged cardiac silhouette similar to a pericardial effusion. When the left ventricle is involved the radiological signs are those of pulmonary venous and arterial hypertension secondary to mitral insufficiency and cardiomegaly is not as marked. The electrocardiogram shows nonspecific, low-voltage QRS complexes and may indicate right atrial enlargement in the form of tall peaked "P" waves.

Hemodynamics

Cardiac catheterization demonstrates the combination of restricted filling and incompetence of the A-V valves. The right atrial pressure is elevated, with prominent systolic waves and steep "X" and "Y" descents. In the severe obliterative cases, the pressures in the right atrium, right ventricle, and pulmonary arteries may be identical and an intracardiac electrocardiogram may be required to locate the position of the tricuspid and pulmonary valves. A dip and plateau ("square root") type of pressure pulse is frequently present in both ventricles. These hemodynamics differ, however, from those found in constrictive pericarditis in that

1. The end-diastolic pressures tend to be equal in both ventricles in constrictive pericarditis whereas they are disparate in restrictive cardiomyopathy.
2. The early diastolic pressures in constrictive pericarditis are frequently at zero, but above zero in restrictive cardiomyopathy.
3. Pulmonary hypertension is much more likely in restrictive cardiomyopathy than constrictive pericarditis. These differences are related to unequal involvement of the ventricles in restrictive cardiomyopathy.

The diagnosis can be established by angiography, which demonstrates an enormously enlarged right atrium and obliteration of the apex of the right ventricle. The same findings are reality detectable by endocardiography. When the ventricular cavity is small, endomyocardial biopsy of the right ventricle may be useful by demonstrating an excess of fibrous tissue, a finding that is highly suggestive of endomyocardial fibrosis. In those forms of this syndrome where significant cardiomegaly is absent, distinction from constrictive pericarditis may be impossible. The only means of making the diagnosis is then by exploratory thoracotomy.

As in congestive cardiomyopathy, where the etiology of the disease is unknown, treatment is highly unsatisfactory and can consist only of palliative administration of digitalis and diuretics.

Hypertrophic Cardiomyopathy

Hypertrophic cardiomyopathy (Fig. 15.7) is recognized as a relatively common disease that frequently masquerades as valvular aortic ste-

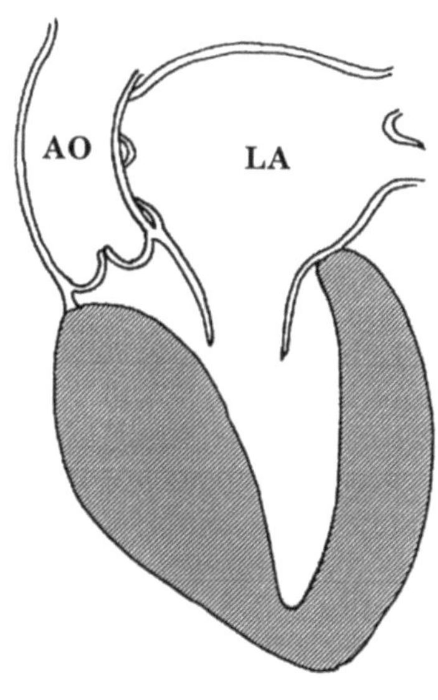

FIGURE 15.7. Diagrammatic representation of the heart in hypertrophic obstructive cardiomyopathy in which there is marked left ventricular hypertrophy and disproportionate involvement of the septum.

nosis, mitral regurgitation, or ischemic heart disease. Since congestive cardiac failure supervenes in approximately 10% of cases it must also be differentiated from the other cardiomyopathies. Early studies recognized the disorder only when muscular outflow obstruction was evident and this has influenced the nomenclature (e.g., "obstructive cardiomyopathy," "hypertrophic obstructive cardiomyopathy," "idiopathic hypertrophic subaortic stenosis," and "muscular subaortic stenosis"). Since it is now appreciated that the nonobstructive form predominates, the term "hypertrophic cardiomyopathy" is preferable.

Definition

Hypertrophic cardiomyopathy is an idiopathic disease of heart muscle, not associated with any other condition. It may involve both ventricles but usually only the left ventricle is affected. In the left ventricle the disease may manifest as symmetric or asymmetric hypertrophy. When the right ventricle is hypertrophied it is usually symmetric in nature. The disease is transmitted as an autosomal dominant trait.

Pathology

Grossly, the characteristic picture is one of asymmetrical septal hypertrophy. In the normal heart, the ratio of thickness of the septum to free wall averages 0.95, whereas ill hypertrophic cardiomyopathy this ratio exceeds 1.3. The left ventricular cavity is usually flattened and sigmoid in shape and the endocardium of the left ventricular outflow tract is nearly always thickened by fibrous tissue. These plaques result from friction with the anterior leaflet of the mitral valve, which is also thickened. This process is accentuated by the more anterior position of the mitral valve apparatus in relation to the ventricular septum. Subendocardial scarring of the papillary muscles of the left ventricle is a frequent finding that is unrelated to coronary artery disease since these vessels are widely patent in the majority of patients.

The characteristic histological abnormality is the presence of numerous foci where the myocardial architecture is disorganized. These regions are composed of cells arranged in whorls with bundles of muscle cells irregularly arranged and coursing in various directions. These foci are interspersed among areas where muscle cells are hypertrophied, but normally arranged. These abnormalities are highly characteristic, but not absolutely diagnostic, of hypertrophic cardiomyopathy and milder forms occur in other conditions.

Pathophysiology

The hypertrophied left ventricle exhibits abnormalities of systolic and diastolic function.

Diastolic Abnormalities

Elevation of left ventricular end-diastolic pressure is characteristic and is a result of decreased compliance. The "a" wave is prominent because atrial systole is important in filling the hypertrophied ventricle. Abnormalities of filling are readily detected by echo Doppler.

Systolic Abnormalities

Left ventricular systolic function is hyperdynamic and the chamber empties almost completely in early systole. Approximately one-third of patients have a systolic gradient between the body of the left ventricle and its outflow tract. In many cases a resting gradient is absent but obstruction may be provoked by physical or pharmacologic maneuvers that (1) increase myocardial contractility or (2) decrease ventricular volume by reducing pre- or afterload.

The gradient occurs at the time of anterior mitral leaflet–septal apposition when the anterior leaflet moves forward (SAM). Whether the gradient is a result of true obstruction or a result of a Venturi effect, whereby the anterior mitral leaflet is sucked into the outflow tract of an empty ventricle, is still debated, but it seems that obstruction is a genuine feature.

Clinical Features

In the first two decades, the condition is frequently asymptomatic. It may be discovered by screening of relatives of affected members of a family, routine physical or electrocardiographic examination.

The onset of symptoms is usually in the third and fourth decade. Exertional dyspnea, angina pectoris, fatigue, and dizziness predominate. Syncope and congestive cardiac failure are fortunately infrequent because they carry a poor prognosis.

Physical Exam

This usually discloses an easily recognized combination of clinical signs. The pulses are brisk and jerky. The apical impulse is typical of left ventricular hypertrophy and is frequently preceded by a palpable atrial contraction. A late starting crescendo–decrescendo midsystolic ejection murmur is best heard along the left sternal border in the third and fourth intercostal spaces and radiates poorly toward the neck. When mitral regurgitation is present an additional pansystolic murmur is present at the apex. The second sound is usually single but occasionally may be paradoxically split.

Auscultation

Cursory auscultation may suggest the diagnosis of ventricular septal defect or mitral regurgitation, but a more common difficulty is the distinction from aortic valve disease. The localization of the murmur at the lower left sternal border and the absence of an aortic ejection click or early diastolic murmur are features that strongly favor the diagnosis of hypertrophic cardiomyopathy.

The accuracy of auscultation is enhanced by noninvasive bedside maneuvers because the obstruction of left ventricular outflow is dynamic. Squatting and hand grip soften the murmur. This is because the gradient decreases following an increase in systemic arterial pressure and left ventricular volume and a reduction in left ventricular ejection velocity. Conversely, the Valsalva maneuver, the administration of amyl nitrite, and the occurrence of a spontaneous premature ventricular contraction intensify the murmur by increasing the gradient (Fig. 15.8). This follows a decrease in the arterial pressure and left ventricular volume and an increase in the left ventricular ejection velocity. In most cases, the administration of amyl nitrite and the observation of the effects of prompt squatting are the only maneuvers required. However, it is important to remember that mitral insufficiency is frequently associated; the effect of squatting may then be confusing because this maneuver may accentuate the murmur of mitral insufficiency.

The Electrocardiogram

This provides important clues to the diagnosis and almost invariably demonstrates severe left ventricular hypertrophy with repolarization change. Frequently there are deep abnormal "Q" waves found in Leads II, III, and AVF and the left precordial leads—a combination that is sufficient to suggest the diagnosis, particularly in the young (Fig. 15.9).

Occasionally, the typical findings of the Wolff–Parkinson–White syndrome are observed. Left axis deviation and left bundle branch block are occasionally seen but bifascicular and complete heart block are extremely rare.

Arrhythmias occur frequently. Atrial fibrillation and supraventricular tachycardias are a result of atrial distension because of high left ventricular end-diastolic pressure. Nonsustained ventricular tachycardia is common and usually asymptomatic.

The Chest X-Ray

This may be normal. It may demonstrate left ventricular hypertrophy but this correlates poorly with the gradient and symptomatology. The aorta is usually normal. Significant enlargement in the ascending portion would be a point in favor of valvular aortic stenosis. Left atrial enlargement and Kerley B lines are seen in advanced cases, particularly when there is atrial fibrillation.

Echocardiography

The 2D technique is the most useful technique because it shows the extent and severity of hypertrophy. It demonstrates whether involvement is symmetric or asymmetric and distin-

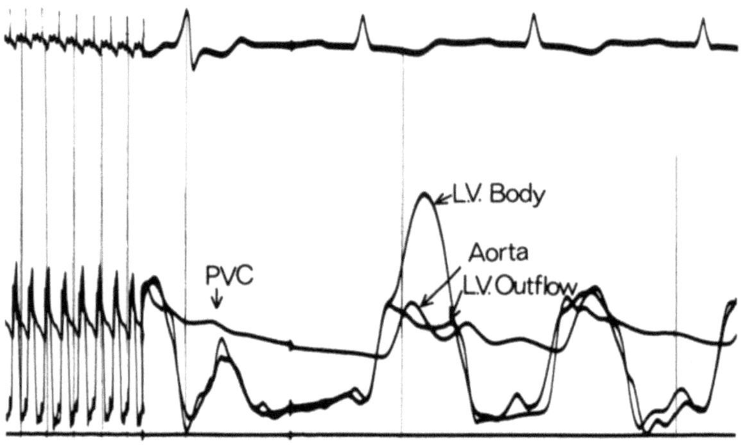

FIGURE 15.8. The effect of a premature ventricular contraction (PVC) in hypertrophic obstructive cardiomyopathy. Following the postectopic pause there is the development of an intracavitary gradient, which disappears with the next beat. There is no gradient across the aortic valve.

guishes between the usual upper septal involvement compared to the rare midcavity or apical obstruction. The small diastolic dimension is quite characteristic.

The M-Mode technique demonstrates that the obstruction to the left ventricular outflow tract is a result of systolic anterior movement of the anterior mitral leaflet called "SAM." The timing of SAM correlates with the other parameters of obstruction, such as the midsystolic dip in the arterial pressure pulse and the onset of the murmur (Fig. 15.10). The demonstration of SAM and an increased septal to posterobasal left ventricular wall ratio (in ex-

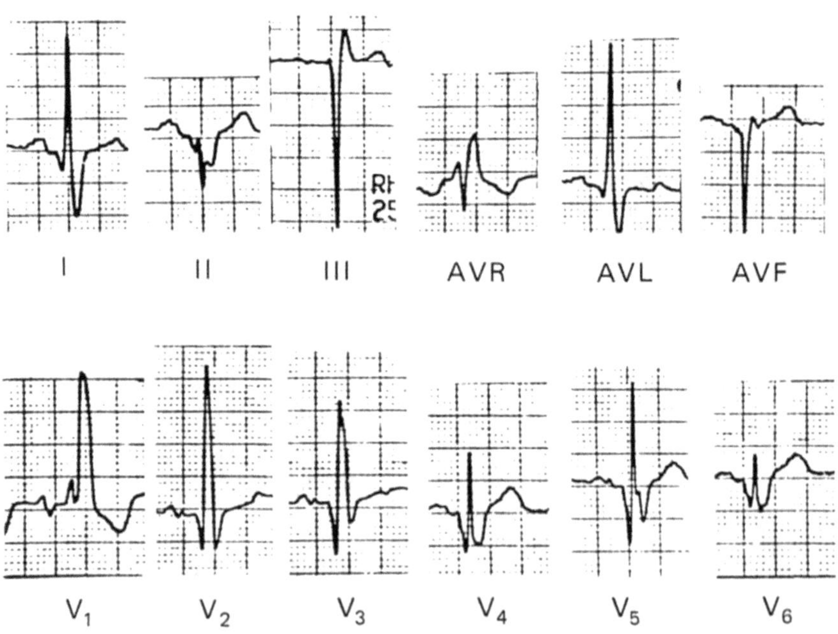

FIGURE 15.9. The electrocardiogram in hypertrophic cardiomyopathy (see text).

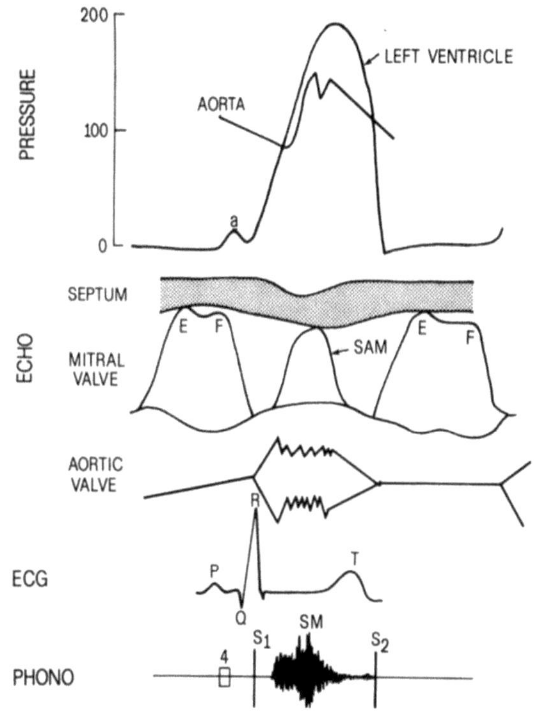

FIGURE 15.10. Simultaneous intraaortic and left ventricular pressures, echocardiogram, electrocardiogram, and phonocardiogram in IHSS demonstrating that "SAM" corresponds with the peak of the systolic murmur, the onset of the aortic gradient, and the posterior indentations in the aortic valve echo.

cess of 1.3/1.0) are practically pathognomonic findings.

Cardiac Catheterization

This is helpful in demonstrating that the obstruction is subvalvular and that the gradient is spontaneously or pharmacologically labile. Gradients may also be detected in the right ventricle in approximately one-sixth of patients. The left ventricular end-diastolic pressure is abnormally elevated, reflecting decreased ventricular compliance.

Left ventricular angiography demonstrates gross thickening of the left ventricular wall and a smaller than normal cavity. During systole, the cavity may be almost completely obliterated and the anterior leaflet of the mitral valve

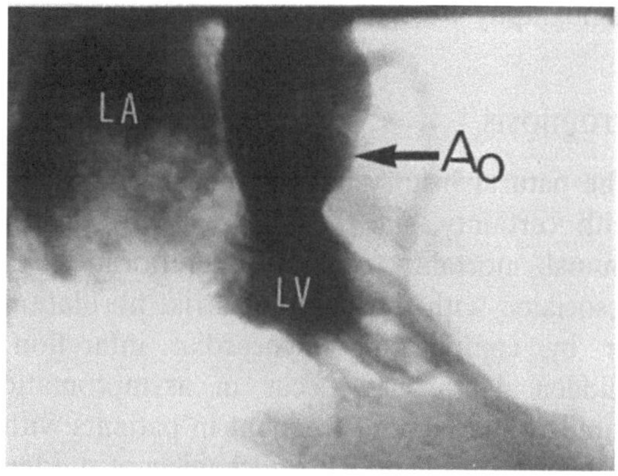

FIGURE 15.11. Left ventricular cineangiogram in IHSS demonstrating gross left ventricular hypertrophy, cavity obliteration, and mitral insufficiency.

may be pulled forward into the outflow tract, findings that are best observed in the lateral view (Fig. 15.11). There is an unusual group where the obstruction is in the midcavity (Fig. 15.12). Mild mitral regurgitation is present in approximately one-half of the patients and is a result of distortion of the papillary muscles. Because the chest pain experienced by these patients is indistinguishable from that of occlu-

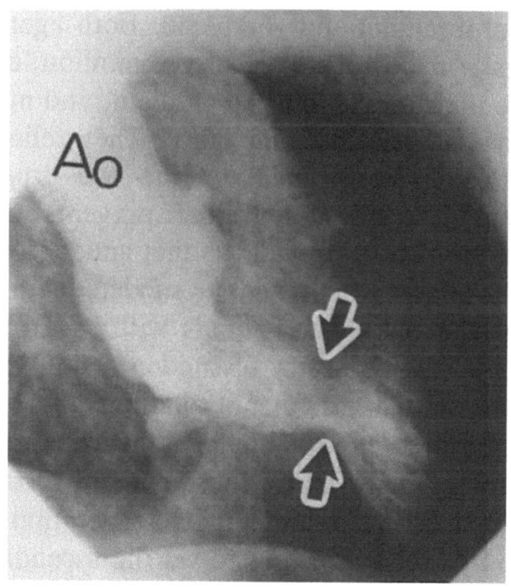

FIGURE 15.12. Left ventricular cineangiogram demonstrating midcavity obstruction (arrows) in hypertrophic cardiomyopathy.

sive coronary artery disease, selective coronary angiography is essential.

Prognosis

The natural history has not been established with certainty but there appears to be an annual mortality of 4%. Deterioration is associated with the onset of atrial fibrillation or by complicating myocardial infarction. Sudden death may occur in asymptomatic subjects and is more frequent in patients with little or no gradient. The mechanism of sudden death is presumed to be a ventricular dysrhythmia.

Management

Many patients are asymptomatic and require no treatment. However, competitive sport should be prohibited in subjects with a family history of sudden death, those with high grade obstruction, and left ventricular hypertrophy.

Symptomatic patients will obtain relief when outflow tract obstruction and/or ventricular compliance is improved. The mainstays of treatment are (1) β-adrenergic blockers, (2) calcium channel blockers, and (3) surgery.

Most experience with medication has been with propranolol and verapamil. Both agents decrease myocardial oxygen consumption, decrease the exercise-induced gradient, and may improve ventricular compliance. They relieve chest pain and dyspnea. Of the two drugs, propanolol is the safer. Neither prevents sudden death. There is evidence that amiodarone may be effective in preventing sudden death in a high-risk subset of patients with recurrent syncope, family history of sudden death, and out of hospital ventricular fibrillation.

Surgical resection of the left ventricular outflow tract is reserved for those patients refractory to medical treatment. The operation is made by excision of muscle via the ascending aorta. The mortality is in the vicinity of 5% and major complications include ventricular septal defect, heart block, and mitral regurgitation. The alternative procedure of mitral valve replacement has favorable hemodynamic effects, abolishes mitral regurgitation, but has all the disadvantages of a prosthetic valve. Like medical treatment, surgery does not decrease the risk of sudden death.

Additional Reading

Abelmann WH: The challenge of cardiomyopathy. J Am Coll Cardiol 13:1219–1239, 1989.

Ainger LE: Heart disease in congenital rubella syndrome. Cardiol Dig 2:21, 1967.

Braunwald E, Morrow AG, Cornell WP, et al.: Idiopathic hypertrophic subaortic stenosis. Clinical, hemodynamic and angiographic manifestations. Am J Med 29:924, 1960.

Buja LM, Ferrans VJ, Roberts WC: Drug induced cardiomyopathies. Adv Cardiol 13:330, 1974.

Chesler E, Joffe HS, Beck W, Schrire V: Tetralogy of Fallot and heart failure. Am Heart J 81:321, 1971.

Chew C, Ziady GM, Raphael MJ, Oakley CM: The functional defect in amyloid heart disease: The "Stiff Heart" syndrome. Am J Cardiol 36:438, 1975.

Frank S, Braunwald E: Idiopathic hypertrophic subaortic stenosis. Clinical analysis of 126 patients with emphasis on natural history. Circulation 37:759, 1968.

Goodwin F, Oakley CM: The cardiomyopathies. Br Heart J 34:545, 1972.

Hirschman SZ, Hammer GS: Coxsackie virus myopericarditis. A microbiological and clinical review. Am J Cardiol 34:224, 1974.

Kirschberg GJ: Trichinosis presenting as acute myocardial infarction. Can Med Assoc J 106:898, 1972.

McIntosch, CL, Maron BJ. Current operative treatment of obstructive hypertrophic cardiomyopathy. Circulation 78(3):487, 1988.

McKenna NJ and Camm, AJ. Sudden death in hypertrophic cardiomyopathy: Assessment of patients at high risk. Circulation 80:5; 1989.

Oakley CM, Olsen EGJ: Editorial: Eosinophilia and heart disease. Br Heart J 39:233, 1977.

Popp RL, Harris DC: Ultrasound in the diagnosis and evaluation of therapy of idiopathic hypertrophic subaortic stenosis. Circulation 40:905, 1969.

Rosenbaum MB: Chagasic myocardiopathy. Progr Cardiovasc Dis 7:199, 1964. Theologides A, Kennedy BJ: Toxoplasmic myocarditis pericarditis. Am J Med 47:169, 1969.

16 Pericarditis

The decline in the incidence of tuberculosis and control of bacterial infections with antibiotics has made pericarditis uncommon. There are many causes of pericarditis—in some cases it is the primary process dominating the clinical picture whereas in others it is one of the manifestations of a general disease such as systemic lupus erythematosus. The most common causes are idiopathic (or viral), uremic, neoplastic, and acute myocardial infarction. A physician's individual clinical experience will depend on the age group and social circumstances of patients in their area of practice. In an elderly American population, pericarditis is diagnosed clinically in approximately one in one thousand cases and the commonest causes are malignancy followed by uremia and myocardial infarction. In less privileged communities tuberculosis may still be prevalent.

Etiology

1. *Infections*
   a. Bacterial: *Staphylococcus*, *Pneumococcus*, *Meningococcus*, *M. tuberculosis*.
   b. Viral: Coxsackie, Echo, Ebstein–Barr.
   c. Fungal: histoplasmosis, nocardiosis, blastomyocosis, echinococcosis.
   d. Parasitic: amebiasis, toxoplasmosis.
2. *Connective Tissue, Hypersensitivity, and Autoimmune Diseases*
   a. Collagen diseases: systemic lupus erythematosus, polyarteritis nodosa, scleroderma.
   b. Acute rheumatic fever.
   c. Rheumatoid arthritis and ankylosing spondylitis.
   d. Postmyocardial infarction, postpericardiectomy syndromes.
   e. Drug-induced: hydralazine, procaine amide, penicillin, phenylbutazone.
3. *Bleeding into the Pericardium*
   a. Trauma: penetrating and nonpenetrating.
   b. Dissecting aortic aneurysm.
   c. Hemorrhagic diathesis: leukemia, reticuloses, scurvy.
   d. Anticoagulants.
4. *Myocardial Infarction*
5. *Malignant Disease and Reticuloses*
6. *Miscellaneous*: uremia, radiation, sarcoidosis, myxedema, amyloidosis, acute idiopathic pericarditis.

Septic Pericarditis

The incidence of acute bacterial pericarditis has decreased steadily during the past 30 years because improved social conditions and the advent of antibiotics have reduced the occurrence of predisposing infections such as pneumonia and osteomyelitis. The causative organisms were generally staphylococci, streptococci, and pneumococci, which reach the pericardium by hematogenous spread from a septic focus such as osteomyelitis or pneumonia.

Septic pericarditis is caused by different bacterial flora because of hospital-resistant strains, immunosuppression because of drugs, lymphoma, or AIDS, and preexisting pericardial effusion. These organisms include methicillin-resistant *Staphylococcus aureus*, gram-negative bacilli, and anerobes. Infection may follow cardiac surgery, pericardial aspiration, extension of aortic root endocarditis into the pericardial sac, and also hemotogenous spread.

In children, the responsible organisms are *Hemophilus*, *Staphlyococcus aureus*, and *N. meningitidis*. The predisposing illnesses are pharyngitis, pneumonid, otitis media, endocarditis, and arthritis.

The clinical course is fulminating. The mortality rate is 50% even with complete pericardial drainage and appropriate intravenous antibiotics. The most important reason for this poor outlook is failure to suspect the condition in debilitated patients with overwhelming systemic infection.

Tuberculous Pericarditis

This is by far the commonest cause of pericarditis in the underprivileged races, and is now rare in Britain and the United States. Men are affected more frequently than women and the disease may occur at any age. The infection usually reaches the pericardium from mediastinal lymphadenitis; associated pulmonary tuberculosis is rare. Organisms are isolated from the pericardial fluid in only 10% of cases, even when there are severe constitutional symptoms.

Pericardial effusion is the commonest mode of presentation, with or without tamponade. Tamponade is often severe and may be produced by a serous, serofibrinous or hemorrhagic effusion. In a little over a third of the cases, the effusion is absorbed with complete resolution. In the remainder, fusion of the parietal and visceral pericardium results in intense constriction. In aggressive infection, constriction may occur as early as 4 weeks after infection, but this usually takes many weeks. Sometimes it is difficult to be certain whether fluid is still present, since loculation is common.

A characteristic course in countries where tuberculosis is endemic starts with a large effusion with cardiomegaly and little evidence of cardiac constriction. The heart shadow then decreases in size and signs of constriction become apparent even when the heart is still moderately enlarged (*effusive constrictive pericarditis*). Sometimes, caseous constriction is the presenting feature. In a minority of patients, there is a mild initial illness with few signs of cardiac involvement, then signs of chronic constriction develop insidiously over a course of months or years.

Intensive antituberculous therapy is essential and includes streptomycin, 1 g daily for at least 3 months, ethambutol, 15 mg/kg/day, and isoniazid 300 mg daily for 12–24 months. Pericardial aspiration should be performed as long as fluid can be easily removed and no more than 500 ml should be aspirated on each occasion.

Early surgery for constriction greatly reduces morbidity and mortality and the operative risk is small. Surgery is not advised during the stage of effusion unless there is uncontrollable tamponade. The prognosis for tuberculous pericarditis with intensive medical therapy and early surgical intervention is good. Complete recovery is the rule in approximately 90% of cases, but when the process has infiltrated the myocardium this may be delayed for a period of many months. The electrocardiogram often remains permanently abnormal.

Acute “Idiopathic” Pericarditis

In those countries where tuberculous and pyogenic pericarditis have become infrequent the acute “idiopathic,” “benign,” or “nonspecific” type has emerged as the most frequent variety. The condition is probably of viral etiology and the Coxsackie and Echo groups may be responsible. In the absence of myocarditis the differential diagnosis from tuberculous pericarditis may be difficult.

Dry or effusive pericarditis may occur and late development of calcific constriction is reported with increasing frequency. Young men are most commonly affected and a preceding upper respiratory infection is often a feature. The illness itself commences abruptly with fever, malaise, and precordial pain. Pericardial friction rub, leukocytosis, and a raised sedimentation rate are found. Pericardial effusion is serous or hemorrhagic and bacteriologically sterile. Pleural effusion is not infrequent. The condition usually settles without treatment within a few weeks. However, relapses are common in the ensuing months or years. Steroids are highly effective in treating recurrent episodes but in obstinate cases with persistent effusion, pericardiectomy may be necessary.

Fungal Pericarditis

Following the introduction of antibiotics and immunosuppressive therapy, opportunistic fungal pericarditis has now emerged more frequently. Histoplasmosis and blastomycosis may affect the pericardium and there may be a close resemblance to tuberculous pericarditis. Cultures of aspirated pericardial fluid and pericardial biopsy are necessary to make the distinction.

Amebic Pericarditis

The usual cause is extension from amebic hepatitis in the left lobe. Rarely, spread may also occur from the right lobe or disease may reach the pericardium from amebic lung abscess. Prior to actual rupture, pericardial irritation by a liver abscess leads to a serous effusion. This heralds rupture of amebic pus into the pericardial sac. Suppurative amebic pericarditis may occur insidiously, but occasionally rupture is rapid and catastrophic.

There are three modes of presentation: (1) Hepatic: This occurs when the primary presentation is that of a liver abscess, followed by deterioration in the patient's general condition and development of signs of a pericardial effusion. (2) Cardiac presentation: The presentation is one of pericarditis with effusion. In this case the causative liver abscess is inconspicuous. Chest pain, left shoulder and arm pain, and pericardial rub combined with tenderness over the liver usually suggest the correct diagnosis. However, sometimes the diagnosis only becomes obvious after aspiration of typical amebic pus from the pericardial sac. (3) Cardiac tamponade.

The most useful diagnostic aids are the amebic gel-diffusion test, a high and immobile left leaf of the diaphragm detected by fluoroscopy, or CT scan. The diagnosis can be confirmed only by pericardiocentesis. Optimal treatment includes adequate drainage of the pericardial sac and at least two antiamebic drugs, preferably metronidazole, and dihydroemetine. Constrictive pericarditis is an occasional complication.

Autoimmune States

Drugs

Pericarditis may develop as part of the lupus erythematosus-like syndrome. Hydralazine and procaine amide have been particularly implicated. Phenylbutazone and streptomycin are also known to produce pericarditis.

Postcardiotomy Syndrome

This syndrome occurs in approximately 30% of patients undergoing any form of cardiac surgery. After a latent period of 2 to 3 weeks there is fever, pericarditis, pleuritis, and pneumonitis with a marked tendency to relapse. Dry pericarditis, or pericarditis with effusion may occur. The illness is self-limited, varies in intensity and duration, but usually lasts only 2 to 4 weeks. Treatment with nonsteroidal antiinflammatory drugs and analgesics such as aspirin is all that is usually necessary. Steroids induce prompt relief but should be reserved for severely affected patients since relapse may occur when they are discontinued and dependency may result. The condition must be distinguished from the postperfusion syndrome seen after open heart surgery, which is probably a result of cytomegalic virus infection. The clinical picture of the latter closely resembles that of glandular fever with pyrexia, skin rash, splenomegaly, and atypical, monocytes in the peripheral blood. The Paul–Bunnell reaction, however, is negative.

Myocardial Infarction

The usual type of pericarditis occurs within the first week in at least 20% of cases of transmural myocardial infarction. It is a result of pericardial irritation by adjacent infarcted myocardium and does not complicate subendocardial infarction. Less commonly, an autoimmune reaction may produce pericarditis 2 weeks to a few months after the ischemic episode (Dressler syndrome). It behaves very similarly to the postcardiotomy syndrome and treatment is the same with nonsteroidal antiinflammatory drugs. Occasionally steroids may be required for relapse. Anticoagulants should be avoided because of the risk of hemopericardium.

Collagen Diseases

Systemic lupus erythematosus is a well-recognized cause of pericarditis, which may be the presenting symptom. Dry or effusive pericarditis may occur and be readily confused with idiopathic benign pericarditis. Arthralgia, anemia, hypertension, skin rashes, and urinary abnormalities are suggestive of systemic lupus. Laboratory findings include a false-positive Wasserman reaction, leukopenia, lupus cells in the blood, raised gamma globulin, and the presence of free antinuclear antibody.

Pericarditis may complicate scleroderma and polyarteritis nodosa. Generally, other signs and symptoms of these diseases will be present.

Rheumatoid Arthritis

Granulomatous pericarditis is a complication of rheumatoid arthritis and ankylosing spondylitis leading to effusion and occasionally constriction. Aortitis and aortic insufficiency may be associated and occasionally there is invasion of the septum, producing heart block.

Rheumatic Fever

This is an important cause of pericarditis, almost invariably associated with severe pancarditis and valvular involvement. Rheumatic pericardial effusion is usually clear, straw-colored, and sterile. Cardiac tamponade is rare and the fluid usually resorbs rapidly in response to salicylate or steroid therapy. Chronic constrictive pericarditis is never rheumatic in origin but an adherent pericardium with flecks of calcification is not uncommon.

Malignant Pericarditis

Neoplastic pericarditis is usually secondary to malignancy of the bronchus, breast, or kidney. The condition is also not uncommon in Hodgkin's disease and other lymphomas. Primary tumors of the pericardium are rare and usually a result of mesothelioma following asbestos exposure.

Metastases may produce a large hemorrhagic effusion or severe constriction when tumor encases the heart. Malignant cells may be found in 85% of cases of aspirated pericardial fluid.

The management of neoplastic pericardial effusion depends on the type of malignancy and condition of the patient. Commonly, pericardial disease is a preterminal event. Palliation can be obtained by subxyphoid pericardiotomy. Partial pericardiectomy (pericardial window) through a left thoracotomy should be reserved for patients who have a better prognosis and are likely to respond to chemotherapy or radiation.

Uremia

Prior to the introduction of hemodialysis, pericarditis complicated renal failure in about 50% of cases and was frequently a preterminal event. Uremia produces a fibrinous, often hemorrhagic inflammation that may lead to tamponade, and constriction in some cases.

Symptomatic pericarditis that occurs before initiation of dialysis will respond to repeated hemodialysis. Many patients who develop pericardial effusion, who are regularly dialyzed will also respond to intensification of the dialysis regime. Those who do not will require drainage either by subxyphoid pericardiotomy or pericardial window. Pericardiocentesis is associated with a high risk of intrapericardial hemorrhage.

Trauma

This produces two forms of pericarditis. One is a direct result of trauma with hemorrhage into the pericardial cavity and formation of hemopericardium. If associated myocardial or valvular injury is absent, complete recovery is the rule, although chronic constriction may develop. The combination of traumatic ventricular septal defect and constrictive pericarditis is not uncommon. The physical signs are those of the ventricular septal defect and the constriction may easily be missed; disproportionate systemic venous congestion provides the clue. The second type is a form of recurrent pericarditis allied to the postcardiotomy and postmyocardial infarction syndromes, which may also result in chronic constriction.

Cholesterol Pericarditis

Effusions containing cholesterol crystals may occur in myxedema, hemorrhagic, or constrictive pericarditis from tuberculosis, or there may be no obvious cause. Signs of chronic tamponade may develop and surgical resection of the pericardium may be required.

Myxedema

Effusions with a high protein content are frequent in untreated myxedema. Myxedema must always be excluded in any patient with a chronic, asymptomatic, pericardial effusion. Cardiac tamponade does not occur.

Radiation Pericarditis

This usually follows treatment for Hodgkins disease, lymphoma, and breast cancer. The incidence of pericarditis depends on how much of the heart is included in the field of radiation, the dose, and the duration of treatment. Radiation is a common cause of effusive-constrictive pericarditis and also may result in myocarditis and premature coronary atherosclerosis.

Clinical evidence of pericarditis may occur during, or shortly after treatment, but is more usually delayed for approximately 1 year. The presentation is one of acute pericarditis with some effusion.

In about 50% of cases there is evidence of tamponade, which may require drainage. Some of these patients will require pericardiectomy because of severe constriction. The prognosis following pericardiectomy is poor in comparison to cases of pericardiectomy performed for other diseases. This is because of underlying myocardial damage and severe thickening of visceral pericardium.

Any of the preceding causes of pericarditis may produce one of the following syndromes:

1. Acute pericarditis without effusion.
2. Pericarditis with effusion with or without tamponade.
3. Constrictive pericarditis.
4. Calcific pericarditis without constriction.

Acute Pericarditis Without Effusion

Pathologically, there is a fibrinous exudate with inflammatory reaction involving visceral and parietal layers. Epicardial irritation is responsible for the clinical and electrocardiographic manifestations.

Clinical Features

Pain is very common but not invariable. It is present in approximately 60% of cases and, characteristically, is stabbing in quality, aggravated by respiration, coughing, body movements, and swallowing. The intensity and quality vary from a dull ache to agonizing, severe pain simulating myocardial infarction. Usually, it is present in the front of the chest, but occasionally may radiate to the neck, arms, and back. The pain may be entirely upper abdominal, simulating an abdominal emergency. True pleuritic pain is frequently associated. The pain is often alleviated by leaning forward. Constitutional symptoms are associated with the underlying cause and viral pericarditis is frequently preceded by an upper respiratory infection.

The pathogonominc rub of pericarditis is scratchy and may have three components as the heart moves with atrial systole, ventricular systole, and ventricular diastole. It is heard in at least 50% of cases. It may be present continuously or intermittently, for days or weeks, but occasionally may last for only a few hours. It is best heard along the left sternal border and at the xiphoid area during held expiration, with the patient leaning forward. The rub may vary markedly with respiration and in some cases may best be heard during moderate inspiration. It is accentuated by pressure with the bell or diaphragm and sounds more superficial than other heart sounds. In contradistinction to a pleural rub the pericardial rub continues to be audible when respiration is held.

Electrocardiogram

This is abnormal and a characteristic evolution is frequently found. ST segment elevation in the limb and precordial leads subsides before T wave inversion develops. A return to normal is usual, but occasionally T wave inversion may be permanent. When these characteristic changes are present they are highly specific and greatly assist in diagnosis.

Radiology and Echocardiography

There is no abnormality unless fluid develops. The differential diagnosis involves those conditions producing anterior chest pain; this includes myocardial infarction, dissecting aortic aneurysm, pulmonary embolism, and acute pleurisy. The most common difficulty is the distinction between acute pericarditis and myocardial infarction. In most cases, a careful history will make the distinction. Additionally, a pericardial rub occurs early in pericarditis but late in the course of myocardial infarction. Any evidence of cardiac failure favors myocardial infarction. The presence of pathologic Q waves favors myocardial infarction but does not exclude Coxsackie myopericarditis. Serum enzymes are elevated in both conditions but the presence of abnormal quantities of the CPK-MB fraction strongly suggests myocardial infarction.

Pericardial Effusion Without Tamponade

This occurs when the inflammatory process is accompanied by exudation of fluid. The effusion may be serous, purulent, or hemorrhagic. A hemorrhagic pericardial effusion may be found in any type of pericarditis but heavy blood-staining is particularly associated with tuberculosis. Rarely, the effusion is hazy with a characteristic shimmering sheen when held up to the light due to the presence of cholesterol crystals.

Clinical Features

1. Pain is of three types: (a) typical pericardial pain as described above; (b) a dull heavy oppressive pain resulting from distention of the pericardial sac; and (c) pain due to hepatic distention.
2. Dyspnea: Contrary to classical teaching this is an early and frequent sign, usually present only with effort. In large effusions orthopnea is marked, and there may be paroxysmal nocturnal dyspnea.
3. Compression of surrounding structures frequently produces cough, which aggravates the dyspnea. Hoarseness and dysphagia are uncommon.
4. Constitutional symptoms associated with the underlying disease may be present.
5. Pericardial friction rub is audible in more than half the cases at some stage of the illness even in the presence of a massive effusion.
6. Cardiac signs indicating the presence of an effusion are dullness to percussion most

commonly detected to the right and left of the sternum and only rarely beyond the apex beat. Usually, the apex beat is impalpable. The heart sounds are frequently muffled and occasionally a third sound is audible.

Compression of the left lung produces dullness and bronchial breathing at the base posteriorly ("Ewart's sign"), but generally this is not helpful in diagnosis, as it may be found in patients with a dilated heart in the absence of a pericardial effusion.

The Electrocardiogram

The changes seen in acute pericarditis with ST segment elevation are not usually seen. The most common pattern is one of low voltage in the standard leads with flattening or inversion of the T waves in most leads. Alternation of the P wave and the entire QRS complex is uncommon, but pathognomonic of tamponade.

Radiology

This always shows generalized cardiac enlargement, which may be indistinguishable from cardiomegaly seen in congestive cardiomyopathy. Fluoroscopy to detect diminished pulsation is an unreliable method of making the diagnosis. Usually the lung fields are not as congested and upper lobe pulmonary venous distention is not as prominent as those seen in congestive cardiac failure. Pleural effusions are common and are a result of high filling pressures.

Echocardiography

This is the most sensitive test for the diagnosis of pericardial effusion. Small effusions may be evident only in systole as an echo-free space between the two layers of pericardium. Larger effusions are present throughout the cardiac cycle, both anteriorly and posteriorly. Massive effusions may be associated with excessive motion of the heart ("swinging heart"), which may be associated with electrocardiographic alternans (R waves alternating in height). Small posterior effusions may be mimicked by the space behind heavy mitral annular calcification, when the latter is mistaken for the pericardial echo.

Pericardial Effusion With Tamponade

Definition

This is present when sufficient fluid accumulates in the pericardium to raise the intrapericardial pressure above the filling pressures of the ventricles resulting in impaired diastolic filling and reduced stroke volume.

Pathophysiology

Normally, intrapericardial pressure is several mm Hg lower than the end-diastolic pressure in the ventricles. When intrapericardial pressure rises with accumulation of pericardial fluid, the transmural pressure gradient is lost and diastolic filling is hampered. Initially, an adequate stroke volume may be compensated for by sympathetic induced tachycardia and vasoconstriction. This eventually fails as intrapericardial pressure rises and further impedes diastolic filling, leading to reduction of stroke volume, hypotension, and death.

The abnormal dynamics of ventricular filling are demonstrable by echocardiography and by the *right atrial pressure pulse*: As intrapericardial pressure rises, diastolic compression and even collapse of the right atrium and ventricle are observed by echocardiography. The equivalent hemodynamic finding is absence of the "y" descent in the right atrial pressure tracing. During *systole*, the cardiac volume decreases abruptly as the ventricles eject, and venous return increases sharply producing a rapid "x" descent. Following opening of the A-V valves in early *diastole*, the high intrapericardial pressure abolishes ventricular filling and the "y" descent is therefore absent.

Early in tamponade, right atrial and ventricular collapse occurs only in early diastole. Eventually, the right-sided chambers are collapsed throughout diastole so that the ventricles can fill only during ventricular systole (i.e., during the period represented by the "x" descent)—hypotension and shock then ensue. The hemodynamics will be aggravated by hypovolemia, which lowers the right sided pressures.

Pulsus Parodoxus

This results from exaggeration of the normal inspiratory increase in velocity of venous inflow, increase in right ventricular size, and a smaller increase in left ventricular size. During tamponade these changes are exaggerated and inspiration results in a disproportionate increase in right ventricular dimension so that the septum bulges into a much smaller underfilled left ventricle. The filling pressures and aortic flow on the left side fall and the arterial pressure drops producing the paradoxical pulse.

Pulsus paradoxus can occur only when there is inspiratory increase in venous return and right ventricular filling. This is why Kussmaul's sign (inspiratory increase in right atrial and jugular venous pressure) is never found in cardiac tamponade, but is characteristic of constrictive pericarditis. Inspiration cannot increase venous return through the thickened noncompliant pericardium and the jugular venous pressure therefore rises. Pulsus paradoxus is frequently observed in emphysema where the excessively negative intrathoracic pressure grossly exaggerates right ventricular filling. Pulsus paradoxus may be *absent* when tamponade occurs in the presence of severe left ventricular hypertrophy. This is because high left ventricular end diastolic pressure does not allow equal compression of the two ventricles.

Clinical Features of Tamponade

Causes

Neoplastic disease, idiopathic pericarditis, uremia, myocardial infarction (receiving anticoagulants), and cardiac perforation are the common causes of tamponade.

Symptoms and Signs

These depend on the rapidity with which fluid accumulates: The sudden addition of 200 ml or less of fluid (e.g., cardiac perforation, rupture of dissecting aneurysm) into a tense pericardial space results in rapid fall in cardiac output, tachycardia, pulsus paradoxus, and a rise in venous pressure. Tachypnea, restlessness, and precordial pain are characteristic. Unless relieved, the condition is rapidly fatal.

When tamponade develops slowly, the patient complains of dyspnea, chest pain, and weakness. The cardinal physical findings are (1) elevation of the jugular venous pressure with prominent "x" and absent "y" descents, (2) tachypnea, (3) tachycardia, (4) pulsus paradoxus, (5) soft heart sounds, and (6) hepatomegaly.

Diagnosis

Echocardiography

This is an invaluable test. The absence of an effusion excludes tamponade except for those loculated effusions which occur post-operatively and may cause cardiac compression. Both M-mode and 2D techniques provide evidence of diastolic compression of the right ventricle and right atrium, which occur early in tamponade.

Cardiac Catheterization

This may be accomplished at the bedside even in seriously ill patients using a Swan-Ganz catheter and arterial line. It establishes the diagnosis and severity of tamponade. The important findings are (1) equilibration of mean right atrial, right ventricular end-diastolic, and mean capillary wedge pressure, (2) characteristic waveform of right atrial pressure, and (3) pulsus paradoxus.

Treatment

Pericardial Drainage

When the clinical situation is critical, pericardiocentesis is the procedure of choice. When there is time, surgical subxyphoid pericardiotomy is a safer alternative.

Pericardiocentesis in the hands of an inexperienced operator may be complicated by laceration of a coronary artery or ventricular fibrillation. The safety of the procedure may be enhanced by using a needle connected to the electrocardiograph, monitoring the changes in the ST-T segment. Detection of current of injury indicates contact of the needle with the myocardium and is an indication for immediate withdrawal. The usual sites for pericardiocentesis are (1) the *subxiphoid approach*, where the needle is inserted into the angle between the left costal margin and xiphoid process and is directed toward the right shoulder; and (2) the *cardiac apex*, with the needle directed toward the midthoracic spine. When bloody fluid is withdrawn, failure to clot indicates that this has not been withdrawn from one of the cardiac chambers.

Two-dimensional echocardiography is useful in guiding pericardial aspiration. Introduction of a small pigtail catheter over a guide wire allows continuous drainage. Blind-needle aspiration of the pericardium can probably be justified only in patients in extremis, in an emergency room for example.

Constrictive Pericarditis

Etiology

The cause of constrictive pericarditis is variable depending on socioeconomic circumstances of the community. In the United States it is attributed most often to acute idiopathic or viral pericarditis, trauma, radiation, rheumatoid arthritis, or chronic renal failure. In countries where tuberculosis is endemic this is by far the commonest cause.

Pathology

Classically, the heart is encased in dense calcified fibrous tissue incorporating all the layers of the pericardium. Fibrosis is particularly marked in the atrioventricular groove. Occasionally, fibrosis in the atrioventricular rings is sufficiently severe to produce mitral or tricuspid stenosis ("annular constrictive pericarditis") with the appropriate murmurs evident on clinical examination. Fibrotic bands may also extend across the outflow tract of the right ventricle producing high grade infundibular stenosis, which requires careful distinction from congenital pulmonary valve stenosis.

Pathophysiology

Uniform constriction of all chambers impedes filling and results in equalization of diastolic pressures. The classic "square root sign" or "dip and plateau" contour of the ventricular pressure pulse reflects the abnormal pattern of ventricular filling. The rapid rise in pressure after the early diastolic dip is a result of rapid early filling, which suddenly stops when the noncompliant pericardium will not allow the volume of the ventricle to increase further (Fig. 16.1).

These changes are reflected in the atrial pressure pulses (and jugular venous pressure). A rapid "y" descent corresponds to the early diastolic dip; the "x" descent is retained so that the waveform resembles that of an "M" or "W." Kussmaul's sign (increase in the jugular venous pressure with inspiration) reflects a fundamental difference from the hemodynamics of cardiac tamponade. In constrictive pericarditis respiratory changes in intrathoracic pressure are not transmitted to the pericardial space and cardiac chambers because of the adherent pericardium. During inspiration the right atrial and jugular venous pressures rise (Fig. 16.2).

Kussmaul's sign is not specific for constrictive pericarditis; it may also occur in restrictive cardiomyopathy and other forms of severe congestive heart failure where there is also restriction to diastolic filling.

Clinical Features

The symptomatology depends to a large extent on the chronicity of the process.

Abdominal symptoms: Swelling of the abdomen due to hepatomegaly is nearly always a

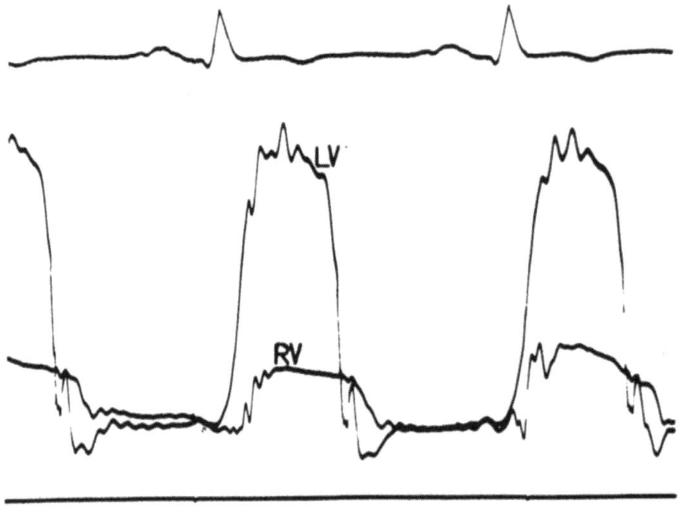

FIGURE 16.1. Simultaneous left and right ventricle pressure tracings. There is equalization of diastolic pressure.

prominent symptom. In long-standing cases, ascites is severe and often disproportionate to the degree of dependent edema. An increase in abdominal girth may be the only symptom in a patient who is otherwise relatively well.

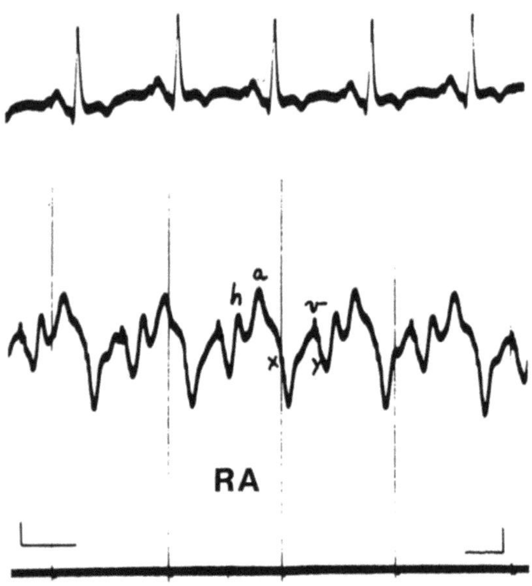

FIGURE 16.2. The right atrial pressure in constrictive pericarditis showing rapid "x" and "y" descents.

Dyspnea is usually slight but becomes severe when ascites and pleural effusions accumulate. Contrary to conventional teaching, orthopnea and paroxysmal nocturnal dyspnea occur because of left atrial hypertension.

Pleuritic pain and cough are not uncommon and are related to pleural effusions.

Signs of Constriction

Jugular Venous Distention

This is always present showing the "M" pattern. Kussmaul's sign is frequent.

Pulse Pressure

The *pulse pressure* is reduced and paradoxus is absent. Atrial fibrillation occurs in up to a third of the patients.

Hepatomegaly

This is almost invariably present and the liver is firm to palpation. Ascites is frequent.

Cardiac Signs

The apex beat is usually impalpable, but occasionally a thrusting early diastolic impulse is present just to the left of the sternal border. In association with the other physical signs it is pathognomonic of constriction. When incorrectly timed it has been mistaken for the systolic lift of right ventricular hypertrophy; it reflects the abnormal pattern of ventricular filling in early diastole. On auscultation, an early third sound, often palpable, may be detected ("pericardial knock").

Analysis of the second sound is critical in diagnosis because it has a diagnostic feature in pericardial constriction. There is an abrupt, short-lived, wide-splitting of the second sound at the onset of inspiration. The splitting is widest at the onset of inspiration and then narrows to become single again after one or two beats. It is produced by sudden shortening of left ventricular systole due to the reduction in ventricular filling. It occurs when the left atrial pressure suddenly drops at the onset of inspiration.

The Electrocardiogram

An abnormal tracing is present in virtually every case. Low-voltage, widespread flattening and inversion of T waves with bifid P waves are characteristic. Atrial fibrillation is quite common in the chronic form. In approximately 5% of cases a pattern of severe right ventricular hypertrophy associated with right axis deviation may be encountered. This pattern is almost certainly related to cardiac distortion and displacement of the cardiac vectors since right ventricular pressure is only mildly elevated and the tracing normalizes after pericardiectomy.

Radiologic Examination

A normal or near normal-sized heart in the presence of marked venous distention or heart failure is suggestive of constrictive pericarditis or restrictive cardiomyopathy. Calcification of the pericardium is diagnostic but its incidence varies from 30 to 70% of cases in different series. Other signs of lesser value are absent of diminished pulsation, absence of pulmonary congestive, and straightening of the cardiac border.

CT and MRI Scan

These techniques demonstrate pericardial thickening and dilatation of the cavae and hepatic veins. Their chief use is in the differentiation from restrictive cardiomyopathy.

Echocardiography and Radionuclide (MUGA) Studies

Their chief use is in demonstrating a normal left ventricular ejection fraction characteristic of uncomplicated constrictive pericarditis. In cardiomyopathies the left ventricular ejection fraction is depressed but not always so. The 2D echo is helpful in excluding amyloidosis and restrictive cardiomyopathy with cavity obliteration.

Cardiac Catheterization

This documents elevation and equalization of filling pressures. In the typical case the difference in filling pressures does not exceed 6 mm HG. The right atrial pressure shows the typical contour and the mean pressure does not decrease normally with inspiration or may show Kussmaul's sign.

Effusive–Constrictive Pericarditis

This is characteristically encountered in active tuberculous pericarditis where there are signs of both tamponade and constriction. It may also occur in neoplastic, radiation, and septic pericarditis.

The symptoms are much the same as those with constriction. Examination discloses pulsus paradoxus and raised jugular venous pressure with prominent "x" and "y" descents. Chest X-ray shows an enlarged cardiac silhouette like that of pericardial effusion but the EKG shows low-voltage-like constrictive pericarditis.

The clue to diagnosis is persistent signs of constriction following adequate pericardial drainage with the right atrial waveform showing prominent "x" and "y" descents.

The management consists of pericardial drainage and antituberculous therapy when indicated. Should hemodynamics not improve, pericardiectomy is indicated.

Calcific Pericarditis Without Constriction

This condition is discovered during routine radiological examination, which demonstrates linear pericardial calcification. There are no symptoms and the cause is usually obscure.

Differential Diagnosis of Constrictive Pericarditis from Restrictive Myocardial Diseases

With the advent of echocardiography, CT and MRI scan, and endomyocardial biopsy the distinction between congestive cardiomyopathy and effusive and constrictive pericarditis is no longer a problem.

However, it is still difficult to separate congestive pericarditis from restrictive myocardial diseases. The distinction is vital because pericardiectomy is one of the most satisfying operations in terms of cure. Idiopathic restrictive cardiomyopathy, endomyocardial fibrosis, amyloid disease, and hemochromatosis may closely resemble congestive pericarditis. Points of differentiation are as follows:

1. *Clinical*: There may be few helpful clues since raised systemic pressure, Kussmaul's sign, edema, and hepatomegaly are common to both entities. However, murmurs of mitral and tricuspid regurgitation and gallop rhythm are strong pointers against constrictive pericarditis.
2. *Electrocardiogram*: Tracings in congestive pericarditis show low voltage and a normal or rightward QRS axis. Left axis deviation favors myocardial damage rather than constrictive pericarditis.
3. *Chest X-ray*: Calcification of the pericardium favors constrictive pericarditis but unfortunately is not always present.
4. *Echocardiography*: This may be diagnostic in amyloid disease by demonstrating severe symmetric thickening of the walls of the left ventricle with characteristic bright appearance of the echoes-so-called "sparkling granularity." Thickening of the walls of the left ventricle is also seen in hemochromatosis. Endomyocardial fibrosis is characterized by obliteration of the left ventricular cavity (see Fig. 15.6). In constrictive pericarditis the walls of the left ventricle are of normal thickness and typically the ejection fraction is normal.
5. *Left Ventricular Systolic Function*: In the uncomplicated case of constrictive pericarditis in a young person, the left ventricular ejection fraction is normal. In restrictive cardiomyopathies and amyloid disease the left ventricular ejection fraction is frequently depressed.
6. *CT and MRI Scan*: These are diagnostic when they show thickened pericardium.
7. *Cardiac Catheterization*: Equilibration of the filling pressures to within 6 mm Hg is characteristic of constrictive pericarditis. When the pressures differ by more than 6 mm Hg, restrictive cardiomyopathy is likely present. In restrictive cardiomyopathy, the left ventricle is usually more severely affected so that pulmonary hypertension is frequent. Pulmonary artery pressure of more than 50 mm Hg strongly favors restrictive cardiomyopathy rather than constrictive pericarditis.
8. *Endomyocardial Biopsy*: This is a safe technique and frequently diagnostic of infiltration in amyloid disease and hemochromatosis. In restrictive cardiomyopathy the biopsy will show extensive fibrosis.

Should all these tests fail to make distinction between the two entities, exploratory thoracotomy is justified.

Pericardiectomy

This involves stripping the pericardium from apex to base of both ventricles as completely as possible. Resection from the atria and vena cavae is unnecessary. The results in patients early in the disease without myocardial damage is gratifying and the mortality is about 1%. The life expectancy postoperatively is normal.

When the disease is long-standing, operative mortality may be as high as 40%. This is because of myocardial damage and difficulty in obtaining a complete removal of the thickened calcified pericardium. Hepatic damage, protein-losing enteropathy, and inanition add to the risk.

Additional Reading

Armstrong TG, Lewis BS and Gotsman MS: Systolic time intervals in constrictive pericarditis and severe primary myocardial disease. Am Heart J 85:6, 1973.

Chesler E, Mitha AS, Matisonn RE: The ECG of constrictive pericarditis—Pattern resembling right ventricular hypertrophy. Am Heart J 91:420, 1976.

Horowitz MS, Schultz CS, Stinson EB, et al.: Sensitivity and specificity of echocardiographic diagnosis of pericardial effusion. Circulation 50:239, 1974.

Robinson J, Brigden W: Recurrent pericarditis. Br Med J 2:272, 1968.

Schamroth L, Blumsohn D: The significance of left axis deviation in heart disease of the African. Br Heart J 18:153, 1956.

Schrire V: Experience with pericarditis at Groote Schuur Hospital, Cape Town. S Afr Med J 33: 810, 1959.

Schrire V: Pericarditis (with particular reference to tuberculous pericarditis). Aust Ann Med 16:41, 1967.

Spodick DH: Acute cardiac tamponade—pathophysiology, diagnosis and management. Prog Cardiovasc Dis 10:164, 1967.

Spodick DH: Differential diagnosis of acute pericarditis. Prog Cardiovasc Dis 14:192, 1971.

Weir EK, Joffe HS: Purulent pericarditis in children: An analysis of 28 cases. Thorax 32:438, 1977.

Wood P: Chronic constrictive pericarditis. Am J Cardiol 7:48, 1961.

17
Ischemic Heart Disease

In the developed areas of the western hemisphere at least one-half of all deaths are attributable to cardiovascular disease and three-quarters of these are a result of coronary atherosclerosis. During the last century these countries have witnessed a tremendous improvement in life expectancy calculated from the time of birth, chiefly because of the conquest of infectious diseases. However, for individuals who have already reached the age of 40, the improvement in life expectancy has been less dramatic because of their predisposition to coronary artery disease. In the United States, 500,000 deaths are a result of ischemic heart disease and one-half of these occur suddenly.

Despite the magnitude of the problem, there has been an encouraging decline in mortality since 1978. This is related to changes in the way of living with reductions in cholesterol levels and smoking. Additionally, the advent of prehospital resuscitation, coronary care units, and coronary artery bypass surgery has contributed to improved outcome for patients with ischemic heart disease.

Anatomy of the Coronary Arteries

The coronary arteries (Figs. 17.1 and 17.2) arise from the left and right aortic sinuses, respectively. The main left coronary artery passes behind the base of the pulmonary artery and is a short vessel, approximately 2 cm in length. It bifurcates into anterior descending and circumflex branches. The anterior descending artery runs in the interventricular groove curving around the apex of the heart to supply the anterior walls of both ventricles and anterior portion of the ventricular septum; its diagonal branch is fairly constant in position and supplies the anterolateral aspect of the left ventricle. The circumflex artery runs along the left atrioventricular groove, giving off several obtuse marginal branches that supply the lateral wall of the left ventricle.

The right coronary artery passes beneath the right atrial appendage along the right atrioventricular groove to the back of the heart. The conus branch runs anteriorly across the right ventricular outflow tract whereas the SA nodal branch courses posteriorly. The acute marginal and right ventricular branches supply the right ventricle. In 90% of subjects the right coronary artery is "dominant," giving rise to the posterior descending artery with its A-V nodal branch, which supplies the inferior aspects of both ventricles and posterior portion of the ventricular septum.

There is considerable variation in size, position, and area of supply of the coronary vessels. In 10% of hearts, for example, the left coronary artery is said to be "dominant" because the circumflex branch crosses the crux to continue posteriorly as the posterior descending artery, thus supplying the inferior aspect of

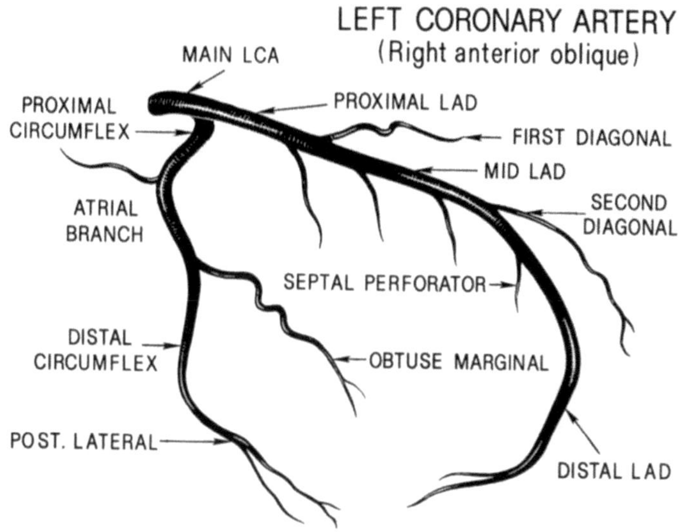

FIGURE 17.1. The anatomy of the left coronary artery in the right anterior oblique position.

both ventricles and the posterior portion of the ventricular septum, and also giving rise to the A-V nodal artery. The term "dominant" is frequently used to describe coronary angiograms and can be misleading. "Right coronary dominance" does not mean that most blood supply to the heart is from the right coronary artery, only that it gives off the PDA and A-V nodal artery. The left coronary artery provides the main blood supply to the myocardium (Figs. 17.1 and 17.2).

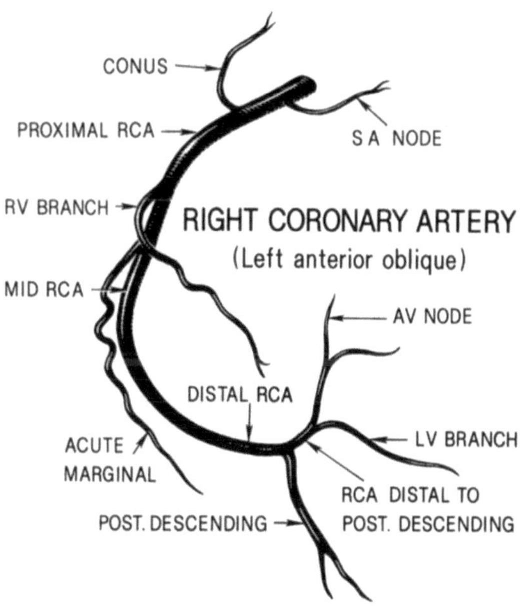

FIGURE 17.2. The anatomy of the right coronary artery in th left anterior oblique position.

Pathology of Coronary Atherosclerosis

Atherosclerotic lesions are essentially focal and confined to the epicardial branches of the coronary arteries; for reasons not understood, the intramyocardial portions of the coronary arteries are spared. In cross section, lesions are either circumferential, leaving a central lumen, or eccentric, producing a slit-like lumen. The eccentric lumen has important implications for the coronary angiographer: high-grade stenosis will be missed when the angiographic view is at right angles to an eccentric lesion because the greatest width may equal that of the original lumen; the narrowing is detected only by an end-on view.

The most common site of atherosclerotic involvement is that portion of the right coronary artery between its acute marginal and posterior descending branches, in the region known as the "crux." Next in order of frequency is the proximal one-half of the left anterior descending artery. The third most frequent site of disease is that segment of the right coronary artery between its origin and the marginal branch. Atherosclerotic lesions are characteristically multiple and frequently involve more than one artery. In general, the previously held concept that the disease becomes progressively less severe distally along the course of an artery is untrue, and in many instances a distal lesion may be more severe than a proximal one. This has important surgical connotations. Among patients with angina pectoris, involvement of only one vessel is unusual. In three-quarters of such patients, two-, three-, and even four-vessel (including the left main coronary artery) involvement is found in over three-quarters of coronary angiograms.

Histologically, the atheromatous plaque consists of an accumulation of lipid-laden macrophages in the intima. The initial narrowing of the lumen may be aggravated subsequently by an overlying fibrous reaction, a hemorrhage into the atherosclerotic plaque, and/or superimposition of thrombus. When a plaque reduces the lumen to less than 70% of its original size, there is sufficient impediment to flow to produce a pressure gradient. Small intercoronary branches arising proximal to the lesion can enlarge and help supply flow distally. This collateral flow can occur at the expense of flow to the remaining unobstructed vessels (i.e., coronary steal). With time, these collateral vessels may develop in size adequate enough to supply segments of vessels distal to an area of complete occlusion. Visualization of collaterals by coronary angiography provides important information for potential surgical bypass grafting distal to an obstruction.

Etiology

As noted above, the atherosclerotic lesion is the primary pathologic event, and appears to be a result of lipid infiltration of the intima. Subsequent thrombosis within the vessel should be regarded as a complication of the primary process.

The contention that coronary atherosclerosis is a result of dietary-induced hypercholesterolemia is supported by a wealth of epidemiologic evidence. Excessive consumption of fat from animal sources, particularly saturated fats, raises the blood cholesterol. Thus, coronary atherosclerosis is extremely common among Caucasions in the United States, Finland, Western Europe, and Australasia. It is rare in the Far East and Africa. The Chinese of Taiwan and the Japanese are rarely affected in their native countries, but when translocated to an American environment where there is heavy cholesterol intake, the risk of coronary atherosclerosis is increased. Indeed, serum cholesterol level is probably the best predictive value for risk of developing coronary atherosclerosis. The data indicate that there is no clearly defined "normal" level for serum cholesterol. There is evidence to suggest that risk for myocardial infarction increases exponentially with serum cholesterol concentration. The previously accepted upper limit of normal of 250 mg/100 ml for serum cholesterol is too high. A total level of under 200 mg/100 ml with the LDL level less than 130 mg% and the HDL level more than 35 mg% is more desirable.

In the majority of patients with clinically evident coronary artery disease and elevated serum cholesterol levels, lipoprotein electrophoresis is not essential. However, this should be performed when there is evidence of a genetically determined disorder of lipid metabolism (e.g., family history, xanthomata, abdominal pain, lipemia retinalis, and hepatosplenomegaly).

Surveys have shown a striking increase in the prevalence of coronary atherosclerosis. When hypertension and hypercholesterolemia coexist. In Taiwan and in the South African black population where hypertension is extremely common, coronary atherosclerosis is rare because of the infrequency of associated hypercholesterolemia. The mechanism whereby hypertension accelerates the development of atherosclerosis is not clear. Perhaps it does so by facilitating the infiltration of lipids into the arterial wall, or by mechanically damaging the arterial wall and thus predisposing to lipid deposition. The control of hypertension has not yet been shown to have a beneficial effect on the course of coronary atherosclerosis although there does appear to be such an effect with cerebral atherosclerosis.

There is a definite tendency for coronary atheroma to manifest with a familial predisposition, but it has not been possible to clearly separate true genetic factors from nutritional risk factors operative in the same family. Therefore, at the present time, in the absence of a genetically determined variety of hyperlipidemia, it would be premature to conclude that subjects whose parents were affected by the disease are at increased risk.

Certain other factors should be mentioned, though their relative roles may be obscure. Exercise has been held to be important in preventing atheroma since the disease occurs more frequently in sedentary subjects than in manual laborers. The evidence is inconclusive because it is difficult to separate lack of exercise itself from the other risk factors such as diet. The Finns are heavy manual laborers but consume a very high cholesterol diet and have one of the highest incidences of myocardial infarction.

Obesity is risk factor in univariate analysis. However, because it is frequently associated with hypertension, diabetes, and hypercholesterolemia, it is a nonsignificant factor by multivariate analysis. Multivariate analysis allows the assessment of the independent effects of each risk factor.

Most studies incriminate three major risk factors—serum total cholesterol, cigarette smoking, and hypertension. However, these do not provide a completely accurate risk profile for all groups of patients with ischemic heart disease. When the three major risk factors are combined with several less important factors such as genetic background, diabetes, obesity, physical activity, and emotional makeup, it is possible to predict development of ischemic heart disease more accurately. Tension, anxiety, and emotional factors have also received a great deal of attention. The so-called Type A behavior pattern (characterized by a strong sense of urgency, indulgence in excessive competitive activity, and marked drive) has been thought to be associated with a greater incidence of coronary heart disease. Unfortunately, determining the role of stress is hampered by lack of objective means of measurement.

Clinical Manifestations of Ischemic Heart Disease

For clinical purposes the manifestations of coronary atherosclerosis are described as clearly defined entities. However, these syndromes may be difficult to relate to the actual coronary artery pathology because identical atherosclerotic lesions (with or without concomitant thrombosis) may be responsible for either sudden death, myocardial infarction, or stable or unstable angina; or there may be no symptoms at all. Furthermore, the clinical symptoms do not progress in orderly sequence from stable to unstable angina to acute myocardial infarction and eventually to chronic heart failure. In fact, the most common presentation of coronary atherosclerosis is sudden unexpected death in the absence of myocardial infarction.

Angina Pectoris

Angina pectoris is produced by transient myocardial ischemia when oxygen demand exceeds supply. The exact mechanism for production of pain is uncertain, but the stimulus is carried by sympathetic nerves that accompany the coronary arteries and then proceed to the upper cervical sympathetic ganglia, entering the spinal cord with the upper four or five thoracic spinal nerves, ultimately reaching the thalamus. Ischemic pain is referred to the distribution of the upper five thoracic spinal nerves but is qualitatively different from somatic pain.

Blood flow to the left ventricle through the coronary arteries occurs mainly during diastole, because in systole the intramyocardial pressure exceeds aortic systolic pressure. The major factors that determine the amount of oxygen consumed by the myocardium are (1) the heart rate, (2) the state of myocardial contractility, and (3) systolic wall stress on the myocardium. The systolic wall stress on the myocardium is proportional to the height of systolic pressure and the radius of the ventricle. By the Law of Laplace, the tension that a myocardial fiber must develop to maintain a given pressure increases as the radius of the ventricle increases. Therefore, myocardial oxygen requirements are significantly greater in patients who have dilated left ventricles. In normal individuals, the heart size (and therefore ventricular radius) decreases during exercise, and there is a proportionate reduction in myocardial fiber tension and oxygen requirement. In patients with ischemic heart disease, atherosclerotic lesions limit the ability of myocardial blood flow to increase in response to demands of tachycardia, increased blood pressure, and inotropic stimulation of the myocardium. These effects are aggravated among patients with left ventricular failure where the radius of the left ventricle remains large, or even increases during exercise.

During an ischemic episode myocardial contracility is impaired in the ischemic area and hypokinesis and dyskinesis may be observed angiographically, by echocardiography, or by direct visualization at the time of operation. Frequently, there is also evidence of acute left ventricular failure. Accompanying the pain, patients frequently experience dyspnea because of reduced compliance of the ischemic ventricle. Elevated left ventricular filling pressure produces a passive rise in the pulmonary capillary pressure, stiffening of the lungs and, interstitial pulmonary edema. Frequently, there is systemic hypertension during the attack.

Stable Angina Pectoris

The diagnosis of angina pectoris is heavily dependent on the patient's history and is, therefore, very subjective. The temperament and psychological makeup and reaction to pain of the patient must be individually and carefully assessed. Descriptions depend on the patient's powers of observation, intelligence, and knowledge. Additionally, evaluation of a patient's history is greatly dependent on the skill of the physician in eliciting and defining symptoms. Even with the most artful questioning of an intelligent cooperative patient, there should be no illusions about the possibility of diagnostic error. Correlations of clinical diagnosis with coronary angiography indicate inaccurate diagnosis of angina pectoris in at least 6% of patients, and this figure will be even higher if the history is taken from an unintelligent or uncooperative patient by an inattentive physician.

The classical description of the pain is one of a squeezing, vise-like pressure located in the upper two-thirds of the chest, in the midline behind the sternum. It may be described as choking, aching, or burning in quality. The pain comes on gradually, reaches a maximum, persists for a few minutes, and then gradually subsides. It rarely lasts more than 15 minutes except when it is unstable. It is not sharp in the sense of "stabbing," "pricking," or "knife-like." Victims may clutch their chest, indicating a sensation as if gripped by a band or vise. The pain extends to both arms and to the hands, wrists, and fingers, which frequently feel numb, especially on the inner aspects; not infrequently it radiates down the left arm only. Occasionally, it is felt in the back, and may also radiate very widely to include the jaw or upper abdomen. The pain need not be central, but may be felt parasternally on the left, or even in the left arm, or jaw only. It is usually not felt in the left breast or axilla. Patients frequently experience a vague sensation in the arms, often referred to as a lameness, which may or may not be associated with the more typical ischemic pain.

The most significant feature of angina pectoris is the circumstances under which pain occurs. It is usually provoked by effort or emotional stress, such as anger or excitement. Heavy meals or walking uphill in the cold against the wind are particularly provocative. The pain or discomfort usually forces the patient to halt or slow down before it subsides after a few minutes; occasionally it will diminish despite continued exercise (the "breakthrough" phenomenon). Usually the pain does not last for more than 15 minutes and rarely longer than half an hour, unless infarction has occurred. In some patients angina is predictable and reproducible and directly related to the amount of effort undertaken. More usually, however, the occurrence of attacks is variable because of emotional and other factors, so that assessment of efficacy of any specific form of therapy is difficult. The inconsistency of angina is in fact highly diagnostic. Some days patients can walk miles without pain and at other times they cannot manage 100 yards. There may be a circadian pattern, with the pain often occurring early in the morning, for example, while shaving or other mild physical activity, and then disappearing for the rest of the day.

The importance of emotional tension is well exemplified by angina provoked by driving an automobile, where continuous electrocardiographic monitoring has shown frequent ST segment depression and increased excretion of urinary catecholamines. Other factors apart from emotion may be responsible for the extreme variability with which attacks are provoked: The underlying atherosclerotic process may fluctuate in its severity and rate of progression, collateral channels may be established, or active vasoconstriction or coronary spasm may contribute. Moreover, some episodes of ischemia may occur without symptoms ("silent ischemia"), and up to 25% of patients with acute myocardial infarction will fail to have symptoms.

In some patients paroxysms of pain are accompanied by extreme anxiety, a fear of impending death (angor animi), and local chest wall tenderness. With progression of the disease, angina may occur with less exertion and also at rest. Attacks occurring during sleep may be related to dreaming, when there is marked fluctuation in blood pressure and an increase in cardiac output, but in patients with severe angina, nocturnal symptoms may be due to a primary decrease in coronary blood flow.

Angina pectoris is strikingly relieved by sublingual nitroglycerin. The response occurs within 1 to 2 minutes, and this consistent relief by nitroglycerine is of considerable diagnostic help. When it takes more than 5 minutes for chest pain to be relieved by nitroglycerin, the pain is generally not angina. When angina is a result of obstructive cardiomyopathy nitroglycerine may aggravate the episode. It should be remembered that administration of nitroglycerine may relieve the pain of esophageal spasm.

Diagnosis

The diagnosis is made primarily by the history, but is supported by stress electrocardiography and radionuclide perfusion studies when necessary. Examination during an attack will usually show pallor and sweating with a raised blood pressure. Tachycardia is often present and a fourth heart sound, a murmur of mitral insufficiency (due to papillary muscle dysfunction), may appear, or become accentuated during the attack. Between episodes of pain, the physical examination is frequently unremarkable. Abnormal physical signs may be detected when ventricular damage has occurred; such as dyskinetic precordial pulsation, paradoxical splitting of the second heart sound, and third or fourth heart sounds.

Conditions other than coronary obstruction can contribute to or cause angina pectoris, usually by increasing oxygen demand. It is important to exclude hypertension, anemia, diabetes mellitus, and thyroid disease, which may be aggravating factors. Congenital, rheumatic, or senile aortic stenosis may cause angina but are readily recognized by auscultation. Syphilitic aortitis with coronary ostial stenosis is now an exremely rare cause of angina, which may be suspected clinically by hearing the early diastolic murmur of aortic insufficiency.

Angina is a frequent presenting symptom of obstructive cardiomyopathy, and a careful search for this condition should be made, particularly in young patients. Important clues are the jerky pulses, clinical and electrocardiographic evidence of severe left ventricular hypertrophy, and loud fourth sound. It is not infrequent for the systolic murmur of obstructive cardiomyopathy to be labeled "innocent" or "functional," or a result of papillary muscle dysfunction, particularly because the murmur varies in intensity and may even disappear spontaneously. Nitroglycerine may exacerbate symptoms in these patients by reducing coronary perfusion pressure without decreasing left ventricular pressure, which remains high because of the outflow obstruction.

Differential Diagnosis

Psychogenic Chest Pain (Da Costa's Syndrome, Neurocirculatory Asthenia)

Left chest pain associated with anxiety, or hyperventilation syndrome is frequently confused with angina pectoris. Women are affected more frequently than men. The pain is stabbing in nature, variable, not strictly related to effort, lasts longer than typical angina, and does not respond promptly to nitroglycerine. Hyperventilation may be obvious during an interview, and symptoms such as sighing respiration, paraesthesia, and fatigue frequently coexist. For reasons unknown, hyperventilation may depress the ST segments at rest, and even more so following a stress test.

The clinical diagnosis of an anxiety state or hyperventilation syndrome is usually fairly readily made, but in some instances coronary arteriography is a necessary and justifiable procedure to resolve the problem. The chest pain associated with mitral valve prolapse is psychogenic and frequently aggravated by excessive medical attention—subjects should be reassured that they have a minor abnormality of their mitral valve, which is unlikely to have any serious complications.

Hiatus Hernia and Reflux Esophagitis

Heartburn is generally an easy symptom to recognize, particularly when there is a history of regurgitation of acid fluid. Frequently, symptoms are relieved by antacids or ingestion of milk. Occasionally, however, symptoms of esophagitis are described as a pressure-like constricting pain occurring across the central chest, often radiating to the back. The most important diagnostic investigation is cine-esophagography, which demonstrates reflux of barium from the stomach into the esophagus across an incompetent esophageal sphincter. The Bernstein acid-infusion test whereby 0.1 N hydrochloric acid is infused into the lower esophagus in an attempt to reproduce the patient's symptoms may also be of diagnostic value.

Esophageal Spasm

When there is diffuse spasm of the esophagus, the symptoms may be suggestive of coronary artery disease particularly when the discomfort is relieved by nitroglycerine. The quality of the pain may closely mimic angina pectoris, but is not usually related to exertion. The diagnosis is made by a history of attacks following ingestion of food, and radiological demonstration of esophageal spasm.

Neurological and Muscular Causes of Chest Pain

Cervical rib, the scalenus anticus syndrome, and a first thoracic rib are varieties of thoracic outlet syndrome in which there is neurovascular compression affecting the upper limbs. The neurological and vascular symptoms are usually confined to the upper limb, but occasionally anterior chest pain may occur and simulate angina pectoris. Objective evidence of neurological and vascular impairment may be present or become obvious by extension and rotation of the head and neck. Pain is usually precipitated by movement of the neck, shoulder, arm, or chest and by coughing and sneezing. Exercise stress testing is negative and there is no response to nitroglycerin.

Chest Wall Pain

Pain and tenderness of the chest wall of unknown etiology are fairly common. The pain may be elicited by pressure on the affected area and by movement of the chest. The pain is of long duration and is not relieved by nitroglycerin. Pain, swelling, and tenderness of the costochondral joints of unknown etiology occurs in Tietze disease, which is self-limited, but local anesthetic infiltration may be required for relief.

Diagnostic Testing

Electrocardiogram

The resting electrocardiogram is a useful and inexpensive test for the evaluation of patients with angina pectoris. The presence of pathologic Q-waves strongly suggests the diagnosis of previous myocardial infarction and this is helpful in supporting a diagnosis of angina. However, it should be remembered that pathological Q-waves may occur in other conditions such as hypertrophic cardiomyopathy, muscular ventricular septal defect, and the Wolff–Parkinson–White syndrome. In fact, when a young patient complains of chest pain, the diagnosis of hypertrophic cardiomyopathy can be strongly suspected from the electrocardiogram when there is the combination of deep Q-waves and QRS voltage of severe left ventricular hypertrophy.

In general, electrocardiographic evidence of a Q-wave infarction correlates fairly well with the location of the involved coronary artery. Thus, an anterior infarction pattern (V1 to V4) signifies left anterior descending disease and an inferior infarction (leads II, III, and AVF) is usually a result of right coronary occlusion. Involvement of the left circumflex coronary artery is more difficult to identify because this may be associated with a pattern of inferior or lateral myocardial infarction. It should be noted that the resting electrocardiogram may be normal in up to one-half of patients with stable angina pectoris. When the QRS complex is normal in a patient with angina it may suggest limited disease, such as single vessel disease in the absence of previous myocardial infarction. However, two and even three vessel coronary artery disease may also be associated with a normal electrocardiogram. In the individual patient, therefore, the presence of a normal electrocardiogram does not mean that severe coronary artery disease is absent. Left bundle branch block among patients with angina pectoris carries an adverse prognosis because it is often associated with severe left ventricular damage from extensive previous myocardial infarction.

The resting electrocardiogram is most helpful when it documents transient ST segment depression during episodes of chest pain. This is most likely to occur when a patient has been admitted to a clinic or hospital for evaluation. Under these circumstances, every effort should be made to record a 12-lead electrocardiogram whenever chest pain occurs.

Exercise Testing

Exercise testing is of limited value as a screening test to predict the presence or absence of coronary artery disease in asymptomatic patients with few risk factors. This is because of the high frequency of false positives when the pretest likelihood of disease is low. However, exercise testing yields important information about the severity, prognosis, and treatment in patients with an established diagnosis of angina pectoris and assists in the diagnosis of ischemic heart disease in those with chest pain and multiple risk factors.

The goal of exercise testing is to induce temporary myocardial ischemia while constantly monitoring the heart rate, electrocardiogram, and blood pressure. At maximum exercise, the following important information should be available:

1. The presence or absence of angina.
2. The appearance of the patient (pallor sweating, anxiety, dyspnea, nausea).
3. The double product (heart rate × peak systolic blood pressure).
4. ST segment and T-wave changes.
5. Dysrhythmias.

The *double product* is a good clinical index of myocardial oxygen consumption. Generally, the lower the double product at the time of onset of ischemic, changes on the EKG, the lower the coronary flow reserve and the more severe the coronary artery disease. A high double product (more than 28,000) at the onset of a positive test generally indicates mild ischemia and less extensive disease.

Interpretation of the double product must take other factors into account: Drugs such as β-blockers, through their negative inotropic and chronotropic effects, increase the capacity for physical exercise by delaying the point at which the coronary flow reserve is depleted. Thus, patients will exercise longer to reach the same double product and angina, or may not reach that double product at all. Obviously, patients who have angina at a relatively high double product are most likely to achieve successful control of angina with medical treatment. Physical conditioning also plays a role in the interpretation of the results. A deconditioned person without coronary disease may attain a high double product very rapidly whereas a physically fit person may exercise much longer to achieve the same blood pressure and heart rate: The double product carries the same significance in terms of coronary flow reserve for both individuals, yet one is capable of much more physical work. An "early positive" test has often been described in terms of time on the treadmill (e.g., Stage I of the Bruce Test, or five mets). For the reasons given above this is of less value in assessing coronary flow reserve and severity of disease then the double product. Time on the treadmill and energy expenditure (mets) are more useful measures of exercise capability for purposes of cardiac rehabilitation and assesment of disability.

Severe exercise-induced ischemia (i.e., "early positive") is suggested by one or more of the following:

1. ST segment depression at a double product of less than 14,000.
2. Two millimeters or more of horizontal or down sloping ST segment depression.
3. Persistence of ST segment depression for 5 minutes or more after completion of exercise.
4. Hypotension during exercise.
5. Dyspnea and S3 gallop.

The occurrence of exercise-induced hypotension (20 mm Hg or more) is an ominous finding and when combined with ST segment depression often signifies left main coronary artery disease, frequently associated with left ventricular dysfunction.

Abnormalities of the resting electrocardiogram may preclude exercise electrocardiography. These abnormalities include digitalis-induced ST segment depression, the pattern of left ventricular hypertrophy and strain, Wolff–Parkinson–White syndrome, or left bundle branch block. These abnormalities almost invariably result in false-positive depression of the ST segment. Under such circumstances, exercise testing with concomitant radionuclide flow studies are more sensitive and more specific for myocardial ischemia.

Exercise Radionuclide Angiography

This test involves labeling red blood cells with radioactive technetium and then having the patient exercise on a bicycle in the supine position. Repeated measurements of left ventricular ejection fraction are obtained at rest and with increasing workloads. Normally, ejection fraction rises as exercise proceeds. Failure of the ejection fraction to rise, or an actual fall, signifies left ventricular disease such as cardiomyopathy, ischemia, or left ventricular hypertrophy. A fall in ejection fraction accompanied by a new wall motion abnormality (dyskinesis) signifies the onset of ischemia and both are very specific for coronary artery disease. However, the results of the test must be interpreted with caution when atrial fibrillation or ventricular ectopy is present since these dysrhythmias interfere with the ability of the computer to reconstruct a typical cardiac cycle when time averaging the radioactive counts.

Stress Thallium-201 Myocardial Perfusion Imaging

Thallium-201 is a potassium analog that when given intravenously is taken up so avidly by myocardial cells that the amount taken up in a region of the heart is proportional to the flow to that region. Thallium injected at the peak of exercise and images obtained immediately and again several hours later in a normal heart show uniform distribution both at peak exercise and later at rest. Ischemic areas are demonstrated by defects during exercise (regions receiving proportionately less flow) that "redistribute" after recovery (i.e., at at rest demonstrate equal perfusion). Infarcts are evident by defects that are present during exercise and recovery. Thallium scintigraphy is more sensitive than exercise electrocardiography, but is expensive. False positives may occur in the presence of left bundle branch block or WPW. The test is useful in quantitating and localizing the extent of myocardial hypoperfusion. Multiple redistribution defects, with abnormal lung uptake and transient left ventricular dilatation, suggest severe left ventricular disease.

For selected patients who are unable to exercise because of intermittent claudication or physical handicaps, dipyridamole-thallium testing is a useful procedure. Intravenous dipyridamole decreases coronary flow resistance producing a "coronary steal" so that myocardium supplied by stenotic coronary arteries then become relatively ischemic, demonstrated by reversible defects on scanning. Among patients with severe coronary artery disease, the sensitivity of this study exceeds 90%, and the specificity is 75%.

TABLE 17.1. Prognosis in patients treated nonsurgically in the early 1970s.

Status	Annual mortality (%)
Normal LV[a] function	
1-, 2-, or 3-vessel disease	1.6
1-vessel disease	0.6
2-vessel disease	1.6
3-vessel disease	3.6
LMCAD	10 (for first 2 years)
Abnormal LV function	
1-, 2-, or 3-vessel disease	8.4
1-vessel disease	3.5
2-vessel disease	5.6
3-vessel disease	6–11.5
LMCAD	20 to 25 (for first 2–3 years)
Normal or abnormal LV function and 1-, 2-, or 3-vessel disease	4.3
Congestive heart failure and 1-, 2-, or 3-vessel disease	12.4
Progressive chest pain	Increased incidence of death and nonfatal myocardial infarction at almost all levels of vessel involvement and state of LV function
Treadmill exercise test (Bruce protocol)	
Low risk	1-year mortality 1%
Negative test or stage IV and/or heart rate ≥160 beats/min	4-year mortality 7%
High risk	1-year mortality 15%
Positive test in stage I or II	4-year mortality 37%
Positive test plus maximal	1-year mortality 20%
Positive test plus maximal heart rate <120 beats/min	4-year mortality 69%

[a]LV, left ventricular; LMCAD, left main coronary artery disease

From Rahimtoola SH: Coronary bypass surgery for chronic angina—1981: A perspective. Circulation 65:225–241, 1982. By permission of American Heart Association.

Management of Patients with Stable Angina Pectoris

Each patient with angina pectoris presents an individual problem and there are no algorithms that substitute for sound clinical judgment. The management of a sedentary man of 70 years of age with associated medical conditions such as obstructive airways disease is very different from that of a 45-year-old construction worker. Once a clinical and social profile has been formulated, treatment is designed to relieve symptoms with as few side effects as possible, and to improve life expectancy. Based on evidence from randomized trials for coronary artery bypass surgery and survival studies of patients treated nonsurgically (Table 17.1) certain generalizations are in order:

1. Left ventricular ejection fraction is the most important prognostic factor determining survival.
2. With normal left ventricular function the prognosis for single-vessel disease is good (90–100% survival at 5 years) but becomes progressively worse for two- and three-vessel disease, and is worst for left main disease, which has a grave outlook. With abnormal left ventricular function and/or congestive heart failure the outlook is significantly worse in all categories.
3. The mortality is higher when there is severe exercise-induced ischemia at a low double product.
4. When the prognosis is judged to be poor (based on the number of diseased vessels, poor left ventricular function and early posi-

tive stress tests) patients benefit more from coronary artery bypass surgery than medical treatment.

It follows that the indications for coronary angiography among patients with *stable* angina pectoris are (1) abnormal left ventricular function at rest, (2) a stress test (exercise electrocardiogram, exercise radionuclide angiography, or thallium test) that demonstrates onset of ischemia or left ventricular dysfunction at a low double product or, (3) symptoms so severe that the quality of life is greatly impaired despite medical treatment. The angiographic findings will help define both the patients prognosis and the risk of intervention, major factors in determining subsequent management. Coronary angiography is also indicated for diagnosis when symptoms are atypical, or the results of noninvasive tests are equivocal.

Medical Treatment

General Management

Strong psychological reassurance is important to avoid unnecessary restriction of activity and/or early retirement from work. It may, however, be necessary to modify the patient's activities with common sense avoidance of overwork, worry, and anxiety.

Although *obesity* is not a contributing factor in the genesis of atherosclerosis, it does increase the workload of the heart and aggravate angina pectoris. A weight reduction program should be instituted to bring the patient to within the desired normal weight range. *Cigarette smoking* is a potent risk factor, and patients should be encouraged to quit.

Exercise is important in treatment because it has a beneficial psychological effect and avoids introspection and hypochondriasis. It has a conditioning effect on the heart by decreasing the heart rate for any level of exercise, thus reducing the pressure rate product enabling the patient to perform at increased workload before reaching the ischemic threshold. However, although exercise improves the general sense of well being and exercise tolerance there is still no definite proof that it prolongs life span or the need for surgery in patients with angina pectoris.

General medical conditions such as anemia, thyrotoxicosis, tachycardia, and hypoxia increase myocardial oxygen needs and may aggravate or actually precipitate angina. These conditions should be adequately treated. Although control of hypertension has failed to affect the mortality from coronary artery disease, blood pressure control is important for treating the symptoms of angina pectoris. Some of the drugs, utilized for the treatment of angina pectoris, such as calcium channel and β-blockers, are quite effective at lowering blood pressure.

There are data to support treatment of *elevated cholesterol* levels in patients with coronary artery disease. Evidence favors some reduction in cardiac mortality and regression of coronary artery lesions in those patients with high serum lipid levels who successfully improve their lipid profile. Although there may not be much wisdom in treating elderly patients with hypercholesterolemia and extensive coronary artery disease, it seems justified to reduce high cholesterol levels in younger patients suffering from angina pectoris.

The first step is dietary, with a reduction in the consumption of animal and saturated fats, and a switch to unsaturated vegetable oils. Dietary modification should aim at a total cholesterol of less than 200 mg%, an LDL cholesterol of less than 130 mg%, and a HDL cholesterol level of more than 35 mg%. When dietary modification fails drug treatment should be employed.

The major drugs available to lower LDL cholesterol are bile acid sequestrants, nicotinic acid, and lovastatin.

Bile Acid Sequestrants

These reduce LDL cholesterol depending on the dose administered. Since these agents are not absorbed, most adverse effects are limited to the gastrointestinal tract. Nausea and constipation are the most common side effects. In high dosage they can cause malabsorption, and this includes the fat-soluble vitamins. Two preparations are available: cholestyramine and colestipol. Selection of one drug over another largely depends on each patient's preference. The recommended dose of cholestyramine is 4 g taken one to six times daily, and for colestipol 15–30 g in divided doses two to four times daily.

Nicotinic Acid

The mechanism of action of nicotinic acid has not been established. Generally, it produces a 10–15% decrease in LDL cholesterol level. The main adverse effect of nicotinic acid is facial flushing, often accompanied by severe pruritus. Treatment is usually started with small doses (100–250 mg one to three times daily) immediately following meals, and gradually increased every week to total dose of 3 g/day (1 g t.i.d.).

Lovastatin

This drug partially blocks the synthesis of cholesterol, lowers the LDL level, and increases the HDL cholesterol level. Generally, it is well tolerated, but may produce temporary disturbance in liver function, and more importantly rhabdomyolysis. Rhabdomyolysis is more likely to occur when lovastatin is used in combination with nicotinic acid or immunosuppressive therapy. Preferably, the drug should be used only when it is a single agent for cholesterol control.

Drug Therapy for Angina Pectoris

There are three classes of drugs available for the control of angina pectoris. These are nitrates, β-adrenergic blockers, and calcium channel antagonists.

Nitrates

Nitroglycerin is the cornerstone of treatment and still the most effective remedy for curtailing an attack of angina pectoris. The drug acts predominantly through its venodilator effect thereby reducing preload, decreasing the ventricular volume, and increasing ventricular compliance. This has the effect of reducing myocardial wall tension and the oxygen demands of the myocardium, an effect that is enhanced by a concomitant, but lesser reduction in the peripheral vascular resistance (afterload). The hemodynamic and therapeutic effect is most pronounced in the standing position, and this may be responsible for the occasional occurrence of postural hypotension, particularly in patients who are volume depleted by diuretics. Nitrates dilate both large and small coronary vessels, provided there is sufficient smooth muscle within the vessel wall, and they also dilate normal coronary arteries.

Following the administration of sublingual nitroglycerin, peak plasma levels are reached in approximately 2 minutes after the tablet has dissolved. Patients should be instructed to carry nitroglycerin at all times. Tablets more than 4 to 6 months old have reduced potency and eventually become ineffective. Tablets of 0.2–0.6 mgm. are allowed to melt sublingually, or chewed, until there is relief of angina. Side effects include throbbing headaches and transient hypotension and patients should be warned about the latter possibility, especially during hot weather or following a hot bath. Nitroglycerin may also be administered in the form of a spray. The advantages are that the spray is stable, easy to administer, and preferred by some patients over the sublingual tablets.

Long Acting Nitrates

Chemical forms include various preparations of nitroglycerin, isosorbide dinitrate, pentaerythritol tetranitrate, or isosorbide-5-mononitrate. These can be given orally, sublingually, or transcutaneously. Isosorbide dinitrate in a dosage of 10–30 mg favorably effects hemodynamics and is also of prophylactic and therapeutic value. A single oral dose generally lasts for 3 to 6 hours but may last up to 8 hours. Chewable isosorbide dinitrate has a faster onset of action (similar to sublingual nitroglycerin), but is of shorter duration of action. Nitrates may also be effectively delivered through the skin in the form of an ointment or as a transdermal patch that can provide predictable blood levels for longer time periods. The efficacy of transdermal nitroglycerin (15-

TABLE 17.2. Dosage and pharmacodynamics of β-blocker drugs.

Drug	Daily dose (mg)	Frequency	Cardio-selective	Lipid solubility	Primary route of elimination
Propranolol (Inderal)	160–480	2–4	No	High	Hepatic
Atenolol (Tenormin)	50–200	1	Yes	Low	Renal and hepatic
Metoprolol (Lopressor)	100–200	2–3	Yes	Intermediate	Hepatic
Timolol (Blocadren)	20–40	2	No	Low to intermediate	Hepatic and renal
Nadolol (Corgard)	40–320	1	No	Low	Renal and biliary
Acebutolol (Sectral)	400–1200	2–4	Yes	Low	Hepatic and renal
Pindolol (Visken)	7.5–22.5	3	No	Intermediate	Renal and hepatic

105 mg for 24 hours) taken as sustained therapy may be compromised by the development of tolerance. This tolerance is not easily overcome by increasing the dose and can also occur with other preparations if they are given in higher doses repeatedly over 24 hours. For this reason a nitrate-free interval of at least 8 hours (usually at night) is often recommended. A relatively common side effect of all nitrate preparations is headache, which can be minimized by starting at low dosages and increasing gradually, depending on the patient's response. Administration of a mild analgesic following commencement of treatment is frequently helpful. Nitrates should probably not be administered to patients who have chronic recurrent migraine.

β-Adrenergic Blockers

β-Adrenergic blocking agents (Table 17.2) have proved to be highly effective in the treatment of angina pectoris and are frequently used as first-line therapy. Approximately 75% of patients will have satisfactory relief of their symptoms with these drugs alone.

Myocardial β-receptors are predominantly β_1, whereas those in the smooth muscle of blood vessels and the bronchi are β_2. Blockade of β_2 (vasodilator) receptors results in unopposed α-adrenergic stimulation and vasoconstriction. β_1-Blockade has a negative inotropic effect (reduced myocardial contractility) and a negative chronotropic effect (slowing of the heart rate). These drugs should be used with caution in patients who have severely impaired left ventricular function, particularly if combined with other negative inotropic agents. "Cardioselective" β-blockers are those that block β_1-receptors alone. However, in large doses this selectivity is lost and bronchospasm may still occur. It is advisable, therefore, not to use the drugs in patients who have significant bronchospastic airway obstruction, Raynaud phenomenon, or severe peripheral vascular disease. Propanolol and Metropolol are lipophilic and cross the blood–brain barrier more easily, contributing to occasional neurologic side effects such as fatigue, depression, and nightmares. Hydrophilic β-blockers (Atenolol) are less penetrating in the central nervous system and have a longer duration.

β-Blockers are most effective when angina is clearly related to exertion. They produce resting bradycardia, and decrease both heart rate and catecholamine response to exercise. An adequately treated patient will exercise longer on the treadmill to reach the maximum double product, or the patient will stop from fatigue at a lower double product. The choice of a particular drug will largely depend on the patient's tolerance and cost, since the clinical response to various preparations is much the same. The usual β-blocking dose of propranolol is 240 mg daily, Metropolol 100 mg daily, and Atenolol 100 mg daily. The therapeutic efficacy should be tested on the treadmill or with an informal evaluation of monitoring the heart rate during exercise. An adequate response is reduction in the frequency of attacks and blunting of the heart rate and blood pressure response to exercise.

The important side effects produced by β-blockers are (1) exacerbation of congestive

TABLE 17.3. Dosage and pharmacodynamics of calcium entry blockers.

Calcium antagonist	Dose (mg)	Vasodilation Coronary	Vasodilation Peripheral	Conduction Heart rate	Conduction SA node A-V node	Myocardial contractility
Verapamil	80–160 tid	↑	↑	0/↓	↓	↓
Diltiazem	30–90 q6h	↑	↑	0/↓	0/↓	↑ ↓
Nifedipine	10–40 tid	↑	↑ ↓	0/↑	0	0
Nicardipine	20–40 tid	↑	↑ ↓	0/↑	0	0

heart failure, (2) severe sinus bradycardia, (3) hypotension, and (4) aggravation of angina and myocardial infarction when treatment is stopped suddenly. So-called "up-regulation" of β-receptors due to increased number or sensitivity exaggerates the response to endogenous catecholamines when β-blockers are withdrawn. Withdrawal should be treated with a rapid acting intravenous β-blocker such as esmolol, given as a bolus of 3 to 5 mg followed by maintenance of 6 to 20 mg until oral treatment can be resumed.

Calcium Antagonists

By preventing the entry of calcium into cells, these agents diminish contractility of cardiac and vascular smooth muscle (Table 17.3). Reduction in myocardial contractility and afterload makes these agents highly suitable for chronic treatment of angina pectoris. Other effects include depression of automaticity of the SA node and depression of conduction through the A-V node. The effect of a particular agent depends on the balance struck between these direct effects and reflex activation of the baroreceptors. Moreover, some of the agents vary considerably in their chemical structure, and may alter calcium kinetics at different intracellular sites.

Nifedipine and Nicardipine

These two closely related calcium antagonists are quite potent for reducing afterload and increasing coronary blood flow by relaxing smooth muscle. There are minimal effects on SA and A-V nodal conduction. The reduction in peripheral vascular resistance produces a baroreceptor-induced tachycardia that may make them very effective in combination with a β-blocker. They may also be useful in patients with bronchospasm and Raynaud phenomenon. The powerful vasodilator effect accounts for a relatively high incidence of side effects, such as facial flushing, hypotension, and ankle edema, which may be marked. When a rapid effect is required, a nifedipine capsule may be broken and the liquid swallowed. Nifedipine is also available in a sustained release preparation that may produce fewer side-effects by having a more stable serum level.

Diltiazem

This is in widespread use because of a very low side-effect profile. It relaxes smooth muscle in the coronary and peripheral vessels, increasing coronary blood flow and reducing afterload. It has significant negative inotropic effects. It depresses both SA and A-V nodal automaticity and conduction, and should be used cautiously with a β-blocker since bradycardia may be profound. The daily dose is 120 to 360 mg daily given in three divided doses.

Verapamil

This was the first calcium channel blocker available for clinical use. It has a pronounced negative inotropic effect. Like Nifedipine and Diltiazem it increases coronary blood flow and decreases afterload. It also has a major effect in slowing conduction through the A-V node. For these reasons it should be used with great caution when the left ventricular ejection fraction is less than 35%. The usual dose is 360 to 480 mg/day in three divided doses.

Combination Treatments

Certain combinations of two drugs may be useful and results are predictable from the individual actions.

1. β-Blocker and Nitrates. Nitrates lower the preload, which counteracts the increase in left ventricular volume and pressure produced by β-blockade. The β-blocker in its turn counteracts the tachycardia produced by nitrates.
2. β-Blocker and Nifedipine. The β-blocker counteracts the reflex tachycardia induced by Nifedipine and this is an effective antianginal combination.
3. Verapamil or Diltiazem and a β-Blocker. This is an effective combination for the relief of angina provided the ejection fraction is more than 35%. The hazards of this combination are severe sinus bradycardia, congestive heart failure, hypotension, syncope, and left ventricular failure. Intravenous Verapamil should be used only rarely and with great caution in a patient who is β-blocked. (Intravenous calcium may counteract the adverse effects of Verapamil in an emergency.)
4. Nifedipine, β-Blocker, and Nitrates. This form of triple therapy does *not* have any particular efficacy. The vasodilator effects of Nifedipine and nitrates may produce profound fatigue, dizziness, and syncope. Because of increased potential for side-effects, plus unproven efficacy compared to optimal double therapy, all three classes of the antianginals should rarely be used together.

Revascularization Procedures

Percutaneous Transluminal Coronary Angioplasty (PTCA)

Balloon dilatation of coronary arterial stenoses is an alternative to surgical revascularization. It has a place somewhere between medical and surgical treatment. When there is severe angina, with objective confirmation of myocardial ischemia, dilatation of a single lesion that has optimal angiographic features will yield an excellent result. There is currently a great wave of enthusiasm for this procedure. However, it should be remembered that we do not yet know from adequately controlled trials how cost effective and efficacious PTCA is in comparison to surgical and even medical treatment.

Indications

Generally accepted indications for PTCA include

1. Angina pectoris unresponsive to medical treatment.
2. Poor patient compliance or intolerance of medical treatment.
3. Patients with an optimal lesion who are either very young or very old with single vessel disease. It is obviously desirable to avoid thoracotomy in the elderly. In young patients, where progression of coronary disease and subsequent surgery is quite likely, PTCA is also a tempting initial treatment.
4. As a palliative procedure when there is severe general medical disease (neoplastic, pulmonary, and renal, etc.).
5. As an alternative to a second operation among patients with angina and previous cardiac operations (cardiac valve replacement, coronary artery bypass surgery).

Results

The ideal coronary artery lesion for balloon dilatation has the following characteristics: (1) less than 1 cm long, (2) not calcified, (3) no thrombus, (4) distal to the coronary ostium, and (5) away from branch points, (6) in a straight segment of artery, and (7) subtotal occlusion. When these features are present the initial success rate (decreasing the stenosis to less than 50%) should be more than 90%, the incidence of nonfatal myocardial infarction less than 4.5%, and the mortality rate less than 1%. Stenosis may be expected to reoccur in one-fourth to one-third of lesions within approximately 6 months. Because of their smaller vessels, the results are not as good in women. Conversely, high-risk lesions are long, calcified, involve a branch point, or are situated in an angulated (more than 45°) segment of an artery. The risk will increase (1) when more than one vessel is dilated, (2) when the operator is inexperienced, or (3) where facilities for emergency coronary artery bypass surgery are not readily available.

The decision to refer a patient for PTCA is not always easy. The prognosis for patients with single-vessel disease treated medically is excellent in precisely those cases where the angiographic characteristics of the lesion make the patient an ideal candidate for PTCA. However, tight stenosis proximal to the first septal perforator branch of the left anterior descending coronary artery places a large area of myocardium in jeopardy and revascularization is superior to medical treatment. This lesion has an excellent prognosis when treated by left internal mammary artery grafting. To dilate this lesion involves a careful consideration of some of the factors mentioned (i.e., skill of the surgical vs the PTCA operators, age, concomitant diseases, etc.). Decisions to dilate multiple lesions become even more problematic.

Coronary Artery Bypass Surgery

Unlike PTCA there is clear evidence that coronary artery bypass surgery (CABS) improves long-term survival in certain patients with chronic stable angina pectoris. Also, for patients intolerant of medication or unsuitable for PTCA, CABS provides better relief of symptoms than medical treatment for at least 5 years after operation. Thereafter, the percentage of patients who remain asymptomatic decreases progressively, and the reoperation rate and the use of medications increase concomitantly.

In order of importance, the survival of medically treated patients depends on two factors: (1) left ventricular function and (2) the severity of coronary artery disease. These factors act synergistically, in that left ventricular dysfunction is more evident as the severity of coronary disease increases. The most lethal combination is that of left main coronary artery disease and left ventricular dysfunction (Table 17.1).

Since a major impact of surgery is to improve survival it is important to recognize those groups in which this effect is most clear-cut.

Left Main Coronary Artery Disease

Mortality among medically treated patients with more than 70% stenosis of this vessel is approximately 30% at 18 months and 50% at 3 years. The survival is better when the stenosis is less severe (i.e., less than 50%).

Other factors indicating an adverse prognosis among patients with more than 70% stenosis are (1) chest pain with minimal exertion or at rest, (2) history of congestive heart failure, (3) resting EKG abnormalities, (4) cardiomegaly on chest X-ray, (5) positive exercise test at a low double product, (6) elevated left ventricular end-diastolic pressure, (7) left ventricular dysfunction, and (8) concomitant right coronary artery stenosis.

With surgical revascularization several studies demonstrate that approximately 85–90% of patients will be alive at 4 years compared to 60% treated medically.

Three-Vessel Disease

Most major studies show a slight improvement in life expectancy with surgical treatment for stable angina in three-vessel disease, especially if there is concomitant left ventricular dysfunction (ejection fraction between 35 and 50%).

Two Vessel Disease

Surgery appears to offer an advantage over medical treatment when one of the vessels involved is the left anterior descending coronary artery poximal to the first septal perforator branch. Otherwise, the results of surgical and medical treatment are much the same.

Single-Vessel Disease

CABS offers no advantage for survival compared to medical treatment.

Risks of Coronary Artery Bypass Surgery

Mortality

With improvement in technique, major centers have an average mortality of 1 to 3% per annum. Predictors of mortality include (1) poor left ventricular function (depressed left ventricular ejection fraction, past or present congestive heart failure, cardiomegaly on chest X-ray, persistant S3 gallop, elevated left ventricular end-diastolic pressure, or regional wall motion abnormality by echocardiogram, angiogram, or radionuclide angiogram), (2) age, (3) female gender, (4) unstable angina, and (5) evolving myocardial Infarction.

Perioperative Myocardial Infarction

This has also decreased in incidence with increasing surgical experience. Nevertheless, most centers experience an incidence of approximately 10% and in most cases this is a result of early vein graft or internal mammary artery occlusion.

Graft Occlusion

Early graft occlusion (within the first week) is a result of thrombosis, and occurs in 10–15% of cases. It results from poor runoff or technical difficulty with the anastamosis, factors that predispose to adhesion of platelets. The incidence can be dramatically decreased by the administration of aspirin 325 mg daily given immediately *after* operation via nasogastric tube. Aspirin given before operation increases bleeding and the number of reoperations required to control bleeding.

Three years after operation only 65% of venous grafts are patent. Late occlusion is a result of intimal hyperplasia, which is probably caused by damage inflicted to the wall by high arterial pressure. Internal mammary grafting appears to be the surgeons choice for treating proximal left anterior descending lesions.

Unstable Angina Pectoris (Preinfarction Angina, Acute Coronary Insufficiency, Crescendo Angina, Impending Myocardial Infarction)

Unstable angina pectoris is characterized by the sudden, recent onset of recurrent angina, or a dramatic recent change in pattern of established angina. The term should not be used to describe the quite common variations in angina with weather, amount of activity, and so on that commonly occur as described in the previous section. Attacks of unstable angina usually last more than 15 minutes, occur more than twice daily, are provoked by minimal activity, and also occur at rest. Among individuals with stable angina pectoris the occurrence of anemia, arrhythmias, infection, thyrotoxicosis, hypertension, or hypotension may cause angina to become unstable. In the typical case of unstable angina pectoris, however, the condition manifests itself in the absence of the aforementioned precipitating clinical factors.

Pathophysiology

It seems likely that the onset of unstable angina is initiated by rupture of an atheromatous plaque. Within the plaque varying degrees of hemorrhage and thromboses are evident. Aggregation of platelets on the plaque precedes formation of thrombus. It is not known why the plaque ruptures, but when it occurs myocardial ischemia is induced.

Thrombosis plays an important role in the pathogenesis of unstable angina. Thrombus is frequently found in pathologic specimens and may be observed angiographically. Fibrinolysis of the thrombus may account for resolution of unstable angina.

Prognosis

The natural history of unstable angina has not been clearly delineated but the mortality is significantly higher than that of the stable variety where the death rate is about 4% per year and the incidence of myocardial infarction about 5% per year. Some studies with clearly defined criteria for unstable angina indicate an incidence of myocardial infarction of approximately 25% and a mortality rate of approximately 15% within 1 year of onset. It is possible that unstable angina may be more common than generally realized, because many patients with acute myocardial infarction experience premonitory symptoms suggestive of unstable angina within 2 months prior to the event.

Myocardial infarction is most likely to occur within the first few hours of the onset of unstable angina. After 3 months the incidence is much the same as for patients with stable angina.

Clinical Presentation

The typical presentation is one onset of new angina, or aggravation of previous angina. The attacks are more frequent, more severe, longer, and may not be relieved by nitroglycerin. The electrocardiogram does not show new Q waves, but ST segment depression and T wave depression are common during pain, with ST segment elevation occurring less frequently. Findings are frequently transitory and every effort should be made to obtain a record during pain. Changes may also be observed in the absence of pain—indicative of "silent ischemia." Serum enzymes are normal.

Treatment

At least 75% of patients will respond to medical treatment of unstable angina in a coronary care unit. The efficacy of aspirin has been proved beyond doubt. Given in a dose of 325 mg daily, there is a 50% reduction in the death rate, and incidence of nonfatal myocardial infarction from 3 months to years after the initial episode. There is evidence to suggest that heparin may also be efficacious. Calcium channel and β-blockers are frequently used, but their efficacy is not as well established as aspirin. Intravenous nitroglycerin is frequently effective in relieving pain, and morphine should be used as required.

Patients who do not respond to initial medical therapy should have coronary angiography to assess the feasibility of surgical revascularization or PTCA. In high-risk patients (i.e. those with left ventricular dysfunction and two- or three-vessel disease), it is likely that the outcome is more favorable with revascularization. If the patient improves with initial therapy, decisions regarding subsequent invasive intervention can be more circumspect, and involve all those considerations previously discussed for patients with stable angina pectoris.

Prinzmetal's or Variant Angina

Angina not clearly related to exercise or stress, associated with transient elevation of the ST segments on EKG that return to normal with subsidence of the pain, is known as Prinzmetal's angina. In this author's experience the condition is rare. Although the pain is unrelated to effort or emotion, the quality is similar to that of the usual form of angina, and is promptly relieved by sublingual nitroglycerin. During the episode there are impressive electrocardiographic changes that include marked ST segment elevation much like that occurring during a typical transmural myocardial infarction. These changes are frequently observed in the inferior leads because of the frequency of involvement of the right coronary artery. The electrocardiographic abnormalities have also been noted to occur spontaneously without subjective sensation of pain among patients with variant angina. Ventricular arrhythmias and temporary A-V block may also occur.

The pathogenesis of Prinzmetal's angina is undoubtedly related to coronary spasm, which may be visualized by coronary angiography either occurring spontaneously, or provoked by the intravenous injection of ergonovine malleate. This drug should be used only when the coronary arteries are angiographically normal, or near normal, because of the danger of inducing myocardial infarction. Coronary spasm occurs with equal frequency with angiographically normal coronary arteries with fixed obstructive lesions. The cause of coronary artery spasm is unknown, but could be a result of α-adrenergic stimulation, or a deficiency of endothelial relaxant factor.

The management of variant angina is with nitrates and calcium channel blockers. Both classes of drugs are coronary vasodilators and the effects may be additive. They produce a striking reduction in the frequency of episodes of pain.

In those patients with variant angina and angiographically normal coronary arteries, β-blockers and aspirin may actually aggravate the condition. The deleterious effect of β-blockers is through unopposed α-adrenergic induced vasoconstriction; that of aspirin is through inhibition of the coronary vasodilator prostaglandin I_2.

The prognosis for patients with variant angina is not clear. Before the advent of calcium channel blockers, sudden death, myocardial infarction, and dysrhythlnias were frequent. Calcium channel blockers are so effective in reducing the attack rate that it is likely that the prognosis is much the same as that for stable angina pectoris.

"Silent" Myocardial Ischemia

Among patients with coronary atherosclerosis, not all episodes of acute myocardial ischemia are accompanied by angina. Some patients never experience pain despite clear evidence of myocardial ischemia, and up to one-fourth of patients suffering acute myocardial infarction do not experience pain. Silent ischemia may be detected during an exercise test or by Holter electrocardiography. ST segment depression detected during 24-hour Holter recording signifies myocardial ischemia. This has been confirmed by studies of myocardial perfusion (positron emission tomography and exercise thallium studies) and by hemodynamic monitoring.

Obviously, most episodes of silent ischemia have been detected in patients with stable angina pectoris because this population is more likely to be investigated. The frequently in the rest of the population is unknown. Whether silent ischemia is more common in diabetics is still the subject of debate. Episodes of ischemia are more frequent shortly after awakening in the early morning, the time at which there is the peak incidence of acute myocardial infarction. Most episodes occur with a normal heart rate. Episodes may also be induced by mental stress or smoking.

Among patients with clinically manifest ischemic heart disease, episodes of ST segment depression, whether painful or painless, have the same prognosis. As such, patients with episodes of silent ischemia should be treated in the same way as patients with stable angina pectoris, and they will respond to the same antianginal medication. When silent ischemia is detected in patients without other manifest evidence of ischemic heart disease, management is more problematic. Such patients may be discovered, for example, when Holter recordings are used for detection of arrhythmias. Subsequent evaluation will likely depend first on results of risk factor assessment and noninvasive testing. Therapy designed to decrease the frequency or duration of episodes of silent ischemia in such patients appears attractive but studies supporting efficacy are lacking.

Myocardial Infarction

Pathology

Myocardial infarction is necrosis of heart muscle caused by prolonged ischemia. Although atherosclerosis is invariably present, the occurrence of acute coronary occlusion by thrombosis is often the precipitating acute event. Sudden total occlusion of a vessel can cause transmural infarction (i.e. involving the entire thickness of the ventricle). If arterial occlusion is subtotal or recanalization occurs early, or there is some collateral flow, damage may be limited to the subendocardium. The subendocardium is more "at risk" for infarction because myocardial perfusion is from epicardium to endocardium by penetrating branches of the main epicardial coronary arteries. Although subendocardial infarction has been associated with non-Q wave infarction by EKG (and Q waves with transmural infarction) this clinical pathologic correlate has not held up to close scrutiny.

Myocardial infarction is usually restricted to the left ventricle, but in approximately one-third of patients with inferior myocardial infarction there is involvement of the right ventricle. Isolated right ventricular infarction occurs in about 3% of cases of myocardial infarction at autopsy, usually in patients with pulmonary hypertension and right ventricular hypertrophy.

The *location* of the infarction depends on the vessel involved. Occlusion of the left anterior descending coronary artery results in infarction of the anterior wall, ventricular septum, lateral wall, and anterolateral papillary muscle. Occlusion of a dominant right coronary artery results in infarction of the inferoposterior wall, inferior septum, and posteromedial papillary muscle; the same region would be affected when the circumflex coronary artery happens to be dominant and the right coronary artery congenitally small. The extent of the infarction depends on the blood supply (if any) from collateral circulation and the amount of myocardium at risk, which of course is greatest when an occlusion is proximal.

Angiography early in the course of acute transmural myocardial infarction has shown occlusion of approximately 90% of infarct-related vessels by thrombus. Thrombosis appears to be the final event following plaque rupture, platelet adhesion, and coronary vasospasm. Recanalization can occur due to spontaneous thrombolysis, and this increases in frequency with time.

In the early stages of acute infarction the gross and histological appearances of the myocardium may be normal, even though electrocardiographic and enzymatic evidence of myocardial infarction is irrefutable. Following the initial stages of necrosis there is leukocytic infiltration of the involved area, followed by removal of muscle fibers. Muslce fiber removal leads to thinning of the myocardium and, after 3 weeks, scar formation is evident.

During the first week following myocardial infarction, *rupture of the heart* with hemopericardium is a major cause of mortality. Rupture of the free wall is strictly a complication of transmural infarction and usually occurs at the periphery adjacent to healthy muscle. Rupture may also, however, involve the ventricular septum and the papillary muscles.

Mural thrombus may develop on the endocardium of the infarct and is a potential source for systemic emboli. Thrombus as a result of stasis may also occur at the apex of the left ventricle when there has been heart failure.

Overlying an area of transmural infarction, *pericarditis* is a frequent complication. This is of the fibrinous variety, and is without serious complications until organization occurs. Rarely, there will be rupture of friable vessels in epicardial/pericardial granulation tissue leading to hemorrhage and tamponade. The risk of hemorrhagic pericarditis is greater among patients who have received anticoagulant drugs.

The amount of damage from myocardial infarction is quite variable, and can be graded angiographically. In addition to determining the size and location of the injury, the severity of resultant muscle dysfunction can be graded as mild, moderate, or severe hypokinesis, akinesis (no movement with systole), dyskinesis (bulging with systole), or aneurysm (bulging even in diastole).

Aneurysm formation may complicate the acute and late stages of myocardial infarction. In the usual instance, the wall of an aneurysm is composed of elements of infarcted left ventricular myocardium and represents bulging of a weakened wall. There is a gradual widening of the left ventricular cavity and thinning of the left ventricular wall in the area of the aneurysm. Residual muscle fibers can usually be identified even in those cases where the wall consists predominantly of fibrous tissue. By definition, therefore, this common type of left ventricular aneurysm is a *true* aneurysm. These aneurysms are frequently lined by mural thrombus. Rupture of a true aneurysm is rare because there is adequate fibrous tissue, and there is a buttressing effect of the thickened pericardium.

Uncommonly, myocardial infarction may be complicated by the formation of a *false* aneurysm (Figs. 17.3 and 17.4). In contrast to a true aneurysm, a false aneurysm is a thin-walled fibrous sac in which myocardial elements cannot be identified. They are frequently saccular, sharply demarcated from the wall of the left ventricle, and have small ostia. These aneurysms are essentially organized pericardial hematomata that result from rupture of the left ventricular wall. Prior to rupture, a pericaridal reaction overlying the infarcted area is sufficient to prevent a free escape of blood into the pericardial space: The contained pericardial hemorrhage subsequently organizes to produce a fibrous-walled aneurysm. Understandably, these aneurysms tend to occur early in the course of myocardial infarction and, unlike true aneurysms, have a great propensity for rupture.

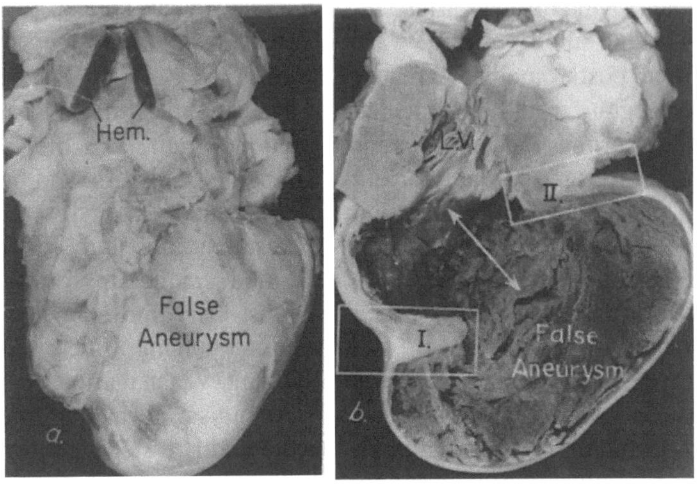

FIGURE 17.3. False post-infarction aneurysm. (a) External view of the heart. There is a prominence of anterolateral aspect of the left ventricle produced by a false aneurysm. Contained in the pericardial adhesions of the base of the heart is an encapsulated hematoma (HEM). (b) coronal section through the heart. The junction between the infarcted region of the left ventricle and the aneurysm is indicated by the arrows. Rupture of the cardiac wall is evident within each rectangular area. Reprinted, with permission, from Chesler E, et al.: False aneurysms of the left ventricle following myocardial infarction. Am J Cardiol 23:76, 1969.

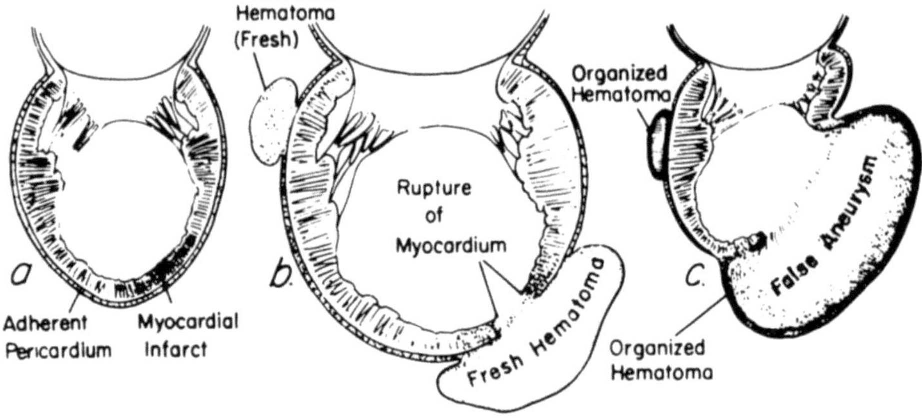

FIGURE 17.4. Diagrammatic representation of the pathogenesis of the false aneurysm in Figure 17.3. In the initial stage of myocardial infarction (a) there are adhesions of the pericardium over the left ventricle. In (b) rupture of the left ventricular wall produces a hematoma communicating with the left ventricular cavity and also a localized pericardial hematoma at the base of the heart. (c) The state in which the fresh hematoma has become organized to form a false aneurysm while the edges of the perforation of the left ventricle have retracted; the localized pericardial hematoma has become organized. Reprinted, with permission; from Chesler E, et al.: Am J Cardiol 21:72, 1968.

Clinical Presentation

Myocardial infarction usually presents as a sudden acute incident in an apparently normal subject, more frequently at rest than during effort. Occasionally, surgery, trauma, hemorrhage, or almost any cause of hypotension can be precipitating factors. Although most cases are apparently unheralded, careful questioning will occasionally elicit a history of premonitory vague ill-health, dyspnea, new unstable angina, or conversion from stable to unstable angina. Early awareness of these worsening prodromes is important in the prevention of early sudden deaths in myocardial infarction.

Pain

This usually dominates the picture. The quality and description are the same as for angina, but are more severe in myocardial infarction, lasting more than 30 minutes and frequently persisting for hours. It may be so intense that it is unresponsive to large doses of morphine. It is continuous and crushing in nature, and is frequently accompanied by restlessness, and vasomotor symptoms such as sweating, faintness, vomiting, and abdominal distension.

Shock

This is manifest clinically by hypotension, clammy, moist skin, agitation, confusion, and, in some instances, unconsciousness. Evidence of metabolic acidosis may be present in advanced cases.

Acute Pulmonary Edema

This may dominate the picture so that pain is obscured by the respiratory distress. The onset of dyspnea may be sudden with cough, hemoptysis, and frothy sputum in severe cases.

Cerebrovascular Syndrome

Hemiplegia is the most common manifestation of compromised cerebral blood flow, but symptoms of vertebrobasilar insufficiency may also occur. Cerebrovascular manifestations occurring at the onset, or early after myocardial infarction, are usually a result of reduced cerebral perfusion in patients with concomitant cerebral atherosclerosis, whereas hemiplegia occurring later is usually a result of embolism from left ventricular mural thrombosis.

Silent Infarction

Painless cardiac infarction undoubtedly occurs, but the frequency is in dispute. The presence of old and even recent infarction without a history of pain is recognized fairly frequently on routine electrocardiography. Some studies indicate a 30% incidence of silent myocardial infarction. Certain reservations, however, are still in order. Symptoms may be present, but misinterpreted as gastrointestinal in origin, or chest cold, or even denied altogether. During an actual attack, pain may be overshadowed by shock, syncope, or pulmonary edema. Following recovery, complete amnesia for pain may be present.

Physical Examination

Physical examination reveals a patient in severe pain who is restless and sweating. When shock dominates the picture, the patient is listless, prostrate, with a gray, ashen color, and there are signs of peripheral circulatory failure, such as cyanosis, mottled skin, and cold extremities. Episodes of unconsciousrless may be a result of vasovagal disturbance in response to pain and fear, a Stokes–Adams attack, or profound shock. When left ventricular failure is dominant the patient is propped up, dyspneic, and coughing up frothy blood-stained sputum.

Jugular Venous Pressure

Mild distension is often present initially, but usually subsides unless frank congestive failure supervenes. A positive Kussmaul sign is an important clue to the diagnosis of right ventricular infarction: The typical findings in right ventricular infarction include (1) transmural inferior or posterior myocardial infarction, (2) normal lung fields clinically and radiologically, and (3) right ventricular third or fourth heart sounds.

Pulses

The rate is rapid in the presence of heart failure and is difficult to palpate when shock and associated vasoconstriction are present. Arrhythmia of any type may occur.

Blood Pressure

Except in shock, the blood pressure is usually maintained or even high initially, but may fall to very low levels after a day or two, even in previously hypertensive patients. After a week or two, there is a gradual return to normal. Occasionally, in hypertensive patients the blood pressure is permanently reduced to normal. This is not necessarily due to massive infarction of the left ventricle, or associated with signs and symptoms of reduced cardiac output. It is most likely a result of a permanent fall in the peripheral vascular resistance.

The Heart

In the absence of hypertension or congestive failure the heart size is normal but dyskinetic areas may be palpable. The heart sounds are normal in intensity except when there is hypotension, when they are soft. A presystolic gallop rhythm is almost invariable, but an audible third sound is less frequent. A pericardial friction rub is heard in about a sixth of the cases, irrespective of the site of infarction. It occurs a few days after the infarction, is characteristically transient, and often lasts for only a few hours. If the rub persists for several days, or disappears and then recurs, a false aneurysm or the postmyocardial infarction syndrome should be suspected.

General Findings

Fever is mild, to at most moderate, occurring within 1 to 2 days and lasting a few days. Rarely, high fever (105°F) and prolonged pyrexia occur, usually with an extensive infarction. Recrudescence, or persistence of fever suggests the postmyocardial infarction syndrome. Leukocytosis is usually moderate, beginning within a few hours and subsiding within a few days. The *sedimentation rate* does not rise until the second or third day and remains elevated for several weeks.

Glycosuria usually indicates associated diabetes, but occasionally may be transient ("stress diabetes"). Carbohydrate metabolism may return to normal only after 3 months.

When there is marked reduction in the cardiac output, arterial and tissue hypoxia produce *metabolic acidosis* with resultant increase in the blood lactate concentration. Sympathetic stimulation during infarction causes increased blood and urinary concentrations of epinephrine, norepinephrine, and their breakdown products. Shortly after myocardial infarction the plasma concentrations of cholesterol and triglycerides drop precipitously, and preinfarction levels may be reached only 3 months later.

Diagnosis

The clinical diagnosis is confirmed by the electrocardiographic changes and enzyme studies.

The Electrocardiogram

This may be normal if obtained very early after the onset of infarction. When abnormal Q waves develop they generally do so within a few days, whereas T wave inversion may be delayed for a few days to several weeks. Daily tracings are required to detect serial changes. When systematically performed, the EKG signs at infarction are found in approximately 80% of cases. Nonspecific ST-T wave changes must be interpreted with caution because they may be a result of coincidental hypertension or other forms of heart disease. Conduction defects, such as left bundle branch block, or the presence of a permanently implanted pacemaker, may also obscure the diagnosis. Additionally, the electrocardiograms of the Wolff–Parkinson–White syndrome, pulmonary emphysema, left anterior hemiblock, and severe left ventricular hypertrophy are characterized by very poor, or absent R waves in the anterior precordial leads, findings that closely mimic the pattern of anterior myocardial infarction. The following patterns are commonly encountered:

1. *Q wave infarction.* Significant Q waves with T wave inversions anteriorly (leads I, AVL, and precordial leads) or diaphragmatically (AVF, leads II and III).
2. *Non-Q wave infarction.* Persistent ST segment depression with T wave inversion in the left ventricular surface leads, and leads I and II, with elevation in AVR.
3. *Ischemic changes.* T wave inversion in the left ventricular surface leads, with or without ST segment change, which are less specific findings than (1) and (2).
4. *Bundle branch block.* Myocardial infarction is readily recognizable in the presence of right bundle branch block, but left bundle branch block often masks evidence of infarction.
5. *RV infarction.* Elevation of the ST segment in the right sided precordial leads may confirm RV infarction complicating cases of inferior infarct (Q-waves in II, III, and AVF).

Cardiac Enzymes in the Diagnosis of Acute Myocardial Infarction

The *serum glutamic oxalacetic transaminase (SGOT)* level becomes elevated within 8–12 hours of myocardial infarction, reaching a peak within 12 to 36 hours and persisting for 2 to 5 days. This test is positive in over 95% of cases of clinically evident myocardial infarction associated with pathological Q waves on the electrocardiogram. Unfortunately, the test is not very specific and congestive cardiac failure may be associated with raised levels, particularly in the presence of hepatic disease. Myocarditis, paroxysmal tachycardia, dissecting aneurysm, pancreatitis, liver disease, and skeletal muscle disease are other causes of elevated levels. For these reasons it is no longer a routine measurement.

Creatinine Phosphokinase (CPK)

Elevated levels appear in the serum within 6 hours, reach a peak within 24 hours, and return to normal 4 days after myocardial infarction. The total serum CPK activity can also be elevated by skeletal muscle damage produced by intramuscular injection, alcoholic intoxication, and convulsions, so isoenzymes are used to be more specific for myocardial damage. The MB isoenzyme is found largely in cardiac muscle, although smaller amounts are found in skeletal muscle. Cardiac operations, PTCA, and cardioversion with more than 400 J may increase the level. Only extensive damage to skeletal muscle, usually readily evident clinically (e.g., severe crush injuries, rhabdomyolisis, hypothermia) will elevate the MB fraction. In the appropriate clinical setting, therefore, elevation of the MB fraction above four units usually indicates myocardial necrosis.

Lactic Acid Dehydrogenase (LDH)

This appears after 24 hours and reaches a peak 3 to 6 days following an infarct. Elevated levels may persist for up to 14 days. It is most useful, therefore, in patients seen late (more than 48 hours) following the onset of chest pain. Total LDH activity is increased in hemolysis, blood dyscrasia, pulmonary infraction, and various forms of liver disease as well, so it is quite nonspecific. There are five LDH isoenzymes, but heart muscle contains a preponderance of LDH1. Thus, elevation of LDH1 or an LDH1/LDH2 ratio of more than 1 in the absence of hemolysis is presumptive evidence of infarction.

In general, the magnitude of rise of serum enzymes (particulary CPK) correlates with the extent of myocardial necrosis, but this is difficult to apply to an individual patient. Among patients with subendocardial infarction where there is minimal elevation of the serum enzymes, a good prognosis does not necessarily apply since it is now known that patients with an uncompleted infarct are at high risk for a subsequent fatal event.

Echocardiography

Two-dimensional echocardiography is a useful diagnostic tool in evaluating patients with confirmed or suspected myocardial infarction. It provides a useful estimate of overall left ventricular function and detects abnormalities of wall movement. It is more sensitive and spe-

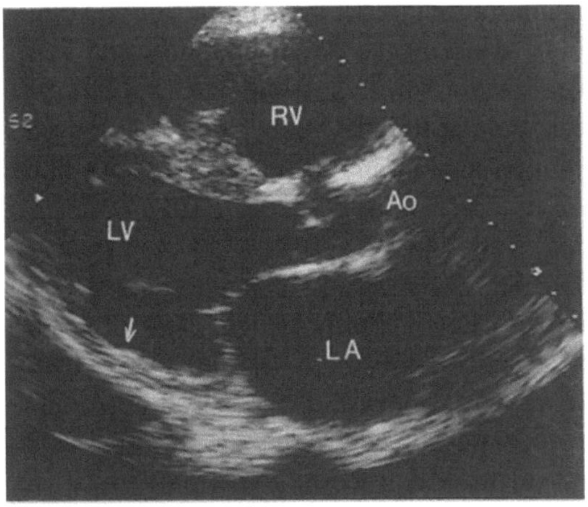

FIGURE 17.5. Two-dimensional echocardiogram showing inferior myocardial infarction and left atrial enlargement.

cific for detecting anterior, as compared to inferior myocardial infarction (Fig. 17.5). Importantly, it rapidly excludes pericarditis and other conditions such as aortic dissection that mimic myocardial infarction. It can also be used to help diagnose mural thrombus, present in up to 50% of anterior transmural infarcts.

Radionuclide Techniques

These are rarely required and are expensive. Technetium-99 pyrophosphate (TCPP) is taken up by infarcted myocardium as a "hot spot." Scans using this tracer are usually positive 1 to 3 days after infarction. In the occasional late case, where enzyme changes are inconclusive, echocardiography is technically unsatisfactory, and electrocardiography is difficult to interpret (e.g., bundle branch block), TCPP scanning may be useful.

Differential Diagnosis

Pulmonary Embolism

When there is occlusion of the peripheral branches of the pulmonary artery, pain is usually pleuritic, associated with hemoptysis and a pleural rub—the diagnosis is therefore relatively easy. When the main pulmonary arteries are involved, however, the pain may be indistinguishable from that of myocardial infarction. Dyspnea is the most frequent and outstanding symptom of massive pulmonary embolism, occurring suddenly and without pulmonary congestion. The electrocardiogram, serum enzymes, and radioactive lung scan are most helpful in diagnosis, but occasionally pulmonary angiography may be required.

Pericarditis

The pain frequently differs from that of myocardial infarction in that it is made worse by coughing, deep breathing, swallowing, and extension of the neck. Early detection of a pericardial friction rub, slowly resolving ST elevation with domed ST segments on the electrocardiogram, and absence of a significant rise in the serum enzyme changes help confirm this diagnosis.

Dissecting Aneurysm

The pain is usually acute and tearing and reaches an early crescendo. Back pain radiating down the legs and loss of peripheral pulses are suggestive clinical features. Electrocardiographic changes are usually absent. Roentgenography of the chest may reveal widening of the nediastinum. Echocardiography, aortic angiography, computerized tomography, or nuclear magnetic resonance imaging will establish the diagnosis. It should be remembered that dissection can, on rare occasion, involve the right coronary ostia and produce concomitant myocardial infarction.

Spontaneous Pneumothorax

Sudden onset of unilateral chest pain associated with severe dyspnea are the usual presenting features. Crunching systolic sounds in the involved side of the chest and decreased breath sounds, and the radiological findings are diagnostic.

Spinal and Chest Conditions

Spondylitis, cervical disc, herpes zoster, pleurisy, diaphraglnatic hernia, Bornholm disease, and Tieteze syndrome may all simulate myocardial infarction. Mediastinitis resulting from rupture of the esophagus may be diagnosed clinically by the detection of crepitus in the subcutaneous tissues of the neck and over the anterior chest wall. This diagnosis can be confirmed by chest roentgenography demonstrating the presence of mediastinal air. Muscular disorders of the thorax and shoulder, bursitis, arthritis, and tendonitis may occasionally cause confusion.

Abdominal Conditions

Peptic ulcer, acute cholecystitis, acute pancreatitis, and incarceration of a diaphragmatic hernia may produce a confusing clinical picture, but the electrocardiogram is usually the most helpful distinguishing feature. Rarely, electrocardiographic findings of ischemia and even of infarction have been found in acute pancreatitis without cardiac involvement at necropsy. Enzyme changes, particularly the CPK-MB, are of great value.

Anxiety states and functional disorders are a very frequent cause of chest pain but a carefully taken history combined with an electrocardiogram will lead to the correct diagnosis.

Shock and Syncope

If a patient presents in shock, distinction must be made from acute surgical emergencies and other causes of acute peripheral circulatory failure produced by blood loss, sepsis, torsion, bowel obstruction, or perforation of an abdominal viscus. Syncope may be caused by an arrhythmia, and in some cases the arrhythmia may be due to acute myocardial infarction. Myocardial infarction should be considered if patients presenting with significant supraventricular or ventricular tachyarrhythmias, or with advanced degrees of heart block even if syncope is not a component of the history.

Course and Complications

Shock

Cardiogenic shock exists when cardiac output is inadequate to maintain normal organ perfusion. Additional hemodynamic findings include elevation of left ventricular filling pressure (measured as the left ventricular end-diastolic or the pulmonary artery wedge pressure) and low systolic blood pressure (less than 90 mm Hg). Urinary output is diminished (less than 20 ml/hour), and there are often signs of impaired cerebral perfusion such as confusion, agitation, or even coma. Clammy, moist skin and metabolic acidosis are frequent accompanying features. The prognosis for cardiogenic shock is extremely poor despite the most active medical therapy, with a mortality rate of 80 to 95%.

Rupture of the Heart

This occurs in approximately 8% of patients dying of myocardial infarction and is a cause of sudden death, or of shock unresponsive to treatment. Usually, rupture supervenes on the third or fourth day following the onset of myocardial infarction and is more common among women. The most common variety of rupture involves the free wall of the left ventricle and fatal hemopericardium is the result. The usual site of rupture is at the periphery of the infarct, adjacent to healthy muscle, which suggests that the tear is the result of a shearing action. There are no physical signs or electrocardiographic findings that predict impending rupture.

Rupture of the Venticular Stepum

This can occur with either anterior or inferior infarction and results in sudden heart failure. A loud systolic murmur provides clinical evidence of the condition, but can be confused with acute mitral insufficiency. The prospect for survival is poor even with aggressive medical and surgical treatment.

Rupture of a Papillary Muscle

When one of the heads of a papillary muscle ruptures, acute massive mitral insufficiency ensues, and the outlook is determined by the magnitude of the infarct involving the left ventricular wall. When left ventricular function is reasonable, these patients are candidtates for prosthetic valve replacement. Rupture of the entire body of the papillary muscle is incompatiable with survival.

The clinical distinction between rupture of the ventricular septum and a papillary muscle may be difficult. In both conditions a systolic murmur may be audible at the left sternal border. A Swan-Ganz catheter placed in the pulmonary artery will detect a rise in oxygen saturation in the case of ruptured venticular septum but not in the case of mitral insufficiency. Doppler-echocardiography with color flow is invaluable in making the distinction.

Acute Pulmonary Edema

If damage is extensive, pulmonary edema usually supervenes shortly after the acute episode of myocardial infarction. It is frequently associated with shock, and is often fatal. Shortness of breath may be a presenting symptom of acute infarction and, when severe, may obscure the characteristic pain. Significant arrhythmias are frequently associated.

Congestive Cardiac Failure

Mild left ventricular failure is frequently found early after infarction. It is best recognized by routine radiologic examination, which demonstrates upper-lobe pulmonary venous engorgement. Basal rales, gallop rhythm, and tachycardia are later manifestations. Secondary right heart failure occurs days later and indicates a worse prognosis. Chronic congestive failure often results, especially with repeated infarctions.

Arrhythmias

Almost any type of arrhythmia may be encountered, but ventricular premature systoles are the most frequent. Paroxysmal tachycardia, atrial fibrillation, and heart block occur frequently.

Embolism and Thrombosis

Systemic embolism arising from mural thrombus within the left ventricle is an occasional cause of sudden death. Usually cerebral embolism is the event of greatest clinical significance, but any systemic artery may be involved. Pulmonary embolism from peripheral venous thrombosis is a hazard in patients immobilized for prolonged periods.

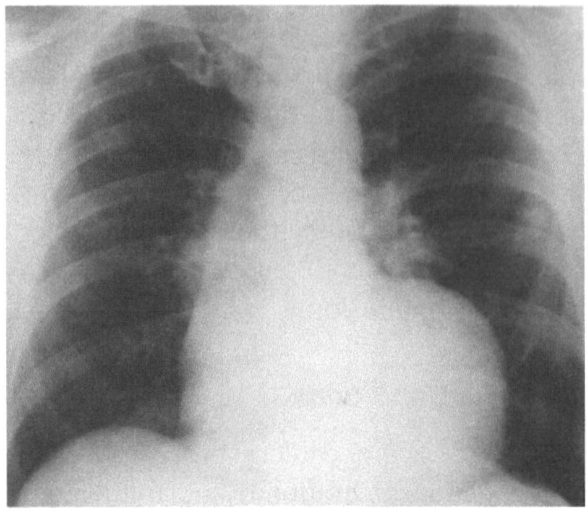

FIGURE 17.6. X-ray of the chest showing large post-infarction left ventricular aneurysm.

Left Ventricular Aneurysm

The presence of an aneurysm can often be suspected by precordial palpation, which detects a dyskinetic ectopic impulse. Persistent ST segment elevation is a suggestive electrocardiographic feature. Roentgenography frequently, but not invariably, demonstrates a bulge on the left cardiac border with calcification involving the wall of the aneurysm or its contained mural thrombus (Fig. 17.6). When more than 25% of the left ventricle is involved by an aneurysm, congestive cardiac failure is likely. Aneurysms can occasionally be the source of recurrent episodes of ventricular tachycardia.

When there is clinical suspicion of a left ventricular aneurysm, two-dimensional echocardiography can confirm the diagnosis, and left ventricular and coronary angiography should be considered. The information obtained will demonstrate whether there is sufficient left ventricular function to allow resection of the aneurysm, and also whether bypass grafting is required at the same procedure. Occasionally, the results of aneurysmectomy are gratifying, but in the many instances the cause of death is recurrent myocardial infarction or protracted congestive cardiac failure.

Postmyocardial Infarction (Dressler) Syndrome

This syndrome has been attributed to a hypersensitivity reaction in which necrotic cardiac muscle forms the antigen. The condition is allied to the postpericardiotomy syndrome. It usually has its onset 2 weeks after the initial episode of infarction, although it may be delayed for up to 3 months. Pericardial pain occurs and varies from a continuous dull ache to a severe crushing substernal pain radiating to the neck, shoulders, and arms. The temperature is usually elevated and undergoes gradual defervescence. A persistent pericardial friction rub is important evidence, and pleural effusion with pulmonary involvement is frequent. In rare instances, recurrent episodes of pericarditis occur over a period of months, or even years, causing considerable morbidity. The condition generally responds to conservative measures and salicylates. Occasionally, steroids are necessary but there is a danger of relapse when they are stopped, and there is also a risk of steroid dependency.

Prognosis

Although the association of Q wave infarction with transmural infarction and non-Q wave infarction with nontransmural infarction, respectively, is questionable, there are clinical correlates with development of Q waves that can be helpful.

Q Wave Infarction

Prognosis in the individual case is hazardous because the complications are unpredictable. At least one in three patients die during the acute attack. Of these, half are dead within 1 hour, two-thirds within 24 hours, and three-quarters by the first week. Thus, patients accommodated in hospital are a select group (having survived long enough to get there), and they have an average mortality of approximately 15%. If the patient survives an acute myocardial infarction the risk of suffering another infarct is eight times the normal risk, and more than 50% will die with repeated infarction.

Once a patient has survived 5 years after an acute attack without further incident, the natural life expectancy begins to approach that of the general population, matched for age and sex. The survival rate at 10 years is approximately 30%. Mortality increases with advancing age. The most important predictor of long-term mortality is global left ventricular function. The 1 year mortality is less than 5% when the ejection fraction is above 40%, but above 50% when the ejection fraction is 20% or less.

Arrhythmias occurring early in the course of myocardial infarction reflect electrical instability and if adequately treated do not necessarily carry an adverse long-term prognosis. Similarly, when it occurs early congestive cardiac failure is not as ominous prognostically as when it occurs late. The electrocardiographic changes are of limited prognostic help, but the development of left or right bundle branch block and complete heart block are unfavorable signs.

Non-Q Wave Infarction

Lack of Q waves usually indicates less myocardial necrosis, and left ventricular function is relatively well preserved. The immediate mortality is lower (8%), but there is a higher recurrence rate. Thus at 3 years the mortality is the same as that for Q wave infarction. Non-Q wave infarctions are also complicated by a higher incidence of postinfarction angina.

Treatment of Myocardial Infarction

Prehospital Care

The demonstrated success of the coronary care unit in preventing early electrical deaths shortly after the onset of myocardial infarction has led to the development of prehospital care. This has been provided in the form of mobile coronary care units, paramedic teams, and mobile ambulances operating from a base hospital. In some instances, the service has been provided by the local fire deparment, and in other communities by cooperating general practitioners. Because 20% of patients with acute myocardial infarction die within 2 hours, often before reaching a medical facility, and because the annual mortality from coronary artery disease in the United States is approximately 600,000, the costs involved both in terms of finance and effort are logistically justified. The services are less likely to impact on those deaths that are due to "pump failure" but can be clearly effective in those patients who suffer ventricular fibrillation. The two major difficulties in the institution of such a program are the delay in calling for help on the part of the victim and the expense of the program. Resuscitative measures provided by these various emergency teams certified in Advanced Cardiac Life Support (A.C.L.S.) include closed chest massage, endotracheal intubation, electrical defibrillation/cardioversion, intravenous antiarrhythmias, analgesics, or sympathomimetric as indicated by the patient's clinical status and cardiac rhythm.

Hospital Care

Ideally, the victims of myocardial infarction should be admitted directly to a coronary care unit, thus avoiding the administrative delays characteristic of the admissions department of most general hospitals.

The Uncomplicated Case

This includes those patients who are (1) hemodynamically stable with a systolic blood pressure above 100 mm Hg, (2) have no evidence of pulmonary edema, and (3) are electrically stable in sinus rhythm.

Oxygen

This should be given routinely since most patients have mild to moderate degrees of hypoxia because of ventilation–perfusion mismatch. Hypoxia predisposes to dysrhythmias and is also associated with larger sizes of infarctions.

Nitroglycerin

Nitrates are often helpful in relieving pain because they are coronary vasodilators and also decrease left ventricular preload. There is evidence that they reduce infarct size, and therefore the mortality of acute myocardial infarction. Nitroglycerin should be given cautiously to patients with inferior myocardial infarction because it may produce, or aggravate hypotension and/or bradycardia. Nitrates should not be given at all to patients with right ventricular infarction because of their extreme sensitivity to a decrease in right ventricular preload.

Sublingual nitroglycerin is given in doses of 0.2 to 0.6 mg. Should pain persist the drug may be given intravenously, starting at an infusion rate of 10 μg/min, increasing by 10 μg every 5–10 minutes until pain disappears or until there is a significant decrease in systolic blood pressure (at least 10%, but not below 95 mm Hg). The maximum dose is 200 μg/min. Nitrates cannot be expected to relieve all pain if there is ongoing myocardial necrosis, and analgesics should be added as needed.

Analgesia

Morphine remains the drug of choice and should be given i.v. in doses of 2–5 mg every 30 minutes until pain is controlled. The drug not only relieves pain and anxiety but also reduces preload and afterload. The most common side-effects are nausea and vomiting. Occasionally, it results in hypotension and bradycardia, effects that may be relieved by i.v. fluids and atropine.

Thrombolytic Therapy

Occlusion of a coronary artery by thrombus leads to progressive myocardial necrosis within 20 to 30 minutes. Approximately 60% of patients show evidence of acute coronary occlusion (ST segment elevation) on admission to a hospital (Fig. 17.7). Numerous trials have demonstrated that early thrombolysis-induced reperfusion reduces infarct size and decreases mortality. The most striking benefit is seen in patients under the age of 65 with early extensive anterior myocardial infarction. Based on recommendations of the American College of Cardiology and the American Heart Association (Patients without Contraindications to Thrombolytic Therapy: Recommendations for Administration of Thrombolytic Therapy

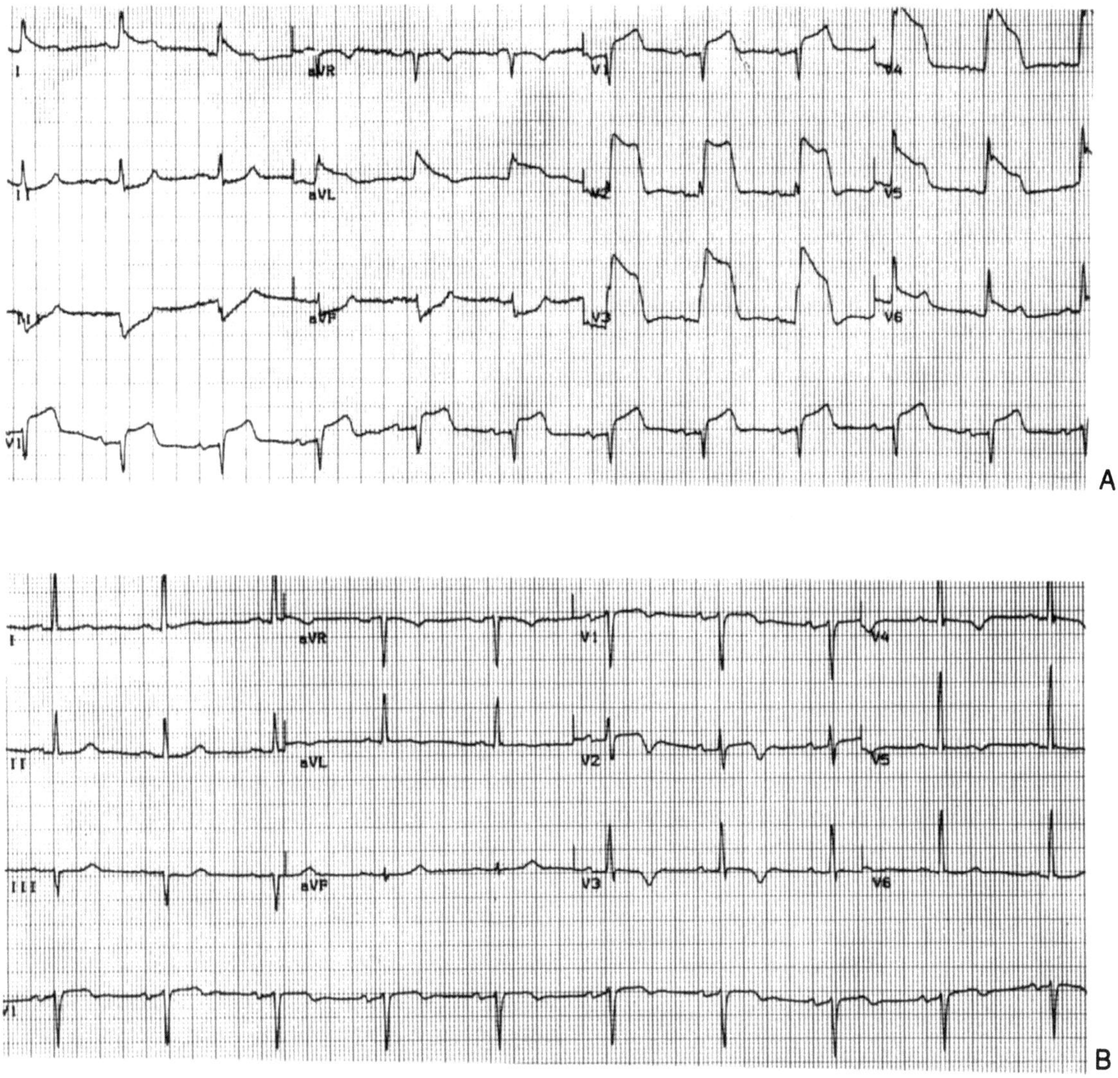

FIGURE 17.7. EKGs in hyperacute myocardial infarction before lytic therapy (A) and 1 hour later (B).

to Patients with Myocardial Infarction) the following are the indications and contraindications for treatment:

Class I: Usually indicated, always acceptable, and considered effective:

1. Patients less than 70 years of age who present with chest pain consistent with the diagnosis of acute myocardial infarction and at least 0.1 mV of ST segment elevation in at least two contiguous ECG leads in whom treatment can be initiated within 6 hours of pain onset.

Class IIa: Weight of evidence in favor of usefulness/efficacy:

1. Patients between 70 and 75 years who present with chest pain consistent with the diagnosis of acute myocardial infarction and at least 0.1 mV of ST segment elevation in at least two contiguous ECG leads in whom treatment can be initiated within 6 hours of pain onset.
2. Patients with acute myocardial infarction more than 6 hours after symptom onset, but with a "stuttering" pattern of pain.

3. Patients who suffer clinically apparent reinfarction in the days after administration of thrombolytic therapy.

Class IIb: Not well established by evidence, may be helpful and probably not harmful:

1. Patients who present with chest pain consistent with the diagnosis of acute myocardial infarction and at least 0.1 mV of ST segment elevation in at least two contiguous EGC leads in whom treatment can be initiated between 6 and 24 hours after pain onset.
2. Patients more than 75 years of age who present with chest pain consistent with the diagnosis of acute myocardial infarction and at least 0.1 mV of ST segment elevation in at least two continguous ECG leads in whom treatment can be initiated within 6 hours of pain onset where the impending infarction is extensive.
3. Patients who present with chest pain consistent with the diagnosis of acute myocardial infarction with ECG changes less profound than 0.1 mV of ST segment elevation in two contiguous leads who can be treated within 24 hours.

Class III: Not indicated, may be harmful: Patients who have had chest pain when

1. Treatment cannot be initiated within 24 hours of onset of chest pain and pain has not recurred.
2. Chest pain onset is known and has receded.
3. The cause of the chest pain is unclear.

Contraindications to thrombolytic therapy: The major side-effect of all thrombolytic agents is hemorrhage. The contraindications to thrombolytic therapy include the following: Absolute Contraindications:

1. Active internal bleeding.
2. Suspected aortic dissection.
3. Prolonged or traumatic cardiopulmonary resuscitation.
4. Recent head trauma or known intracranial neoplasm.
5. Diabetic hemorrhagic retinopathy or other hemorrhagic ophthalmic condition.
6. Pregnancy.
7. Previous allergic reaction to the thrombolytic agent (streptokinase or APSAC).
8. Recorded blood pressure greater than 200/120 mm Hg.
9. History of cerebrovascular accident known to be hemorrhagic.

Relative Contraindications*:

1. Recent trauma or surgery more than 2 weeks; trauma or surgery more recent than 2 weeks, which could be a source of rebleeding, is an absolute contraindication.
2. History of chronic severe hypertension with or without drug therapy.
3. Active peptic ulcer.
4. History of cerebrovascular accident.
5. Known bleeding diathesis or current use of anticoagulants.
6. Significant liver dysfunction.
7. Prior exposure to streptokinase or APSAC (this contraindication is particularly important in the initial 6- to 9-month period after streptokinase or APSAC administration and applies to reuse of any streptokinase-containing agent, but does not apply to rt-PA or urokinase).

Thrombolytic Drugs

Streptokinase. This agent has enjoyed the largest experience. It should be given once only because of the potential for allergic reactions (human plasma contains antibodies to streptokinase). Despite lack of clot selectivity, bleeding is uncommon if invasive procedures are avoided. Another potential complication is hypotension when the drug is given rapidly. Anaphylactic reactions may occur in rare instances.

Compared to rt-PA the action of streptokinase is time dependent so that after 4 hours its efficacy has dropped to less than 30%. Importantly, it is approximately one-tenth the cost of rT-PA. The dose is 1.5 million units over 1 hour.

---

*From guidelines for the early management of patients with acute myocardial infarction. JACC 16:249–92, 1990. Reproduced with permission of American College of Cardiology.

Recombinent Tissue Plasmogen Activator (TPA). This drug is clot-selective and has more thrombolytic effect than streptokinase. The fibrinolytic effect of TPA is short because of its short half-life. It does not produce resistance, and does not induce hypotension or allergy. The dose is 60 mg in the first hour intubated with a 6 to 10 mg bolus, followed by 20 mg over the second and third hours.

Anisoylated Plasminogen Streptokinase Activator Complex (APSAC). This differs from its parent compound, streptokinase, in that the 30 mg dose is given as a single bolus of 5 units. Its duration of action is longer and there is a much smaller incidence of hypotension.

Complications of Thrombolysis

The leading complication is intracranial bleeding. With streptokinase the risk is 1 to 10 per 1000 patients and with rt-PA it is 5 to 10 per 1000.

Immediate Results of Thrombolytic Therapy

When rt-PA or streptokinase is given within 2 hours after the onset of pain, patency of the infarct-related artery will be restored in approximately 70% of cases. Thrombolysis restores patency but there is still the potential for platelet adhesion and recurrent thrombosis at the site of the ruptured plaque. Reocclusion occurs in 20% of cases. For these reasons, heparin is given in a bolus of 5000 units followed by 800 units hourly so that the activated partial thromboplastin time is prolonged to 1.5 to 2 times the control value. Aspirin is of proven benefit, and should be initiated immediately in a daily dose of 160 mg. Heparin should be stopped after 3–4 days, but aspirin may be continued indefinitely. Routine PTCA following successful thrombolysis of an infarct-related vessel has not improved outcome, and the risks of complication from the procedure are increased.

Antiplatelet and Anticoagulation Therapy

Heparin. Heparin can be considered, even when lytic therapy has not been used (patients presenting greater than 24 hours after pain for example). Low-dose subcutaneous heparin (5000 units every 12 hours) started within 8 hours of acute myocardial infarction and continued for 10 days reduces the incidence of deep vein thrombosis. The risk of deep vein thrombosis is higher in elderly patients and in those with congestive heart failure and cardiogenic shock.

High-Dose Subcutaneous Heparin. The incidence of left ventricular mural thrombus is increased among patients who are not anticoagulated. Heparin (12,500 units q12h) should be given as soon as possible to patients with large anteroseptal myocardial infarction and in patients with heart failure, and should be continued for at least 10 days. When echocardiography identifies a large area of dyskinesis (with or without thrombus) oral warfarin should be given for 3 months if there is no significant contraindication.

Aspirin. The incidence of early recurrence or extension of infarction may be significantly reduced by aspirin given in a dose of 160 to 325 mg daily. There is also convincing evidence that aspirin reduces the rate of reinfarction.

β-Blockers. Several studies have demonstrated that starting treatment intravenously and continuing orally for 2 to 3 years reduces the mortality from myocardial infarction. Those patients already receiving a β-blocker at the time of myocardial infarction should have the treatment continued in intravenous form. The intravenous route is also the preferred way of treating those patients who have continuing ischemia.

Those patients considered to have a good prognosis following myocardial infarction may not require long term β-blocker therapy because the adverse effects of treatment outweigh any small benefits. Included in this group are patients with single- or two-vessel disease, good left ventricular function, no dysrhythmia, and a negative stress test.

Contraindications to β-blockers include severe left ventricular failure, bronchospastic obstructive airways disease, heart rate less than 60 beats/min, systolic blood pressure less than 100 mm Hg, atrioventricular block, and clinical signs of peripheral circulatory failure. These drugs should be used with caution in brittle diabetics and patients receiving calcium channel blockers.

Commonly used preparations are

1. *Metropolol*: 15 mg is given i.v. slowly over 15 minutes followed by 50 mg orally q6h for 48 hours, and then changed to 100 mg b.i.d.
2. *Atenolol*: 5 mg is given i.v. over 5 minutes followed 10 minutes later by an additional 5 mg. This is followed in 10 minutes by 50 mg orally then 50 my 12 hours later. The maintenance dose is 100 mg daily.
3. *Esmolol*: This is a useful intravenous preparation whose effects are reversible in less than 10 minutes after stopping the infusion. The dose must be titrated to achieve the required hemodynamic and antidysrhythmic effects.

Calcium Channel Blockers

Unlike β-blockers these drugs do not reduce the mortality of acute myocardial infarction. They are, however, useful in the treatment of postinfarction angina.

Evaluation and Prognosis After Myocardial Infarction

Following recovery from relatively uncomplicated myocardial infarction certain clinical characteristics may point to an adverse long-term prognosis: (1) advanced age, (2) female gender, (3) hypertension, (4) diabetes, (5) cigarette smoking, (6) left ventricular dysfunction evidenced by cardiomegaly or clinical exam or X-ray, persistent S3 gallop, high levels of CK enzymes, or persistent atrial fibrillation.

Those of patients who leave the hospital free of the above indicators should be further assessed for the most important determinants of long-term survival (i.e., left ventricular dysfunction and evidence of myocardial ischemia).

Myocardial Ischemia

Most patients with uncomplicated myocardial infarction are discharged after 7 to 10 days. If exercise testing is employed before discharge, submaximal testing protocols should be used (5 mets on a modified Bruce or Naughton protocol).

A more cost-effective strategy is to use a symptom-limited maximal exercise test at 3 weeks in patients who are low risk by the aforementioned clinical indicators. This provides more prognostic information and a better assessment of residual functional physical capacity. Patients who are able to exercise beyond 7 mets (Stage Il of Bruce protocol) and achieve a double product of more than 20,000 have a 98% survival rate at 1 year. Those who have a positive test (1 mm of ST segment depression at less than 5 mets or at a double product of less than 20,000, or a drop in blood pressure of 15 mm Hg or more, or a 3 beat run of ventricular tachycardia, or develop angina) are candidates for coronary angiography. Ischemia at 5 mets signifies inability to carry out household activities and is a criterion used by Social Security Administration to determine cardiac disability.

When resting EKG abnormalities (left bundle branch block or ST wave abnormalities) make interpretation of stress electrocardiography difficult, an exercise radionuclide ventriculogram or thallium test is an alternative even though more expensive. Radionuclide ventriculography provides important information about left ventricular function (i.e., left ventricular ejection fraction at rest and end-systolic volume, at rest and with exercise). A drop in ejection fraction accompanied by a wall motion abnormality at a low double product signifies a large area of ischemic myocardium. Similarily, thallium will demonstrate a large area of reversible ischemia and pulmonary uptake when the left ventricle fails because of severe ischemia.

Management of Complicated Myocardial Infarction

Tachyarrhythmias

Atrial Dysrhythmias

Sinus tachycardia may be a result of pain, anxiety, hypovolemia, hypoxia, or left ventricular failure. Treatment should be directed at these causes. Intavenous β-blockers are useful provided there is no severe left ventricular failure.

The treatment of atrial flutter, fibrillation, and ectopic tachycardia depends on the clinical condition of the patient. When there is pulmonary edema, hypotension, and/or shock, cardioversion should not be delayed. Intravenous Digoxin is useful for converting atrial fibrillation and flutter or controlling the ventricular response to these dysrhythmias. Intravenous verapamil or intravenous β-blockers are used to control the ventricular response to atrial fibrillation provided there is no evidence of left ventricular failure. Intravenous procainamide may be used for cardioversion or for preventing recurrence of dysrhythmias.

Ventricular Dysrhythmias

Early

Ventricular Ectopy. This is almost universally present early in the course of acute myocardial infarction. When premature beats are frequent (more than 6/min) or exhibit the R on T phenomenon, or occur in runs of 3 or more successive beats and when multifocal, they may presage ventricular fibrillation. However, ventricular fibrillation occurs in 50–60% of cases without these "warning" dysrhythmias.

Lidocaine is effective in abolishing or controlling ventricular premature beats but evidence that it decreases in-hospital mortality is lacking. This is probably because electrical cardioversion of primary ventricular fibrillation in the coronary care unit is so effective. Lidocaine is usually given in an i.v. bolus of 1 mg/g up to a maximum of 100 mg, followed by an infusion of 1.5 to 3.5 mg/min.

Ventricular Tachycardia. This complicates up to·15% of cases of acute myocardial infarction and is frequently nonsustained. When sustained it is accompanied by shock and pulmonary congestion and requires immediate electrical cardioversion. In the more hemodynamically stable patient, lidocaine can be tried first.

Accelerated Idioventricular Rhythm. Usually the ventricular rate is less than 80 beats/min and there is no hemodynamic compromise. This dysrhythmia is usually transitory and does not require intervention.

Ventricular Fibrillation. Primary ventricular fibrillation is responsible for most of the deaths occurring in the first hour after the onset of acute myocardial infarction. Most episodes are correctable even before the patient reaches hospital. Resuscitation should follow an organized protocol (see p. 158). When ventricular fibrillation complicates congestive heart failure, follows prolonged hypotension, or complicates drug toxicity, the prognosis is much worse (secondary ventricular fibrillation). Prevention of ventricular dysrhythmias is of great importance. Electrolyte abnormalities, particularly hypokalemia, should be corrected. Alcohol abuse, malnutrition, diuretics, aminoglycosides, and cisplatin may produce hypomagnasemia and ventricular tachycardia. Two to four grams of magnesium sulphate should be infused intravenously to correct hypomagnasemia.

When ventricular tachycardia and ventricular fibrillation are recurrent, lidocaine should be infused; if this fails, intravenous procanamide should be substituted. Bretyllium tosylate is frequently effective in preventing recurrent ventricular fibrillation.

Late

Late in the course of myocardial infarction, and following discharge, couplets of ventricular premature beats and runs of nonsustained ventricular tachycardia, particularly when associated with left ventricular dysfunction, are predictors of increased risk for sudden death. Identifying such patients is not easy. Of the 5 to 15% of patients who die suddenly after discharge only one in four will have such dysrhythmias detected by Holter recording. Programmed ventricular stimulation is unsuitable for general use because inducible ventricular tachycardia may be found in as many as 40% of unselected patients who are at low risk for sudden death. Signal average electrocardiography may prove to be useful in identifying those patients without late potentials and little risk for late dysrhythmias.

Those patients who have sustained ventricular tachycardia or fibrillation late in the course of their hospital stay or following discharge should be aggressively investigated. They require programmed ventricular stimulation and guided antidysrhythmic therapy to suppress the dysrhythmia. If this technique fails surgical ablation is the next step.

Bradyarrhythmias

Sinus and Junctional Bradycardia

These dysrhythmias occur in up to 40% of cases of acute myocardial infarction and in most instances the infarction is inferoposterior. The pathogenesis is ischemia of the lower portion of the interatrial septum rather than ischemia at the sinus node. This results in reflex bradycardia and hypotension (Bezold–Jarisch reflex), which is responsive to atropine.

Relief of pain and hypovolemia will correct most cases of sinus bradycardia. When sinus or junctional bradycardia is complicated by hypotension, atropine (0.5 to 2 mg) is an effective treatment.

Conduction Abnormalities

New conduction abnormalities occur in up to 25% of patients. Their management and prognosis are directly related to the site of infarction and involvement of the conducting system.

Inferoposterior infarction involves the conduction system *proximal* to the bundle of His. In such cases the disturbance is usually transient first and second-degree A-V block (Wenckebach). Progression to complete A-V block is uncommon. When it occurs, the progression is slow and the idioventricular rhythm is stable at 40 to 50 beats/min. For these reasons the management of conduction disturbances complicating inferoposterior myocardial infarction is conservative, and most cases will respond to repeated injections of atropine. Temporary pacing should be reserved for those occasional cases resistant to atropine, where the escape rhythm has a wide QRS complex or there are pauses of more than 4 seconds. In more extensive infarction accompanied by hopotension and congestive heart failure, pacing is useful when bradycardia does not respond rapidly to atropine.

Anterior myocardial infarction involves the *distal* conducting system (below the bundle of His). When complete heart block occurs the idioventricular focus is slow and unstable. Bundle branch block, bifascicular block, and complete A-V block occur in 15 to 20% of patients. Temporary pacing is indicated when there is (1) new bundle branch block, (2) new bifascicular block, (3) Mobitz Type II block, (4) second-degree A-V block, and (5) complete A-V block.

When complete heart block complicates anterior myocardial infarction the mortality is at least 75%. The advent of prophylactic or therapeutic pacing for heart block complicating anterior myocardial infarction has made little impact on the long-term prognosis because most patients die of acute or chronic pump dysfunction rather than the bradyarrhythmia. For the same reason, prophylactic insertion of a temporary pacemaker in the presence of right bundle branch block, with or without left anterior or posterior hemiblock or left bundle branch block, is of doubtful or marginal value because of the poor ultimate prognosis. In any event, few of these patients do in fact ultimately develop complete heart block. When complete A-V block persists in a case of anterior myocardial infarction a permanent pacemaker should be inserted.

Shock

Cardiogenic shock, a dreaded complication of myocardial infarction, has a mortality rate of 80 to 90%. As previously discussed, the diagnosis depends on the blood pressure, urinary output, mental state, and skin changes. Although this assessment is valuable, effective management of the various causes can be accomplished only by invasive monitoring. The majority of patients with shock have a low cardiac output and high left ventricular end diastolic pressure with some degree of pulmonary edema. Correction of the high filling pressure so as to provide the optimal cardiac output requires continuous monitoring of intracardiac pressures. Before inserting this catheter and using an arterial line, the role of thrombolysis should be defined. If thrombolysis is to be used the catheter should be not placed in the subclavian or internal jugular veins but rather in an arm vein where it can be compressed. Swan-Ganz catheters should not be left in place for more than 5 days because of the risk of infection.

Invasive monitoring of hemodynamics will facilitate detection of factors other than loss of functioning myocardium, which may produce a fall in output and the clinical syndrome of shock.

Hypovolemia

This is a frequent complication of myocardial infarction often precipitated by the routine administration of powerful diuretics. Vomiting induced by opiates can be an important contributing factor. The condition is difficult to recognize clinically because reflex vasoconstriction can help maintain jugular venous pressure near normal. Measurement of the hemodynamic parameters will show a low cardiac output, a normal or low left ventricular filling pressure (pulmonary capillary wedge pressure), and a low right atrial pressure. Under these circumstances patients should be tested for volume responsiveness by administrating bolus infusions of 50 to 100 ml of saline or dextran. When the patient has volume responsive shock these bolus injections will produce an improvement in peripheral perfusion without much change in the right atrial pressure. The infusion may be continued until the left atrial pressure reaches 18–20 mm Hg so as to maintain an adequate left ventricular filling pressure but still be well below a level that would promote pulmonary edema. When, however, cardiac output remains low despite a left ventricular filling pressure in this range, cardiac dysfunction is the primary component.

Pump Failure

The hemodynamic findings are characterized by (1) cardiac index of less than 2.5 litres/min/m^2, (2) pulmonary capillary wedge pressure of more than 15 mm Hg, and (3) variable arterial pressure.

Arterial Pressure Less Than 90 mm Hg

When arterial pressure is low despite correction of reversible factors such as hypovolemia or drug effects, this is classic cardiogenic shock with a grim prognosis. Attempts should be made to correct hypotension pharmacologically: when the systolic blood pressure is less than 80 mm Hg, norepinephrine should be infused until the blood pressure is 80 to 90 mm Hg. This should be followed by dopamine in high dose of 5 to 15 μg/kg/min to promote vascoconstriction. If the blood pressure rises sufficiently, dobutamine (2.5 to 5 μg/kg) should be added. This low dose of dobutamine increases cardiac output and decreases systemic vascular resistance and pulmonary capillary wedge pressure without affecting renal perfusion and blood pressure.

If pharmacologic support fails, intraaortic balloon counterpulsation should be considered. This improves circulatory hemodynamics and is accomplished by introducing a balloon holding 30 cm^3 of carbon dioxide into the aorta via the femoral artery. The balloon is inflated mechanically by a signal triggered from the R wave of the electrocardiogram. It is deflated immediately prior to left ventricular systole so that the left ventricle ejects against a low resistance. It is then reinflated after the aortic valve shuts, thus raising the aortic diastolic pressure, thereby improving coronary blood flow. The total effect is to increase left ventricular stroke volume, improve coronary perfusion, and decrease the peripheral vascular resistance. Without coronary reperfusion, however, the expected survival is still only 10%. For this reason, intraaortic balloon support is usually limited to use in those patients felt to be candidates for corrective procedures. This will avoid having machine dependent patients who cannot be weaned from support. There is early but uncontrolled evidence which indicates that PTCA may improve survival in selected cases.

General measures in the treatment of cardiogenic shock include correction of acid–base abnormalities and hypoxia. Positive end expiratory pressure ventilation may be necessary to control pulmonary edema.

Arterial Pressure More Than 90 mm Hg

In these patients with left ventricular failure the systemic pressure is high enough to permit afterload reduction as the first line of treatment. Sodium nitroprusside, in doses of 20 to 400 μg/min, should be administered until the wedge pressure is reduced by approximately 50%, provided systemic arterial pressure is maintained in the region of 80 to 90 mm Hg. Reduction in systemic vascular resistance improves peripheral perfusion, increases urinary output, decreases the wedge pressure, and relieves pulmonary congestion.

Whereas nitroprusside is a more powerful arteriolar vasodilator, nitroglycerin is a more potent venodilator and also dilates the epicardial coronary arteries. Thus, early in the course of myocardial infarction when ischemia is prominent, nitroglycerin may be the better choice.

Should nitroprusside or nitroglycerin fail to adequately improve cardiac output, dobutamine may be added in doses from 5 to 20 mg/kg/min. This drug improves cardiac output, decreases pulmonary wedge pressure, and promotes renal perfusion without significant peripheral vasoconstriction. If dopamine is used in the patient with adequate blood pressure, it should be kept at low doses (less than 5 mg/kg/min), where it has a selective renal vasodilator effect and its positive inotropic effects can help improve cardiac output without significant peripheral vasoconstriction. Higher doses increase afterload and should be used only if necessary to maintain adequate blood pressure.

Right Ventricular Infarction

Occasionally, shock may supervene when infarction involves the posterior left ventricular wall, the contiguous posterior portion of the ventricular septum, and the adjacent right ventricular wall. This syndrome of right ventricular infarction may be suspected when, in the presence of an electrocardiographically located inferior myocardial infarction, there is elevation of the jugular venous pressure with Kussmaul's sign, hypotension, and evidence of heart block. Echocardiography may be helpful in demonstrating an enlarged right ventricle, and right sided precordial EKG leads can show ST elevation.

Normally, the main purpose of the right ventricle is to simply provide an adequate filling pressure for the left ventricle. The left ventricular filling pressure, or wedge pressure is therefore slightly higher (14 mm Hg) as compared to the right ventricular filling pressure (right atrial pressure of 8 mm Hg). Infarction of the right ventricle may produce a discrepancy in relationship between the right and left ventricular hemodynamics, with right atrial pressure equal to, or higher than the wedge pressure. This alteration between the normal gradient of right and left ventricular filling pressures suggests diseases involving the right ventricle (infarction) or the pulmonary vascular bed (thromboembolism). When there is reason to suspect the presence of right ventricular infarction, shock may be successfully combated by volume expansion, to help maintain normal left ventricular filling pressure.

Intravenous fluids should be given rapidly until the right atrial pressure and pulmonary capillary wedge pressure are more than 20 mm Hg and the blood pressure is stable: dobutamine may also be required. Venodilators and diuretics should be withdrawn. Occasionally, hypotension does not respond to volume infusion and dobutamine, in which case intraaortic balloon counterpulsation should be considered. When heart block is a complication, A-V sequential pacing is much more effective than ventricular pacing for several reasons. An appropriately timed atrial contraction increases the right ventricular preload and cardiac output in a ventricle that has lost its compliance. Also, atrial systole is transmitted to the pulmonary artery in a right ventricle that has decreased or absent systolic function.

Surgical Treatment of Complications of Myocardial Infarction

Rupture of the Ventricular Septum

When this is complicated by pulmonary edema, cardiogenic shock, or congestive heart failure, repair should be undertaken immediately. Stabilization prior to operation involves balloon counterpulsation, mechanical ventilation, afterload reduction, inotropic drugs, and diuretics. The operative mortality is high but the long-term results can be good.

In those patients who are stable following

rupture, operation may be delayed for a few days only. This semielective approach avoids the possibility of sudden catastrophic extension of the original smaller tear.

Rupture of a Papillary Muscle

Partial rupture of a papillary muscle leads to catostrophic mitral regurgitation. Complete rupture is fatal within minutes. Usually, it is the posteromedial muscle that is supplied by the posterior descending coronary artery that is involved. The clinical presentation may be indistinguishable from rupture of the ventricular septum. The distinction is made by color flow Doppler echocardiography, Swan-Ganz catheterization, and angiography.

Patients should be stabilized prior to surgery as in the case of ventricular septal rupture. Operative treatment may involve mitral valve replacement, or mitral valve repair and coronary artery bypass surgery, depending on the findings in the individual case.

False Aneurysm

Free wall rupture usually occurs within the first 14 days of myocardial infarction and is much more common in women. Few patients survive rupture long enough for surgical treatment and there are few clues to the diagnosis. A persistent pericardial friction rub may lead to repeat chest X-ray, and, more importantly, to 2D echocardiography. The characteristic findings with the latter technique are a thin-walled saccular aneurysm with dyskinetic pulsation whose ostium is narrow with sharp margins. When a false aneurysm is discovered it should be resected as soon as possible because of the high risk of rupture.

Cardiac Rehabilitation

Rehabilitation should start soon after myocardial infarction since there are obvious early benefits. Early ambulation, use of a commode, and self-exercise programs under supervision of a physical therapist should be undertaken prior to a predischarge submaximal exercise test. Concomitant patient education is an important part of most programs to provide understanding of the disease and encourage life-style changes that may be necessary to promote medical compliance and risk factor information. The advantages include diminished incidence of thromboembolism and hypostatic pneumonia, improved psychological status and sense of well being, and possibly an earlier return to work.

Outpatient cardiac rehabilitation and exercise programs under supervision carry a low risk of complications but are expensive. Long-term prospective trials to test the efficacy of these programs will probably never be available because of the large study population required, difficulties with long-term follow-up, and avoidance of dropouts and noncompliance.

Nevertheless, metaanalysis (a form of statistical analysis that evaluates pooled data from multiple studies) indicates that long-term exercise programs may reduce mortality from reinfarction by 25%. Exercise training increases the maximal work capacity. Also, the heart rate and blood pressure product are both lowered, thus improving myocardial oxygen demand: The effect is to delay the onset of myocardial ischemia so that the incidence of ST segment depression and thallium defects during exercise testing is diminished.

These potential benefits should not obscure the potential risks among patients recovery from a large myocardial infarction. Those who have dangerous dysrhythmias, severe hypertension, aortic stenosis, or cardiac failure should have appropriate modifications to their program.

Additional Reading

Braunwald E (ed): "The Myocardium: Failure and Infarction." HP Pulishing Co., New York, 1974.

Chatterjee K, Parmley WW: The role of vasodilator therapy in heart failure. Prog Cardiovasc Dis 19:301, 1977.

Gerlsini GG: Coronary artery spasm and angina pectoris. Chest 68:709, 1975.

Guidelines for the early management of patients with acute myocardial infarction. A report of the American College of Cardiology/American Heart Association Task Force on assessment of diagnostic and therapeutic cardivascular procedures (subcommittee to develop guidelines for the early management of patients with acute myocardial infarction). JACC 16(2):249–292, 1990.

Guidelines for percutaneous transluminal coronary angioplasty. A report of the American College of Cardiology/American Heart Association task force on assessment of diagnostic and therapeutic cardiovascular procedures (subcommittee on percutaneous transluminal coronary angioplasty). JACC 12(2):529–545, 1988.

Guidelines for exercise testing. A report of the Joint American College of Cardiology/American Heart Association Task Force on assessment of cardiovascular procedures (subcommittee on exercise testing). Circulation 74(3):653A–666, 1986.

Kannel WB: Some lessons in cardiovascular epidemiology from Framingham. Am J Cardiol 37:269, 1976.

Kannel WB, Feinleib M: Natural history of angina pectoris in the Framingham study. Am J Cardiol 29:154, 1972.

Killip T III, Kimball JT: Treatment of myocardial infarction in a coronary care unit. Am J Cardiol 20:547, 1967.

Lesch M, Gorlin R: Pharmacological therapy of angina pectoris. Mod Concepts Cardiovasc Dis 42:5, 1973.

Mclntosh HD, Garcia JA: The first decade of aorto-coronary bypass grafting, 1967–1977. A Review. Circulation 57:405, 1978.

Meltzer LE, Kitchell JB: The incidence of arrhythmias associated with acute myocardial infarction. Prog Cardiovasc Dis 9:50, 1966.

Pantridge JF, Adgey AAJ, Geddes JS, Webb SW: "The Acute Coronary Attack." Grune & Stratton, New York, 1975.

Pantridge JF, Geddes JS: A mobile intensive care unit in the treatment of myocardial infarction. Lancet 2:271, 1967.

Roberts WC, Buya LM: The frequency and significance of coronary arterial thrombi and other observations in fatal acute myocardial infarction. A study of 107 necropsy patients. Am J Med 52:425, 1972.

Russek HI: Natural history of angina pectoris. Am J Cardiol 35:590, 1975.

Stamler J: Epidemiology of coronary heart disease. Med Clin North Am 57:5, 1973.

Swan HJC, Forrester JS, Danzig R, Allen HN: Power failure in acute myocardial infarction. Prog Cardiovasc Dis 12:568, 1970.

Symposium on Myocardial Ischelnia, Mayo Clinic. Proc. Feb–May 65, 1990.

Vlodaver Z, Edwards JE: Pathology of coronary atherosclerosis. Prog Cardiovasc Dis 14:256, 1971.

18 Hypertension and Hypertensive Heart Disease

Definition

Blood pressure in excess of 140/90 mm Hg is the accepted criterion for the diagnosis of hypertension. At first, this definition may appear somewhat arbitrary because of fluctuations of readings even in "normal" persons. Yet, persistent readings of 140/90 or more are associated with increased risk and this is therefore an acceptable cut-off point. So-called "labile hypertension" describes the condition in which blood pressure readings are occasionally greater than 90 mm Hg. Because of the natural variability in pressures, and uncertainty as to whether such individuals eventually become permanently hypertensive, they should be labeled "borderline hypertensive" and have readings checked annually. Diastolic blood pressure of 90 to 104 mm Hg is regarded as mild, 105 to 114 as moderate, and 115 or more, as severe hypertension.

Epidemiological studies have shown that hypertension is one of the most common cardiovascular disorders in most population groups. It is particularly common and severe in the black population of various countries. It has been estimated that 10% of the population in the United States suffers from hypertension with its attendant complications of heart failure, uremia, atherosclerosis, and stroke. The risk of cardiovascular complications increases continuously as the systolic and diastolic pressures rise.

Measurement of Blood Pressure

Accurate measurement of the blood pressure is crucial, particularly when office readings are only mildly elevated. Casual office readings are frequently significantly higher than ambulatory recordings and those recorded at home. Since the treatment of mild hypertension is not without side effects, repeated office and home measurements should be made; the frequency depends on the diastolic blood pressure: When the pressure is 90 to 95 mm Hg follow-up should be at 3 months and for 96 to 104 mm Hg follow-up should be at 1 month. When the blood pressure is 160/104 or more the patient should be promptly assessed for secondary causes of hypertension and target organ damage.

The blood pressure cuff should fit properly and should be wide enough to transmit pressure uniformly to the brachial artery. The air bladder in the cuff should encircle 80% of the upper arm and the cuff should be wide enough to cover two-thirds of the length between the elbow and the shoulder.

Measurements should be made with the patient seated with the arm supported at the level of the heart. The blood pressure should be recorded in each arm and the higher reading should be taken as the true blood pressure. The diastolic reading should be taken at the point where the sounds disappear. After readings have been taken in the seated position, measurements should be made after 2 minutes standing to test for orthostasis.

Whether diastolic hypertension is *secondary* to some identifiable cause, or essential without an identifiable cause, it may behave in *benign*, *accelerated*, or *malignant* fashion. However, the term "benign" hypertension is something of a misnomer since persistent diastolic hypertension is associated with all the vascular complications in the vulnerable organs, namely the eyes, heart, kidneys, and brain. It is papilledema, rather than the height of the blood pressure that specifically categorizes malignant hypertension. Accelerated hypertension implies a sudden increase in the level of hypertensive readings, or symptoms suggestive of malignant hypertension but without actual papilledema.

Complications of Hypertension

The Heart

Systolic overload of the left ventricle results in concentric left ventricular hypertrophy, elevation of the left ventricular end-diastolic, left atrial, and pulmonary arterial pressures resulting in congestive cardiac failure. There is a predisposition toward coronary atherosclerosis that results in angina pectoris and myocardial infarction.

The Aorta

Cystic medial necrosis is commoner in hypertensive as compared to normotensive subjects in the same age groups. The combination of hypertension and medial necrosis of the aorta may lead to *dissecting aneurysm*. Aneurysms may also result from extensive atherosclerosis particularly in the abdominal aorta; they are usually situated just below the renal arteries. Widespread embolism of aortic atheromatous material may involve the small arteries of the lower extremities producing a clinical picture resembling polyarteritis medosa (cholesterol embolism).

Systemic Arterioles

The earliest change is medial hypertrophy and this is followed by intimal thickening. In malignant hypertension the intimal thickening is of the concentric type producing the so-called "onion-peel" thickening. These changes involving the arterioles are observed in the entire systemic circulation including the kidney myocardium, pancreas, brain, and retina.

The Kidneys

The changes are primarily a result of the arteriolar lesions described above. Nephrosclerosis is a result of arterial insufficiency and is characterized by hyalinized glomerulae, tubular atrophy, and increased fibrous tissue. Renal infarction may result from embolism emanating from thrombus within the left ventricle, or occlusion of the renal artery by dissecting aneurysm.

The Brain

Cerebral infarction may occur because of thrombosis or embolism. Carotid artery occlusion, produced by dissecting aneurysm or by thrombus superimposed on atherosclerotic plaque, may produce strokes or transient ischemic attacks. Cerebral hemorrhage may follow rupture of an intracerebral vessel, and subarachnoid hemorrhage may follow rupture of a congenital aneurysm of the circle of Willis.

Causes of Hypertension

Primary (Essential) Hypertension

In 95% of cases of hypertension there is no obvious cause and *essential* hypertension is said to be present.

The mathematical equation for blood pressure is simple: blood pressure = cardiac output times peripheral resistance. However, there is a wide variety of factors that influence both items in the equation: The cardiac output is influenced by (1) cardiac factors such as myocardial contractility and heart rate that is under baroreceptor regulation. (2) Renal function regulates blood volume through sodium and potassium metabolism, which in turn is influenced by mineralacorticoids (aldosterone etc.).

The peripheral vascular resistance is regulated by (1) the sympathetic nervous system, (2) local autoregulatory factors, and (3) humoral factors [e.g., angiotension and catecholamines (vasoconstrictor) and prostaglandins (vasodilator)]. The interplay of all these factors is not understood. Furthermore, there are racial, genetic, and gender differences. Hypertension is more common and most severe in black men, whereas white women have the most benign proynosis.

Secondary Hypertension

In the remaining 5% of cases, there is hypertension secondary to an identifiable cause of which chronic renal disease is the commonest (4% of all cases of hypertension). Renovascular disease, primary aldosteronism, Cushing syndrome, oral contraceptives, and coarctation of the aorta combined cause only 1% of all cases of hypertension.

Renal Hypertension

Renal Parenchymal Disease

In pyelonephritis, infection produces a reduction in the mass of functioning renal tissue, and scarring leads to perivascular fibrosis and vascular distortion. The resultant renal ischemia activates the renin–angiotensin system, producing hypertension. Sodium retention by the damaged kidney may also be an important contributing factor. Thus, patients with salt-losing pyelonephritis do not develop hypertension, whereas most patients with salt retention do. Sodium retention leads to an increase in extracellular fluid volume, increased venous return and increased cardiac output which provokes peripheral vasoconstriction and an increase in peripheral resistance which may be maintained even though the cardiac output returns to normal.

Renal Arterial Hypertension

Renal arterial hypertension (the Goldblatt kidney) is the classic situation where impairment of renal blood flow leads to systemic hypertension. The pressor substance released by the ischemic juxtaglomerular apparatus is renin, which interacts with plasma α_2-globulin to produce inactive angiotensin I. Angiotensin I is converted to the highly active vasopressor substance angiotensin II by a converting enzyme. Any cause of renal artery stenosis leads to an increase in renin secretion from the affected kidney and this may be detected in the renal vein. Renin in turn stimulates the adrenal cortex to secrete aldosterone leading to sodium retention, expansion of the blood volume, and hypertension.

Adrenal Hypertension

Primary aldosteronism induces sodium retention and potassium excretion by its action on the renal tubules. The sodium-retaining effect of the glucocorticoids is responsible for hypertension in Cushing syndrome. In the adrenogenital syndrome deoxycorticosterone is responsible for sodium retention and resultant hypertension.

Coarctation of the Aorta

The cause of the hypertension is most likely related to the aortic constriction itself.

Oral Contraceptives

The hypertension is related to the estrogen content of the pill. These drugs should be discontinued for a period of 6 months before an adequate assessment of hypertension can be made.

Pheochromocytoma

This chromaffin tumor produces paroxysmal and sustained hypertension by secreting catecholamines.

Clinical Features

Symptoms

Hypertension itself is probably not responsible for symptoms other than headache and epistaxis. Dizziness, fatigue, and palpitation are a result of anxiety and develop once the patient has been informed of his condition. Occipital headache is associated with severe hypertension, particularly the malignant type. It is often present when the patient wakes in the morning and tends to disappear during the day. It is relieved by hypotensive therapy.

Cardiovascular manifestations include dyspnea on effort, orthopnea, paroxysmal cardiac dyspnea, pulmonary edema, angina pectoris, and dissecting aneurysm as described elsewhere. Central nervous system manifestations are produced by infarction and hemorrhage with resultant strokes, epilepsy, subarachnoid hemorrhage, and coma. Interference with vision due to retinopathy is common. Hypertensive encephalopathy is associated with severe headache, vomiting, epileptic attacks, and coma. Renal manifestations include nocturia, renal pain and uremic drowsiness, vomiting, and coma.

Clinical Evaluation

This is directed at determining whether hypertension is *essential* or *secondary* and determining the extent of vascular disease.

The History

Diastolic hypertension in patients under 25 years of age is strongly suggestive of the secondary type. Essential hypertension usually manifests itself between the ages of 25 and 50 and a strong family history is frequent. A history of drug ingestion (oral contraceptives or steroids) is of obvious importance. Renal parenchymal disease is suggested by a history of repeated genitourinary infection, renal stones, hematuria, and instrumentation of the urinary tract. Paroxysms of headache, palpitation, perspiration, nervousness, and tremor suggest the presence of pheochromocytoma. Weight loss also suggests the latter diagnosis, whereas weight gain suggests Cushing syndrome. Hypokalernic muscle weakness is suggestive of primary aldosteronism.

Physical Findings

The height of the blood pressure varies considerably from patient to patient, and in the same patient at different stages of the disease. Occasionally, hypertensive readings disappear following an episode of myocardial infarction. Malignant hypertension is nearly always associated with a diastolic pressure of 120 mm Hg or more. The femoral pulses should be carefully palpated for radiofemoral delay and if necessary the blood pressure should be measured in the legs, where it is normally higher than in the arms.

The heart exhibits features of left ventricular hypertrophy with a thrusting displaced apex. A presystolic gallop is an extremely common finding. Later, evidence of right ventricular enlargement and failure appear with a diastolic gallop and murmur of functional tricuspid insufficiency. Occasionally, an early diastolic murmur of aortic insufficiency may be present.

The Retina

Examination of the *fundi* is the most important. The arteriolar walls are normally invisible; narrowing of the arteries and arterioles is due to thickening of their walls, since the column of blood in the vessel lumen is what is normally seen with the ophthalmoscope. Narrowing of the arteries is best assessed by comparing an artery to its accompanying vein, which is only slightly larger than the artery (grade I retinopathy). If the artery is much smaller than the vein, the vessel wall is thickened and sclerotic. Other evidence of vascular involvement includes tortuosity of the vessels, disappearance of the veins at the arteriovenous crossings (A-V nipping), and alteration in the light reflex. These changes in the vessels have been referred to as grade II retinopathy. Grade III retinopathy indicates the presence of hemorrhages, and/or exudates, in the fundi. Superficial hemorrhages are streaky or flame-shaped, whereas deep hemorrhages are round. Exudates may be fluffy, hard white patches, dots, or star-shaped, especially around the macula. The presence of papilledema indicates grade IV retinopathy, and therefore malignant hypertension.

The electrocardiogram is an important guide to the presence and degree of left ventricular hypertrophy. When definite evidence of left ventricular hypertrophy is present this forms a valuable guideline to the severity of hypertension and the effects of treatment. The presence of a normal electrocardiogram is a good prognostic indicator when hypertension has been long-standing. Other electrocardiographic features observed are the findings associated with myocardial infarction, left atrial enlargement, and conduction defects such as left bundle branch block.

Echocardiography, when affordable, is the best method for detecting left ventricular hypertrophy.

Radiology does not contribute much to the diagnosis of hypertension other than the specific findings associated with coarctation of the aorta. Enlargement of the cardiac silhouette is a late finding at which time cardiac failure is evident clinically. Prominence of the ascending aorta may be the result of hypertension or atherosclerosis and this sign is, therefore, not very specific.

Routine Laboratory Studies

Tests for Renal Function

Urinalysis

This is important in the evaluation of primary and secondary renal involvement. Examination should be made of a fresh midstream early morning specimen. The presence of bacteria, casts, and red and white blood cells points to pyelonephritis.

Serum Creatinine

A normal reading excludes a diagnosis of renal parenchymal disease. The test also aids in the monitoring of patients with essential hypertension. It should be remembered that the serum creatinine only exceeds the normal value when the glomerular filtration rate has decreased by 50%. Therefore, the test has limitations in detecting early nephrosclerosis.

Blood Chemistry

Serum sodium and potassium are relevant to the diagnosis of aldosteronism, and the blood glucose for diabetes. Measurement of serum cholesterol (total and HDL) may be indicated in high-risk subjects.

More extensive investigation to detect the secondary forms of hypertension is required when diastolic hypertension is severe, accelerated, or malignant when hypertension is sustained in young people and when there is clear documentation of the sudden onset of severe hypertension in previously normotensive individuals.

Secondary Causes of Hypertension

Renal Arterial Disease

Approximately 1% of all cases of hypertension are attributed to renal artery stenosis. In 60% of these cases obstruction of either the main renal artery or its branches is a result of atherosclerosis. Usually, the obstruction involves the orifice or proximal 1 to 2 cm of the renal artery. When the arterial lumen is reduced by 60%, the pressure drop is sufficient to stimulate renin production. Occasionally, renal artery obstruction is complete, yet renal function and renin production are maintained via collateral vessels.

Fibromuscular dysplasia accounts for 40% of cases of renal artery stenosis; it affects women more commonly than men. Other unusual causes are renal artery aneurysm, dissection of the aorta, aortic arteritis, and compression of the renal arteries by tumors and cysts.

Mechanisms of Hypertension

Hypotension distal to an obstruction in the renal artery stimulates the juxtaglomerular apparatus to secrete renin. Renin acts on a plasma globulin, angiotensingin, to release angiotensin I, which is converted to angiotensin II by angiotensin-converting enzyme (ACE). Angiotensin II is not only a powerful vasoconstrictor but also a major stimulus to aldosterone production. Aldosterone stimulates sodium reabsorption by the renal tubule leading to expansion of the plasma volume.

Clinical Features

Hypertension of recent origin and of rapid progression, especially in a relatively young individual without a family history, or with recent renal vascular accident is suggestive of the diagnosis. Frequently, there is a history of pain in the loin, especially if hematuria has occurred, a history of trauma to the back or abdomen, or a sudden increase in the degree of hypertension, particularly the development of accelerated or malignant hypertension.

Careful auscultation of the upper abdomen and back should be practiced in every patient with hypertension, since murmurs are frequently found in renal arterial disease. Murmurs in the midline are usually unimportant, especially in the elderly. Significant murmurs are heard lateral to the midline, anteriorly, or in the flank. The murmur starts in systole after the first sound and runs to, or beyond, the second sound. These characteristics are found over any artery that is critically narrowed producing hypotension beyond the area of stenosis.

Diagnostic Tests

Contrast angiography is the definitive test for renal artery stenosis. This may be made by selective catheterization of the renal arteries via the percutaneous femoral artery route. Digital subtraction angiography is less morbid for the patient but does not supply the same precise anatomic definition.

The functional significance of an angiographically observed stenosis may be assessed by split renal function tests, which involve individual ureteric catheterization and analysis of the urine from each kidney. This shows decreased urine and sodium excretion and increased creatinine excretion on the involved side. In unilateral renal artery stenosis, bioassay of plasma renin activity of venous blood from the affected kidney reveals one and one-half times the value for the normal side.

Screening tests such as intravenous pyelography, isotope renography, and assay of peripheral renin activity (PRA) lack sensitivity and specificity. However, measurement of PRA before and after one 50 mg dose of Captopril shows promise as a highly sensitive and specific screening test. Venous blood is sampled 1 hour after administration of the drug. Patients with renal vascular hypertension show (1) a stimulated PRA of more than 12 ng/ml/h or more, (2) an absolute increase of 10 ng/ml/h, and (3) a 150% increase in PRA (or 400% increase if baseline PRA is less than 3 ng/ml/h).

Pheochromocytoma

These tumors are usually benign and arise from chromaffin tissue. Approximately 90% arise in the adrenal medulla. The extramedullary sites involve the sympathetic chain, the chest, the organ of Zuckerkandl, and the urinary bladder. Tumors may be found in the thorax, testes, ovaries, and neck (carotid body). Tumors involving the adrenal glands are bilateral in about 10% of cases. Less than 10% of pheochromocytomas are malignant.

Clinical Features

Pheochromocytomas are found in approximately 1 in 200 hypertensive patients. The effects of a pheochromocytoma are related to the release of epinephrine and norepinephrine. The two important clinical presentations are (1) paroxysmal hypertension and (2) sustained hypertension. Paroxysmal hypertension is the more easily recognized manifestation since patients are more symptomatic. Sudden spontaneous attacks of paroxysmal acute hypertension develop, which usually increase in frequency and severity and ultimately lead to persistent hypertension, with or without paroxysmal increases in pressure. Paroxysms may be provoked by tricyclic antidepressents, β-blockers, steroids, and manual manipulation. The paroxysms are a result of the sudden release of catecholamines into the circulation. The usual symptoms are headache, palpitation, severe sweating, anxiety, vomiting, and substernal constricting pain. During episodes of profound hypertension, pulmonary edema or cerebrovascular accident may occur. On examination, the striking feature is the presence of hypertension, often severe, associated with sweating and pallor. The heart rate depends on which of the catecholamines is secreted in the greater quantity. When hypertension is sustained, pheochromocytoma is more difficult to diagnose since the features are those of benign or malignant hypertension.

Features that suggest pheochromocytoma are excessive sweating, raised temperature, elevated BMR, glycosuria, and hyperglycemia. Weight loss is frequent and thyrotoxicosis is often suspected. Orthostatic hypotension is found in some patients. Occasionally an abdominal mass is palpable.

Tests for Pheochromocytoma

Biochemical

Measurement of norepinephrine and epinephrine in the urine is a highly sensitive method for detecting the presence of pheochromocytoma. Additionally, the urinary secretion of the metabolites of catecholalnirles [e.g., metanephrine and vanillyl mandelic acid (VMA)] are increased. Measurement of total metanephrines is the most sensitive (99%) and measurement of VAMA is almost as sensitive (90%). Measurement of urinary metanephrines as a screening test followed by measurement of urinary fractions of catecholamines is an effective diagnostic combination. There are many factors and drugs that may interfere with these results. However, their usefulness may be enhanced by collection of urinary specimens after a typical "spell."

Tumor Localization

CT scanning will identify 90% of tumors when they are in the field of scan. Magnetic resonance imaging (MRI) may be more useful in pregnancy and for tumors located outside the adrenals.

Treatment

The hazards of surgical treatment can be minimized by adequate preoperative pharmacological preparations so that the patient is normotensive at the time of operation. The α-adrenergic receptors should be blocked with phenoxybenzamine several days prior to the operation. This controls the vasoconstrictor effect of catecholamines and avoids sudden peripheral dilatation following removal of the tumor. β-Blockade with propranolol may also be necessary to control tachycardia and arrhythmias. The surgeon should be prepared to explore the entire abdominal cavity since the tumors may be multiple. Phentolamine should be given intravenously to control blood pressure rises produced by handling the tumor. Vasodilators such as sodium nitroprusside should be available for hypertensive reactions that are not responsive to phentolamine. The blood volume is frequently decreased because of prolonged hypersecretion of catecholamines, and blood transfusion or plasma and volume expanders may be required during and after the operation.

Primary Aldosteronism

This rare cause of hypertension is the result of an aldosterone-secreting adenoma or idiopathic hyperplasia of the adrenal cortex. Primary aldosteronism is responsible for approximately 1% of cases of hypertension. An adenoma is present in one-third, and hyperplasia is present in the remaining two thirds of these cases.

Clinical Features

Hyperaldosteronism results in potassium depletion, sodium retention, alkalosis, and renin suppression. Symptoms are attributable to the electrolyte abnormalities and include muscle weakness, fatigue, and polyuria. Hypertension is moderate to severe, but malignant hypertension with papilledema is very rare. Despite sodium retention, edema is characteristically absent unless there is complicating congestive cardiac failure.

Diagnosis

The combination of hypertension and hypokalemia should suggest the possibility of hyperaldosteronism.

The diagnosis is made by demonstrating (1) hypokalemia with inappropriate potassium loss, (2) suppressed plasma renin activity, and (3) a nonsuppressible aldosterone level. Hypokalemia may be spontaneous or induced by diuretics. A 24-hour urinary potassium, upright plasma renin activity (PRA) and aldosterone concentration (PAC) should be measured. When the 24-hour urinary potassium exceeds 30 mg/h, the PRA is less than 3 mg/ml/hr, and the ratio of PAC/PRA is more than 20, hyperaldosteronism is likely.

The diagnosis of primary aldosteronism is confirmed by an aldosterone suppression test: All drugs (e.g., spironalactone, diuretics, estrogen, and ACE inhibitors) that interfere with the renin–angiotensin–aldosterone axis are stopped. Sodium chloride may be administered as an intravenous infusion over 4 hours or by oral loading over 5 days. Hypokalemia is corrected by oral potassium supplementation. A positive test consists of failure of suppression of aldosterone excretion in the urine and the presence of low upright PRA.

The distinction between adrenal adenoma and adrenal hyperplasia in primary aldosteronism may be made by adrenal CT scanning. When an adenoma larger than 1 cm is detected, unilateral adrenalectomy should be recommended. When microadenomas (less than 1 cm) are detected by CT scan further evaluation is made by posture studies: patients with hyperplasia have a postural increase of more than 33% over baseline whereas adenomas show no change. Treatment is by pharamacologic inhibition of aldosterone using spironalactones. Diuretics such as triamterene and amiloride that act on the distal tubule (independent of aldosterone) to conserve potassium are also useful.

Treatment of Hypertension

The ideal form of treatment is operative intervention and cure of those forms of secondary hypertension such as unilateral renal ischemia, pheochromocytoma, or primary aldosteronism. Unfortunately, this applies only to a small fraction of the population of hypertensive people.

When there is evidence of hypertensive vascular disease, treatment is mandatory and relief of cardiac failure and regression of retinopathy is common clinical experience. In untreated malignant hypertension, death is invariable within 2 years and the efficacy of antihypertensive therapy is proven beyond dispute. When diastolic hypertension exists without vascular disease, priority for treatment should be given to black patients, young patients, and those with a strong family history of hypertension or myocardial infarction.

Currently, there is no drug available that provides effective control of blood pressure without side-effects. Many patients with hypertension are asymptomatic and have no evidence of cardiac, renal, or cerebral involvement. However, initiation of life-long treatment and medical supervision in such cases can be justified because there is clear-cut evidence of the long-term benefits of such treatment. The Veterans Affairs Cooperative Study and several other studies have clearly demonstrated that antihypertensive therapy is effective in reducing cardiovascular morbidity and mortality, chiefly from stroke, heart failure, and renal failure when hypertension is adequately controlled.

The original studies demonstrated these benefits with diastolic pressures above 104 mm Hg; later work showed similar findings with pressures between 90 and 104 mm Hg. Data from insurance companies show increasing morbidity and mortality with systolic hypertension but evidence that treatment improves the outlook is lacking. Similarly, a reduction in the mortality from coronary artery disease has yet to be demonstrated.

Compliance is a major problem in treating asymptomatic people with mild to moderate degrees of hypertension. Patients will need to be convinced that the side-effects of the various medications are in their long-term interest. Improved continuity of care and more time spent with the patient may be provided by nurse practitioners in special hypertension clinics rather than by busy internists.

General Measures

These are worthwhile adopting in all patients with hypertension before resorting to drug treatment. They may be all that is needed in some patients with mild hypertension.

Alcohol Restriction

Excessive drinking contributes to poor compliance with medication. Alcohol may also lead to persistent hypertension, presumably through the release of catecholamines.

Contraceptive Pill

The incidence of hypertension increases with the length of use. The mechanism is through renin–aldosterone-mediated expansion of the blood volume. In cases of mild to moderate hypertension, the pill should be avoided for 3 months before instituting other treatment.

Weight Reduction

There is a definite relationship between obesity and hypertension. Weight reduction may normalize the blood pressure. The goal should be reduction to within 15% of the ideal body weight.

Drug Therapy

The choice of drug therapy falls into the following sequential categories.

Diuretics

Oral Diuretics

The precise mechanism of action is unknown, but induction of a negative sodium balance thereby reducing blood volume, cardiac output, peripheral vascular resistance, and arterial pressure is a likely mechanism. Permanent lowering of peripheral vascular resistance may be a result of reduction in intracellular sodium and water in the walls of blood vessels.

Diuretics are usually used as "first-line" therapy since they are often all that is needed in cases of mild hypertension. Also, they augment the effects of other antihypertensive drugs and reduce the salt-retaining effects of some agents such as minoxidil. Diuretics have been discussed in the chapter dealing with angina pectoris. The various groups and an example in each group is summarized below.

Thiazide Diuretics

There is little difference in the various preparations. Hydrochlorathiazide is the most frequently used in a dose of 25 to 100 mg daily. The maximum effect is reached in 14 days.

Loop Diuretics

These are particularly useful when hypertension is complicated by heart failure. Also, when there is renal failure, large doses of loop diuretics retain their diuretic potency whereas thiazides do not. The most commonly used preparation is furosemide 20 to 180 mg daily. Loop diuretics are not more effective than the thiazides in controlling hypertenison.

Potassium Sparing Diuretics

Spironolactone antagonizes aldosterone and is an effective antihypertensive drug. The dose is 50 to 100 mg daily. Triamterine and amiloride are usually used in combination with a thiazide to counteract the loss of potassium in the urine.

Diuretics may induce hypokalemia, hyperuricemia, and hyperglycemia, which may require adjustment of medication or potassium supplementation. Hypokalemia may predispose to digitalis toxicity and also enhance the

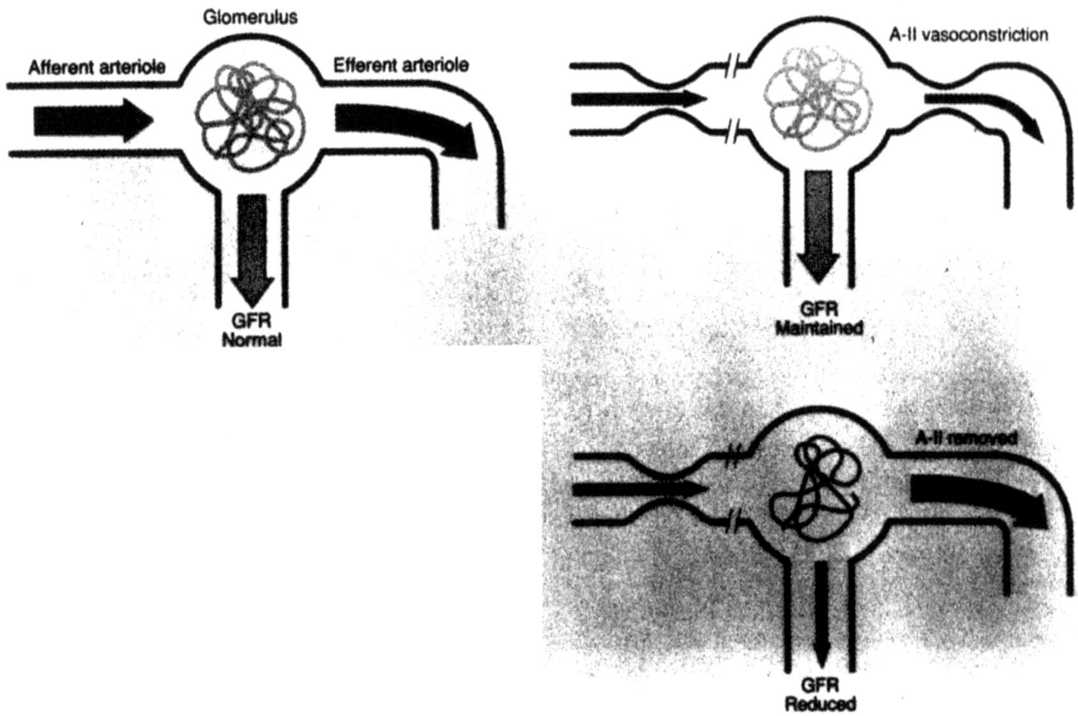

FIGURE 18.1. The effects of ACE inhibitors on renal function in the presence of renal artery stenosis. Glomerular filtration rate (GFR) is maintained by high intraglomerular pressure through angiotension II-mediated constriction of efferent arteriole. When A-II vasoconstriction is removed by ACE inhibitor, GFR is reduced and renal failure ensues. Reprinted, with permission, from Nally JV: The Captopril tests: a new concept in detecting renovascular hypterten-sion. Cleveland Clinic J Med 56(4):395–401, 1989.

proarrhythmic effect of various antidysrhythmic drugs.

ACE Inhibitors

Following diuretics these are frequently used as the next step in therapy. They reduce the peripheral vascular resistance and are therefore particularly useful when there is complicating congestive heart failure. They are generally well tolerated and serious side effects are rare. They may precipitate renal failure in patients with bilateral renal artery stenosis or unilateral stenosis in a solitary kidney (Fig. 18.1). Hypotension may occur when there is high plasma renin activity or when there is hypovolemia induced by diuretics. Neutropenia and skin rashes are rare. There is a risk of hyperkalemia when ACE inhibitors are used with potassium supplements, spironolactone, and when there is impaired renal function. The dosages are Captopril, 25 to 300 mg daily given b.i.d.; Enalaporil, 2.5 to 4 mg daily given b.i.d.; and Lisinopril, 5 to 40 mg given once daily.

β-Adenergic Blockers

Their actions are described in the text dealing with the treatment of angina. They are standard second line treatment such as ACE inhibitors and calcium channel blockers. Their efficacy is enhanced when there are associated conditions such as angina, hypertrophic cardiomyopathy, and supraventricular tachycardia, which are in themselves responsive to β-blockade. They are contraindicated when there is cardiac failure, severe asthma or obstructive airways disease, severe peripheral vascular disease, sinus bradycardia, and brittle diabetes.

Although β-blockers lower the blood pressure in the same manner (reduced cardiac output, decreased renin production, decreased peripheral vascular resistance) there are individual differences. Lipophylic preparations (metropolol, inderal, timolol) cross the blood–brain barrier. They are metabolized in the liver and have a plasma half-life of 6 hours. They may produce fatigue and depression. Hydrophylic preparations (atenolol, acebutolol, and nadolol) are less likely to cause fatigue and depression since they do not cross the blood–brain barrier. They are excreted by the kidney and their dosage must be reduced in renal failure. The "cardioselectivity" of metropolol, atenolol, and acebutolol is lost at high dosage and β_1- and β_2-receptors are equally blocked. Similarly, intrinsic sympatheticomimetic activity (ISA) is not of much practical importance. β-Blockers with ISA (pindolol and acebutolol) show this effect at rest and may counteract sinus bradycardia; during exercise they have the same negative inotropic effect as the other β-blockers.

Calcium Channel Blockers

By reducing the peripheral vascular resistance these agents are effective treatment for hypertension. Like β-blockers they have a beneficial effect on coexisting conditions (exertional and vasospastic angina, Raynaud phenomena, reentrant tachycardia).

All calcium channel blockers have a negative inotropic effect and should not be used when there is heart failure or a seriously depressed left ventricular ejection fraction. Nifedipine and nicardipine are powerful vasodilators that reflexly stimulate the sympathic nervous system. These effects include tachycardia, flushing, headache, and edema of the feet, which may be severe. Verapamil has a powerful negative chronotropic effect and may precipitate all grades of A-V block. The combination of verapamil and a β-blocker should be used with great caution because of the negative inotropic and chronotropic effects. Nifedipine and nicardipine can usually be safely used with a β-blocker which counteracts the reflex tachycardia. All calcium channel blockers (but especially Verapamil) intefere with digitalis excretion and may precipitate toxicity.

Vasodilators

When diuretics, β-blockers, and calcium channel blockers, and ACE inhibitors fail in treating hypertension, vasodilators are third-line choice.

Hydralazine (Apresoline)

This drug has a direct action on vessels producing peripheral vasodilatation, reducing the peripheral vascular resistance and elevating the heart rate and cardiac output. Renal blood flow is increased by hydralazine. Because it has a cardiac stimulatory effect it should be used with caution when there is evidence of congestive cardiac failure. On its own, its antihypertensive effect is mild but it has a potentiating effect with other drugs such as diuretics and propranolol: When large doses are used (over 300 mg per day) the most important toxic effect is an illness closely resembling systemic lupus erythematosus, including LE cells in the peripheral blood. The condition is potentially fatal and may require administration of steroids. Other side-effects include headache, anorexia, nausea, and nasal congestion. Usually the dosage of hydralazine should not exceed 50 mg four times daily.

Prazosin (Minipress)

This drug produces direct relaxant effect on vascular smooth muscle and a peripheral adrenergic sympatholytic effect. Despite its vascular relaxing effect, it does not produce peripheral venous pooling, change in the cardiac output, or tachycardia.

The drug is fairly well tolerated apart from mild nausea and light headedness in a small proportion of patients. The chief side effect is postural hypotension, which is dose related and most likely to occur when patients are volume depleted by diuretics. It can be avoided by starting with doses of 1 mg at night. Usually, the maximal dose does not exceed 20 mg/day given in two to four divided doses.

Minoxidil

This has a vasodilator effect on arteriolar smooth muscle similar to that of apresoline, and produces a reflex tachycardia and increase in cardiac output. It is, however, more potent than hydralazine. It should be used with caution in the presence of angina pectoris, which it may aggravate because of the tachycardia and increase in cardiac output. The oral dose is in the range from 2 to 40 mg/day, but because of a tendency for sodium restriction to occur, it should be used in conjunction with a diuretic.

Centrally Acting α-Blockers

α-Methyldopa (Aldomet)

This drug may produce its antihypertensive effects by producing a false neurotransmitter that interferes with the synthesis of norepinephrine, thus reducing peripheral vascular resistance. It may also decrease the release of renin from the kidneys. It has little or no effect on the heart rate or the cardiac output. Aldomet is not a powerful antihypertensive drug but its hypotensive effect is potentiated by diuretics. Side effects include transient drowsiness, dry mouth, nausea, depression, fever, disturbance of hepatic function, and hemolytic anemia. The drug is contraindicated therefore in depressive states and liver disease. Although the incidence of hemolytic anemia is uncommon, many patients develop a positive Coomb's Test. The usual dose is 250 mg two to four times a day.

Clonidine (Catapres)

The hypotensive action of this drug is produced by inhibition of outflow from the sympathetic centers in the central nervous system to the heart and peripheral vessels. It is an effective drug in mild and the more severe forms of hypertension and its use is enhanced by simultaneous diuretic therapy. The use of clonidine is characterized by a unique withdrawal syndrome when discontinued abruptly and the blood pressure may not only revert to pretreatment readings but there may also be a hypertensive crisis. The latter is related to sympathetic overactivity and should be treated by reinstitution of clonidine or the use of an α- or β-blocker. It should not be used in unreliable patients. Clonidine is given as 0.1 mg b.i.d. to a maximum of 0.8 mg daily.

Guanabenz

The action is similar to aldomet and clonidine and it also shares the potential for a withdrawal syndrome. It has the advantage of producing less salt retention and less edema. The usual dose is 4 mg daily with a maximum of 64 mg daily.

Peripheral Adrenergic Antagonists

Guanethidine (Ismelin)

This drug inhibits the release of norepinephrine at the neurone terminals. It does not act as a ganglion blocker, hence the unpleasant effects due to parasympathetic inhibition are avoided. It decreases the cardiac output, peripheral resistance, and heart rate. The drug is a potent hypotensive agent and it should be used with caution in patients with cardiac and vascular insufficiency. The response is most marked in the upright position and it has a prolonged duration of action. The addition of thiazides increases the antihypertensive response in the supine position and reduces the dose requirements of guanethidine. Tricyclic antidepressant drugs prevent the concentration of guanethidine at its site of action and antagonize its antihypertensive effects. The side effects are orthostatic hypertension and syncope. Guanethidine is particularly effective in the ambulant patient but it is advisable to start with a small dose of 10 mg daily, increasing by 5 to 10 mg daily at weekly intervals until the effective dose is reached—generally 30 to 60 my daily. Patients are advised to sleep propped up on pillows. The blood pressure must always be checked in the lying and standing position and after exercise. The latter is particularly important as hypotension on effort may result from overdosage and produce syncope. Side-effects include diarrhea and failure of ejaculation in the male.

Rauwolfia Compounds

These have a central and peripheral action, depleting the body stores of norepinephrine and reducing the blood pressure in the supine and upright position. Maximum effectiveness is reached after 2 to 3 weeks of therapy. Reserpine (Serpasil) is the móst commonly used preparation in a dose of 0.1 to 0.5 mg daily. Side-effects are not uncommon and include nasal stuffiness, dizziness, drowiness, increased appetite, and weight gain. Serious symptoms include insomnia, salt retention, and severe depression. Catecholamine depletion may occur and this may precipitate cardiac failure in patients with compromised cardiac function. This group of compounds is most useful in the treatment of cases of mild to moderate hypertension.

Combination Drug Treatment

Despite the confusing variety of drugs, many patients will respond to a simple program. Approximately 50% of patients can be controlled with one drug alone. Many physicians use the stepped-care approach advocated by the National Committee on Detection, Evaluation and Treatment of High Blood Pressure. When nonpharmacological approaches fail to control hypertension the first move is to prescribe a diuretic, β-blocker, calcium antagonist, or ACE inhibitor. If this is insufficient, a combination of these may be efficacious. For example, an ACE inhibitor and a diuretic is highly effective: Diuretics increase renin levels, which enhances the effect of ACE inhibitors, and a diuretic-induced hypokalelnia is decreased by the ACE inhibitor. Should this combination fail, a third drug may be added.

Treatment of Hypertensive Emergencies

Encephalopathy, fulminating heart failure, cerebral hemorrhage, and severe hypertension complicated by intractable angina may require urgent treatment.

Intravenous Sodium Nitroprusside

This may be the ideal drug for treatment of a hypertensive emergency. Its action on the resistance vessels, without effect on the heart or sympathetic nervous system, is immediately reversible. It is administered in a dose of 1 μg/kg/min, with constant monitoring of arterial pressure. When used for prolonged periods the blood thiocyanate levels should be checked because toxicity may appear when this is in excess of 12 mg percent.

Diazoxide

This is a nondiuretic benzothiadiazine, related to the thiazide diuretics, which dramatically lowers the blood pressure within 1 to 2 minutes when given intravenously in a dose of 250 to 350 mg. The duration varies from 1 to 18 hours, and this dose may be repeated. The site of action is on the smooth muscle of the arteriolar wall so that it usually does not produce pronounced postural falls in blood pressure. Its chief use is for the rapid reduction of the blood pressure in an emergency.

Trimethaphan (Arfonad)

This is an extremely rapidly acting ganglion blocking agent with brief duration of action. Tolerance develops rapidly but it gives an opportunity for slower but longer acting preparations to become effective.

Reserpine

This is one of the most reliable drugs but takes 1 or 2 hours to act, whether given intravenously or intramuscularly. Usually, 3 mg is given intramuscularly, repeated every 4 to 6 hours, depending on the blood pressure response. Its main disadvantage is that it produces somnolence and this may interfere with clinical observation of the hypertensive encephalopathic state.

α-Methyldopa (Aldomet)

When given intravenously in a dose of 250 mg to 1 g, a satisfactory hypotensive response is obtained in 1 to 4 hours and this may last up to 18 hours.

Labetolol

This is a combined α- and β-blocker. Given intravenously it is effective within 5 to 10 minutes. The dose is 20 to 80 mg by intravenous bolus every 10 minutes followed by an infusion of 2 mg/min.

When faced with a desperately ill patient in acute pulmonary edema or with dissecting aneurysm where immediate control of hypertension is required nitroprusside, diazoxide, or trimethaphan is the drug of choice. Intravenous furosemide may be administered with any of these drugs and is particularly useful when there is pulmonary edema.

Additional Reading

Guyton AC, Coleman TE, Fourcade JC et al.: (1969) Physiologic control of arterial pressure. Bull NY Acad Med 45:811, 1969.

Page IH: Arterial hypertension in retrospect. Circ Res 34:133, 1974.

Pickering G: Hypertension: Definition, natural histories and consequences. Am J Med 52:570, 1972.

Symposium on Hypertension: Mayo Clin Prac 64:1533–1552, 1989; 65:67–72, 1990. The 1988 Report of the Joint National Committee on Detection, Evaluation and Treatment of High Blood Pressure: Arch Int Med 148: 1023–1038, 1988.

Veterans Administration Cooperative Study Group on Antihypertensive Agents (Freis E.D., Chairman): I. Results in patients with diastolic blood pressures averaging 115 to 129 mm Hg. JAMA 202:1028, 1967; II. Results in patients with diastolic pressures averaging 90 to 114 mm Hg. JAMA 213:1143, 1970.

19
Diseases of the Aorta

Cardiovascular Syphilis

Syphilis is nearly always acquired through sexual contact and the cardiovascular system is affected soon after the initial invasion by the spirochete. However, a latent period of 15 to 25 years is characteristic before the results of cardiovascular syphilis become manifest. In rare cases, clinical heart disease may appear within as little as a year or two. Men are more commonly affected than women and the peak incidence is between the ages of 35 and 50.

The introduction of penicillin has made the disease uncommon but hopes that it would disappear entirely have been premature. Certainly in less advanced populations, syphilis is an important cause of cardiovascular morbidity and mortality.

The brunt of the disease falls on the ascending aorta, which is involved throughout its thickness. Thus, the infection is introduced into the aorta via the lymphatics of the adventitia, resulting in endarteritis and scarring. Destruction of the media produces weakening and thinning of the aortic wall with subsequent dilatation or aneurysm. Involvement of the intima produces scarring and proliferation, which is unimportant in itself in the large aortic lumen, except that atheroma formation and calcification is promoted. The coronary ostia are situated at the site of election of the disease and narrowing, and eventual occlusion of the ostia produces a pathologic and clinical syndrome associated with coronary insufficiency. The inflammatory process does not involve the aortic cusps directly. Weakening and dilatation of the valve ring lead to separation of the cusps at the commisures resulting in aortic insufficiency. The aorta is never involved in congenital syphilis.

Involvement of the myocardium is rare. Occasionally, gummata develop, but these are unimportant except when the septum is involved and the conducting tissue affected. Complete heart block may then result. Syphilitic cardiac aneurysms are of historic interest only.

Clinical Features

Latent Syphilis

Syphilitic aortitis is usually asymptomatic. An accentuated A_2 may be heard and there may be radiologic evidence of dilatation or calcification of the ascending aorta. Positive serologic tests for syphilis confirm the diagnosis.

Coronary Disease

Angina pectoris, rarely cardiac infarction, cardiac aneurysm, or sudden death may result from involvement of the coronary ostia. Aortic insufficiency is nearly always associated. The diagnosis is based on the presence of associated aortic valve disease and positive serology. The condition should be suspected when angina pectoris is encountered in young men, and when severe angina pectoris is associated with disproportionately mild aortic insufficiency. The diagnosis can now be made with certainty by coronary angiography and successful palliative surgical treatment may be achieved by endarterectomy of the coronary ostia, or by saphenous vein bypass grafting.

Aortic Insufficiency

The presenting symptoms may be those of coronary insufficency or of left heart failure. Because of coronary ostial stenosis, angina and cardiac infarction is far commoner than in rheumatic aortic insufficiency. Pain on effort is quite indistinguishable from angina of atherosclerotic origin, but nitroglycerin is often less effective. Attacks of angina decubitus are not infrequent.

The physical signs are the same as those of rheumatic aortic insufficiency. Pure insufficiency without any stenosis is the rule. Loud systolic murmurs may be present because of the large stroke volume. Because of the unfolding and dilatation of the ascending aorta, the murmurs are frequently better heard to the right of the sternum. In advanced cases a basal systolic thrill conducted into the vessels of the neck may be encountered, but again this is the result of high flow. An apical Austin–Flint murmur is generally audible and this may have presystolic accentuation. The first heart sound is usually soft, and this with the absence of an opening snap helps in the distinction from rheumatic heart disease. Occasionally, a musical ("cooing-dove") diastolic murmur is produced by eversion or detachment of an aortic cusp. Syphilis is the commonest cause of this type of murmur, which again may be better heard to the right of the sternum.

The presence of aortic disease radiologically is helpful in establishing the diagnosis. Aneurysmal dilatation or calcification of the ascending aorta may be present. Evidence of syphilitic disease elsewhere (e.g., tabes dorsalis), positive serology (75% of cases), and a raised sedimentation rate are all helpful.

Differential Diagnosis

Rheumatic Aortic Insufficiency

This is the commonest cause of pure insufficiency, apart from syphilis, and differentiation at any stage may be difficult or impossible. The disease is usually encountered in the younger age group, however, and the serology is negative.

Infective Endocarditis

This usually supervenes on a rheumatic or a congenital bicuspid valve: rarely, are normal valves affected. Infective endocarditis rarely may involve the aortic leaflets in syphilitic aortitis.

Aneurysms of the Sinuses of Valsalva

These may produce aortic insufficiency by traction on the valve cusps. The diagnosis is difficult, when the aneurysm is intact because the presentation is one of pure aortic insufficiency without any helpful distinguishing features. The diagnosis should be thought of when aortic insufficiency presents in adolescence in the absence of a history of rheumatic fever. When the aneurysm perforates into the right ventricle or the right atrium, a continuous murmur usually obscures the early diastolic murmur and aortic insufficiency is recognized only at cardiac catheterization.

Marfan Syndrome

This produces dilatation of the ascending aorta and the valve ring resulting in aortic insufficiency (Figs. 19.1 and 19.2). Frequently, the usual physical stigmata of Marfan syndrome (the slender body build, arachnodactyly, high-arched palate, depressed sternum, pectus excavatum, dislocation of the lens) are absent and the presentation is one of isolated aortic valve disease. The diagnosis may be suggested by the X-ray showing marked dilatation of the ascending aorta. Not uncommonly, however, the condition is recognized only at operation when the aorta is found to be abnormally thin because of the underlying medionecrosis.

Hypertension and Atherosclerosis

This may occasionally be associated with mild aortic insufficiency, particularly when hypertension is uncontrolled. The murmur may disappear when the blood pressure is controlled.

Ankylosing Spondylitis

This produces an aortitis closer to the aortic valve than syphilis. Scarring of the leaflets and aortic regurgitation are a result. In 50% of cases there is extension of the inflammatory process into the ventricular septum producing varying degrees of heart block.

Syphilitic Aortic Aneurysm

This involves the ascending aorta and the arch with equal frequency. Less commonly, the descending aorta is involved, and least commonly the abdominal aorta. It is not unusual for the aorta to be involved at more than one site in the same patient. Syphilitic aneurysms are usually saccular (fusiform aneurysms of the aorta are a result of atherosclerosis). The clinical presentation is dependent on compression of the adjacent structures and therefore varies with the portion of aorta involved.

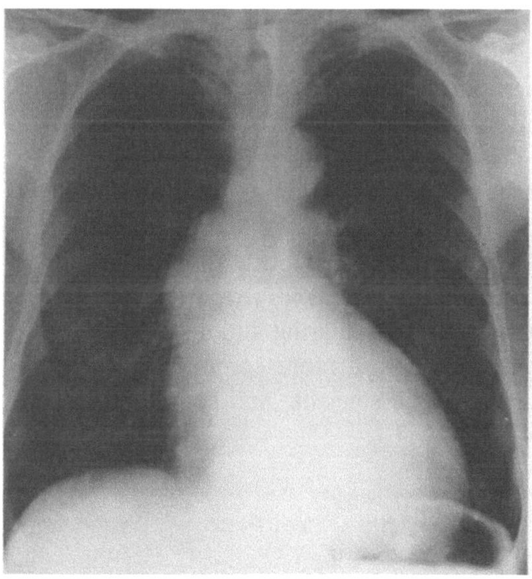

FIGURE 19.1. Chest X-ray showing aneurysm of ascending aorta in case of Marfan syndrome.

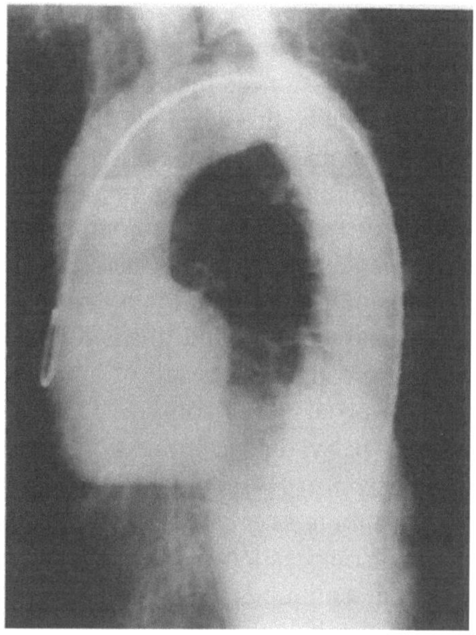

FIGURE 19.2. Aortic angiogram demonstrating a large saccular aneurysm of the ascending aorta with marked aortic insufficiency in a case of Marfan syndrome.

Aneurysms of the Ascending Aorta

This has been termed the "aneurysm of signs." Compression of the superior vena cava produces distended nonpulsatile neck veins, with dilated collateral venous channels when the obstruction is complete. When obstruction is incomplete, pulsation may persist and the anastamotic vessels may not be prominent. Edema in the drainage area of the superior vena cava may be marked, with suffusion, edema, and cyanosis of the face, neck, and upper limbs. Occasionally, the outflow tract of the right ventricle is involved producing hemodynamically significant pulmonic stenosis with the appropriate physical signs. Compression of the right main bronchus and lungs produces respiratory complications. Erosion of the sternum produces a superficial pulsating mass on one or other side of the sternum. The pulsating tumor gradually erodes through the surrounding tissue and points beneath the skin. Rupture through the skin or perforation into the superior vena cava, or into a bronchus, is usually a terminal event.

Aneurysm of the Arch of the Aorta

This is known as the "aneurysm of symptoms" because of compression of the trachea, bronchi, and nerves, which produce the appropriate symptoms. Dyspnea, hoarseness, dysphagia, and pain are prominent. Pulmonary complications secondary to large airway compression are frequent, leading to bronchiectasis, lung infection, and hemoptysis. Initially, a dry "brassy" cough is characteristic and this is followed by a productive cough as a result of infection. Recurrent laryngeal nerve compression leads to vocal cord palsy, and compression of the sympathetic chain to Horner syndrome. Paralysis of the diaphragms is rare. Erosion of the vertebrae and compression of nerves give rise to deep seated continuous bone and root pain. Rupture into the neighboring structures may be a terminal event.

An aneurysm may be suspected clinically by unequal pulses and blood pressures in the upper limbs, the presence of a tracheal tug, or a continuous murmur suggesting rupture into the right heart chambers. Not infrequently, an aneurysm is first detected by chest X-ray, and therefore must be distinguished from neoplasms, cysts, retrosternal goiter, thymic, and lymphatic gland enlargement. Expansile pulsation demonstrated by fluoroscopy is helpful but this is not always present because of extensive laminated thrombus. Linear calcification of the aneurysmal sac is a helpful sign. The ultimate diagnosis is usually established by aortic angiography.

Aneurysms of the Descending Thoracic Aorta

These are usually detected on routine chest radiography since they generally reach a large size before producing symptoms. Compression of the lungs produces cough, dyspnea, and pulmonary infection. Erosion produces bone pain and swelling of the left posterior chest wall.

Aneurysms of the Abdominal Aorta

Less than 5% of syphilitic aneurysms involve the abdominal aorta. Their clinical presentation is similar to that of the more common atherosclerotic aneurysm to be discussed later.

Treatment

Antisyphilitic treatment should be given as soon as the disease is recognized. Positive serology is present in most cases of aneurysm, but treatment should be administered even if a syphilitic etiology is suspected but not proven. Herxheimer's reaction following administration of penicillin is rare. Benzathine penicillin G should be given in a dose of 2.4 million units weekly for three successive weeks. When there is allergy to penicillin, tetracycline 500 mg four times daily for a period of 1 month may be administered.

Dissecting Aneurysm of the Aorta

Aortic dissection arises as a consequence of cystic medial necrosis. The intima is torn, most frequently in the ascending aorta, producing hemorrhage that cleaves the layers of the aortic wall. The entire length of the aorta may be involved although the separation of the layers frequently does not encircle the whole circumference of the aorta. Alternatively, weakening of the aorta results in a localized saccular aneurysm, of which medial necrosis is the commonest cause.

Cystic medial necrosis is a frequent component of Marfan syndrome, but is also observed in the aorta of apparently normal elderly people. In the latter group the superimposition of the hydraulic stress of hypertension predisposes to intimal tearing and dissection. Aortic dissection is also more common during pregnancy, aortic stenosis, and coarctation of the aorta.

Classification

DeBakey has classified aortic dissection on the basis of the site of the intimal tear and the extent of the dissection. In Type I, the tear occurs in the ascending aorta distal to the aortic

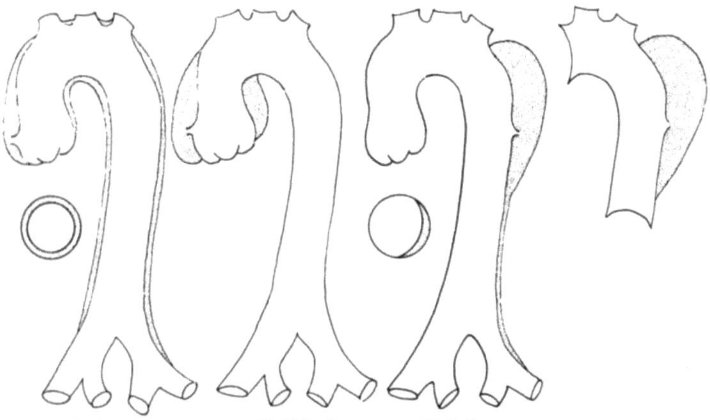

FIGURE 19.3. Dissecting aneurysm of the aorta. In Type 1 the rupture hematoma completely surrounds the aorta extending a variable distance down the descending aorta. In this diagram it extends to the bifurcation. In Type 2 the hematoma stops at the innominate artery. In Type 3 the dissection starts just beyond the origin of the left subclavian artery to involve a variable length of aorta but does not usually completely surround the aorta. After DeBakey et al., J Thor Cardiovasc Surg 49:130, 1955, with permission.

sinuses and extends to involve the aorta through its whole length. In Type II only the ascending aorta is involved (Fig. 19.3). In Type III the tear is located below the origin of the left subclavian artery and extends a variable distance down the thoracic and abdominal aorta.

The Stanford classification is simpler and more practical. Stanford Type A includes Types I and II of DeBakey. Type A dissections are more lethal and require surgery for correction. They account for approximately 70% of cases. Type B (DeBakey Type III) has a better prognosis and may respond to medical treatment.

Clinical Presentation

The most common presentation is one of an acute cardiac catastrophe resembling myocardial infarction with severe pain, shock, and death within 48 hours. Less commonly, the disease is subacute and patients may survive for months or years, and this is particularly likely to occur with a Type III dissection.

Pain is the commonest symptom, and is characteristically sudden, tearing, or crushing. It is indistinguishable from myocardial infarction, located in the center of the chest, but radiates through to the back. The pain is often maximal at the onset. Severe abdominal pain radiating to the lower back may be present. In as many as a third of patients pain may be absent. The pain of aortic dissection is so severe that it is one of the few pains not relieved by morphine.

Involvement of the peripheral arteries is responsible for hemiplegia when the carotids are affected. When the limb vessels are involved there is pain in the affected limb, parasthesia, coldness, vascular insufficiency, and absent pulses. Occlusion of the anterior spinal artery results in paraplegia, girdle pain, and other neurologic syndromes. Renal involvement produces pain in the lumbar region, hematuria, and renal failure. Occlusion of the abdominal arteries produces a picture resembling an acute surgical emergency such as cholecystitis, pancreatitis, and intestinal obstruction. Rupture into the lung produces the picture of pulmonary infarction, pneumonia, or pleural effusion.

Hypertension and cardiomegaly are frequent. An aortic diastolic murmur of recent origin strongly suggests dissecting aneurysm

(Types I and II). This is not necessarily due to a tear in the aortic valve but can be caused by distortion, so that surgical repair of the dissection may restore normal function without necessitating valve replacement. Pericardial friction rub and tamponade are uncommonly encountered clinically, since in most cases dissection into the pericardial sac is instantaneously fatal.

A normal electrocardiogram is often invaluable in differentiating the condition from myocardial infarction. When the coronary arteries themselves are dissected, however, the clinical and electrocardiographic changes are exactly the same as those of myocardial infarction. Radiologically, the findings are very similar to those of a syphilitic aneurysm with widening of the supracardiac shadow, straightening of the aortic arch, and compression of the surrounding structures. A diagnostic finding is a double aortic knob, or widening of the aortic wall, the calcified intima being separated from the lateral border by a centimeter or more. A sudden increase in the size of the aorta is highly suggestive of the diagnosis. Left ventricular hypertrophy may be present, and pleural effusion is not uncommon. However, these findings are not reliable in diagnosis.

Diagnosis

Aortography

Aortography demonstrates the true lumen filled with angiographic contrast material, which is frequently compressed by the hematoma contained in the media. Often the contrast material can be identified entering the false channel through the intimal tear. The technique provides important information about aortic insufficiency and involvement of the coronary arteries and branch vessels off the aorta. The entry and reentry sites into the intima are frequently observed. The sensitivity of the procedure is about 80% and the specificity about 95%. The disadvantages of aortography are that it is invasive and requires a large volume of iodine-containing dye which is contraindicated when renal function is impaired.

Echocardiography

The transthoracic technique yields good images of the aortic arch but poor images of the retrocardiac and descending aorta. Transesophageal echocardiography provides excellent images of the retrocardiac and descending aorta but poor images of the arch. A combination of the two techniques yields excellent information. Echo Doppler is also able to detect pericardial effusion and aortic regurgitation.

In expert hands the sensitivity and specificity of the technique are superior to that of aortography. The disadvantages are the difficulty in imaging large patients.

Computed Tomography

CT scans are more accurate than aortography in the diagnosis of dissection. It is also very useful in demonstrating blood in the pericardium, pleural space, and mediastinum. It can image the entire aorta in 30 to 60 minutes and there is no interference with life support equipment. The technique is therefore ideal for use in cricitally ill patients.

Like other imaging techniques CT makes the diagnosis by detecting the flap in the 2-lumina aorta. It is the most sensitive technique demonstrating calcification of the intima—medial displacement of which is a sure sign of dissection.

Disadvantages of CT include use of large volumes of iodinated dye, and radiation exposure that limits the number of follow-up examinations.

Magnetic Resonance Imaging (MRI)

MRI does not require the use of contrast and is therefore ideal for use in allergic patients and in those with abnormal renal function. With the use of spin-echo MRI, the intimal flap is seen as a line separating the true and the false lumina. It is superior to other imaging techniques in visualizing the intimal flap and easily distinguishes between Type A and B dissections. However, it cannot, visualize the coronary arteries and can be used to study only stable patients. Metallic objects including metallic cardiac prosthesis preclude the use of MRI.

Prognosis

The prognosis for aortic dissection is poor; only 25% of patients survive 14 days and only 10% survive one year. The prognosis is much better for those cases where the dissection occurs distal to the arch (Type III). The heavy mortality associated with Type I and II (Stanford Type A) occurs because of involvement of the aortic valve, coronary arteries, and the brachiocephalic vessels.

Treatment

For Type A treatment is surgical and indications for acute intervention are (1) severe aortic regurgitation, (2) hemopericardium, (3) cardiac tamponade, (4) occlusion of branches of aorta, (5) bleeding into the left pleural space, (6) uncontrollable pain, and (7) continuing dissection.

The treatment of Type B dissection is medical in contrast to Type A since these patients are frequently hypertensive. The systolic blood pressure should be reduced to 120 mm Hg as soon as possible using nitroprusside or trimethaphan intravenously. Oral propranolol or guanethidine may be given additionally. Medical failure is indicated by expansion of the aneurysm and rupture. These should be treated with immediate operation.

Emergency surgery for all types of dissections is associated with a high mortality of up to 50% whereas that for elective procedures is approximately 12%. When patients are seen for the first time, 14 or more days after the acute event, surgery is indicated only if complications such as aortic insufficiency, progressive enlargement of the aneurysm, or evidence of vascular insufficiency is present.

Surgical Technique

The aim of surgery is to prevent rupture of the aneurysm, which is the principal cause of mortality. The principles of repair, using cardiopulmonary bypass, are to open the aneurysm widely and transect the distal aorta. A preclotted woven dacron graft is placed in the aortic lumen and all layers of the aorta included in the anastomosis proximally and distally. Aortic valve replacement may be necessary for aortic regurgitation.

Arteriosclerosis of the Aorta

Arteriosclerosis leads to widening and the elongation of the aorta throughout its length, with kinking and tortuosity involving the abdominal portion in particular. Loss of elasticity, rigidity, and calcification result in loss of recoil, which is reflected by systolic hypertension and a large pulse pressure. With the elongation of the aorta and kinking of its branches, the right carotid artery in particular is looped back on itself presenting as a pulsating tumor in the right side of the neck, often mistaken for an aneurysm—the so-called "kinked carotid." This is found particularly in elderly women with hypertension and arteriosclerosis. Unless complications occur, aortic arteriosclerosis produces no symptoms, but is frequently recognized radiologically as tortuosity on dilatation of the aorta or by the formation of a fusiform aneurysm, which may have to be differentiated from syphilis or dissecting aneurysm. Dilatation of the aortic valve ring may produce aortic insufficiency. Lack of compliance of the arteriosclerotic vascular system of the elderly patient produces a rapid rate of rise of the carotid pulse even in the presence of severe aortic stenosis and this may cause diagnostic confusion.

Thoracic Aneurysms

Despite the fact that the overwhelming majority of arteriosclerotic aneurysms are abdominal, arteriosclerosis has become a more common cause of thoracic aneurysm than syphilis, tending to involve the arch and descending segments. These aneurysms are fusiform and when sufficiently large may produce all the complications mentioned in the previous section dealing with syphilitic aneurysm.

Rupture of thoracic atherosclerotic aneurysms occurs in approximately 50% of patients. The indications for operation are (1) diameter exceeding 6 cm, (2) severe hypertension, (3) symptoms attributed to the aneurysm, and (4) progressive enlargement while under observation.

Abdominal Aortic Aneurysms

Ninety-eight percent of all abdominal aortic aneurysms are situated below the renal arteries and they may extend into the iliac arteries. They frequently remain silent until they rupture and this is responsible for death in 4 per 1000 elderly people.

Abdominal aneurysms are frequently detected during a routine clinical examination as a pulsatile mass, or by routine radiography which demonstrates curvi-linear calclification in the wall. Ultrasound is not only useful in the initial diagnosis of abdominal aortic aneurysm but also in their follow-up (Fig. 19.4). Echocardiography is almost 100% sensitive and specific in diagnosis and can precisely measure the size. Aneurysms more than 5 cm are likely to rupture and should be resected. Sudden pain in the back or abdomen suggests the presence of rupture into the retroperitoneum and should be operated upon immediately. Aneurysms less than 5 cm should be followed by echocardiography every 4 to 6 months.

The prognosis for this condition is poor; only one-third of patients survive 5 years. In the absence of severe symptomatic coronary artery disease the operative mortality should be less than 5% in experienced surgical hands.

Aortic Atherosclerosis

Even when extensive, this produces no obstruction to the lumen of the aorta. Complications arise from superimposed thrombosis and embolism. Small thrombi break off from atheromatous plaques and lodge in the abdominal vessels or organs, or the lower limbs.

Cholesterol Embolism

Rarely, atheromatous ulcers may discharge cholesterol debris that blocks multiple small vessels particularly in the lower limbs. The skin and the kidney are also affected leading to a picture closely resembling polyarteritis nodosa with petecchial hemorrhages on the trunk and lower extremities, renal failure, and high ESR. The condition usually occurs spontaneously, but may also follow cross-clamping of the aorta during surgery.

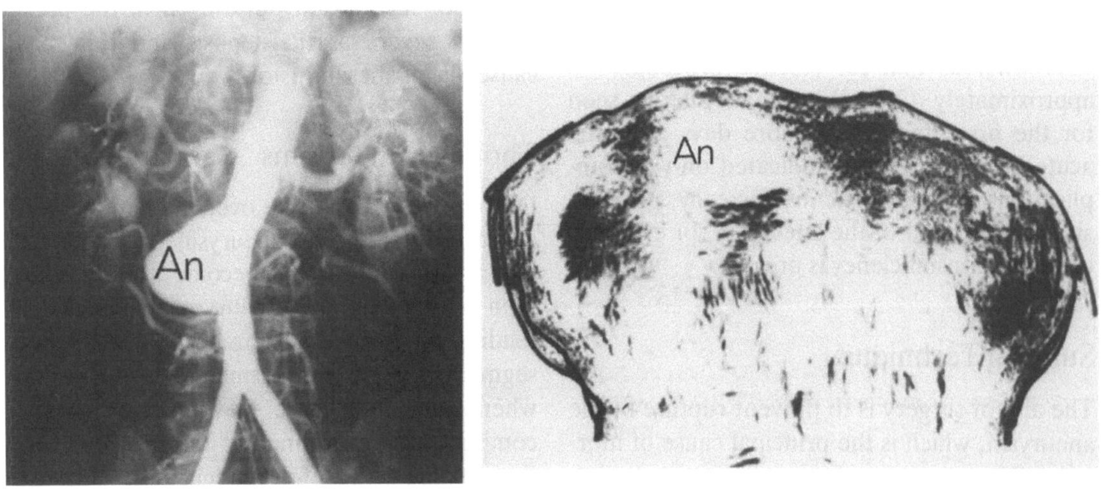

FIGURE 19.4. Atherosclerotic aeurysm of descending aorta just below the origin of the renal arteries detected by ultrasound (A) and by aortography (B).

LeRiche Syndrome

Progressive atherosclerotic occlusion of the aortic bifurcation leads to claudication of the lower back and thighs, impotence, and absence of the femoral pulses. It is usually possible to differentiate this condition from congenital coarctation and aortitis, but occasionally angiography will be necessary.

Aortic Arch Syndrome

Progressive occlusion of the brachiocephalic vessels by atherosclerosis leads to the so-called "aortic arch syndrome" or "reversed coarctation." The condition may also be produced by syphilitic aortitis, dissecting aneurysm, and congenital abnormalities associated with a severe preductal coarctation and a patent ductus arteriosus. Under these circumstances, the femoral pulses are more readily palpable than the carotids and arm pulses.

Aortic Arteritis: "Pulseless" or Takayasu Disease

The syndrome of arteritis of the aorta and its major branches was first documented by the Japanese ophthalmologist, Takayasu, who drew attention to the eye manifestations in afflicted young women. The condition is most common in children and young adults, affecting women particularly. It is encountered in most countries of the world, particularly the Far East, India, and Africa. The etiology is unknown.

Pathologically, there is focal or diffuse loss of muscular and elastic tissue, with extensive fibrosis of the media and destruction of the elastic lamina affecting the larger elastic arteries. Recently involved areas show a fibrolastic proliferation with ingrowth of new capillaries resembling granulomas. Narrowing of the arterial lumen is produced by gross fibrotic intimal thickening and proliferation, with organization and superimposed thrombosis. Premature atherosclerosis is a common result and this is often associated with hypertension. Calcification of the atheroma produces linear shadows seen on the chest X-ray. When the media is weakened, dilatation of the wall leads to aneurysm formation. The inflammatory process also leads to obliteration of the lumen because of superimposed thrombosis. The lesion is extensive but patchy, so that several vascular territories are simultaneously affected, but to varying degrees. Combinations of stenosis and aneurysm formation are encountered.

The most common symptoms are a result of hypertensive heart failure. Hypertension is a result of renal artery involvement or obstruction of the aorta proximal to these vessels.

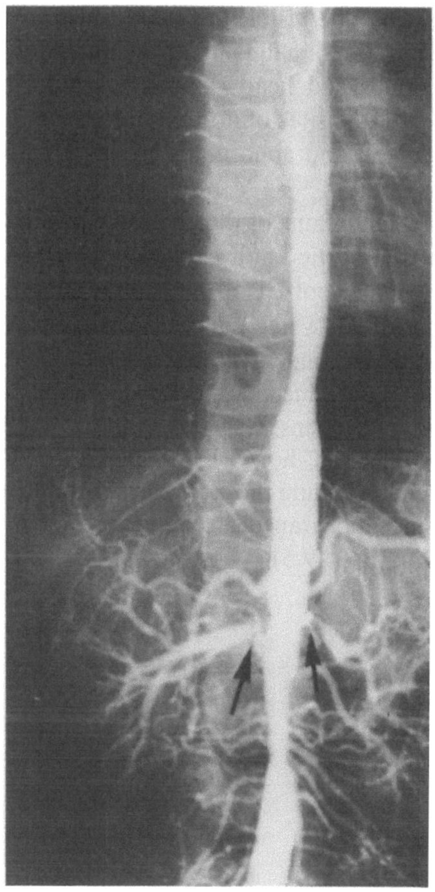

FIGURE 19.5. Lower thoracic and abdominal aortogram in idiopathic aortitis demonstrating the "rat-tail" appearance at the level of the diaphragms, stenosis of the origin of both renal arteries (arrows), and narrowing of the aorta below the level of the renal arteries.

Central aortic hypertension is often present, but may not be detected because of occlusion of the subclavian arteries. Other symptoms include syncope, epilepsy, hemiplegia, and aphasia when there is cerebral involvement. Claudication of the upper limbs and motor weakness reflect subclavian artery involvement.

The diagnosis must be made from syphilis and other causes of the aortic arch syndrome and from peripheral vascular disease and hypertensive heart disease. Occasionally, the picture of congenital coarctation is closely mimicked. Evidence of diffuse arterial involvement is often present and, most importantly, the site of coarctation and the related murmur is unusual. Dilated anastomotic intercostal arteries may be visible over the lower chest. There is marked inequality of the pulses of the upper limbs and head vessels, murmurs and thrills over the sites of arterial narrowing, fundal changes, and abnormally sensitive carotid sinuses.

Roentgenograms of the chest are invaluable in that the aortic knob is clearly defined and the left upper border of the cardiac silhouette is not formed by the enlarged left subclavian artery, as in congenital coarctation. The disease may produce fusiform dilatation and saccular aneurysms anywhere in the aorta. The sites of election, however, are the aortic arch and the descending thoracic aorta, producing a "rat-tail" appearance at the level of the diaphragm (Fig. 19.5).

The prognosis is variable. Death is usually a result of cerebral involvement or heart failure. The condition may be compatible with many years of life when there is adequate development of collateral channels. Occasionally, bypass grafts between the proximal and distal aorta have been required for palliation.

Additional Reading

DeBakey ME, Henly WS, Cooley DA, Crawford ES, Beall AC: Surgical management of dissecting aneurysm of the aorta. J Thorac and Cardiov Surg 49:130, 1965. Erb BD, Tullis IF: Dissecting aneurysm of the aorta. Circulation 22:315, 1960.

Gotsman MS, Beck W, Schrire V: Selective angiography in arteritis of the aorta and its major branches. Radiology 88:232, 1967.

McKusick VA: The cardiovascular aspects of Marfan's syndrome: A heritable disorder of connective tissue. Circulation 11:321, 1955.

Nakao K, Ikeda M, Kimata S, Niitani H, Miyahara M, Ishimi X, Hishiba K, Takeda Y, Ozawa T, Matsushita S, Kuramochi M: Takayasu's arteritis. Circulation 35:1141, 1967.

Rich C, Webster B: The natural history of uncomplicated syphilitic aortitis. Am Heart J 43:321, 1952.

Schrire V, Asherson A: Arteritis of the aorta and its major branches. Q J Med 33:439, 1966.

Wheat MW, Jr.: Treatment of dissecting aneurysm of the aorta: Current status. Prog Cardiovasc Dis 16:87, 1973.

20
Cor Pulmonale

Cor pulmonale is the term used to describe hypertrophy and dilatation of the right ventricle as the result of lung disease. Although the causes of cor pulmonale are diverse, they have as their common effect, the production of alveolar hypoxia producing pulmonary arterial vasoconstriction and/or an anatomical reduction of the pulmonary vascular bed. When these changes are severe and bilateral, *pulmonary arterial hypertension* develops and this is responsible for the pathogenesis of cor pulmonale. Passive pulmonary arterial hypertension secondary to left atrial hypertension (e.g., left ventricular failure or mitral valve disease) and hyperkinetic pulmonary hypertension secondary to left-to-right shunts (ASD, VSD etc.) are specifically excluded from this definition. Malfunction of the lungs may not only be because of parenchymal disease but also a result of failure of the bellows action of the chest or ventilatory drive by the central nervous system.

Clinical Findings

Generally, it is not difficult to make a diagnosis of pulmonary hypertension at the bedside with the assistance of the electrocardiogram and chest X-ray. An exception applies when there is chronic obstructive airways disease (COPD) in which case precordial palpation and auscultation are seriously compromised by the barrel shaped chest.

The jugular venous pressure shows prominent "a" waves and when there is tricuspid regurgitation "cv" waves, which become more prominent with inspiration. Systolic pulsation of the liver may also be present. Precordial palpation eliclts a left parasternal lift and, in advanced cases, pulmonic valve closure can be felt.

The chief auscultatory feature is the accentuated sound of pulmonic valve closure, which may be louder than that of aortic valve closure. The second sound becomes narrowly split even on deep inspiration. A pulmonic ejection click often followed by a short scratchy ejection systolic murmur signifies dilatation of the main pulmonary artery. A localized early diastolic murmur occurs when there is pulmonic insufficiency. The murmur of tricuspid regurgitation is present when there is right ventricular failure and this is usually accompanied by a loud third sound. Prior to the occurrence of right ventricular failure, a loud S4 is the auscultatory counterpart of the large "a" wave in the jugular venous pressure.

Central cyanosis will occur when there is a right-to-left shunt across the patent foramen ovale and the differentiation from congenital heart disease may then require cardiac catheterization.

The Electrocardiogram

This provides evidence of right atrial and right ventricular overload, which must be considerable for changes to occur, particularly in the case of COPD. The important findings are (1) right axis deviation (more than 90°), (2) P pulmonale, (3) reversal of the normal ratio of R/S of 1/3 in lead V1, and (4) T wave inversion and ST segment depression in leads V1–3.

The Chest X-Ray

The leading findings are (1) enlargement of the main pulmonary artery and its proximal branches and (2) "pruning" (attenuation) of the peripheral pulmonary arteries.

Echocardiography

This is not helpful in the presence of COPD because hyperinflated lungs preclude good imaging. In other cases of pulmonary hypertension the test is useful in demonstrating right-sided enlargement and excluding mitral stenosis and other causes of pulmonary venous hypertension. Doppler interrogation of the incompetent tricuspid valve provides a useful assessment of the peak right ventricular and pulmonary artery pressures.

Ventilation–Perfusion Scans

A ventilation perfusion mismatch (i.e., a lobar perfusion defect with normal ventilation) makes pulmonary embolism a likely diagnosis. A normal scan is strong evidence against the diagnosis. Matched defects occur when there is lung disease such as pneumonia and atelectasis.

Cardiac Catheterization

Right-heart catheterization establishes the diagnosis of pulmonary hypertension and excludes congenital heart disease (shunts) and left-sided disease (mitral stenosis, left ventricular failure). Selective pulmonary angiography is the gold standard for the diagnosis of pulmonary embolism.

The causes of cor pulmonale may be conveniently classified as follows:

1. Pulmonary Vascular Disease
   A. Embolism or thrombus.
   B. Idiopathic pulmonary hypertension.
2. Hypoxic Vasoconstriction
   A. Primary pulmonary disease—chronic obstructive airways disease, pulmonary fibrosis, and granulomatosis.
   B. Extrapulmonary disease—hypoventilation because of central nervous system disease, chest cage deformity, muscle weakness, and obesity.

Vascular Disease

Pulmonary embolism is common. Approximately one-third of patients dying of congestive cardiac failure have postmortem evidence of pulmonary embolism; in many it is the immediate cause of death. In the overwhelming majority of cases the source of emboli is venous thrombosis of the deep veins of the legs and pelvis. Venous thrombosis occurs most commonly in congestive cardiac failure, whatever the cause, but especially in rheumatic heart disease with mitral stenosis. Other important causes are surgery, fractures, child birth, or prolonged bed rest from any cause. Carcinoma and blood dyscrasia such as leukemia and sickle cell anemia may also be predisposing factors. Venous thrombosis in the legs may occur without inflammatory reaction (phlebothrombosis) or there may be an aseptic inflammatory reaction (thrombophlebitis). In both circumstances venous thrombosis may propagate up the lower extremities and a piece may break off, lodging as an embolus in the lungs.

It is quite clear from autopsy studies, phlebography, and radioactive fibrinogen uptake tests that the clinical recognition of thrombosis in the deep veins of the legs is poor and is identified in only approximately one-third of patients with the manifestations of pulmonary embolism or infarction.

Pulmonary Infarction

This usually does not follow embolism into a normal lung. The lung is supplied not only by the pulmonary arteries but also by the bronchial circulation, which supplies all the pulmonary structures excluding the alveoli. The bronchial arteries arise from the aorta and anastamose with pulmonary aretery capillaries. Pulmonary infarction will occur when the bronchial circulation is unable to maintain sufficient collateral flow to the pulmonary parenchyma. This will occur in any cause of pulmonary congestion such as left ventricular failure or mitral stenosis. Pulmonary infarction is produced by embolic occlusion of the middle sized branches of the pulmonary artery. There is a tendency to involve the lower lobes where blood flow is normally greater than in the upper lobe. Infarcts are segmental, situated on the periphery of the lungs and involve the pleura, hence the frequency of pleuritis and effusions. The effects on the right heart depend on the size and number of infarcts but in most instances the occurrence of pulmonary infarction is usually a clinically benign event. There is ample evidence that the majority of pulmonary emboli undergo rapid lysis in the pulmonary circulation without infarction or hemodynamic embarrassment. The occurrence of a pulmonary infarct, however, is a clear warning of a dangerous situation where there is venous thrombosis in the legs, even though unrecognized, and that fatal massive pulmonary embolism is a distinct possiblity.

Clinical Picture

Occasionally there are local signs such as pain, swelling, and tenderness of the calves that may point to the presence of phlebothrombosis. Pain on dorsiflexion of the foot (Homan's sign) may be present, or precede the acute episode. A rise in pulse rate or a spike in temperature is frequently present. The infarction itself is associated with dyspnea, tachycardia, pleuritis, pain, and cough. Hemoptysis occurs in about one-third of cases, varying from slight, bright blood-streaking, to massive bleeding. A highly characteristic appearance is a solid jelly-like sputum produced by the presence of altered blood. Signs of pleurisy may be found and there may be a friction rub or effusion. Pulmonary signs include rales and/or bronchial breathing. Constitutional disturbances such as leukocytosis, fever, and raised sedimentation rate are usual. Radiological signs consist of single or multiple pulmonary opacities, characteristic wedge-shaped areas of consolidation, areas of disc-atelectasis, and pleural effusion. Elevation of the leaf of the diaphram is frequently present when the infarct is of significant size.

It is important to appreciate that pulmonary infarction is simulated by pneumonia and pleurisy. Hemoptysis in a patient with mitral stenosis may be a result of acute bronchitis, pulmonary venous hemorrhage, or pulmonary infarction and the distinction is not all that easy.

Laboratory findings include leukocytosis and elevation of the serum bilirubin level. A rise in LDH enzyme is fairly frequent and may be of some diagnostic help provided other causes such as myocardial infarction are not present. The blood gases may provide helpful information. Hyperventilation is almost invariably associated with pulmonary infarction. There is usually a reduction in the arterial p_{O_2}, and p_{CO_2} with respiratory alkalosis. Radioisotope scanning is of limited value when there are areas of consolidation, atelectasis, or pleural effusion. The electrocardiogram does not show any significant changes.

Massive Pulmonary Embolism—Acute Cor Pulmonale

This occurs when emboli liberated from the leg are of sufficient size and quantity to occlude at least two-thirds of the pulmonary circulation. This is so because there is considerable pulmonary vascular reserve; pneumonectomy, for example, does not produce pulmonary hypertension if the remaining lung is normal. Any rapid rise in the pulmonary artery pressure produces systolic overload of a normal right ventricle with elevation in its filling pressure and signs of right-sided heart failure. The cardiac output may fall and peripheral circulatory collapse ensue. Usually, left ventricular failure following pulmonary embolism occurs in those patients with preexisting ischemic left ventricular disease.

Clinical Features

The acute episode is associated with sudden onset of pain, dyspnea, and shock.

Pain

When present, pain is characteristically pressing, heavy, situated behind the center of the chest, and indistinguishable from myocardial infarction. It differs from that of pulmonary infarction, which is pleuritic, and which may precede or follow massive embolism.

Dyspnea

This is a very prominent symptom, sudden in onset, and frequently presents as rapid deep breathing without apparent cause.

Shock

The usual manifestations of hypotension, restlessness, sweating, weakness, and coldness of the extremities are present. Tachycardia, however, is out of proportion to the other signs and cyanosis may be severe because of hypoxia and low cardiac output.

Right Heart Failure

Signs of this develop soon and depend on whether the tricuspid valve maintains its competency or not. Tricuspid insufficiency can be recognized by systolic pulsation of the jugular veins and liver, and a tricuspid systolic murmur. Unrelieved acute pulmonary hypertension is recognized by a right atrial gallop and audible accentuation of pulmonary valve closure. Rarely, a pulmonary systolic murmur is present and this has been attributed to friction between the distended pulmonary artery and the taut pericardium. (Means's murmur).

The Electrocardiogram

This demonstrates important findings: There is frequently right axis deviation of the P wave vector to +90° producing prominent "tented" peaked P waves in leads II and III but isolectric in lead I. The mean frontal plane QRS axis is also frequently deviated to the right and a characteristic $S_1Q_3T_3$ pattern may be present (the pattern of posterior herniblock). Usually, abnormal Q waves are not found in lead II and this helps in the electrocardiographic differentiation from inferior myocardial infarction. A prominent R wave in V1, with S waves in V5 and V6, complete or incomplete right bundle branch block and inverted T wave in leads V1–4 may occur.

The Chest X-Ray

Cardiomegaly produced by right-sided enlargement, distension of the main pulmonary artery, and peripheral oligemia may be found. Abrupt cutoff of major branches of the pulmonary arteries may also be present. Usually, however, these changes are not observed and the main value of the chest X-ray is in excluding conditions such as spontaneous pneumothorax and massive postoperative pulmonary atelectasis, which may mimic acute pulmonary embolism.

Diagnosis

In clinical practice this is generally difficult especially in the presence of congestive cardiac failure. The differential diagnosis includes acute myocardial infarction, dissecting aneurysm of the aorta, cardiac tamponade, and spontaneous pneumothorax. The diagnosis of pulmonary embolism should be suspected immediately when there is unexplained fever, tachycardia, sudden deterioration in congestive cardiac failure, and the presence of hemoptysis or pleurisy.

Lung scans using radioactive fibrinogen may be helpful when they show areas of decreased uptake of radioactivity in the presence of a normal chest X-ray. With the aforementioned proviso, a normal lung scan excludes pulmonary embolism. Pulmonary angiography is invasive and only safe in the hands of a well-trained and equipped laboratory. It should be performed only when the possibility of surgical embolectomy is seriously envisaged. At the bedside, valuable hemodynamic information may be obtained with the use of the Swan-Ganz catheter. Characteristically, there is a modest degree of pulmonary hypertension and a normal wedge pressure.

Treatment

The treatment of the acute episode is directed toward supporting the circulation and preventing death from shock and circulatory failure. If this is successful the majority of pulmonary emboli will undergo spontaneous lysis. The condition therefore may be viewed as a self-limited, provided steps are undertaken to prevent recurrence.

Intravenous morphine is administered for pain, dyspnea, and anxiety. Oxygen by nasal mask or catheter is administered to correct hypoxia. Hypotension should be treated with vasopressor substances such as dobutamine with appropriate monitoring of the systemic arterial pressure, and right-heart pressures with a Swan-Ganz catheter. Intravenous heparin is given in doses of 15,000 units intravenously immediately and repeated four hourly until there is appropriate prolongation of the coagulation time; the dose may then be reduced to 7500 units six hourly.

Pulmonary embolectomy should always be considered in those patients who do not respond to supportive therapy. The mortality for severe pulmonary embolism with acute cor pulmonale is approximately 35% and the majority of deaths occur in less than an hour. In each case, therefore, individual judgment must be made and there are no firm guidelines to predict the exact timing of pulmonary angiography and embolectomy. The operation involves considerable mortality when performed on patients who are in serious shock. It is difficult, however, to predict in the individual patient whether there will be a response to medical therapy or not. In the appropriate circumstances when shock is resistant to medical therapy embolectomy may be life saving and the procedure should be carried out employing cardiopulmonary bypass.

When rapid embolectomy is not feasible, fibrinolytic therapy should be strongly considered. Urokinase produces more complete resolution of emboli in the pulmonary circulation compared to conventional anticoagulation with heparin, but does not decrease mortality. There is an important risk of hemorrhage and invasive procedures such as arterial and venous punctures should be kept to a minimum. Fibrinolysis is absolutely contraindicated when there is active internal bleeding, recent cerebral vascular accident, recent trauma, thoracentesis, paracentesis, and so on. When there is clinical evidence to suggest that there are repeated episodes of pulmonary embolism, particularly when the patient is fully anticoagulated, the inferior vena cava should be interrupted as an emergency procedure. Anticoagulants are the most important aspect of therapy and heparin should be administered for at least 10 days followed by coumadin. In most cardiac patients who have sustained pulmonary embolism, anticoagulation should be maintained indefinitely.

Chronic Pulmonary Embolism

Recurrent pulmonary embolism over months or years leads to progressive obliteration of the pulmonary arterial tree. Repeated showers of small emboli may occur, or small emboli may be combined with massive obstruction of one major pulmonary artery or branch. The condition is most common in young women, particularly after childbirth, but may occur at any age, following peripheral venous thrombosis.

The clinical picture is almost indistinguishable from that of primary pulmonary hypertension described below. A history of venous thrombosis, however, can often be elicited and the leg should always be carefully examined for evidence of this. Phlebography and radioactive lung scans may be helpful in diagnosis. The diagnosis is established by pulmonary angiography and more recently by pulmonary angioscopy, which actually visualizes proximal thrombus. Pulmonary embolectomy, interruption of the inferior vena cava with an umbrella device, and permanent anticoagulation may produce dramatic cure.

Fat Embolism

Fat embolism is most likely to occur following multiple fractures of long bones. Fat is liberated from the traumatized bone marrow into the bloodstream as large globules and is also hydrolyzed to toxic free fatty acids. The result is blockage of the capillaries, and tissue hypoxia chiefly affecting the lungs and brain.

Clinically, there is frequently a latent period of several hours to several days between the time of injury and symptoms. Marked dyspnea, tachycardia, cyanosis, cough, and hemoptysis result from pulmonary involvement. Cerebral symptoms include delirium, convulsions, and paralysis and are ominous signs. Skin petechiae are characteristic. In the absence of specific therapy, treatment is one of ventilatory support.

Air Embolism

Air embolism is usually iatrogenic. Air enters the systemic veins during intraveous infusion, neurosurgical and angiographic procedures when air is contained in the injecting syringe. Acute cor pulmonale with shock and cardiac failure results if sufficient air is introduced very rapidly.

Treatment consists of turning the patient into the left lateral position with the head down so that air is trapped in the apex of the right ventricle rather than the outflow tract. Aspiration of the right ventricle may be necessary and closed chest cardiac massage may be successful.

Miscellaneous Causes of Obstructive Pulmonary Hypertension

Pulmonary hypertension due to bilharzia is produced by obstruction of numerous arterioles by ova and occurs particularly in Egypt; the presence of hepatosplenomegaly is an important clue. Systemic lupus erythematosus, polyarteritis nodosa, and scleroderma are rare causes of diffuse vascular disease. Occasionally, small vessels of the lung are obstructed by tumor emboli and these may arise from a renal, hepatic, or gastric carcinoma or chorioepithelioma. Since the latter occurs in young pregnant woman and may respond dramatically to chemotherapy it is important to consider this entity in a young woman with signs of pulmonary hypertension; usually there are lung opacities to suggest the diagnosis, but this is not invariable.

Amniotic fluid embolism, although rare, is an important cause of maternal death in the peripartum period. Embolic manifestations are produced by the solid material of amniotic fluid but the clinical picture is complicated by disseminated intravascular coagulation. The presentation is one of dyspnea, tachycardia, cyanosis, and shock. Bleeding from various sites is a result of the coagulation abnormality. The treatment is supportive as for other cases of thromboembolism, and the administration of fresh blood or plasma may be required to control hemorrhage.

Primary Pulmonary Hypertension

This is a rare condition usually affecting women in the age group 20 to 40; occasionally it occurs in familial form. The primary pathophysiological disturbance is a marked increase in pulmonary vascular resistance, presumably due initially to vasoconstriction, to be followed sooner or later by organic obstruction and obliteration of the terminal pulmonary arterioles. Severe pulmonary hypertension ith pressures usually at, or just below, systemic levels are found. Right ventricular hypertrophy and ultimately right heart failure develop. The etiology is unknown.

Clinical Features

The symptoms are fatigue, weakness, and reduced effort tolerance, which are a result of the low cardiac output. Syncope on effort and angina occur occasionally and sudden death is not uncommon. Dyspnea and congestive cardiac failure are the rule. Cyanosis is not infrequent and is produced by a right-to-left shunt at atrial level.

The differential diagnosis is from other causes of pulmonary hypertension. Particular care should be taken to exclude mitral stenosis with extreme pulmonary hypertension where the middiastolic murmur may be extremely soft. Echocardiography is extremely helpful. Pulmonary hypertension associated with congenital heart disease may be difficult to distinguish from primary pulmonary hypertension. Usually, the absence of central cyanosis and the presence of a large A wave in the jugular venous pulse are suggestive of primary pulmonary hypertension, but cardiac catheterization may be required.

Prognosis

This is poor. At least 75% of patients are dead at 5 years. The usual cause is right heart failure, pneumonia, and sudden death. Poor prognostic features are pulmonary arterial saturation of 60% or less, systemic saturation of 90% or less, and high pulmonary vascular resistance.

Treatment

There is no effective treatment. Anticoagulants may improve the survival to a small degree. Vasodilators may lower the pulmonary artery pressure but may also quite markedly decrease the cardiac output and systemic pressure and their long-term benefit is not established. Heart–lung transplantation has been successful in a few patients.

Vasoconstrictive Pulmonary Hypertension

In this group of disorders the common denominator is alveolar hypoventilation and hypoxia leading to pulmonary arteriolar vasoconstriction, pulmonary hypertension, and cor pulmonale. The pulmonary arterioles are exquisitively sensitive to alveolar hypoxia and acidosis to which they respond by regional vasoconstriction. Acidosis and hypoxia appear to have a synergistic effect but the exact mechanism whereby the response is initiated is unclear.

Chronic Bronchitis and Emphysema

The basic lesion is obstruction to air flow with maldistribution, resulting in inappropriate mixing of air and pulmonary capillary blood—the so-called ventilation perfusion imbalance. A result of airway obstruction and the structural changes induced by chronic bronchitis, with or without emphysema, there may be a complex disturbance in these ratios. Thus, areas that are ventilated may not be perfused resulting in an increase in the physiological dead space, and wasted ventilation. Areas that are perfused may not be ventilated, resulting in intrapulmonary shunts and hypoxia. In regions with low ventilation–perfusion ratios, hypoxic and acidotic pulmonary arterial constriction occurs. If there are sufficient areas such as these in the lungs, pulmonary hypertension will result.

Hypoxia results in polycythemia and increased blood viscosity and this is often accompanied by an increase in total blood volume. The cardiac output is variable and may be normal, raised, or reduced. Neither the change in blood viscosity nor any increase in cardiac output (which is usually a result of associated fever) or capillary destruction as a result of infection appears to be as important as the hypoxic stimulus to vasoconstriction in the pathogenesis of cor pulmonale.

Right ventricular and right atrial hypertrophy develop in response to pulmonary hypertension and eventually failure may supervene. The large pulmonary arteries show dilatation and atheroma in response to the increased pressure. Left ventricular dysfunction and failure are found in some cases of cor pulmonale, but its mechanism is in dispute; in most cases it appears to be a result of associated coronary artery disease.

The fall in pH and rise in carbon dioxide tension produce vasodilatation of the cerebral vessels, which may result in papilledema, and vasodilatation of the vessels to the extremities, which become warm and pink.

Clinical Features

Because chronic bronchitis and emphysema are so prevalant, cor pulmonale is responsible for up to 25% of cases of congestive cardiac failure. Men are more frequently affected than women and this may well be related to the fact that they are more frequently heavy cigarette smokers. Among patients with chronic obstructive airways disease, a past history of asthma in childhood or adolescence is often present and there is frequently an environmental background of exposure to atmospheric polution or pneumoconiosis.

The earliest symptoms are usually the common "smoker's cough" in the early morning with the production of sputum. Many patients come to accept these symptoms as normal and rarely complain of them. Effort dyspnea soon appears, especially if wheezing is superimposed. In the rare patient, especially in the younger age group, symptoms are of recent origin and progress rapidly. Recurrent attacks of acute bronchitis, particularly in the winter, are associated with pyrexia, constitutional disturbance, and expectoration of mucopurulent sputum. These induce acute distress, intensify hypoxemia, raise the pulmonary artery pressure and precipitate congestive cardiac failure. Cyanosis may be intense, and the patient may present with drowsiness and coma simulating a cerebrovascular accident. These symptoms are a manifestation of carbon dioxide narcosis.

On examination, a characteristic finding is a cyanosed patient sitting upright, breathing rapidly, and wheezing with prolonged expiration. Clouding of conciousness, often associated with confusion, may simulate alcoholism. The eyes are often prominent and the conjunctivae suffused. In some patients, the chest is barrel-shape with the ribs held in the inspiratory position. In most patients, hyperinflation of the chest is absent. The accessory muscles of respiration are always in full action but there is little actual chest movement. The breath sounds are faint, expiration is prolonged, and wheezing, rhonchi, and coarse rales are present. Peripheral vasodilatation is manifested by warm hands, tachycardia, peripheral arterial pulsation, and a full bounding regular pulse. In the later stages vasoconstriction may be present. Clubbing of the fingers usually indicates bronchiectasis or pulmonary suppuration. The jugular venous pressure is elevated.

Examination of the heart is difficult because the emphysematous lung obscures the heart and dampens the sounds. The heart sounds are best heard in the epigastrium where a gallop rhythm and systolic murmur of tricuspid insufficiency may be found. Papilledema is occasionally present. Emphysema displaces the liver downward, but with congestive cardiac failure the size is accentuated by congestion.

Two clinical prototypes have been described—the so-called "blue-bloaters" and the "pink-puffers." *Blue-bloaters* are relaxed and somnolent, often stout with twitching hands (asterixis), cyanosis, and suffused eyes. *Pink-puffers* are tense and anxious, often thin, with steady hands, pink mucosae, and clear, or prominent eyes. Blue-bloaters have a small fixed chest cage, are abdominal breathers, with poor breath sounds, wheezing respiration, rales, and rhonchi. Pink-puffers have a large chest cage, held high with marked thoracic cage movement, poor breath sounds, and few additional sounds in the chest. The heart is clinically enlarged in the blue-bloaters and a gallop rhythm, accentuation of the pulmonary component of the second heart sound, hepatomegaly, and edema are frequent. Pink-puffers, on the other hand, have signs of emphysema and the heart size cannot be detected; the heart sounds are distant and heart failure is uncommon.

Electrocardiography

This shows right axis deviation, clockwise rotation of the precordial leads and low voltage in the limb, and sometimes all leads. The S1, S2, S3 syndrome is frequently present and abnormal left axis deviation beyond $-30°$ is occasionally found. The P wave axis is shifted to the right so that its mean axis is nearer $+90°$ and the P waves themselves are peaked. When significant pulmonary hypertension develops, signs of right ventricular hypertrophy may be found with an RS, or tall R, or an RSR complex associated with inverted T waves in V1. Occasionally, right bundle branch block is found. Paroxysmal atrial tachycardia with 2:1 block, unassociated with digitalis administration, is not infrequent and is a life-threatening arrhythmia.

Radiology

In chronic bronchitis the lung fields are often normal, the diaphram is usually rounded, and the heart normal in size (Fig. 20.1). When heart failure is present, cardiomegaly with a

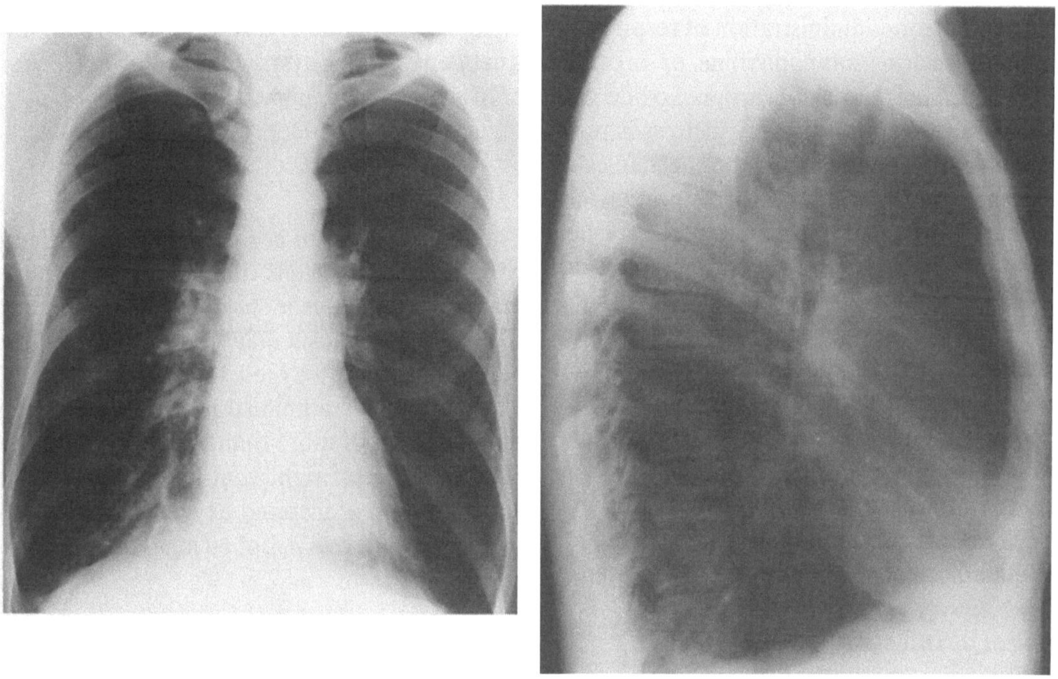

FIGURE 20.1. X-rays of the chest in chronic obstructive airways disease demonstrating hyperinflated translucent lungs, depressed diaphragms, and prominence of the main pulmonary artery.

prominent pulmonary outflow tract is found. The radiological signs of emphysema are notoriously difficult to interpret, except when well advanced. Characteristically, the heart becomes more vertical in position with depressed flat domes of the diaphram and reduced lung markings. In the lateral view, the heart becomes separated from the back of the sternum. The outflow tract of the right ventricle becomes prominent with some tilting up of the apex. The main pulmonary arteries stand out in contrast to the clear lung fields. Enlargement of the right atrium and right ventricle is present, particularly during congestive cardiac failure. A striking feature is the marked cardiomegaly that occurs during an acute episode of cor pulmonale, but which may be completely reversible.

Pulmonary Function Tests

In the typical case, office spirometry will suffice. Characteristically there is a sharp decrease in the FEV_1 and a near normal vital capacity so that the ratio of FEV_1 to FVC is reduced. In a case of established COPD the FEV_1 may be expected to deteriorate by 80–100 cm^3 per annum.

Treatment

Improvement of Oxygenation

Improved ventilation alleviates alveolar hypoxia, relieves pulmonary arterial vasoconstriction, and improves arterial oxygenation and carbon dioxide elimination. Therefore, relief of the obstructive process in the airways is the most important aspect of treatment and prophylaxis of future episodes. Bronchodilators are intensively used and these include aminophylline intravenously, orally, or rectally, and inhalation therapy using nebulized isoethyrine or isoproterenol.

Aspiration of bronchial secretions, encouragement of cough, and softening of sticky exudates are essential to improve the airways. Oxygen is life-saving but must be given with caution by mask or catheter at 2 to 4 liters/min. The simultaneous administration of respiratory stimulants such as aminophylline or nikethamide will reduce the risk of carbon dioxide narcosis. When severe respiratory distress is present due to interference with the mechanics of breathing, mechanical aids to respiration are indicated. This entails intubation of the trachea with intermittent positive pressure respiration, especially in the severely ill, cyanosed, comatose patient. Not only can the patient be adequately oxygenated, but bronchial secretions can be aspirated and secretions thinned with aerosols and liquefying agents. Bronchodilators may be given through a nebulizer. Constant monitoring of the arterial p_{O_2}, pH, and p_{CO_2} is essential so that appropriate correction of metabolic abnormalities may be instituted.

Control of Infection

This is the factor usually precipitating the episode of acute congestive cardiac failure and requires immediate penicillin therapy or broad spectrum antibiotics.

Control of Heart Failure

This is treated with digitalis and diuretics. Though the value of venesection has been debated, it is of undoubted benefit in the polycythemic patient but the hematocrit should not be reduced to less than 45%. Morphia and all other respiratory center depressants are strongly contraindicated—their use may precipitate a fatal outcome.

Arrhythmias are particularly prone to develop in cor pulmonale and are difficult to control. Atrial fibrillation, flutter, atrial tachycardia with 2:1 A-V block, and multifocal atrial tachycardia are common. Predisposing causes are unrelieved hypoxia, pulmonary embolism, hypokalemia, acidosis, and digitalis toxicity. These patients are particularly sensitive to digitalis and some of the arrhythmias are due to this drug. Paroxysmal atrial tachycardia with 2:1 block often complicates cor pulmonale in the absence of digitalis therapy—it should be treated by immediate electrical cardioversion, which may be life-saving.

Multifocal atrial tachycardia may occur spontaneously or follow the administration of digitalis. Verapamil may be effective in the treatment of this dysrhythmia, but correction of hypoxia is more important.

Prognosis

The development of cor pulmonale in patients with COPD shortens life expectancy quite markedly. The 3-year survival rate is less than 50%. The prognosis may be improved by the administration of oxygen 15 to 24 hours daily. The criteria for administration are a p_{O_2} less than 50, p_{CO_2} of more than 55 mm Hg, and clinical evidence of right ventricular failure. The concentration of inspired oxygen should be adjusted to produce a p_{O_2} of 60 mm Hg or more.

Other Pulmonary Diseases

Restrictive Lung Disease

These include the pulmonary fibroses resulting from sarcidosis, asbestosis, radiation, beryl-liosis, carcinomatosis, scleroderma, chronic disseminated histiocytosis, pulmonary alveolar proteinosis, and the Hamman–Rich syndrome (a chronic granulomatous process following an influenzal or bronchopneumonic-like illness). Thickening of the alveolar membrane and an alveolar-capillary block was once postulated, but this concept has now been largely abandoned.

The prime defect appears again to be a ventilation–perfusion inequality and stiff lungs with poor compliance, which results in rapid shallow breathing. Respiratory alkalosis thus develops with a high pH and a low p_{CO_2}. When the hyppxemia becomes severe, pulmonary hypertension supervenes and cor pulmonale results.

Clinical Features

Usually the disease is insidious in onset and may follow a febrile influenza-like illness. Dyspnea is by far the most prominent symptom, characterized by a gross increase in the rate of breathing without the features of obstruction so typical of emphysema. At first, it is noted only on exercise, but as the condition advances it becomes apparent at rest. Thus, the condition can be suspected the bedside, by observing tachypnea at rest, usually with rapid, shallow breathing. Cough is usually present but there is little sputum. Carbon dioxide narcosis does not occur so that mental clarity is preserved. Fatigue and tiredness associated with hypoxia and over breathing are generally present.

On examination, cyanosis is generally absent until the late stages but tachycardia is frequent. Clubbing of the fingers is fairly common. The clinical signs detected in the lungs depend on the cause, but frequently there are only scattered rales. Cardiac examination is therefore easy, and the signs of pulmonary hypertension are frequently appreciated. The electrocardiogram and the chest X-ray usually show more evidence of right ventricular hypertrophy than in emphysema. A diffuse, fine reticular, or granular appearance of the lung fields may be present radiologically (Fig. 20.2).

Treatment

Early in the disease, steroids and immunosuppressive drugs may be helpful. When there is established fibrosis, treatment for heart failure and supplemental oxygen is palliative.

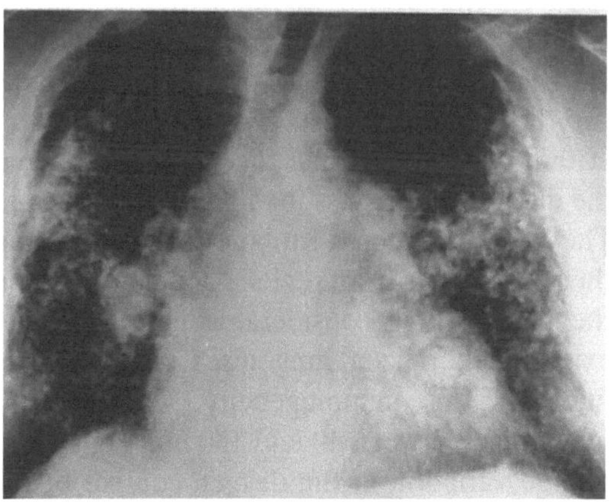

FIGURE 20.2. Chest X-ray in beryllioses showing diffuse pulmonary fibrosis of enlargement of the heart and pulmonary artery.

Extrapulmonary Diseases

Kyphoscoliosis

In kyphoscoliosis the lungs are often normal, but small. The vascular bed is proportionately reduced, probably as a result of limited expansion of the lungs. The mechanics of breathing are ineffective, there is very poor movement and most of the breathing is diphragmatic. Because of the deformed chest and disturbed mechanics, the work of the breathing is increased. This is aggravated by respiratory infections that produce areas of pulmonary collapse. Incomplete resolution of pulmonary infections results in ventilation-perfusion ratio disturbance with resultant venous admixture. The result of all these adverse factors is the development of hypoxia, pulmonary hypertension, and cor pulmonale with cyanosis and dyspnea. It should be emphasized that kyphoscoliosis must be severe to result in the above changes.

Obesity and Pickwickian Syndrome

This syndrome develops in only a small percentage of obese patients so that some inherent fault in their sensitivity to carbon dioxide is likely to be present. An additional factor may be upper airways obstruction due to relaxation of the pharyngeal muscles during sleep.

Characteristically these patients are obese, cyanotic, become drowsy easily, fall asleep during the day, and during sleep may have spasmodic jerking of the limbs. Congestive cardiac failure and respiratory insufficiency may be precipitated by pulmonary infection. Polycythemia may develop and there may be an increased tendency for pulmonary emboli. The proper therapy for the Pickwickian syndrome is weight reduction, which if successful leads to cure of the condition.

Sleep Apnea Syndrome

This refers to abormal respiration during sleep leading to hypoxia and cor pulmonale: (1) *Central apnea* (Ondine's curse) results in stoppage of respiratory effort and air flow due to central nervous system failure. (2) *Obstructive apnea*, characterized by upper airway occlusion, is a result of collapse of the walls of the pharynx, tonsillar and adenoidal enlargement (particularly important in children), falling back of the tongue during sleep, and upper airway narrowing by obesity. (3) *Mixed apnea* is a combination of central and obstructive apnea.

Multiple periods of apnea produce severe hypoxia, pulmonary hypertension, and heart failure with brady- and tachyarrhythmias.

Treatment

Unlike the Pickwickian syndrome, patients with the sleep apnea syndrome are not obese. The most effective therapy is nasal continuous positive airway pressure (CPAP) at night, which holds the upper airway open. Trachyostomy may be needed to bypass pharyngeal obstruction in some cases.

Upper Airway Obstruction in Children

Attention has recently been drawn to the development of severe pulmonary hypertension in young children with obstruction to the upper respiratory passages, usually due to tonsillar and adenoidal hyperplasia. Airways obstruction leads to alveolar hypoventilation, hypoxia, and hypertensive cor pulmonale. The condition is cured by tonsillectomy and adenoidectomy.

Pulmonary Function Test

Only a brief resume of pulmonary function tests and their uses can be given in a volume of this kind.

The prime function of the lung is to exchange gas. The alveolar membrane with an area of 100m^2 has a mean thickness of less than 1 μm. Air is brought to one side of the interface and blood to the other. The air space is connected to the outside by a system of airways that comprises the anatomical deadspace. The blood space is the pulmonary capillary: blood passing through this takes up oxygen and gives off CO_2. The p_{O_2} (partial pressure of oxygen) in the alveolus is about 100 mm Hg and that of mixed venous blood about 40 mm Hg. There is thus a drivihg pressure of 60 mm Hg, rapidly effecting transfer of oxygen from alveolus to blood. The transfer is accomplished in about one-third the available time—there are thus great reserves of diffusion. During exercise even if the blood flows three times as fast through the capillaries there is adequate time for diffusion.

If alveolar hypoxia is present the driving pressure is reduced and the rate of movement of oxygen across the alveolar membrane is slowed. More time is needed for equilibration and on exercise the diffusion defect is exaggerated. The reserves of normal lungs are so great that hypoxemia rarely occurs even when alveolar p_{O_2} is low and oxygen consumption high. At high altitudes, however, the reserves are inadequate and arterial hypoxemia may be present at rest and accentuated with exercise.

"Alveolar capillary block" is a concept coined to account for defective diffusion occurring in diffuse interstitial fibrosis, sarcoidosis, asbestosis, alveolar carcinomatosis, and so on. It has been postulated that the thickened membrane impairs diffusion of gases. This is improbable because the alveolar membrane would have to be thickened at least sixfold, which is unlikely. Evidence has accumulated to show that uneven ventilation and perfusion exist and are responsible for hypoxia.

The normal lungs are not homogeneous. Because of the weight of blood in the upright position there is a much greater blood flow at the bases than the apices, the latter receiving very little blood at rest. Ventilation is greater in the lower zones than the upper zones, but the differences are less than those of perfusion. The ratio between ventilation and perfusion therefore varies from region to region. Even in the normal lung considerable inhomogeneity exists. Generalized lung disease enormously increases this inhomogeneity. Alveolar p_{O_2} may range between 40 and 150 mm Hg so that a large variation in the oxygen content of the blood draining these various lung units exists. In normal lungs in the upright position the major contribution to systemic arterial blood comes from the lung bases, where alveolar p_{O_2} may

TABLE 20.1. Tests of bellows function.

Test	Description	Normal
(a) Respiratory rate at rest		12–16
(b) Tidal volume	Volume of air expired in one ordinary breath at rest	400–600 cm^3
(c) Inspiratory reserve volume	Maximal volume of air that can be inspired at the end of a normal tidal inspiration	2000–3000 cm^3
(d) Expiratory reserve volume	Maximal volume of air that can be expelled at the end of a normal tidal expiration	1000–1500 cm^3
(e) Residual volume	Amount of air in lungs after maximal expiration	1000–1500 cm^3
(f) Total lung capacity	Volume of air in lungs after full maximal inspiration.	4500–6000 cm^3
(g) Functional residual capacity	Volume of air in lungs at the end of a normal expiration	2000–3000 cm^3
(h) Vital capacity	Maximal volume of air that can be expired after maximal inspiration	3500–5000 cm^3
(i) Timed vital capacity FEV_1	Proportion of vital capacity expelled in 1 second	95% expelled in 3 seconds
(j) Maximal breathing capacity	Maximal volume of gas that can be breathed, in 1 minute voluntarily	90–170 liters/min
(k) Dead space	Volume of air in airway from nose to alveoli	
(l) Minute volume	Volume of air expired in 1 minute	4–6 liters

be only 89 mm Hg, whereas the p_{O_2} may be as high as 132 mm Hg in the upper lobes, which are less well perfused. In normal lungs this is unimportant, but in diseased lungs severe hypoxemia may result. This mechanism appears to be responsible for most of the hypoxemia that is encountered in diffuse interstitial fibrosis, as well as emphysema and chronic bronchitis.

One other concept should be considered. Inspired gas does not reach the terminal alveoli directly. The last few millimeters requires diffusion of gases for mixing. Normally the distance is so small that uniform diffusion and gas mixing occur. In diseased lungs dilatation of the smaller airway passages will impair diffusion of gases as in centrilobular type of chronic obstructive lung disease will impair diffusion of gases.

The indices in Table 20.1 except for (e), (f), and (g) can be readily obtained from a spirometric tracing (Fig. 20.3).

The predicted values for normals of given sex, age and height are readily available. Only values outside about 10% of the normal range are considered abnormal. Measurement of the functional residual capacity, from which one can obtain values for the residual volume and total lung capacity, is performed by equilibrating the air in the lungs with a known volume of helium, or by performing a nitrogen washout. By this means one can also obtain information on the distribution of ventilation. The compliance of the lungs is an estimate of their stiffness, and resistance studies measure the amount of friction in the airways.

Abnormal spirograms provide important, though relatively crude, information regarding the nature of the respiratory defect (Fig. 20.4). More refined tests are required for the estimation of (e), (f), and (g), for analyzing distribution of ventilation in the lungs, and intrapulmonary mixing of gases, and for testing of the work of breathing and lung compliance.

The normal range of blood gases at rest is given in Table 20.2. Determination of the blood gases at rest, after exercise, and after inhalation of oxygen provides important information as to the nature and extent of respiratory disease. By virtue of the shape of the

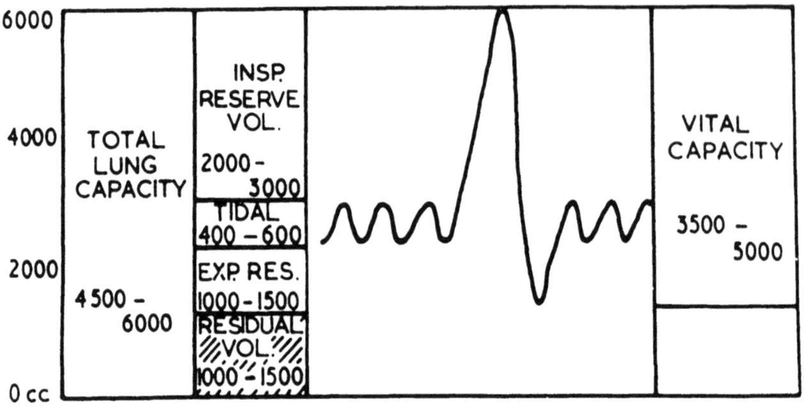

FIGURE 20.3. The lung volumes (see text).

oxygen dissociation curve, significant arterial desaturation does not occur until the oxygen tension has fallen from 102 to approximately 65 mm Hg. Consequently, important lung disease may be present without this being reflected in the arterial saturation. The value of oxygen tension, as opposed to arterial saturation measurements, lies in the early detection of impending respiratory failure, which is of particular assistance when the measurements are made sequentially. In a patient with cyanosis, a raised carbon dioxide content indicates pulmonary disease and excludes a right-to-left shunt as the cause of the cyanosis. The measurement of the uptake of carbon monoxide can be used to test the diffusing capacity or gas transfer rate, employing either a single breath or a steady state technique.

Causes of Hypoxia

Alveolar Hypoventilation

This is defined as ventilation insufficient to maintain the arterial carbon dioxide tension below 45 mm Hg. It is only when this is *severe* in normal individuals that hypoxemia results, with retention of carbon dioxide (hypercapnia) and respiratory acidosis (lowered pH). Breathing of 100% oxygen corrects the hypoxia completely. (After exercise hypoxia may persist or may disappear.) Alveolar hypoventilation is caused by CNS depression (e.g., sedatives), musculoskeletal causes (e.g., polio, kyphoscoliosis), pulmonary disorders (e.g., emphysema, fibrosis, etc.).

Airways Obstruction

This leads to disturbance in the distribution of ventilation and, if severe, may result in ventilation–perfusion imbalance. It is often associated with alveolar hypoventilation. It is commonly found in asthma, chronic bronchitis, and emphysema.

Ventilation/Perfusion Imbalance

Hypoxia with normal carbon dioxide content, or low carbon dioxide due to associated hyperventilation, is the diagnostic finding. Inhalation of oxygen restores normality and exercise intensifies hypoxia. This is characteristically found in diffuse pulmonary fibrosis and pul-

TABLE 20.2. Tests for gaseous exchange

Test	Arterial	Venous
Oxygen saturation	95% or more	65%
Oxygen tension mm Hg	102 – (0.22 × age) mm Hg	33 mm Hg
Carbon dioxide content	50 vol %	54 vol %
Carbon dioxide tension	40 mm Hg ± 5	45 mm Hg
pH	7.4 ± 0.02	7.36

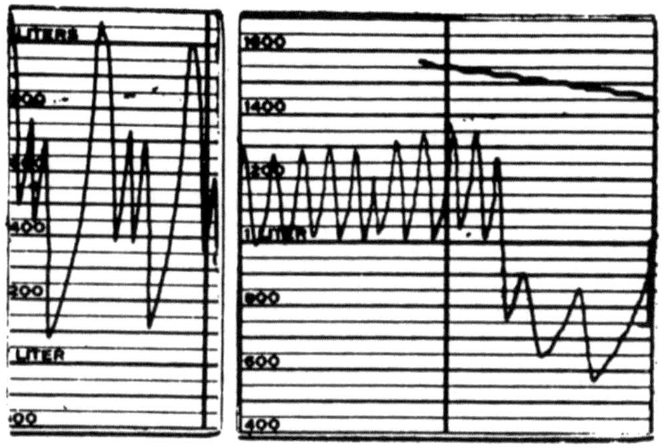

A VC 2120 ml (48% NORMAL) MBC 28 L/m (25% NORMAL)

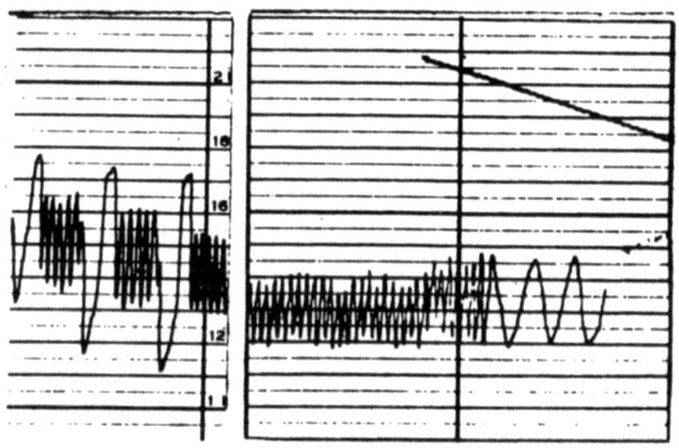

B VC 1320 ml (52% NORMAL) MBC 62 L/m (100% NORMAL)

FIGURE 20.4. Abnormal spirograms in (A) a patient with emphysema demonstrating an obstructive ventilatory defect. Vital capacity is reduced but there is difficulty in moving air in and out of the lungs. Thus, the maximum breathing capcity is much reduced, the timed vital capacity is prolonged because of prolonged expiration, and air trapping is present. After maximum expiration the patient breathes near the top of the inspiratory reserve volume. In (B) a restrictive defect is present because of cardiac failure. The vital capacity and maximum breathing capacity are proportionally reduced and since there is no obstructions air is moved in and out of the lungs normally. Spriograms are read from right-to-left.

monary embolism, but complicates almost any condition affecting the lungs.

Right-to-Left Intracardiac Shunt

Hypoxemia with normal carbon dioxide content is a rule; oxygen does not raise the arterial saturation above 95% and exercise intensifies the hypoxia.

Respiratory Function in Emphysema and Chronic Bronchitis

The disturbance is complex due to (1) airway obstruction, (2) loss of lung elasticity, (3) increased airways resistance, (4) alveolar hypoventilation, and (5) disturbance of ventilation perfusion ratio. Vital capacity is usually low normal or reduced, but the timed vital capacity FEV_1 is grossly abnormal, since the patient requires much more time than normal to move air in and out of the lungs. Maximal breathing capacity is grossly abnormal for the same reason. Spirograms show air trapping, and breathing is shifted to the inspiratory reserve with a reduced inspiratory capacity. Work of breathing is increased; static compliance may be increased but dynamic compliance is usually decreased. Arterial desaturation and hypercapnia are present, aggravated by exercise and corrected by oxygen.

Respiratory Function in Extrapulmonary Disease, Pulmonary Fibrosis, and Extensive Pleural Thickening

Vital capacity is reduced but there is no difficulty in moving air in and out of the lungs, so that timed vital capacity and maximum breathing capacity are normal or only slightly impaired. Ventilation rate is increased, alveolar ventilation and thus gaseous exchange is usually normal, work of breathing is increased, and compliance is abnormal because of "stiff lungs." When bronchospasm and emphysema are superimposed, the features described in airway obstruction above are superimposed.

Respiratory Function in Diffuse Interstitial Fibrosis

Maximal breathing capacity and FEV_1 are not impaired as much as the vital capacity. Work of breathing is increased and the lungs are stiffer than normal. Hyperventilation is present with reduced oxygen tension and the carbon dioxide values are normal or reduced. There is a further fall in oxygen tension on exercise. Although the arterial saturation may return to normal on inhalation of 100% oxygen, the arterial tension does not reach the normal predicted values indicating intrapulmonary right-to-left shunting.

Additional Reading

Burwell CS, Robin ED, Whaley RD, Bickelman AG: Extreme obesity associated with alveolar hypoventilation—A Pickwickian syndrome. Am J Med 21:89, 1965.

Friedberg CK: Pulmonary function tests and the clinical applications. Prog Cardiovasc Dis 1:251, 1958.

Moser KM (ed): "Pulmonary Vascular Diseases." Marcel Dekker, New York, 1979.

Oakley CM, Goodwin JF: Current clinical aspects of cor pulmonale. Am J Cardiol 20:842, 1967.

Oakley CM, Goodwin JF: The current status of pulmonary embolism and pulmonary vascular disease in relation to pulmonary hypertension. Prog Cardiovasc Dis 9:495, 1966.

West JB: Diffusion and impaired gas exchange. Br J Dis Chest 59:185, 1965.

21 Miscellaneous

Preoperative Evaluation of Risk for Cardiac Patients Undergoing Noncardiac Surgery

Ischemic Heart Disease

The prevalence of ischemic heart disease in the American and Westerm European populations is of major proportion. For the first time there are more Americans over the age of 65 than under the age of 25. There is thus a large cohort of people with ischemic heart disease who present for elective surgical treatment for a variety of conditions. In many, the presence of coronary artery disease is already manifest as myocardial infarction, chronic stable angina, congestive heart failure, or previous coronary artery bypass surgery, and a need for preoperative risk assessment is obvious. However, there are also asymptomatic patients with coronary artery disease about to have a major surgical procedure who also require an estimate of operative risk.

The risk for operation depends on, among other things, the magnitude of the procedure. For example, ophthalmic surgery under local or general anesthesia carries little risk in patients with severe coronary artery disease. Contrariwise, resection of an abdominal aortic aneurysm and bypassing of aortoiliac disease has a strong association with severe coronary artery disease, which is responsible for up to 70% of deaths in the postopeative period.

Referral to a cardiologist for preoperative assessment of potential cardiac risk is becoming more frequent, particularly from peripheral vascular surgeons. There is a strong tendency to request the full range of invasive and noninvasive tests to provide the best assessment. There is also a strong temptation to consider, or request, revascularization (coronary artery bypass surgery or PTCA) in an attempt to prevent postoperative cardiac death.

Much of the available information pertaining to estimation of cardiac risk is based on retrospective studies. There are no controlled studies to support prophylactic revascularization in patients about to have major surgical procedures. Despite these limitations it is possible with good clinical history and examination and appropriately indicated tests to formulate an estimation of risk and to plan a therapeutic intervention when necessary. Prospective studies using multivariate discriminant analysis have identified independent predictors of cardiac mortality (Table 21.1). The most important factors are myocardial infarction within the last 6 months and left ventricular dysfunction (S3 gallop or jugular venous distension). This index was derived by Goldman from unselected general surgery patients; it seriousiy underestimates the risk for resection of abdominal aortic aneurysm and for patients with unstable angina pectoris.

Any estimation of risk for elective operation must take into account (1) magnitude and type of the procedure, (2) characteristics of patient population, and (3) local surgical and anesthetic expertise. The risk of perioperative myocar-

TABLE 21.1. Computation of the cardiac risk index.

Criteria[a]	Multivariate discriminate-functions coefficient	"Points"
History:		
Age > 70 years	0.191	5
MI in previous 6 months	0.384	10
Physical examination:		
S3 gallop or JVD	0.451	11
Important VAS	0.119	3
Electrocardiogram:		
Rhythm other than sinus or PACs on last preoperative ECG	0.283	7
>5 PVCs/min documented at any time before operation	0.278	7
General status		
$p_{O_2} < 60$ or $p_{CO_2} > 50$ mm Hg, K < 3.0 or $HCO_3 < 20$ mEq/liter, BUN > 50 or Cr > 3.0 mg/dl, abnormal SGOT, signs of chronic liver disease or patient bedridden from noncardiac causes	0.132	3
Operation:		
Intraperitoneal, intrathoracic or aortic operation	0.123	3
Emergency operation	0.167	4
Total possible		53 points

[a]MI, myocardial infarction; JVD, jugular-vein distention; VAS, valvular aortic stenosis; PACs, premature atrial contractions; ECG, electrocardiogram; PVCs, premature ventricular contractions, p_{O_2}, partial pressure of oxygen; p_{CO_2}, partial pressure of carbon dioxide; K, potassium; HCO_3, bicarbonate; BUN, blood urea nitrogen; Cr, creatinine; SGOT, serum glutamic oxalacetic transaminase. Reprinted, by permission, from Goldman L, et al.: N Engl J Med 57:357–370, 1978.

dial infarction in asymptomatic patients without clinical, electrocardiographic, or radiologic evidence of heart disease is negligible and further testing of such patients is not required. Exercise testing is not indicated because the pretest likelihood of disease is low and the potential for false-positive results therefore high. Also, patients with chronic stable angina and good exercise tolerance with a normal physical examination will tolerate the stress of most noncardiac operations without undue risk.

Patients considered for repair of abdominal aortic aneurysm or grafting of aortoiliac disease who have chronic stable angina pectoris require special consideration because they are at higher risk. They should be regarded as being in the same category as patients with (1) a history of myocardial infarction, (2) severe limiting or accelerating angina, (3) poor effort tolerance, and (4) diabetes. Investigations should follow this protocol:

1. *Left Ventricular Function.* This should be assessed for overall left ventricular ejection fraction and wall motion abnormality by two-dimensional echocardiography or radionuclide studies. The extent of left ventricular dysfunction is a more powerful predictor than a history of myocardial infarction even if the latter occurred within the past 6 months.
2. *Exercise Stress Testing.* If affordable, this should be in conjunction with thallium imaging. Patients with severe intermittent claudication should have thallium testing using dipyrimadole, adenosine, or arm ergometry. Patients with good effort tolerance (more than 7 mets), high double product, and small reversible perfusion de-

fect do not require further testing. Since their coronary artery disease is likely to be mild, the outlook for operation is good. Those patients with poor effort tolerance (less than 7 mets) and large perfusion defects at a low double product should be investigated with coronary angiography.

The decision to embark on coronary revascularization must be made carefully. Depending on the age of the patient, surgical expertise, and so on, the operative mortality for coronary artery bypass surgery lies between 3 and 7%. It has been shown that patients who have successfully undergone coronary artery bypass surgery are at lower risk than those patients who have not had surgery. However, the surgical attrition rate of 3 to 7% may counteract this and may, in fact, include those patients who may have died during general surgery. No trial examining the risks and benefits of prophylactic PTCA before noncardiac operations has been reported.

Therefore, prophylactic coronary artery bypass surgery should be recommended conservatively where the indications are generally accepted anyway. These include (1) left main coronary artery disease, and (2) two- and three-vessel disease with left ventricular dysfunction.

Pre- and Intraoperative Management for Noncardiac Surgical Procedures

Patients with left ventricular dysfunction, history of myocardial infarction, and past or present congestive heart failure should have their treatment maximized before operation. Medications should be continued to the time of operation. This includes β-blockers and antihypertensive medications, since withdrawal may have severe rebound effects. Dysrhythmias should be controlled as adequately as possible. Prophylactic pacing is not required for conduction defects, which are asymptomatic. Swan-Ganz catheterization assists in optimizing hemodynamics before, during, and after operation. Measurement of the wedge pressure during the operation is particularly important in detecting myocardial ischemia and is much more sensitive than the electrocardiogram; a rise in wedge pressure procedes pain and changes in the ST segment. Invasive hemodynamic monitoring carries low risk and should be continued into the postoperative period.

Aortic Stenosis

Asymptomatic patients with severe aortic stenosis (valve area of less than 0.8 cm^2) may undergo noncardiac surgery quite safely. As yet there is insufficient evidence to show that valve replacement improves the life expectancy or operative risk for noncardiac surgery for such patients.

Patients with symptomatic aortic stenosis pose quite a different problem. Signs and symptoms of congestive heart failure, atrial fibrillation, dizziness, and syncope are ominous and the prognosis is less than 2 years. Evidence of severe left ventricular dysfunction (left ventricular ejection fraction of less than 30%) and associated coronary artery disease worsen the prognosis. Aortic valve replacement with these risk factors may carry an operative mortality of up to 25%. Balanced against this is the high mortality for resection of an abdominal aortic aneurysm in such patients. There can be no generalizations that help in the management of this problem. Each case must be decided on its own merit, balancing the risk of noncardiac operations in untreated aortic stenosis, versus valve replacement followed by noncardiac surgery.

Particular care is needed in the management of patients with severe aortic stenosis undergoing noncardiac surgery. Full invasive hemodynamic monitoring is essential. Hypotension must be avoided because this reduces coronary perfusion and impairs left ventricular function. Preload must be high to ensure an adequate stroke volume from the hypertrophied left ventricle. Negative inotropic drugs must be avoided. These patients deteriorate rapidly with the development of arrhythmias, which should therefore be promptly treated.

Mitral Stenosis

Untreated mitral stenosis is becoming rare. Unless noncardiac surgery is urgent, valvulotomy or valve replacement should be performed first. When operation cannot be deferred, avoidance of tachycardia is essential. Reduction of diastolic filling time will result in pulmonary edema. Left atrial pressure should be kept high to maintain flow across the stenotic mitral valve. In those patients with pulmonary hypertension, hypoxia should be avoided because this will precipitate right ventricular failure.

Prosthetic Cardiac Valves

Those patients who have a good result following valve replacement may undergo noncardiac surgery without undue risks. Antibiotic prophylaxis is given as recommended by the American Heart Association. Anticoagulants are discontinued 2 to 3 days before operation and full dose heparinization substituted until 6 hours before operation. Twelve to 24 hours after operation, heparin is resumed until oral anticoagulation is reinstituted 2 days after operation.

Syncope

Syncope is defined as a sudden temporary loss of consciousness and postural tone with unresponsiveness. It is a symptom of many abnormalities and diseases that result in diminished cerebral blood flow through failure of neuroendocrine and cardiovascular homeostasis.

The incidence increases with age. Below the age of 65 years approximately 4% of the general population is affected. Most of these have so-called "isolated syncope" without identifiable cause. Among the elderly the incidence is about 25% and is recurrent in at least one-third of them.

This susceptibility of elderly people is not simply a result of increasing incidence of aortic stenosis, conduction disturbances, and dysrhythmias. Ageing is associated with a continuous decline in baroreflex hemeostatic mechanisms and cerebral blood flow. Elderly patients have a blunted heart rate response to postural change. Also, there is a continuous decline in activity of the renin–aldosterone system with impaired conservation of sodium and blood volume. Thus, many common conditions such as anemia, heart failure, diuretic therapy, hypertensive drugs, diarrhea, and vomiting may be sufficient to further reduce cerebral blood flow and produce syncope in an elderly patient. The causes of syncope are given in Table 21.2.

TABLE 21.2. Causes of syncope.

I. Hypotension
  1. Orthostatic
  2. Neurally mediated
    a. Vasovagal syncope
    b. Carotid sinus syndrome
    c. Postmicturition syncope
    d. Posttussive and postdeglutition syncope
    e. Hypotension-bradycardia syndrome
II. Cardiac diseases
  1. Aortic stenosis
  2. Hypertrophic cardiomyopathy
  3. Atrial myxoma
  4. Severe pulmonary arterial hypertension
  5. Right-to-left shunts
  6. Left ventricular dysfunction (myopathic or ischemic)
III. Cardiac dysrhythmias
  1. Tachyarrhythmias
    a. Supraventricular tachycardia
    b. Ventricular tachycardia
    c. Episodic ventricular fibrillation
  2. Bradyarrythmias
    a. Sick sinus syndrome
    b. Complete heart block

Orthostatic Hypotension

In clinical practice the common causes of hypotension are as follows:

1. *Drugs*. All antihypertensive drugs through their sympathetic blocking effect may induce postural hypotension and syncope. This is aggravated by diuretic-induced hypovolemia and afterload reduction (nitrates, ACE inhibitors).
2. *Autonomic, Peripheral, and Central Nervous System Disorders*. The most common

causes are diabetes, alcoholism, uremia, multiple sclerosis, and amyloid disease.

3. *Deconditioning*. Cardiovascular deconditioning after prolonged illness in elderly patients predisposes to syncope with sudden change in posture.
4. *Pregnancy*. Obstruction of the inferior vena cava by the gravid uterus reduces venous return and cardiac output.
5. *Postprandial Hypotension*. This affects the elderly patients about 1 hour after eating. It is produced by splanchning pooling and failure of reflex vasoconstriction.
6. *Chronic Idiopathic Orthostatic Hypotension*. This syndrome affects elderly men. It is characterized by postural hypotension, postprandial hypotension, impotence, and anhydrosis. There is impaired acceleration of heart rate and peripheral vasoconstriction particularly in response to upright posture. The condition is a result of failure of secretion of norepinephrine at the sympathic nerve endings in the supine and upright positions. (The Shy–Drager syndrome is similar but there are signs of degeneration of the extrapyramidal system and basal ganglia.)
7. *Neurally Mediated Hypotension and Bradycardia*. The common faint (vasovagal attack) is the most frequent cause of syncope, usually triggered by an emotional stimulus. These and other causes of syncope in apparently healthy individuals may be a result of stimulation of ventricular mechanoreceptors. Diminished ventricular volume (hemorrhage, nitroglycerine, catecholamine infusion) stimulates these receptors in the left ventricle enhancing efferent parasympathic activity with resultant reflex peripheral vasodilatation, bradycardia, and even cardiac asystole. The reflex may be provoked by orthostatic tilt and isoprenaline infusion. β-blockers and disopyramide block this response in the laboratory and clinically.

   Other reflex causes of syncope follow micturition, coughing, swallowing, prostatic massage, and tapping the pleural and peritoneal cavities. The *hypersensitive carotid sinus syndrome* exists in the cardioinhibitory form (70%), vasodepressor form, and mixed type. Carotid sinus massage may induce bradycardia and A-V block, or hypotension or combinations thereof.
8. *Cardiac Disease*. The fundamental mechanism is reduction in cardiac output because of reduced stroke volume. This is thought to be the mechanism in hypertrophic cardiomyopathy and left ventricular dysfunction.
9. *Cardiac Arrhythmias*. Arrhythmia-induced syncope may be a result of asystole (complete heart block, sinus arrest in the sick sinus syndrome) or tachyarrythmias (ventricular tachycardia, ventricular fibrillation).

Diagnosis

History

A meticulous history from the patient and bystanders is crucial. Witnesses should be questioned about (1) *onset* (sudden or gradual), (2) *circumstances* (standing upright, emotional upset, micturition, cough, etc.), (3) *recovery* (slow or fast, involuntary movements, incontinence), (4) *appearance* (pallor or cyanosis), and (5) *pulse* (absent, slow, or rapid).

The patient should be carefully questioned about prescribed and self-taken medications. Vasodilators, calcium channel and β-blockers, ACE inhibitors, and diuretics may all be responsible, particularly when taken in combination. Attention should be aimed at distinguishing syncope from the following:

Transient Ischemic Attacks (TIA)

The disturbance of cerebral blood flow tends to produce repetitive deficits (e.g., dysarthria, hemiparesis, hemianopia). Drop attacks are a result of vertebrobasilar insufficiency where the victim falls to the ground but remains conscious.

Epileptic Seizures

Syncope is gradual in onset, brief, without aura, without convulsions, and usually not followed by confusion. Seizures are sudden in onset after a brief aura. Victims are unconscious for a few minutes, injure themselves during convulsions, are frequently incontinent, and are often confused for several hours. The distinction may, however, be difficult without anciliary evidence. Repeated attacks of cardiac asystole may also produce convulsive movements, and severe prolonged mental confusion from anoxic encephalopathy.

Hypoglycemia

This is usually of slow onset with tremor, sweating, and confusion. When unconsciousness supervenes it is prolonged.

Hysterical Attacks

These are frequently in front of an audience, often accompanied by a dramatic fall, which does not result in injury. The vital signs are normal.

Physical Examination

Aortic valve disease, hypertrophic and dilated cardiomyopathy, cyanotic congenital heart disease, and pulmonary hypertension will be evident on clinical examination supported by the chest X-ray and electrocardiogram. Echocardiography will confirm the diagnosis of hypertrophic cardiomyopathy and is also the definitive test for cardiac tumors.

Measurement of the blood pressure standing after at least 3 minutes supine will detect postural hypotension and reproduce symptoms.

Special Procedures

Carotid Sinus Massage

Each carotid sinus should be massaged for 5 to 10 seconds while monitoring the electrocardiogram and the blood pressure. The procedure should be performed with caution in elderly patients with a history of TIA because of the danger of stroke. The *vasodepressor* response is a drop in blood pressure of more than 50 mm Hg. The *cardioinhibitory* response has been defined as a sinus pause of 3 seconds or longer.

Upright Body Tilt

This is the most useful test for diagnosing neurally mediated hypotension and bradycardia. The protocol consists of an upright tilt to 80° for 10 minutes after control supine measurement of arterial pressure and the EKG for a period of 30 minutes. Syncope is rarely provoked in healthy subjects. Among subjects predisposed to neurally mediated syncope, tilt provokes severe hypotension and bradycardia. Isoproterenol infusion may be added to increase the sensitivity of the test. The procedure can be used as a therapeutic test since β-blockers and disopyramide inhibit the left ventricular mechanoreceptors and the ensuing reflex bradycardia and hypotension.

Holter Monitoring and Event Recording

When the electrocardiogram is normal and an arrhythmia suspected, these noninvasive procedures are worthwhile and may detect evidence of a tachy- or bradyarrhythmia.

Signal Averaged Electrocardiography

This noninvasive screening test is cheap and easily performed. If late potentials are not recorded, the likelihood of inducible ventricular tachycardia is extremely low.

Electrophysiology Studies

The role of these studies is difficult to evaluate. They may be useful when there is known heart disease detected by electrocardiography, Holter recordings, and tests of left ventricular function. However, when these tests are normal the electrophysiology study is likely to be negative. Abnormalities detected at the time of the study do not pinpoint the cause because symptoms are so rarely reproduced during such studies.

Treatment

The first step is to treat the primary cause whenever possible. For example, aortic valve replacement, removal of an atrial myxoma, and pacemaker placement for the sick sinus syndrome are highly effective. Tachyarrhythmias should be treated with the appropriate drug or implantation of an automatic implantable defibrillator device.

The treatment of orthostatic hypotension is difficult. Elevating the head of the bed, arising slowly, and use of support hose may help. Increased dietary salt intake and administration of 9α-fluohydrocortisone may expand the plasma volume. Patients with postprandial hypotension should eat smaller, more frequent meals and lie down after each meal. Straining at stool and during micturition should be avoided by appropriate preventive measures.

The cardioinhibitory type of carotid hypersensitivity responds well to an A-V sequential pacemaker. Treatment of the vasodepressor and mixed types is along the lines given above for orthostatic hypotension. Pressor drugs such as ephedrine may be of benefit.

Neurally mediated hypotension and bradycardia diagnosed by positive tilt test should be actively treated since the condition is potentially fatal. Blockade of the left ventricular mechanoreceptors with β-blocker drugs or disopyramide is effective.

High Output States

Thyrotoxicosis

The effect of thyroid hormones on the heart is mediated through a hyperdynamic circulation that results from an increased basal metabolic rate and increased oxygen consumption. The cardiac output is increased and there is peripheral vasodilatation because of the need for increased peripheral blood flow. The hyperdynamic circulation characteristic of thyrotoxicosis is similar to that produced by adrenergic stimulation. Because plasma catecholamine levels are normal, or even low, it has been postulated that thyrotoxicosis sensitizes the myocardium to catecholamines. It seems unlikely that this is the only explanation since β-adrenergic blockade does not always reduce the cardiac output, or cardiac contractility in thyrocardiacs, suggesting that thyroid hormone may have a direct effect on the myocardium.

The excessive demands placed on the heart by thyrotoxicosis, especially in the presence of underlying ischemic heart disease, may eventually lead to heart failure. This is aggravated by a pronounced tendency for the development of arrhythmias, particularly atrial fibrillation.

Clinical Features

The symptoms and signs are due partly to the systemic effects of hyperthyroidism and partly to the specific cardiac manifestations. In Graves disease (diffuse toxic goiter) thyrotoxic symptoms are particularly prominent and include nervousness, tremor, loss of weight despite good appetite, heat intolerance, sweating, diarrhea, oligomenorrhea, muscle weakness, and fatigue.

Characteristically, patients are thin, with staring eyes, lid lag, and exophthalmos. The thyroid is diffusely enlarged. In toxic nodular goiter, the symptoms of thyrotoxicosis are often less pronounced, whereas cardiac manifestations are more prominent, probably because the patients are older. The development of congestive cardiac failure in a young adult, even when frankly thyrotoxic, almost always implies the presence of underlying cardiac disease. In the absence of heart disease, the young patient may tolerate a high cardiac output almost indefinitely without developing symptoms of congestive cardiac failure.

The cardiac symptoms include palpitation because of sinus tachycardia in the young, and paroxysmal tachycardia, atrial fibrillation, or flutter in the elderly. Initially, exertional dyspnea and fatigue do not necessarily imply cardiac involvement but become prominent symptoms once heart failure has developed. In the elderly, angina pectoris is a common complaint.

On examination, signs of peripheral vasodilatation are prominent. The hands are warm and sweaty, the superficial veins are dilated, and tremor is frequent. Tachycardia with a bounding, collapsing pulse is quite characteristic. The apex beat is hyperactive and forceful but usually is not displaced. The heart sounds are snapping in quality and a scratchy ejection systolic murmur may be present in the second left interspace. This scratchy murmur is produced by a dilated pulmonary artery making contact with the pericardium (Mean's murmur). Bruits over the subclavian and carotid arteries are not uncommon. Frequently, a bruit is audible in the enlarged thyroid gland. A third heart sound occasionally followed by a short rumbling middiastolic flow murmur is best heard at the apex.

In young patients the electrocardiogram is usually normal apart from sinus tachycardia. In the elderly, atrial fibrillation, paroxysmal atrial tachycardia, and ventricular arrhythmias are not uncommon. Heart block of varying degrees may occur. Usually this is first degree, with a long PR interval, but rarely it may be complete. Radiologically, the outflow tract of the right ventricle and the main pulmonary artery are prominent and pulmonary arterial pulsations are vigorous. With heart failure, generalized cardiac enlargement develops.

The diagnosis is usually obvious in the presence of frank thyrotoxic manifestations. In the elderly, all of these signs are occult and the presentation is primarily cardiac. The diagnosis should always be considered in the presence of paroxysmal or established atrial fibrillation without obvious cause. Atrial fibrillation is present in almost all cases of thyrotoxic heart failure. The presence of an enlarged thyroid is often of great help, but enlargement may be retrosternal, or the gland may not be recognizably enlarged. When the condition is suspected, an elevated serum thyroxin (T_4) level will clinch the diagnosis. Ideally. the T_3 levels should also be measured to detect the isolated cases of pure "T_3 thyrotoxicosis."

The treatment of thyrotoxic heart disease is directed at the cardiac failure itself and the rapid, safe conversion to euthroidism. Typically, the ventricular response in atrial fibrillation is difficult to control. More digitalis is required to control the heart rate than usual, and the margin between the therapeutic and the toxic dose is narrowed. The addition of proprdnolol promptly reduces the state of adrenergic stimulation, thus providing better control of the atrial fibrillation, also reducing the metabolic demands on the heart. The drug should be used cautiously in the presence of overt heart failure but can be used safely in most instances.

The use of propranolol protects the patient from the adrenergic stimulation of thyrotoxicosis during the time required for antithyroid drugs to block the synthesis of thyroid hormones. Propylthiouracil given in a dose of 200 mg three times a day will achieve this effect. Since the majority of thyrocardiac patients are elderly, the therapy for thyrotoxicosis itself will be the administration of radioactive iodine. This should be given when the course of propylthiouracil is completed to avoid a sudden release of thyroid hormone from the gland following radioactive iodine administration.

Anemia

Since the oxygen-carrying capacity of the blood is reduced in anemia, the cardiac output must be increased to maintain adequate oxygenation of the tissues. This results in a hyperkinetic circulatory state as described with thyrotoxicosis, and tachycardia with peripheral vasodilatation develop. A reduction in the blood viscosity potentiates these effects. The heart is affected as a consequence of chronic work overload and because the coronary perfusate contains insufficient oxygen. The effects on the cardiovascular system are not observed unless the hemoglobin drops below 7g%. Cardiac failure in an otherwise normal heart will not occur unless the hemoglobin is reduced to less than 5 g%. However, cardiac complications may ensue when there is coronary artery disease or left ventricular hypertrophy from any cause.

Clinical Features

Fatigue and listlessness are a direct result of anemia. Angina pectoris is relatively common, especially in the elderly, because of associated coronary atheroma. It may be encountered, however, even in youth when the hemoglobin is less than 5 g%. Tachycardia, dilated peripheral veins, warm hands, collapsing pulse, and raised jugular venous pressure are all a result of raised cardiac output. Dependent edema may be due to cardiac failure with fluid retention, or capillary hypoxia resultant from anemia. The apex beat is frequently displaced and hyperactive and a third sound is frequently audible at this site. Ejection systolic murmurs may arise from the aortic and pulmonic valves as in other high output state.

The electrocardiogram may be normal, or may show nonspecific T wave flattening or inversion. Acute subendocardial ischemia is usually a result of associated coronary artery disease. Radiology demonstrates cardiomegaly, occasionally of massive proportions, with prominence of the right ventricular outflow tract, and the pulmonary arteries. Of special interest is the rapid reduction to normal after treatment. Pulmonary edema or severe congestion generally is the result of an overloaded circulation produced by rapid blood transfusion.

Treatment of the anemia corrects the cardiovascular manifestations. When heart failure is severe, transfusion with packed cells may be required. It is generally safe to transfuse up to 16 cm^3/min to a maximum of 1200 cm^3 in 24 hours. When cardiac failure is present, treatment with digitalis and diuretics along conventional lines is required.

Beriberi

Thiamine deficiency may produce wet or dry beriberi. Dry beriberi manifests with central nervous system disturbances, particularly peripheral neuropathy. The wet form is associated with peripheral vasodilatation, increased cardiac output, and heart failure. In the past the disease was endemic in the Far East, among population groups subsisting largely on polished rice, and was also seen in Japanese and German concentration camps. Elsewhere, sporadic cases are a result of alcoholism or food faddism. The disease is common where alcohol is cheap and economic conditions are poor.

Beriberi is an acute or subacute disease, leading to death or complete recovery, respectively. Even after several episodes of acute cardiac failure, permanent myocardial damage is extremely rare. The acute fulminating form (Shoshin beriberi) produces sudden circulatory collapse, severe acidosis, and death within a few hours or days, unless appropriate treatment is given. Subacute beriberi is much more common and presents as a hyperkinetic circulatory state with heart failure.

Clinical Features

The diagnosis of beriberi should always be entertained in any case of heart failure in an alcoholic where the cause is not readily evident. Symptoms due to chronic alcoholism or malnutrition are frequently present, with anorexia being a prominent feature; vomiting and fatigue are less common. Neurologic symptoms such as paraesthesia and weakness because of peripheral neuropathy, and Wernicke's encephalopathy are occasionally present.

The signs of a hyperkinetic circulatory state are usually manifested by warm hands, tachycardia, collapsing pulses, and raised jugular venous pressure. The heart is almost invariably enlarged, sometimes markedly so, with a triple or quadruple gallop rhythm. Occasionally, atrioventricular regurgitant systolic murmurs are present and tricuspid insufficiency is particularly common. A wide pulse pressure with systolic hypertension is commonly found, but occasionally diastolic hypertension is also present initially, so that hypertensive heart failure may be suspected. It must be emphasized that high output heart failure is not always present. Severe heart failure with a low cardiac output, orthopnea, systemic congestion, and oliguria may occur. Occasionally, right-sided failure dominates the clinical picture and there is disproportionate edema and hepatomegaly.

The electrocardiographic findings are of crucial value in diagnosis. The most common finding is a normal tracing, or one demonstrating right axis deviation with clockwise rotation, when the patient is most severely ill. Less commonly, the initial electrocardiogram shows T wave inversion over the left or right ventricular precordial leads. In either event, daily tracings will show serial changes, either over the right ventricle, the left ventricle, or both. Thus, when the patient has apparently recovered completely, the electrocardiogram may actually be at its worst, showing extensive and deep T wave inversion. The abnormal changes may persist for 24 hours, days, or even weeks following recovery, but complete return to normal is the rule. Radiologically, equally striking serial changes occur. Marked cardiomegaly with a prominent right ventricular outflow and hilar congestion rapidly returns to normal in a week or two following appropriate treatment. The transketolase activity is decreased in the presence of thiamine deficiency and this is a valuable diagnostic test.

Treatment

Thiamine 50–100 mg should be given intramuscularly or intravenously immediately, and this can be repeated daily for several days. In most patients this is quite adequate. However, the response to thiamine may be delayed, and sudden death from pulmonary edema may occur, so that it is well to treat with digitalis and diuretics from the outset. Beriberi is an acute, completely reversible condition and prompt treatment produces most gratifying results.

Arteriovenous Fistula

Arteriovenous fistulae are congenital or acquired. The latter are much commoner and result from penetrating injuries that produce an abnormal communication between an artery and a vein, frequently preceded by a false aneurysm. When a fistula is large, cardiac failure may result from the high output state.

Clinical Features

The pulses are frequently collapsing because of the "runoff" from the arterial to the venous circulation. Suspicion of an arteriovenous fistula should always be aroused when collapsing pulses similar to those of aortic insufficiency are not associated with the characteristic early diastolic murmur. A careful clinical search should be made for the telltale continuous murmur, which may be located in the extremities, abdomen, and neck. Occasionally the arteriovenous fistulae are superficial and therefore palpable. Manual occlusion of the arterial supply to the fistula is frequently followed by a decrease in pulse rate (Branham's sign). Distal to the fistula there may be signs of arterial insufficiency with coolness and pallor. Also, because of the increased venous pressure, there may be venous varicosities and stasis ulcers.

The only treatment for an acquired arteriovenous fistula is surgical excision and this may produce dramatic relief of heart failure with a return to normal heart size.

Congenital arteriovenous fistula may occur at any peripheral arterial site and are frequently multiple. Overgrowth of the affected limb (usually the leg), edema, and ulceration are frequently complications. Continuous murmurs are not as frequently heard in the congenital variety of A-V fistulae because these are usually small and multiple. Arteriography is necessary to demonstrate size and number of fistulous communications.

Paget's Disease of Bone

A high output state may develop in the presence of diffuse active bone involvement, which results in a marked increase of bone blood flow acting like an arteriovenous fistula. The heart may also be involved by metastatic calcification, which involves the annulus of the mitral and tricuspid valves, and the ventricular septum, which may result in heart block.

Liver Failure

In advanced hepatic disease, marked peripheral vasodilatation occurs and there is a high cardiac output. Intrahepatic arteriovenous shunting has been held responsible, The condition is a rare cause of high output failure because most patients die early from the liver disease.

Unknown Causes

A high output state of unknown origin has been described in young people (Gorlin's syndrome). The cardiac output at rest is abnormally elevated and there is a greater than normal increase with exercise. The presentation is of tachycardia, bounding pulses, systolic hypertension, and warm extremities. An ejection systolic murmur is frequently present, best heard at the base and left sternal border. The condition may be difficult to distinguish from IHSS, and in fact may be a variant of the latter condition.

Pregnancy

Pregnancy places a continuous profound increase in the workload of the heart. The cardiac output is increased early in pregnancy and at the twentieth week increases to a peak of 40% above the nonpregnant state. This increase is well within the capacity of the normal heart but may precipitate failure in the diseased heart where the reserve is diminished. Additional risks include infective endocarditis, pulmonary embolism, and an aortic dissection in the case of coarctation of the aorta.

During pregnancy the usual hemodynamic associations of an increased cardiac output are found, and there is tachycardia, full pulse, raised jugular venous pressure, a hyperactive cardiac impulse, triple rhythm, and the frequent occurrence of pulmonary ejection murmur. Edema of the feet is common because of salt and water retention and the effect of uterine pressure on the pelvic veins. A normal pregnant woman frequently complains of dyspnea, palpitation, and swelling of the feet, and this, in conjunction with the signs of high cardiac output, adds to the difficulty of diagnosing cardiac failure in its early stages.

In the presence of heart disease, symptoms usually begin early and heart failure occurs with increasing frequency after the third month, declining in incidence with the drop in cardiac output after the eighth month. Patients with little or no disability (grade 1) usually have an uneventful pregnancy. Where moderate disability (grade 2) exists careful management is required. In the presence of severe disability (grade 3) or cardiac failure (grade 4) energetic therapy, bed rest, and interruption of pregnancy may be required. Labor is generally well tolerated but problems are frequently encountered during the puerperium.

Rheumatic Heart Disease

This is the commonest variety complicating pregnancy, accounting for over 90% of the patients. Prior to pregnancy patients with grade 1 disability should be advised to have their family early. When there is grade 2 disability, pregnancy should be deferred until palliative surgery has been performed. Valvulotomy is indicated for pliable mitral stenosis. In the case of mitral insufficiency (with or without stenosis) and grade 2 disability, valve replacement using a homograft or xenograft is the preferred treatment since anticoagulation is not required. The use of oral anticoagulants results in increased fetal mortality and an increased risk of fetal malformation.

When symptoms develop early during pregnancy, they usually progress and may become urgent at any time, with fatal consequences. When this is the result of mitral stenosis, mitral valvotomy should be recommended, since paroxysmal cardiac dyspnea or fatal pulmonary edema may develop at any time. The results are good from the maternal point of view but there is a fairly high fetal loss. After the sixth month, valvotomy may still be required, but usually pregnancy can be continued without surgery. Mitral valvotomy at term is very rarely required, but when there are urgent indications such as intractable pulmonary edema or hemoptysis, there should be no hesitation in advising urgent operation.

In the case of aortic valve disease, and mitral insufficiency, interruption of pregnancy is advised when these patients are symptomatic during the first trimester. When such patients are seen for the first time during the third trimester, it is generally advisable to allow the pregnancy to continue, and for the obstetrician to decide on the most favorable time to induce labor. Patients seen for the first time, between the second and third trimesters, present the greatest problem and no hard and fast rule can be made. Each patient must be assessed on her own merits.

It is probably better not to operate on pregnant patients using cardiopulmonary bypass until more is known about the effects of this procedure on the fetus. There are, however, a number of reports of successful operations of this type during pregnancy, with dramatic benefit to the mother and no harm to the fetus. In patients who have undergone successful mitral valve replacement, chronic anticoagulation is required during pregnancy. The fetus is therefore prone to the risk of hemorrhage and oral anticoagulation should be changed to subcutaneous heparin during the first trimester and the last 3 weeks of pregnancy. Oral anticoagulation may be recommended following delivery provided breast-feeding is discontinued. The risk to the mother under these circumstances appears to be small, but the fetal mortality rate is high.

Congenital Heart Disease

Most of the common congenital cardiac defects compatible with survival to puberty can be cured by surgery, which is generally advisable if the lesion is suitable. When the patient is seen for the first time during pregnancy, surgery for atrial or ventricular septal defect, patent ductus arteriosus, and pulmonary stenosis can be deferred. In patent ductus arteriosus the diagnosis must not be confused with a mammary souffle audible over the engorged breasts, or with a venous hum. Patients with Tetralogy of Fallot are sometimes advised to have cesarean section, to avoid fetal hypoxia during delivery. Cesarean section is also advised in the case of coarctation of the aorta to reduce the risks of aortic rupture.

Eisenmenger syndrome, whether a result of a shunt at the aortopulmonary, ventricular, or atrial level, is associated with a high maternal mortality rate. Even when such patients are asymptomatic, pregnancy is contraindicated and sterilization should be performed. Death occurs most commonly during labor, or early in the puerperium, and is the result of a syncopal attack or systemic hypertension. This probably follows a reduction in venous return leading to diminished right ventricular output and systemic hypotension.

Essential Hypertension

This is uncommon except in the elderly multipara. The nonpregnant female should be advised to avoid pregnancy because of the increased maternal and fetal risks. When discovered during pregnancy, it should be actively treated since pregnancy aggravates the hypertension and increases the risks for toxemia.

Myxedema

The cardiovascular manifestations of myxedema depend largely on the presence of pericardial effusion. Congestive cardiac failure is extremely uncommon and when it occurs should arouse a suspicion of some other form of associated heart disease.

The clinical features of myxedema are always present. Dyspnea, fatigue, and swelling of the feet are fairly frequent and may suggest cardiac disease, but more usually is a result of the myxedematous state itself.

On examination, bradycardia with a small pulse volume, normal jugular venous pressure, impalpable apex beat, soft heart sounds, and radiological evidence of cardiomegaly are present.

The electrocardiogram shows sinus bradycardia with low voltage nonspecific T wave flattening or inversion in the precordial leads. Most of the cardiac signs are a result of pericardial effusion, which although large, does not produce cardiac tamponade. The effusion has a high protein and cholesterol content. Arrhythmias are extremely uncommon. The diagnosis is obvious once myxedema is recognized and may be confirmed by finding a low serum T_4 level.

Treatment should begin with L-thyroxine 0.025 mg daily, doubling the dose at fortnightly intervals, and a maximum dose of 0.3 mg/day should not be exceeded. A cautious approach is necessary because the administration of thyroid hormone may precipitate intractable angina among patients who have underlying coronary atherosclerosis. When angina is troublesome it may be necessary to add propranolol to the therapeutic regime.

Neurocirculatory Asthenia (Dacosta Syndrome, Cardiac Neurosis, Panic Attacks)

This syndrome is characterized by symptoms that are not attributable to any disease of the cardiovascular system but rather to an underlying anxiety state. The condition is aggravated by fear and may be superimposed on the symptoms arising from organic heart disease.

Dyspnea is a very prominent symptom, often developing after minimal effort. In addition, hyperventilation, associated with frequent sighs, and a feeling of inability to get sufficient air into the lungs. Continued overbreathing results in fatigue and tiredness; the respiratory alkalosis produces circumoral paraesthesia and tingling of the extremities. In severe cases there may be numbness, tetany, dizziness, and even syncope. Palpitation is frequent, drawing the patients attention to the heart and giving rise to further anxiety. Palpitation is particularly prone to occur with slight exertion but may be present at rest.

Left chest pain is the commonest symptom leading to cardiac consultation. The pain is usually sharp, stabbing in quality, situated in the left inframammary region with little radiation. It may be present at any time and is not clearly related to effort. The pain may last for hours and may be associated with chest wall tenderness. Other symptoms include sweating, headache, tremor, diarrhea, and insomnia.

During examination, hyperventilation is frequently evident and abnormal cardiac findings are absent. The electrocardiogram is usually normal, except when pronounced hyperventilation leads to alkalosis and nonspecific ST-T changes, which may mimic ischemia.

The diagnosis of an anxiety state is generally easily made from ischemic heart disease and thyrotoxicosis. The difficulty is to make the diagnosis when the patient does in fact have some form of heart disease. A classic example is the myxomatous mitral (billowing mitral leaflet syndrome), in which all the symptoms described above may be present. There is little doubt that the symptoms attributed to this condition are in fact a result of iatrogenic cardiac neurosis.

Traumatic Heart Disease

The effects of trauma to the heart are of obvious medicolegal significance. Traumatic heart disease is largely a result of penetrating wounds or nonpenetrating trauma. Penetration of the heart may occur following stabbing with any sharp object or as a result of bullet wounds.

There is a fundamental difference between the amount of injury produced by a bullet and that produced by a knife wound. The velocity of travel of a bullet is very much higher than that of a knife wound and therefore there is a much greater release of kinetic energy. Penetration of the myocardium by even a small caliber bullet may result in extensive disruption of the myocardium with a rapidly fatal outcome. Knife wounds, however, are low-velocity injuries that tend to seal spontaneously following removal of the knife.

The commonest clinical presentation of knife wounds is that of *cardiac tamponade*. Pericardiocentesis may be used as an emergency therapeutic measure but the most favorable outcome is obtained by immediate surgical exploration and suture of the myocadial wound. Knife wounds are also complicated by sepsis and a tendency to posttraumatic constrictive pericarditis.

Penetrating knife wounds commonly result in *fistulae* between systemic arteries and veins; or between a systemic artery and a right-sided chamber, producing an intracardiac shunt. When the fistula is of sufficient size, heart failure may be severe and controlled only by surgical repair.

Pericardial constriction may occur in conjunction with a fistula and is often difficult to detect clinically because the murmurs dominate the picture. The presence of constriction should be suspected when disproportionate systemic venous hypertension is present. Patients with traumatic fistulae should always be studied by catheterization and angiography to determine the nature and the size of the defect and associated abnormalities. For example, it is not uncommon to have the combination of a fistula between aorta and outflow tract of the right ventricle, and also a traumatic ventricular septal defect or laceration of the chordae of the mitral or tricuspid valve.

Fistulae are not always clinically evident soon after the actual injury. In many instances, there is the formation of a false aneurysm and the continuous murmur arising from an aorto-pulmonary communication may be audible only some time later. Careful follow-up and repeated examination are therefore essential. The timing of surgical repair will depend on the hemodynamic status of the patient.

Blunt injuries of the heart and pericardium are more common with advancing age because of increasing rigidity of the thorax. There is a wide range of damage that may result from this type of injury. Myocardial laceration may occur in the absence of rib fractures and because of the gross nature of the resultant defect, hemopericardium is frequently fatal within minutes. *Coronary thrombosis* is a rare consequence of nonpenetrating trauma and almost invariably there is well-established coronary atherosclerosis. *Myocardial contusion* usually heals spontaneously but may result in dysrhythmias and rarely, when the necrosis is extensive, to the formation of a false aneurysm. Blunt trauma may also result in laceration of the valves most commonly involving the aortic valve. More usually there is traumatic rupture of the papillary muscles or the chordae tendinae resulting in acute mitral or tricuspid insufficiency. Prompt diagnosis of these lesions has led to successful surgical repair. Blunt trauma to the pericardium may lead to hemopericardium, recurrent pericarditis, and even constriction.

The aorta is not infrequently involved by blunt trauma and the two commonest sites of rupture are just distal to the origin of the left subclavian artery, and the ascending aorta immediately proximal to the origin of the innominate. Aortic rupture is frequently overlooked because of the frequent coexistence of other severe injuries to the abdomen, chest, etc. Chest radiography may be of considerable help in the diagnosis by demonstrating widening of the aortic shadow. The definitive diagnosis is made by aortography, which should not be delayed if aortic rupture is suspected.

Deformities of the Thorax

Deformities of the chest and spine are important for two reasons. First, the skeletal abnormality may interfere with cardiac function and produce cardiac disease. Second, functional disturbances may arise and these may be mistaken for organic cardiac disease.

1. *Organic Disease*. Kyphoscoliosis, when extreme, results in chronic cor pulmonale. Marked sternal depression (pectus excavatum) may result in cardiac displacement and compression. This becomes marked when the anteroposterior measurement of the chest in adults is less than 5 inches. The treatment is surgical for cosmetic and cardiac reasons. The sternal deformity may be associated with Marfan syndrome and a myxomatous mitral valve.
2. *Functional Disturbance*. Certain chest deformities, particularly sternal depression, and the straight back syndrome produce cardiac displacement and thereby give rise to murmurs. The murmurs are usually ejection in type and basally situated. Rarely diastolic murmurs may result. An erroneous diagnosis of cardiomegaly or valve disease may be made with all the consequent psychological trauma to the patient. Electrocardiographic abnormalities (ST segment depression in the diaphragmatic leads) have been described in association with a "suspended heart."

Congenital Subvalvular Left Ventricular Aneurysms

These aneurysms occur in relationship to the aortic and mitral valves. Most cases have been described in African blacks, in whom, because of the rarity of coronary artery disease, constitute the commonest type of aneurysm. The subaortic type occurs subjacent to the intermediate portion of the left coronary cusp of the aortic valve, whereas the submitral type occurs under the posterior leaflet of the mitral valve. The submitral type is the commonest variety.

The clinical presentation is one of heart failure, systemic embolism, angina pectoris, or recurrent episodes of ventricular tachycardia. The murmur of aortic incompetence is present in the subaortic type and that of mitral insufficiency in the submitral type. Submitral aneurysms are larger than subaortic and therefore frequently have abnormal precordial pulsation and a bulge on the cardiac silhouette radiologically (Fig. 21.1). Subaortic aneurysms are not usually recognized radiologically. In both types the electrocardiogram shows evidence of myocardial damage or infarction.

Subaortic and submitral aneurysms arise from a congenital defect in the left ventricular wall, which leads to a false fibrous aneurysm situated in the epicardium. They therefore have a propensity for rupture. The diagnosis should be suspected in an African patient with angina pectoris and electrocardiographic evidence of ischemia. The diagnosis can be confirmed by left ventricular angiography and aortogrophy (Fig. 21.2). The submitral variety is readily amenable to surgical resection in contrast to the subaortic type, where compression of the main stem of the left coronary artery and aortic insufficiency may preclude operative intervention.

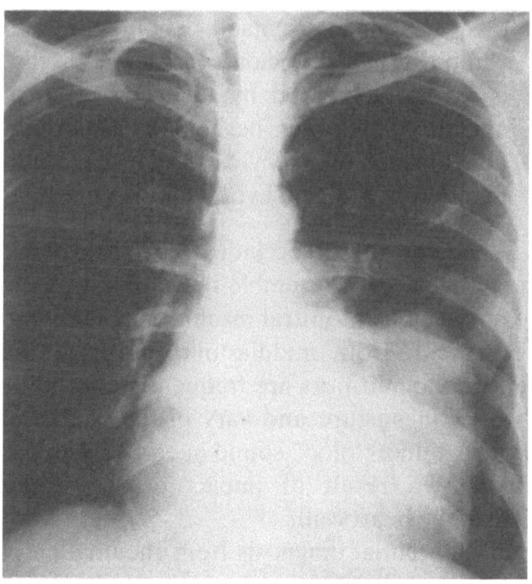

FIGURE 21.1. X-rays demonstrating the typical appearance of a calcified submitral aneurysm in a young African.

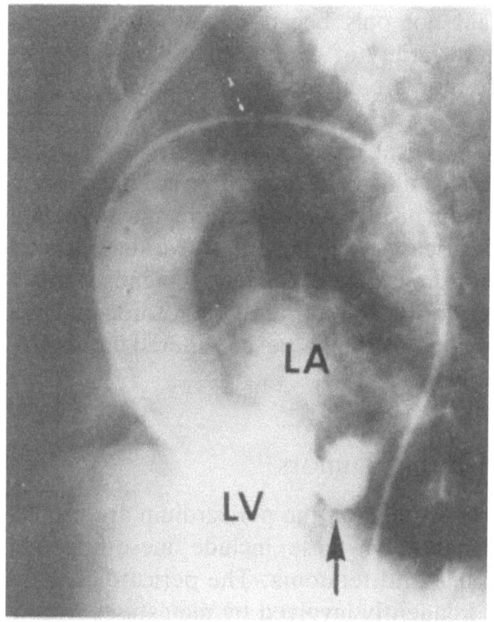

FIGURE 21.2. Left ventricular angiogram demonstrating a small submitral aneurysm (arrow) complicated by mild mitral insufficiency opacifying the left atrium.

Cardiac Tumors

Tumors of the heart are most commonly metastatic from a primary source in the lung, breast, kidney, pancreas, testicle, or melanoma. Usually, the clinical picture is dominated by the malignancy and cardiac involvement occurs as a late and frequently unrecognized complication. Occasionally, however, neoplasms such as bronchial carcinoma may present with cardiac involvement because there is spread by contiguity.

Primary cardiac tumors are 30 times less frequent than the metastatic type and occur in only 0.03% of necropsies. Approximately one-half of these are myxomas, usually found in the left atrium. Left atrial myxomas are thus important not only because they are the commonest variety of cardiac tumor but also because they are amenable to complete surgical cure.

The clinical recognition of primary cardiac tumors is difficult because they are uncommon and their bizarre manifestations may simulate other diseases. The advent of two-dimensional echocardiography has made diagnosis much easier and it is important, therefore, that the possibility of tumor be considered more frequently.

Pericardial Tumors

Primary tumors of the pericardium are usually malignant and these include mesothelioma, sarcoma, and teratoma. The pericardial sac is also frequently involved by metastases from a primary source in the lung or breast and also be infiltration by lymphomas and leukemia.

Malignant involvement of the pericardium usually manifest clinically in one of three ways:

1. Pericarditis with effusion, which is frequently sanguinous and productive of cardiac tamponade. The important differentiation is from tuberculous pericarditis. Examination of the pericardial fluid frequently demonstrates neoplastic cells.
2. The syndrome of pericardial constriction is particularly likely to occur when metastases emanate from lung or breast cancer.
3. The occurrence of atrial flutter or fibrillation, which is particularly prone to occur when the pericardium is invaded directly by a contiguous bronchogenic carcinoma.

Myocardial Tumors

Metastatic tumors are much more frequent than primary tumors and all areas of the myocardium may be involved. Usually they are not responsible for symptoms or signs but the electrocardiogram may show evidence of cardiac infarction. Invasion of the bundle of His and the A-V node may produce heart block and sudden death.

Primary tumors include rhabdomyoma, which is associated with tuberous sclerosis of the brain in 50% of patients. It occurs most commonly in infancy and is frequently responsible for supraventricular and ventricular tachycardia or conduction defects. The clinical diagnosis is suggested by concomitant mental retardation and seizures. Primary mesothelioma of the A-V node occurs more frequently in women and is responsible for complete A-V block and sudden death.

Intracavitary Tumors

Left Atrial Myxoma

These are pedunculated, lobulated tumors attached to the interatrial septum. They are frequently gelatinous and friable, which accounts for their tendency to fragment and form emboli.

Myxomas produced their clinical manifestations in three ways:

1. *Obstruction*. The tumor has a ball-valve effect obstructing the mitral valve and also rendering it incompetent.
2. *Embolism*. These vary in size from the small variety, which simulate bacterial endocarditis, to a large embolus producing major neurologic or systemic deficits.
3. *Systemic Manifestations*. Constitutional symptoms include fever, anorexia, weight loss, arthralgia, Raynaud pehomenon, and clubbing. The suspicion of systemic disease is further increased by the occurrence of anemia (which may be hemolytic), thrombocytopenia, leukocytosis, elevated sedimentation rate, and hyperglobulinemia.

When the tumor occludes the mitral valve the physical signs resemble those of mitral stenosis but signs of mitral insufficiency may also be present. Both middiastolic murmurs and pansystolic murmurs are frequently altered by changes in posture and vary in the course of time. A tumor "plop" sound in early diastole is probably a result of impact of the tumor against the heart wall.

In differential diagnosis from rheumatic mitral stenosis, helpful features are as follows:

1. Positional variation in the auscultatory signs.
2. Absence of an opening snap.
3. Positional syncope.
4. Rapid progression of symptoms, which is disproportionate to the physical examination and radiological and electrocardiographic findings.
5. Intracardiac calcification, which may be demonstrated to be mobile with fluoroscopy.
6. The presence of persistent embolism and petechiae among cases of culture negative "infective endocarditis."
7. The sudden onset of stroke in a young person in sinus rhythm.

The most useful noninvasive test to demonstrate atrial myxoma with a high degree of specificity is echocardiography, which is capable of demonstrating the movable mass. A definitive diagnosis may also be made by selective left ventricular cineangioyraphy, which demonstrates the tumor mass prolapsing from the left atrium into the left ventricle. Nonprolapsing tumors may be demonstrated by forward pulmonary angiography where dye is injected into the pulmonary artery and the left atrium is opacified by follow through—myxomas appear as filling defects.

The treatment for the condition is surgical, which is curative; recurrence is uncommon when complete resection has been performed.

Right Atrial Myxoma

The usual presentation is one of rapidly progressive right-sided heart failure, constitutional symptoms, and occasionally cyanosis produced by right-to-left shunting across the foramen ovale. Attacks of pain in the right hypochondrium and weakness are frequent. Postural aggravation of symptoms may occur as in left atrial myxoma.

The tumor interferes with tricuspid closure producing the hemodynamic, auscultatory, radiological, and electrocardiographic features of tricuspid stenosis and/or regurgitation. The differential diagnosis is from rheumatic tricuspid stenosis, carcinoid syndrome, constrictive pericarditis, and Ebstein disease. The possibility of right atrial myxoma should be entertained in any a case of isolated tricuspid valve disease. The tumor may be visualized by two-dimensional echocardiography and by angiograms performed from the superior vena cava. Treatment is by surgical excision.

Right Ventricular Tumors

Rhabdomyomas, myxomas, and fibromas protrude into the cavity of the right ventricle producing obstruction at infundibular and valve levels. Tumor involvement of the pulmonary valve may produce pulmonary insufficiency. Pulmonary hypertension may follow tumor emboli to the lung.

Left Ventricular Tumors

These do not have the same propensity to produce outflow tract obstruction as do right ventricular tumors. Fibromas are the commonest variety and their presentation is usually with dyspnea, angina, and syncope. The diagnosis should be entertained when these symptoms are combined with evidence of pericardial involvement and arrhythmias.

Additional Reading

Blumgart HL, Freedberg AS: The heart and the thyroid: With particular reference to I131. Treatment of heart disease. Circulation 6:222, 1952.

Burwell CS, Metcalfe J: "Heart Disease and Pregnancy: Physiology and Management." Little Brown, Boston, 1958.

Chesler E: Aneurysms of the left ventricle. Cardiovasc Clinics 188, 1972. DeGroott LJ: Thyroid and the heart. Mayo Clin Proc 47:864, 1972.

Freeman, WK, Gibbons, JR, Shub, C: Preoperative assessment of cardiac patients undergoing noncardiac surgical procedures. Mayo Clinic Proc 64:1105–1117, 1989.

Gilchrist AR: Cardiological problems in young women: Including those of pregnancy and the puerperium. Br Med J 1:209, 1963.

Graettinyer JL, Meunster JJ, Checchia CS et al.: Correlation of clinical and hemodynamic studies of patients with hypothyroidism. J Clin Invest 37:502, 1958.

Moritz AR: Injuries of the heart and pericardium by physical violence. Chapter XII. In Gould SE (ed):

"Gould Pathology and the Heart." Charles C Thomas, Springfield, IL, 1960.

O'Keefe JH, Shub, C, Rettke: Risk of noncardiac surgical procedures in patients with aortic stenosis. Mayo Clin Proc 64, 406–405, 1989.

Sandler G, Wilson GM: The nature and prognosis of heart disease in thyrotoxicosis. Q J Med 28:347, 1959.

Sanghvi LM, Sharma R, Misra SN: Cardiovascular disturbances in chronic severe anernia. Circulation 15:373, 1957.

Schrire V, Grant J: The electrocardiographic changes associated with beri-beri heart disease. S Afr J Lab Clin Med 5:195, 1959.

Symposium on Cardiac Tumors. Am J Cardiol 21:307, 1968.

Index

D

E

I

N

MIX
Papier aus verantwortungsvollen Quellen
Paper from responsible sources
FSC® C105338

If you have any concerns about our products,
you can contact us on
ProductSafety@springernature.com

In case Publisher is established outside the EU,
the EU authorized representative is:
Springer Nature Customer Service Center GmbH
Europaplatz 3, 69115 Heidelberg, Germany

Printed by Libri Plureos GmbH
in Hamburg, Germany